Atlas of FELINE SURGICAL Techniques

Editor
Alberto Barneto

Anna Calvet
Salvador Cervantes
Antonio Peña
Llibertat Real

edra
PUBLISHING

This book was originally published in Spanish under the title:
Atlas de técnicas en cirugía felina

ISBN Spanish edition: 978-84-18706-84-4

Atlas of Feline Surgical Techniques
Alberto Barneto Carmona, Anna Calvet Alemany, Salvador Cervantes Sala, Antonio Peña Rodríguez, Llibertat Real Sampietro

ISBN: 978-1-957260-58-7
eISBN: 978-1-957260-72-3

Book Publishing Manager: Costanza Smeraldi
Paper, Printing and Binding Manager: Paolo Ficicchia
Translation: Chef du Monde SL
Illustrators: David Martín Rubio (www.comunicandoconlatierra.com), Jacob Gragera Artal
Cover: Jacob Gragera Artal
Layout: Raquel Fernández Bermúdez, Nieves Marín Ortiz
Copyediting: Jorge Viejo Adiego

Edra Publishing US LLC
3309 Northlake Boulevard, Suite 203
Palm Beach Gardens, FL, 33403
EIN: 844113980
info@edrapublishing.com
www.edrapublishing.com

edra PUBLISHING

Printed by "Printer Trento" S.r.l., September 2023

Authors

Alberto Barneto Carmona

Degree in veterinary medicine from the Complutense University of Madrid (UCM) in 1989. Postgraduate ESVPS Cert SAS (European School of Veterinary Postgraduate Studies Certificate in Small Animal Surgery) in feline medicine and surgery in 2010. AVEPA-certified in feline medicine and member of the GEMFE/AVEPA (Spanish Feline Medicine Study Group/Spanish Small Animal Veterinary Association) scientific committee until 2019. Head of surgery at Ayavet veterinary clinic in Boadilla del Monte, Madrid, and collaborator at the Diagnosfera specialized center for feline medicine and surgery.

Salvador Cervantes Sala

Degree in veterinary medicine from the Autonomous University of Barcelona (UAB) in 1998. Postgraduate degree in feline medicine and surgery (1999-2001) and more recently feline dentistry (2019) from the ESAVS (European School for Advanced Veterinary Studies). GEMFE/AVEPA-certified in feline medicine and a member of that group's scientific committee. Author of the book *Diseases of Senior Cats and Dogs: Diagnosis and Therapy* (Edra Publishing, 2022) and co-author of the European GRAM (Guidance for the Rational use of Antimicrobials) guide.

Anna Calvet Alemany

Degree in veterinary medicine from the UAB in 1998. Postgraduate SAS-certified degree in soft tissue surgery and traumatology in 2010 from the ESVPS. Head of the surgical team at Barcelona feline clinic since 2016. She has published in international journals.

Antonio Peña Rodríguez

Degree in veterinary medicine from the UCM. GEMFE/AVEPA-certified in feline medicine and a member of that group's scientific committee. European diploma in feline medicine from the ESVPS. Associate of the Surgery Professorship of the Veterinary Department of the UCM. Co-owner of the Lisboa veterinary center in Alcorcón, Madrid.

Llibertat Real Sampietro

Degree in veterinary medicine from the University of Zaragoza, Spain, in 1995. AVEPA-certified in feline medicine. Member of International Society of Feline Medicine (ISFM) since 1996. In 2000, she did a residency at Nine Lives Veterinary Practice for Cats, the first veterinary clinic in the United Kingdom exclusively for cats. She completed three postgraduate courses in feline medicine and surgery at the ESAVS in Zurich, Switzerland, from 1999 to 2001 and a postgraduate course in feline dentistry in Novara, Italy, in 2019. She currently focuses her activity on feline medicine and surgery at Ayavet veterinary clinic in Boadilla del Monte, Madrid.

Preface

You have in your hands one of the few books published to date specifically dedicated to feline surgery.

Some of the authors have been collaborating for several years with the publishing house Grupo Asís Biomedia, especially on works where image played a central role. Even more time, in my case, has been dedicated to feline medicine and surgery. When I was preparing for a surgical procedure, I always found it difficult to understand the anatomical structures and steps in each stage of the procedure. The few books published on feline anatomy did not illustrate the details well either. Only scientific articles had drawings, which were not always good quality but were helpful for understanding. In our experience, to understand a surgical procedure step-by-step, a good illustration is better than a photograph, since the anatomical structures are more clearly differentiated, in addition to being able to highlight, mark, color and even animate the areas that are key to the treatment in each case. And this publisher has great illustrators who are also veterinarians! As they say nowadays, a win-win situation.

Each of the authors of this book have been dedicated to feline medicine and surgery for over 20 years. It is probably the fastest growing veterinary clinical specialty of the last three decades. Cats have entered our lives and our practices with force and are here to stay. This means that works dedicated especially to them have a priori significant popularity.

When we proposed this work, we intended it to be a practical book, useful both for students and surgeons who need to delve deeper into the feline specialty. It was never our aim to write a long and deep treatise on surgery; we do not consider ourselves capable of this, nor would our daily occupations have allowed us to do so. Rather, we prefer to cover interventions for exclusively feline pathologies or, at least, the most frequent ones presented in our hospitals and clinics.

We have tried to give the book a very practical approach. All the things you will read are interventions that we perform in our usual work. The photos and videos are also original (or borrowed from colleagues who are specialists in each case). We preferred a work that was more limited, but that could give you an idea of the problems you may encounter in each intervention and how to resolve them if you want to dedicate yourself to feline surgery.

We have to thank many people around us for their help.

First of all, to all the guardians of our patients and to the cats themselves. They are the very reason for our work. Their patience and trust help not only in their treatment, but also in building the experience from which you can now benefit.

Secondly, to our families, who understand that sometimes the time we steal away from them is invested in beneficial healthcare work.

We also thank our colleagues for their help: those who taught and trained us; those who have shared and discussed their cases with us in lectures and congresses, referring their patients to us. You are all a continual incentive for our work. Of course, we are also grateful for the help of junior veterinarians (who, because of our age, already constitute a very large population...); they are another reason for our existence. With their curiosity and desire to learn, they allow scientific knowledge to continue to be passed on over the years.

And finally, to all the professionals at Grupo Asís Biomedia: Ana Hernández, the first one who believed in the project; Tatiana Blasco, the person who built the solid framework for the book by advising, correcting and structuring each chapter; the illustrators, Jacob Gragera and David Martín, who have successfully captured the ideas, details and corrections to translate them into illustrations that give quality and level to the book and attempt to explain each surgical technique better than many photos.

And the secret is that among this whole chain of important people who have shaped the atlas we present to you most are veterinarians. A profession that, rare in the 21st century, still allows us to cover wide and varied areas of knowledge, all of which are also exciting.

Make a lot of use of the book! If in a few years the atlas has a worn spine, a few loose pages and notes, it will mean that our work and yours has been worthwhile.

Alberto Barneto
Madrid, summer of 2022

Table of contents

2 SKIN SURGERY

3 HEAD AND NECK SURGERY

4 ABDOMINAL SURGERY

Dedication

This book is a collaboration by five friends who are dedicated to feline veterinary medicine. I dedicate it to the other four.
But also, and above all, to Llibertat, the best partner I could have by my side. And to our children, Javier, Darío and Aurora; they are my motivation for each day.
And of course to all the cats, for what they teach us every day as we try to help.
Alberto

To Salvador, my companion and life partner, for pushing me to be better in everything, to Alberto for entrusting me with this project, to my colleagues in feline medicine, who are my cat family, and to my sons, Salva and Albert, for always being understanding, we have not made it easy for them.
Anna

As always to my family, for their unconditional love and infinite patience. To you, the co-authors of this book, I am proud not only to be able to write it with you, but also to be able to call you my friends. Your trust has pushed me to where I am today.
And finally, to my cats, Arnau and Isaac, for all the lessons they have taught me.
Salva

To my parents, always to them. Thank you for your effort and unconditional support, which has enabled me to enjoy this profession and do things like this. I love you.
To my wife, Alicia, and my son, Carlos. Forgive me for all the stolen time, which I will try to repay. Thank you for agreeing to this.
To my associate and friend, José González, for his help in our daily work and because without an anesthesiologist like him we would not have been able to perform so many surgeries. Thank you for your willingness to let me work on projects like this.
Antonio

To Alberto and the cats, who have taught me so much.
Llibertat

1

OVERVIEW

THE FELINE SURGICAL PATIENT 1

Salvador Cervantes

Introduction

The cat as a surgical patient requires special conditions, as it does for a general physical examination. Conditions and materials tailored to its idiosyncrasies help us to respond better and faster to the perisurgical and perianesthetic needs of the feline patient. Clinical veterinarians who work with cats know that "a cat is not a small dog," and this statement is even more true within the surgical environment.

Characteristics of the cat as a surgical patient

A cat has physical, metabolic and behavioral characteristics that will modify our anesthetic protocol design, as well as the surgical protocol and even our operating room layout. These characteristics and their consequences are summarized in Box 1.

Adaptation of the operating room and surgical environment

The environment where sedation, anesthesia and subsequently surgery will be performed on a cat should be quiet and free of noise and odors (especially free of odors from other cats and dogs), with the ability to regulate light intensity and temperature.

Equipment tailored to the size of a cat should always include the following:

- Small-volume syringes, 1 ml or even smaller for cats and kittens under 1 kg (Fig. 1).
- Low-pressure endotracheal tubes with a Murphy eye or supraglottic airway devices (Fig. 2).
- Systems to keep the patient dry and warm, such as hot air or water beds. Some electrical systems may also be suitable so long as precautions are taken to avoid burns. In dental cleaning or dental procedure situations, bubble wrap may be appropriate to prevent heat loss and protect the patient from moisture (Fig. 3).

BOX 1. Physical, metabolic and behavioral characteristics of cats

Small and fearful	Strict carnivores	Predator and prey	Susceptible to oxidative damage	Ability to conceal clinical signs
■ Require tailored equipment and material ■ Prone to temperature loss ■ Prone to overdose ■ Risk of arrhythmias due to catecholamines	■ Fast and limited metabolism ■ Limited response to toxins ■ Low resistance to fasting	■ Concealment of clinical signs such as pain ■ Prone to adrenergic reactions: fight or flight reflex	■ Prone to liver damage ■ Prone to hemoglobin denaturation ■ Sensitive to many drugs and toxins	■ Increased number of sudden deaths ■ Higher proportion of perianesthetic complications ■ Increased occurrence of clinical signs of previously hidden diseases

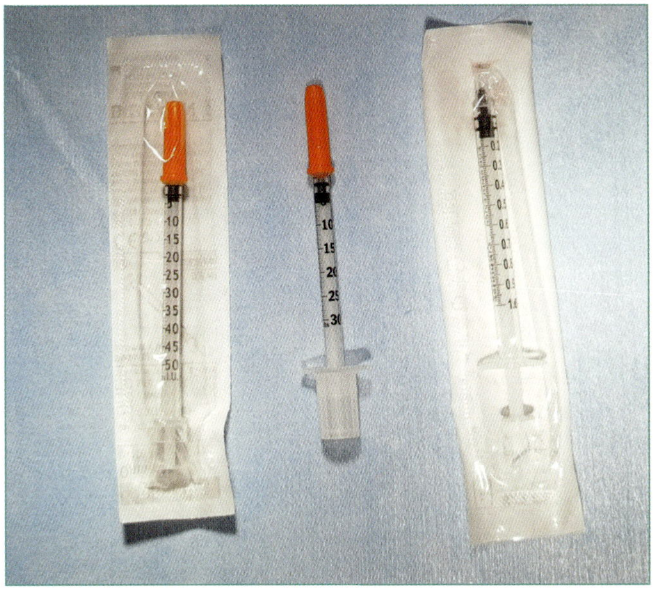

FIGURE 1. Very low-volume syringes for feline anesthetics.

- Often, monitoring the feline patient involves the use of clamps for continuous electrocardiography. For this, alcohol or electrolyte solutions are used that allow cardiac electrical impulses to pass through. However, these substances often contribute to the rapid cooling of the patient. To avoid this extra temperature loss, dry pads can be applied to the palms and soles of those extremities that do not require the use of fluid to allow adequate reception of electrical impulses from the heart (Fig. 4).
- Cats, like all anesthetized patients, require the administration of intravenous fluids for the duration of the anesthesia or sedation. For their administration, drips or flow regulators can be used. However, the use of continuous infusion pumps that allow the administration of a constant volume at rates as low as those needed by feline patients, with minimal error volumes, is becoming more and more widespread (Figs. 5 and 6).

> IV fluid infusion rate during anesthesia (ml/kg/h):
>
> Formula: **$80 \times$ Weight in kg$^{0.75}$**
> (or empirical system: **2–3 ml/kg/h**)
>
> These doses should be reduced in kidney, hypertensive or heart patients.

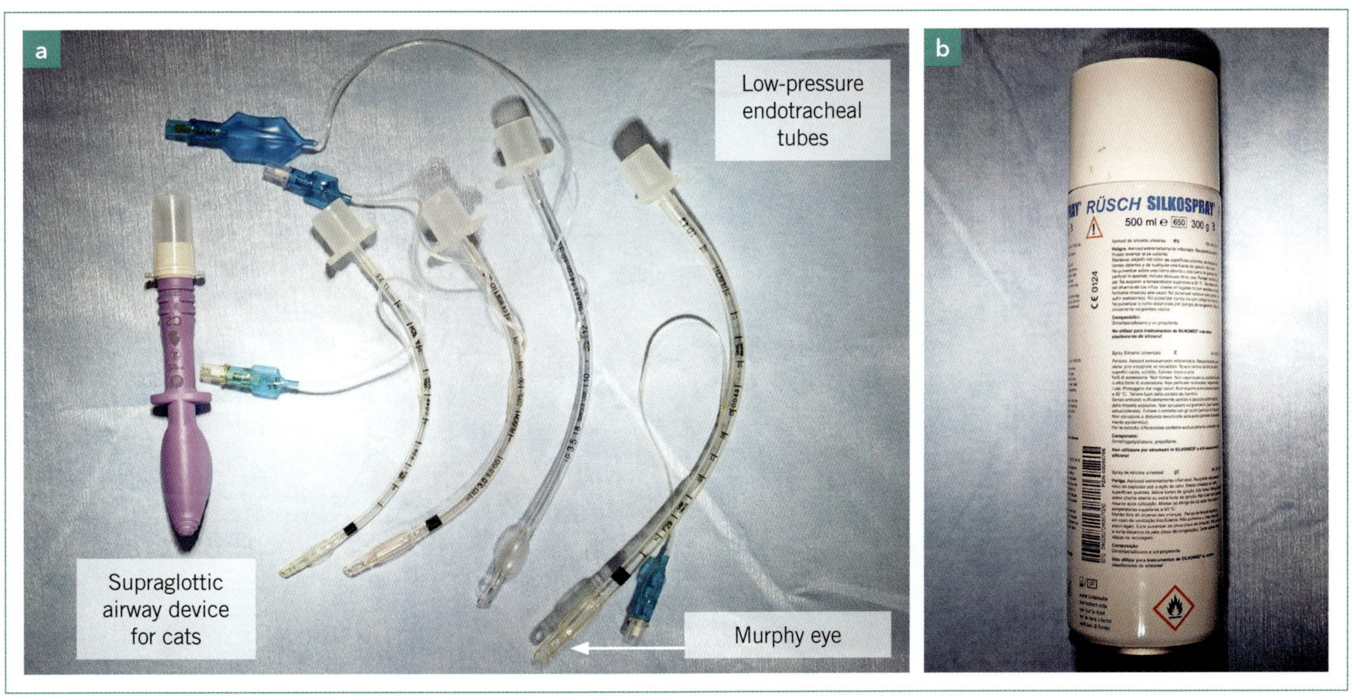

FIGURE 2. (a) Endotracheal tubes and supraglottic airway device for cats. (b) Medical grade silicone spray for endotracheal tubes; its use reduces the need to increase balloon pressure.

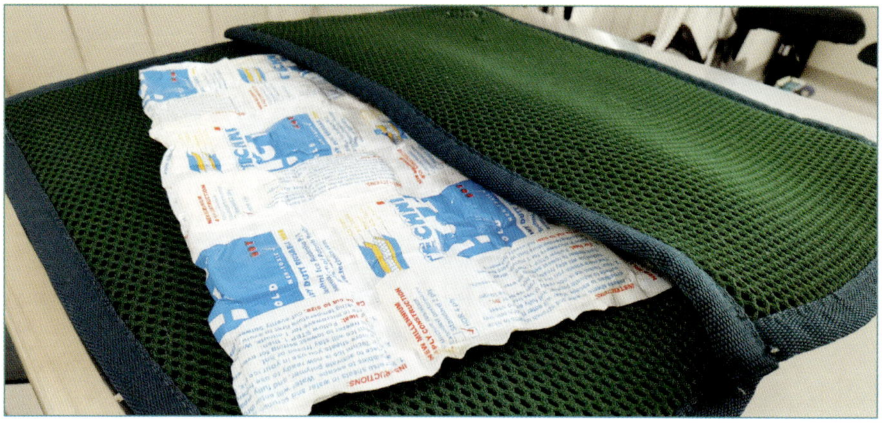

FIGURE 3. Mattress system using heating pads to reduce hypothermia and the risk of burns.

- Finally, anesthetic circuit selection is also important, as open circuits usually contribute to temperature loss by requiring 2 to 4 times the cat's tidal volume to ensure no rebreathing, while semiclosed circuits allow for reduced patient temperature loss with lower oxygen volumes, close to the patient's tidal volume.

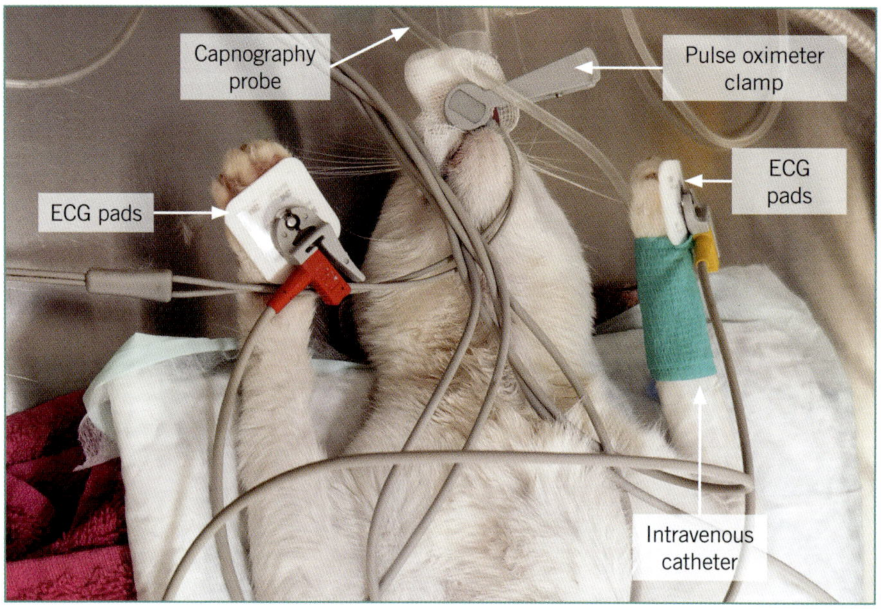

FIGURE 4. Feline patient prepared for ovariohysterectomy. Pad-type electrodes have been used to avoid wetting armpits and groin with alcohol.

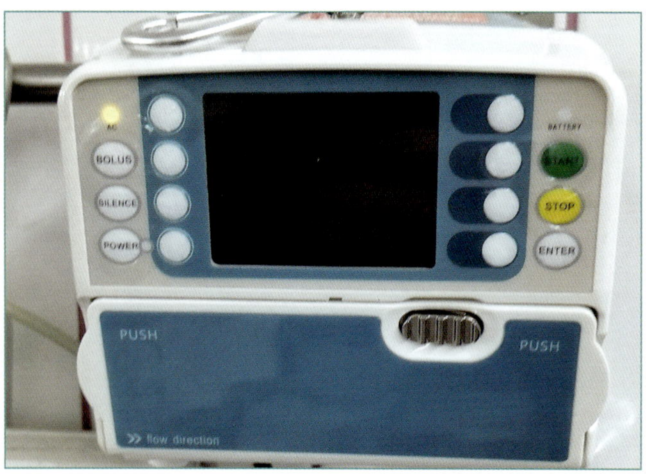

FIGURE 5. Fluid infusion pump for small-sized animals.

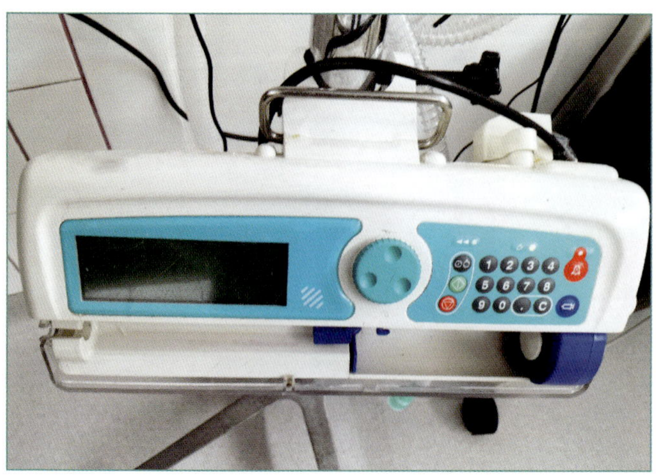

FIGURE 6. Syringe pump for administration of medication and fluids in very small patients.

Perioperative considerations

Fasting and reintroduction of oral feeding

Traditionally, much longer fasting times have been recommended than is currently the case. A cat, due to some of its characteristics, does not tolerate very long fasting times.

This is due in part to its high surface area:body volume ratio, with a high capacity for heat loss. In addition, its liver needs a constant supply of protein to avoid a catabolic state, and requires a continuous supply of external antioxidants to metabolize, among other substances, oxidizing products such as the majority of anesthetics. In addition, we must keep in mind that a normal cat's stomach is usually emptied within 90 minutes of ingestion and that passage through the digestive tract may be complete within 12 hours.

For these reasons, in adult cats **fasting times** of no more than **6–8 hours** are sufficient, while in kittens or diabetic patients fasting is not recommended and they are premedicated with products such as maropitant and/or butorphanol, which have an important antiemetic effect.

Likewise, once the surgery or anesthesia has ended, a small meal of about 10–15 g of dry feed or 30–40 g of wet feed can be administered as soon as the patient recovers its swallow reflex. This will help restore normal blood glucose levels, which are very important for brain metabolism, in addition to providing sufficient glucose to the liver (primarily responsible for the creation of heat and maintenance of normal temperature). Only cats that have undergone interventions where dysphagia may have occurred (laryngeal surgeries or those with neurological involvement) or in which the integrity of the digestive tract has been altered will not be fed orally as soon. However, if they cannot be fed orally within 12 hours of the operation, feeding tubes will be placed so that nutrition is not further delayed (see Ch. 3 "Postoperative care in feline medicine").

VIDEO

Kittens eating after neutering

Reduction of perioperative stress

Cats, due to their hunter/prey dichotomy, can rapidly release large amounts of catecholamines that can delay the action of sedatives and favor the development of cardiac arrhythmias, increasing the risks associated with anesthesia. For this reason, a gentle physical approach should be attempted in all feline patients to reduce the possibility of perioperative stress. Easily stressed patients can be sedated at home by administering gabapentin at a dose of 50–100 mg the night before surgery and 3 hours before being placed in their carrier. Other very interesting recommendations for correct sedation are:

- Conduct it in the presence of the cat's owner.
- Perform it in an area free of odors and noise, with the ability to lower the light level.
- Use cocktails that can be injected not only intramuscularly but also subcutaneously in patients that are more sensitive or experiencing pain.
- Perform it inside the carrier with the cat's blanket or towel impregnated with its own facial pheromones. Or, alternatively, use artificial facial pheromones and calming scents such as catnip or valerian root in sensitive cats.
- After the veterinarian and veterinary assistants have performed the entire preoperative protocol and the injection of sedatives, they will remain at a distance where the patient feels comfortable.

> Only patients with suspected or diagnosed heart disease or those with dyspneic problems should be separated from their owners to be placed in a hyperbaric chamber and properly preoxygenated.

VIDEO

Sedation of a patient after subcutaneous drug administration

Finally, once the anesthetic/surgical procedure is completed, the patient should wake up in a warm environment, without noise or strong odors and with a dim, indirect light source.

Feline patient monitoring and surveillance

Homeostasis is the set of self-regulation phenomena that allow relative constancy to be maintained in the composition and properties of the internal environment of an organism. Without homeostasis, life is not possible; in fact, life is only possible within fairly narrow homeostatic margins. Unfortunately, anesthesia jeopardizes these conditions. The role of the veterinary anesthesiologist is to maintain these conditions during the surgical or diagnostic procedure so that anesthesia can be successfully reversed and the patient returned home without sequelae.

Basic and advanced parameters can be surveilled/monitored. Vital signs are usually the focus of basic surveillance/monitoring and are summarized in Table 1, along with their normal ranges.

In terms of advanced surveillance/monitoring, our discussion can include serum concentrations of substances, perfusion levels or parasympathetic tone estimates. However, such advanced monitoring is available to very few anesthesia professionals and is beyond the scope of this atlas.

For this reason, we decided to focus on those surveillance systems that provide more information, help reduce the most common anesthetic risks and complications, and whose control leads to rapid improvement in our feline patients.

The most important anesthetic complications in the feline species are hypothermia, hypoxia, arterial hypotension and cardiac arrhythmias.

If we want to monitor our feline patients in order to effectively combat these complications, we will need an esophageal or rectal continuous temperature monitor, a curve capnograph, a pulse oximeter and a continuous electrocardiogram monitor. There are several noninvasive, indirect oscillometric devices for reading blood pressure and various invasive, direct reading devices using an arterial catheter. The latter, although much more reliable, are much more complex as they require the catheterization of an artery, a procedure that is not common in clinics or hospitals that do not have the personnel and equipment for it.

In the authors' experience, noninvasive blood pressure monitors integrated into multiparametric systems (Fig. 7) are not as reliable as systems dedicated only to pressure reading, whether or not they are high-definition oscillometric systems. The veterinarian should find a device or brand that guarantees greater repeatability and compare the data obtained with the clinical signs being observed, such as heart rate and the presence of metatarsal, metacarpal and femoral pulses. Although the Doppler system is a validated method, it admittedly requires more work and skill in these cases, as the probe moves relatively easily.

TABLE 1. Vital signs observed in basic surveillance/monitoring

Vital signs	Normal/anesthetic values
Heart rate	110–140 bpm (normal) 80–160 bpm (under anesthesia)
Respiratory rate	20–30 rpm (normal) 8–10 rpm (under anesthesia)
Temperature	38–39°C
Systolic blood pressure	>90 mmHg
Pain	Present (without analgesic) or absent
O_2 saturation	>92%

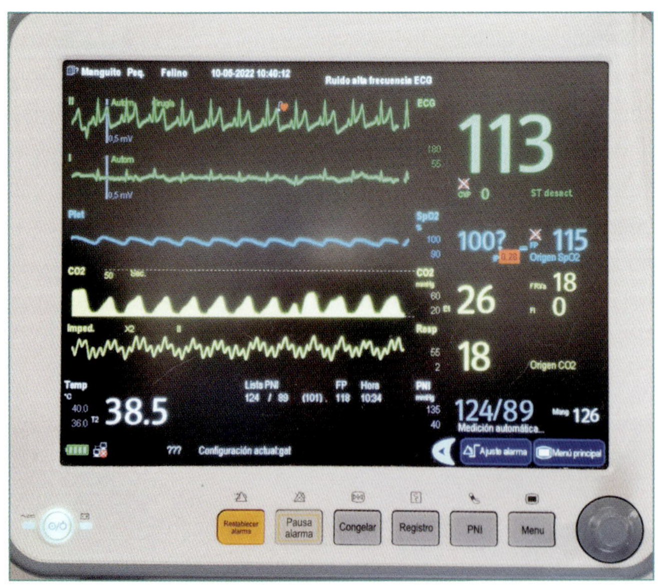

FIGURE 7. Multiparameter monitor used during feline surgery.

Bibliography

Carney HC, Little S, Brownlee-Tomasso D et al.; American Association of Feline Practitioners; International Society of Feline Medicine. AAFP and ISFM feline-friendly nursing care guidelines. *J Feline Med Surg*, 2012; 14(5):337–349.

Davis H, Jensen T, Johnson A et al.; American Association of Feline Practicioners; American Animal Hospital Association. 2013 AAHA/AAFP fluid therapy guidelines for dogs and cats. *J Am Anim Hosp Assoc*, 2013; 49(3):149–159.

Kudnig ST, Mama K. Guidelines for perioperative fluid therapy. *Compend Contin Educ Pract Vet*, 2003; 25:102–111.

Robertson SA. Assessment and management of acute pain in cats. *J Vet Emerg Crit Care*, 2005; 15:261–272.

Wellman M, DiBartola S, Kohn C. Applied physiology of body fluid in dogs and cats. In: DiBartola S (ed.). *Fluid, Electrolyte, and Acid-Base Disorders in Small Animal Practice*, 3rd ed. St. Louis, MO: Saunders Elsevier, 2006; pp. 3–26.

FELINE SEDATION, ANESTHESIA AND ANALGESIA 2

Salvador Cervantes

Introduction

Anesthesia is an intoxication of the central nervous system. All sedation and anesthesia has an inherent risk. Currently, the average feline perianesthetic sedation/anesthesia mortality rate is estimated to be around 0.1%–0.2%. The clinician should be aware of this and properly inform the patient's caregiver. This risk, logically, increases if the patient suffers from hidden diseases, if diseases have been diagnosed but not stabilized, or if the patient has not been properly evaluated.

Phases of anesthesia

Sedation or tranquilization

Period during which the patient receives a dose of a drug or combination of drugs that calms them and allows them to be handled without risk to either the patient or the veterinary team. Among the most common risks for the patient are airway obliteration and more or less marked secretion of catecholamines, which can lead to tachycardia, arrhythmias, hypertension and subsequent cardiovascular destabilization. In diagnostic procedures or when obtaining samples in uncooperative patients, the anesthetic process is usually stopped at this point. Surveillance is usually basic and is often only performed by physical examination.

Drugs commonly used for this phase: α_2-adrenergic agonists, phenothiazines, benzodiazepines and some opioids and anesthetics with sedative effects depending on dose and route of administration (e.g., butorphanol and alfaxalone).

Induction (with intubation)

Period during which the patient is administered a dose of hypnotic anesthetic that allows the adequate anesthetic plane to be reached while, simultaneously, after the application of a local anesthetic in the area of the epiglottis, endotracheal or supraepiglottic intubation is performed. Intubation tubes shall always be lubricated with a biocompatible product that does not damage the tube material. More intensive monitoring is usually started.

Drugs commonly used for this phase: propofol, intravenous alfaxalone and, less frequently, etomidate.

Maintenance

This is the time during which the patient receives a continuous dose of hypnotic to maintain the correct anesthetic plane. Surgical procedures are performed during this period. Throughout this phase the patient is properly monitored.

Commonly used drugs: halogenated gases (e.g., isoflurane and sevoflurane) or intravenous continuous rate infusion (CRI) hypnotic agents (e.g., propofol, alfaxalone and etomidate).

Recovery

This is the phase during which the patient stops receiving doses of the hypnotic agent and begins to regain reflexes and consciousness. It should be noted that almost 75% of perianesthetic deaths occur in this phase. This is due to several factors, but in cats two are perhaps the most important:

- Reduced level of monitoring and surveillance.
- Release of catecholamines due to postsurgical stress as a result of increased consciousness, which can add to an increased sensation of pain in the absence of proper analgesic coverage.

Drugs usually used: during this period it is not necessary to use any drug, since the normal metabolism of the drugs that have already been administered leads to recovery. However, the use of α_2-agonists lead to the administration of reversal agents such as atipamezole for α_2-agonists, flumazenil for benzodiazepines or buprenorphine to reverse the sedative effects of pure agonist opioids.

Characteristics required for all general anesthesia

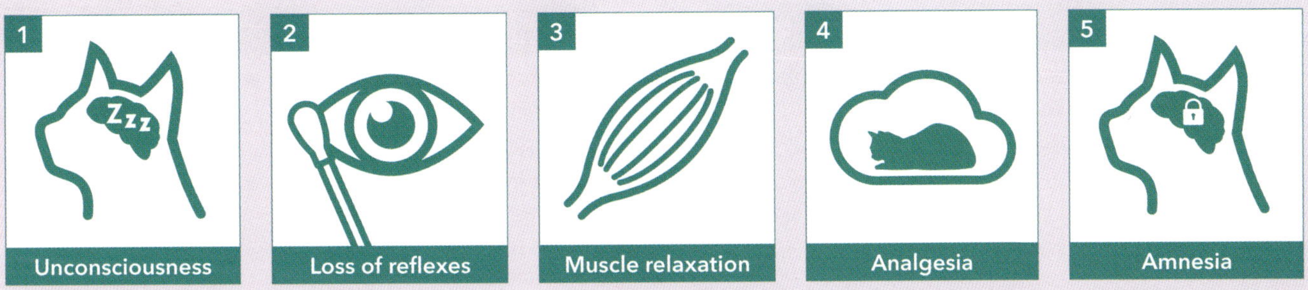

General anesthesia that does not consist of these five characteristics cannot be considered anesthesia, emphasizing that none of them can be left out.

Feline anesthesia and sedation pharmacology

Sedatives

This group includes phenothiazines, α_2-adrenergic agonists and benzodiazepines.

Phenothiazines

The best known and most widely used drug of the group is acepromazine, followed by chlorpromazine.

Advantages and disadvantages of phenothiazines

Advantages	Disadvantages
■ Classified as antihistamines ■ Powerful sedatives (saves 1/3 of the anesthetic dose) ■ Muscle relaxants ■ Antiemetics ■ Desensitize the myocardium to catecholamines, which is why an antiarrhythmic effect is attributed to them	■ Not analgesics ■ Powerful hypotensive agents ■ Do not produce amnesia

α_2-adrenergic agonists

Medetomidine and others such as dexmedetomidine and xylazine are the most commonly used sedatives today.

Advantages and disadvantages of α_2-adrenergic agonists

Advantages	Disadvantages
■ Powerful sedatives (saves up to 3/4 of the anesthetic dose) ■ Muscle relaxants ■ Analgesics (act well on modulation) ■ Can be antagonized (atipamezole)	■ Very emetic ■ Alter cardiac function

Benzodiazepines

This group includes diazepam and also midazolam.

Advantages and disadvantages of benzodiazepines

Advantages	Disadvantages
■ Powerful antiepileptics in cats (anti-convulsant and seizure preventive) ■ Very mild sedatives (save <5% of the anesthetic dose) ■ Muscle relaxants ■ Produce amnesia ■ Do not affect cardiorespiratory function ■ Cause hunger (orexigen)	■ Not analgesics ■ Cause paradoxical excitation (in monotherapy)

Opioids

These may be pure, partial agonist or agonist-antagonist effect opioids.

Pure opioids

The most commonly used are morphine, methadone and fentanyl.

Advantages and disadvantages of pure opioids

Advantages	Disadvantages
■ Powerful analgesics (although not equally effective for all pain) ■ Mild sedatives (dose-dependent effect) ■ Mild muscle relaxants ■ Do not affect cardiorespiratory function (dose-dependent effect)	■ Can cause dysphoria without good sedation ■ Can cause emesis (especially morphine) ■ Cause intestinal stasis and constipation

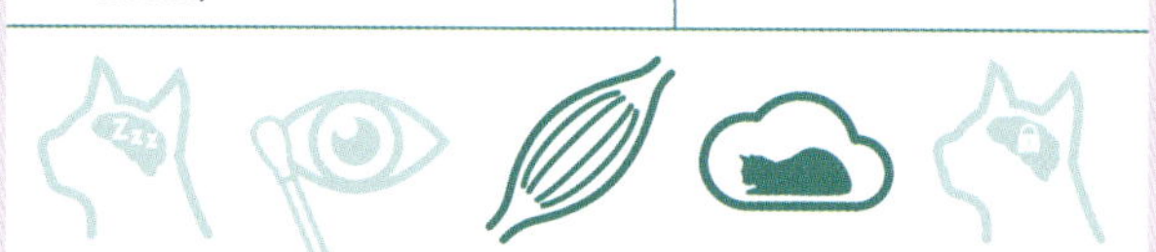

Partial agonist opioids

The main drug in this group is buprenorphine.

Advantages and disadvantages of buprenorphine

Advantages	Disadvantages
■ Analgesic for moderate pain ■ It is very well absorbed by transmucosal and intravenous routes, less so by intramuscular and subcutaneous routes ■ Does not affect cardiorespiratory function ■ Reverses the sedative/cardiorespiratory effects of pure agonists	■ Does not produce sedation, muscle relaxation or amnesia ■ Takes up to 45 minutes to take effect according to some studies ■ Has a ceiling effect and can inhibit other pure agonists from fully taking effect

Agonist-antagonist opioids

Butorphanol and also pentazocine are representative of this group of opioids.

Advantages and disadvantages of agonist-antagonist opioids

Advantages	Disadvantages
■ Analgesics for mild to moderate pain, especially visceral pain ■ They are very well absorbed by all routes and act very quickly ■ Do not affect cardiorespiratory function ■ Have a good sedative effect ■ Offer an important antiemetic effect	■ Their duration is short, between 1 and 4 hours, depending on the dose and what it is used for ■ Require other analgesics for proper analgesia

Dissociative agents

Ketamine is the main dissociative agent used in cats. The combination of tiletamine with zolazepam is also marketed.

Advantages and disadvantages of dissociative agents (ketamine)

Advantages	Disadvantages
■ Short-acting drugs ■ Eliminated by the kidney bound to calcium ■ Effective for musculoskeletal and chronic pain (NMDA antagonist) ■ Can be administered by any route ■ Very broad therapeutic range with different dose-dependent effects	■ Moderate cardiac disturbance ■ Cause muscle spasm effects ■ Increase intracranial and intraocular pressure ■ Poor-quality awakening

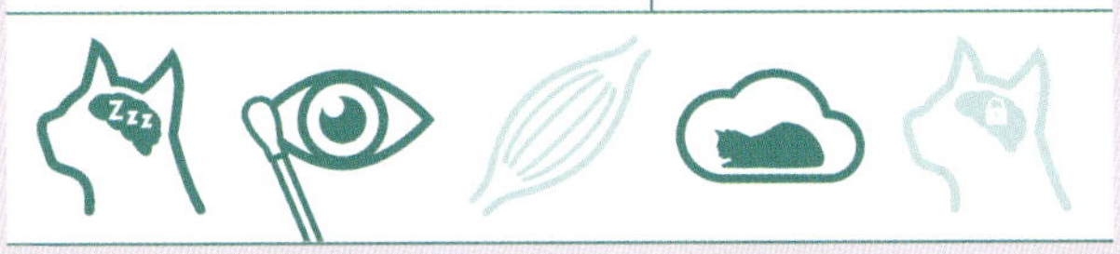

Phenolic agents

The most commonly used is propofol.

Advantages and disadvantages of propofol

Advantages	Disadvantages
■ Ultra short-acting drug ■ Does not accumulate and can serve as an agent for TIVA in the cat if the procedure does not last more than 60–90 minutes ■ Metabolized in the liver and probably in the muscle ■ Near-perfect awakening	■ Marked respiratory and cardiac depression proportional to the dose ■ Irritating if it leaks out of the vein ■ May induce hemolytic anemia in cats

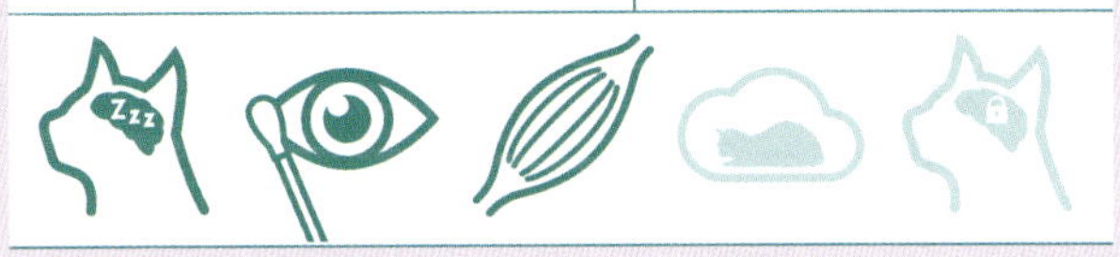

Steroid agents

The typical neuroactive steroid is alfaxalone.

Advantages and disadvantages of alfaxalone

Advantages	Disadvantages
■ Short-acting drug ■ Does not accumulate and can serve as an agent for total intravenous anesthesia (TIVA) in the cat ■ Scant cardiorespiratory depression, although boluses can produce apnea ■ Broad therapeutic range ■ Can be administered intravenously, but also intramuscularly or subcutaneously ■ Orexigenic	■ Patient awakening is not optimal if the effects of sedatives are no longer maintained when the effect of alfaxalone is eliminated

Imidazole agents

The most common imidazole drug is etomidate.

Advantages and disadvantages of etomidate

Advantages	Disadvantages
■ The safest of all anesthetics ■ Short-acting drug ■ Very broad therapeutic range ■ Can be used for TIVA, but it affects glucocorticoid synthesis ■ Does not affect cardiorespiratory function	■ Awakening is not high quality ■ Causes myoclonus during induction and awakening if sedation is not very good

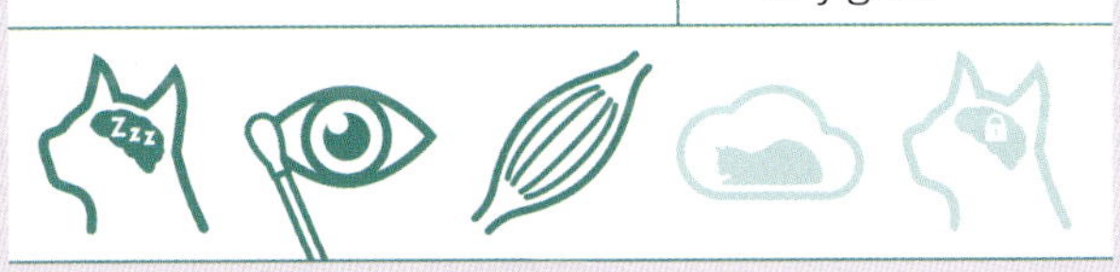

Halogenated agents

The most frequently used inhalation anesthetic is isoflurane.

Advantages and disadvantages of halogenated agents

Advantages	Disadvantages
■ The dose can be very well regulated according to the effect (it is necessary to take into account the sedatives and opioids administered) ■ Allow long anesthesia with almost no cumulative side effects	■ Dose-dependent hypotensive ■ Cause hypothermia

Figure 1 shows an overview of the anesthetic procedure in the feline patient.

Table 1 summarizes the characteristics of the main drugs used in feline anesthesia and sedation (Fig. 2).

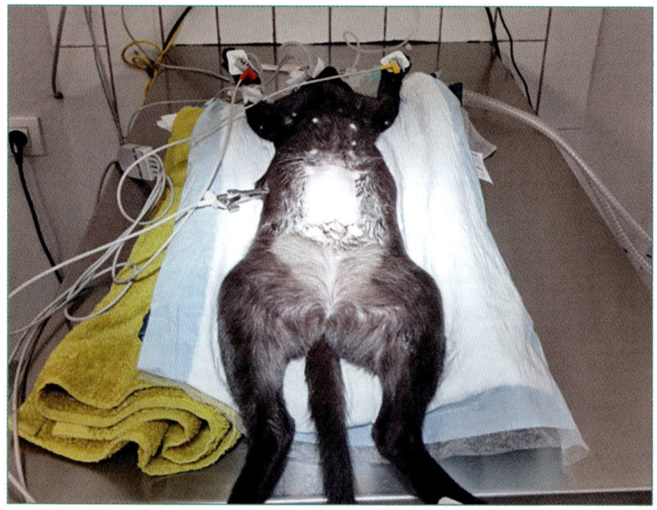

FIGURE 2. Anesthesia and monitoring of a feline patient.

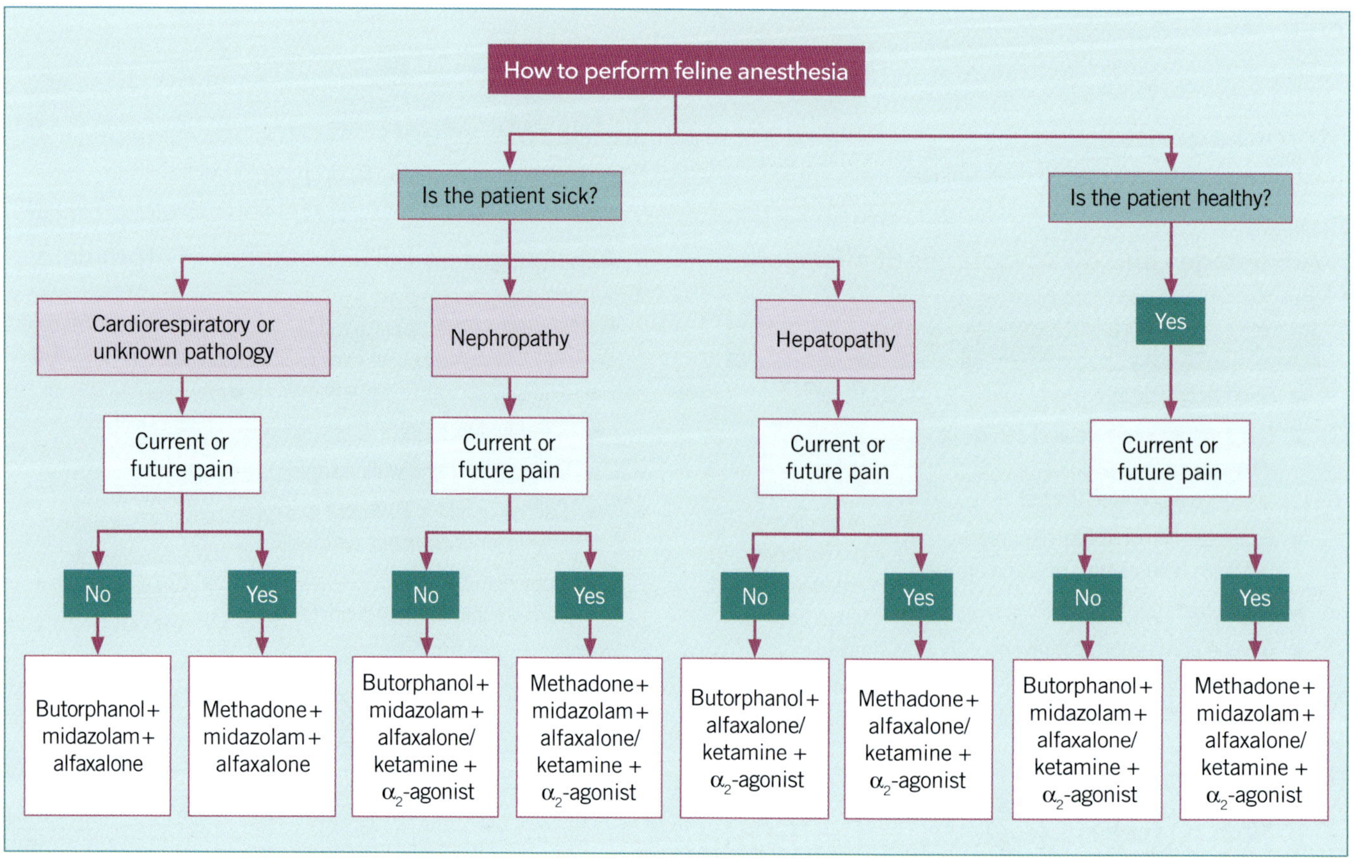

FIGURE 1. Anesthetic protocol in the feline patient.

TABLE 1. Main drugs used in feline anesthesia and sedation

Active ingredient	Dose and route of administration	Dose (ml)	Presentation in solution (%)	Type	Unconsciousness	Analgesia	Muscle relaxation	Amnesia	Reversible	Anti-inflammatory
Acepromazine	0.01–0.1 mg/kg IV, IM or SC	0.002–0.02 ml/kg	0.5% sol.	Phenothiazine	✗	✗	✓	✗	✗	✗
Alfaxalone	1–5 mg/kg IV, IM or SC	0.1–0.5 ml/kg	1% sol.	Anesthetic or sedative according to route of administration	✓	✗	✓	✗	✗	✗
Butorphanol	0.2–0.4 mg/kg IM or SC	0.02–0.04 ml/kg	1% sol.	Opioid	✗	✓	✓	✗	✓	✗
Midazolam	0.2–0.5 mg/kg IM or SC	0.04–0.1 ml/kg	0.5% sol.	Benzodiazepine	✗	✗	✓	✓	✓	✗
Medetomidine	20 µg/kg IM or SC	0.02 ml/kg	0.1% sol.	α_2-agonist	✗	✓	✓	✗	✓	✗
Dexmedetomidine	10 µg/kg IM or SC	0.02 ml/kg	0.05% sol.	α_2-agonist	✗	✓	✓	✗	✓	✗
Methadone	0.1–0.5 mg/kg IM or SC	0.01–0.05 ml/kg	1% sol.	Pure opioid	✓	✓	✓	✗	✓	✗
Ketamine	1–5 mg/kg IM or SC	0.05–0.25 ml/kg	10% sol.	Dissociative anesthetic NMDA antagonist	✓	✓	✗	✗	✗	✗
Bupivacaine	2 mg/kg	0.8 ml/kg	0.25 % sol.	Local anesthetic	✗	✓	✗	✗	✗	✗
Lidocaine	4 mg/kg	0.2 ml/kg	2% sol.	Local anesthetic	✗	✓	✗	✗	✗	✗
Meloxicam	0.2 mg/kg SC, IM or IV	Various	Various	NSAID	✗	✓	✗	✗	✗	✓
Robenacoxib	2 mg/kg SC	0.1 ml/kg	2% sol.	NSAID	✗	✓	✗	✗	✗	✓

Bibliography

Crowell-Davis SL. Benzodiazepines: pros and cons for fear and anxiety. *Compend Contin Educ Pract Vet*, 2008; 30(10):526–529.

McCollum JS, Dundee JW. Comparison of induction characteristics of four intravenous anaesthetic agents. *Anaesthesia*, 1986; 41(10):995–1000.

McConnell J, Kirby R, Rudloff E. Administration of acepromazine maleate to 31 dogs with a history of seizures. *J Vet Emerg Crit Care*, 2007; 17(3):262–267.

Moon PF. Cortisol suppression in cats after induction of anesthesia with etomidate, compared with ketamine-diazepam combination. *Am J Vet Res*, 1997; 58(8):868–871.

Paddleford RR, Harvey RC. Alpha 2 agonists and antagonists. *Vet Clin North Am Small Anim Pract*, 1999; 29(3):737–745.

Tobias KM, Marioni-Henry K, Wagner R. A retrospective study on the use of acepromazine maleate in dogs with seizures. *J Am Anim Hosp Assoc*, 2006; 42(4):283–289.

POSTOPERATIVE CARE IN FELINE MEDICINE

3

Salvador Cervantes

Introduction

The postanesthetic period is undoubtedly one of the most important phases if we seek to minimize perioperative and perianesthetic mortality, since it is in this period that almost 75% of anesthesia-related deaths occur. This phase can be further divided into two subparts, recovery or the immediate postoperative period after anesthesia and the long-term postoperative period. The objectives are different in each period and the strategies used and care provided will also be different.

Recovery or immediate postoperative period

In human medicine, this phase traditionally lasts about 24 hours after surgery. However, in feline medicine, due to the tendency to minimize the patient's time away from home, the authors agree that it is a phase with a variable duration, lasting from the moment the patient wakes up from anesthesia until they arrive back at home. The postoperative objectives in this first phase can be grouped into:

- Awakening management
- Pain control
- Infection control
- Temperature control
- Blood glucose control
- Inflammation control

Awakening management

The objective of this management is to ensure that the patient recovers their reflexes, from the blink reflex to the swallowing reflex; all of them have to return quickly and progressively to ensure that the patient is able to stay within the margins of homeostasis.

Pain control

Postsurgical pain is of no benefit to our patient, delays the return to function and normality, is a risk for the onset of a central sensitization process and can cause arrhythmias due to the release of catecholamines. For these reasons, we will restart or prolong the analgesic methods that were initiated during sedation or anesthetic maintenance to avoid a lack of analgesic coverage.

During this period, pain is usually controlled by various analgesic strategies, the most significant of which are:

- **Opioid analgesics:** pure opioids such as methadone or constant rate infusions of fentanyl are usually administered for severe pain, while partial opioid agonists such as buprenorphine or tramadol are left for the treatment of moderate pain.
- **Local anesthetic nerve blocks:** these blocks can completely eliminate pain sensations for periods ranging from hours to a few days, reducing the need for opioids and allowing for a rapid return to normalcy with high functionality. They can be applied before the surgery starts to obtain the maximum analgesic effect or just after the intervention before awakening the patient. This second option is usually used in surgeries where there is bleeding, since local anesthesia will cause vasodilation and, therefore, more bleeding.
- **Nonsteroidal anti-inflammatory drugs:** these agents are widely used in veterinary medicine and in the last 20 years a couple of "felinized" molecules have appeared that allow the use of these products during the postoperative period. These are meloxicam and robenacoxib, which reduce inflammation, pain and, in the case of meloxicam, control temperature by inhibiting prostaglandin synthesis. These products can only be administered in normotensive and normovolemic patients; without these two conditions we should refrain from administering them, since they can induce acute kidney or pancreatic disease by reducing the production of prostaglandins that ensure blood supply to both organs.

Infection control

Preventing and treating infection is crucial in all surgeries; however, the strategies used depend on the **type of wound** (clean, clean–contaminated, contaminated, dirty). In all interventions we should apply the same techniques for cleaning and disinfecting the surgical site, where shaving followed by the application of a **chlorhexidine-alcohol solution** are usually the methods of choice, since they better combine a fast speed of action with a greater residual effect. Once the surgery is finished, we must disinfect the incision area again and clean it of blood and rests of organic tissues. During the first 24 hours it is important to keep the wound clean, until the fibrin plug that will seal it until it is healed is created. The application of **aqueous solutions of chlorhexidine or stabilized hypochlorous acid** is adequate for this purpose, without causing itching or stinging in the patient that would induce licking.

The use of prophylactic antibiotics is not recommended in clean elective surgeries such as ovariectomies, ovariohysterectomies or castrations. First-choice antibiotics will be administered against the bacteria that mainly proliferate at the site of infection (which will be different according to the type of surgery). Thus, first-generation cephalosporins (e.g., cephalexin, cefazolin, cephalothin or cefadroxil) are indicated to prevent *Staphylococcus* spp. infections, while amoxicillin or amoxicillin with clavulanate will be chosen for *Escherichia coli* infections. In other words, in orthopedic surgery involving implants, cephalosporins will be preferred, while in surgery of the abdominal cavity entailing a solution of continuity of the gastrointestinal or urinary tract, the use of amoxicillin (with or without clavulanate) will be preferred.

> For the optimal application of these antibiotics, it is recommended that an intravenous infusion of these products be started 30 to 60 minutes before the first incision is made.

These drugs should be administered every 2-4 hours until the end of the procedure, but never for more than 24 hours.

Temperature control

Temperature control is a vital issue for all veterinarians who anesthetize cats. This is because hypothermia is one of the most frequent complications suffered by these patients due to their high volume:body surface area ratio. All feline patients, even those that have not undergone surgery but only sedation or anesthesia for a diagnostic procedure (e.g., abdominal ultrasound), are susceptible to hypothermia to a greater or lesser degree. It is for this reason that all cats under sedation/anesthesia will have an assistant in charge of controlling their body temperature until they have recovered normothermia. The most commonly used methods for temperature recovery are hot air heaters, hot water mattresses and infrared lamps (Fig. 1). With any of these methods, it is important to be aware that a patient waking up from anesthesia will not be able to sense thermal sensations correctly, so they may end up with a burn from coming into contact with a heat generator or some surface that has become too hot from being too close to a heat source (Fig. 2).

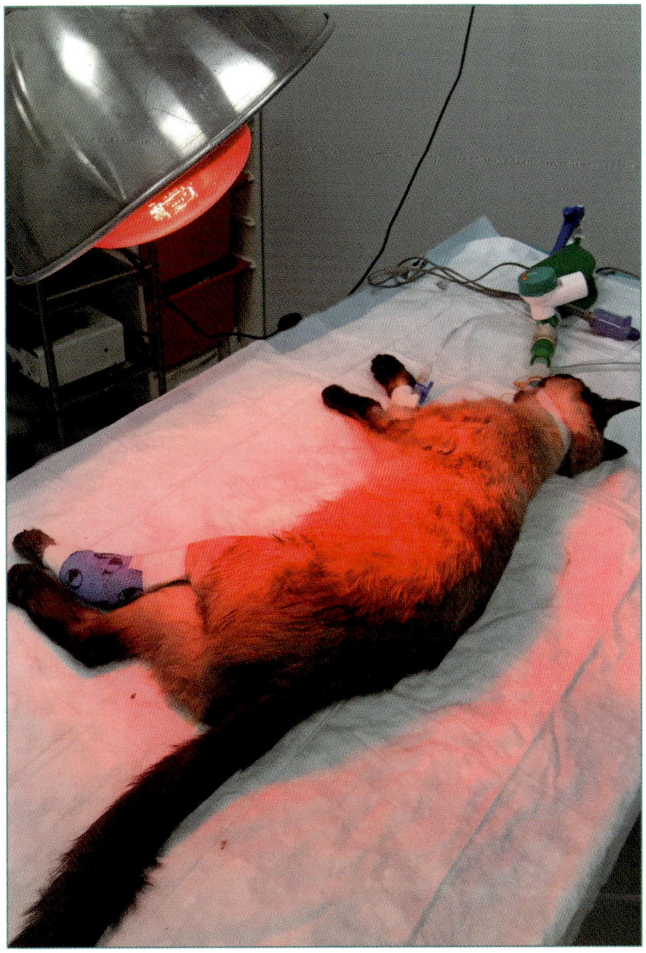

FIGURE 1. Patient during the immediate postoperative period under an infrared lamp to avoid cooling.

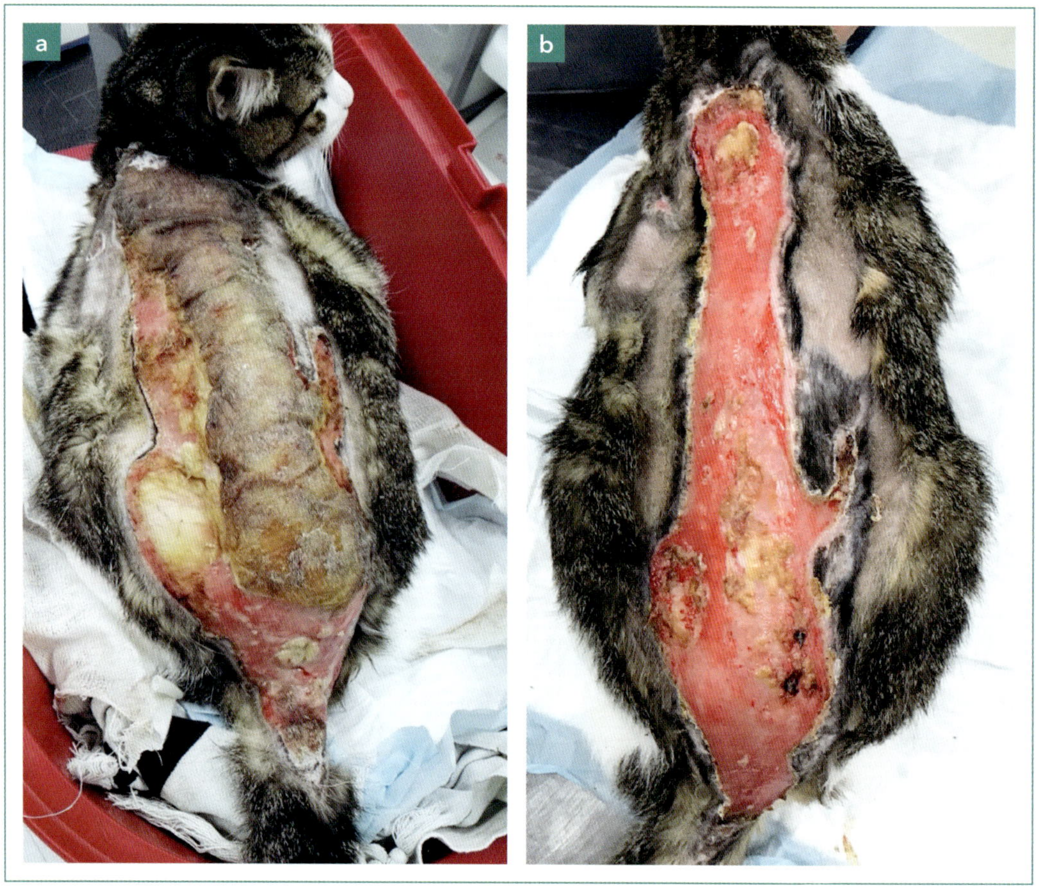

FIGURE 2. (a) Burn caused by an electric mat on a patient during an operation; a few days later the skin began to open up. (b) Result after debridement and granulation tissue growth.

Blood glucose control

Maintaining blood glucose levels and the restoring of intestinal normality is essential in cats, much more so than it is in dogs. This is because cats require an external supply of antioxidants in order to properly metabolize the drugs used during anesthesia. In addition, they are more sensitive to fasting than dogs, which is not in vain evolutionarily as one is a strict carnivore/hunter and the other is considered a carnivore/opportunist. It is for this reason that the authors recommend, except on rare occasions, reducing presurgical fasting times in cats from 12 to 8 hours or even 4 hours in the case of kittens or cats with hyperthyroidism. Similarly, the authors recommend that food be reintroduced quickly after anesthesia. This early reintroduction achieves several objectives: better elimination of the drugs used during the intervention, reduction of oxidative damage, recovery of gastrointestinal motility and physiological normalization of glycemia. Only in the case of surgeries affecting the digestive tract is there a delay in the reintroduction of food, and this delay normally does not go beyond 12 hours.

Inflammation control

For the control of inflammation there are various strategies, from pharmacological (already mentioned during pain control) to mechanical, such as compressive bandages or the application of cold to the affected area. Cold packs should be used only if the patient has already recovered body temperature; otherwise, they may interfere with temperature control and recovery.

Long-term postoperative period

This period lasts from the patient's arrival at home until full functional recovery, if possible. In this phase, some of the postoperative care initiated during the immediate postoperative period is maintained and, additionally, functional recovery control is initiated, central sensitization is countered and body condition and muscle mass are monitored. One of the care elements that is usually prolonged from the previous phase is infection control, which in the case of surgery with stitches is usually maintained until the stitches are removed (e.g., by applying antiseptics every 12 to 24 hours).

Functional recovery control

Although this care may often be seen in a reductionist manner, focused only on prolonging the pain control initiated in the immediate postsurgical stage, it is not. It is true that, for an early functional recovery, the patient should not suffer pain or at least it should be mild and allow them to start working the affected area, but functional recovery also includes active and passive physiotherapy and the application of techniques such as acupuncture, electrotherapy (e.g., transcutaneous electrical nerve stimulation —TENS—), laser therapy, etc.

Pain control

Pain control does not just involve the most immediate perioperative pain. The veterinary surgeon can be seen as one of the main causes of chronic pain, as is the surgeon in human medicine. This is because the long-term control of pain and the role of pain in central sensitization has traditionally been underestimated. If a good postsurgical pain protocol is to be designed, several factors must be taken into account, such as the quality of life obtained after surgery, the level of functional recovery and, finally, the possibilities shown by the patient–owner partnership. It should be added that, in the case of cats, there will often be an "unknown" factor due to a lack of knowledge as to whether the patient can improve a little more. Unfortunately, if this factor is to be ruled out, therapeutic tests should almost always be performed, in which the owner assesses the patient's activity level and quality of life, both before and after treatment. This information will be evaluated by the clinician, who will decide to what extent the patient may be suffering from chronic pain syndrome.

Infection control

Treatment to prevent infection should be carried out from the preoperative period until the stitches are removed or, if surgery has been performed on an infected area, until the area has fully recovered (e.g., osteomyelitis of the maxilla or mandible). For those cases that only require skin care, solutions with 2% chlorhexidine or stabilized hypochlorous acid are highly recommended. In the case of mucous membranes, the same active ingredients can be used but diluted, as in the case of chlorhexidine, which is used at 0.12%.

As far as antibiotics are concerned, it has already been mentioned that antibiotics are only rarely recommended in the immediate postoperative period, and generally only for 24 hours. In cases where infection is a given (e.g., osteomyelitis, oral surgeries) antibiotic treatment may be extended.

Feeding tubes

Cats are very susceptible to anorexia and hyporexia (Box 1). This is because they have difficulty reducing their liver transaminase activity rate in the presence of a reduced protein intake, causing the patient to quickly (about 3 days after the onset of anorexia or hyporexia) suffer the consequences of reduced calorie or protein consumption. For this reason, veterinarians often need to place feeding tubes in patients to avoid clinical signs caused by not ingesting the correct amount of calories and protein.

Enteral versus parenteral feeding

Whenever possible, the veterinarian should choose to administer nutrients by the enteral route because it is more physiological, it maintains the health of the gastrointestinal tract and it is safer and more economical than the parenteral route. In fact, parenteral feeding is not at all common in feline medicine and is reserved for truly exceptional cases.

BOX 1. Causes of anorexia and hyporexia in cats

- Presence of poorly controlled pain
- Presence of nausea or vomiting
- Hospitalization stress
- Offering unfamiliar foods
- Induction or development of food aversion
- Elevated inflammatory cytokine profile
- Medication side effects

When to opt for enteral tube feeding

More and more professionals are opting for the placement of a feeding tube if, after diagnosis and the first phases of treatment, the patient does not manage to ingest enough calories and proteins. And we know that keeping a feline patient in a state of malnutrition is not at all beneficial. Malnutrition increases the length of hospitalization and the chances of patient death, i.e., it increases the morbidity/mortality rate.

Currently, the placement of a feeding tube is part of standard treatment for many clinical conditions where it is known or anticipated that the patient will have difficulty meeting their daily calorie and protein requirements.

Feeding tubes used in cats

There are four types of feeding tubes (Table 1), although three are most commonly used and, of these three, the esophagostomy tube is the most common. When selecting a tube, six important points should be taken into account before deciding on one or another.

Factors for selecting a feeding tube

1. Duration that the tube will be in place, or the time that assisted feeding will be necessary.
2. Type of food required. Narrower tubes such as nasal or jejunostomy tubes are much more restrictive in this regard, as their diameter does not allow for diets that are not very liquid.
3. The pathology to be treated.
4. The presence or absence of disease affecting the nose, mouth, pharynx, esophagus or stomach.
5. The patient's ability to overcome anesthesia. Only nasoesophageal tubes can be placed in unanesthetized cats.
6. Concerns and abilities of guardians, especially if assisted feeding is to be continued in the patient's home.

Nasoesophageal tubes

Nasoesophageal tubes are relatively well tolerated by patients, but above all they tend to be preferred by cat guardians, as they are very economical, do not involve anesthesia or sedation and are easily removable, if necessary.

The great advantage of this type of tube is that they can provide nutritional support quickly and easily. Nevertheless, the clinician must understand that these tubes can only remain in place for a short period of time, and that esophagostomy or gastrostomy tubes will be more appropriate for nutritional treatments that last longer than a week.

However, the most notable disadvantages in hospitalized feline patients are the discomfort caused by the tube and the Elizabethan collar, which is usually mandatory in most cats, or the rhinitis that may occur. Said rhinitis can complicate an already existing respiratory process and cause dyspnea/tachypnea syndrome, resulting in the tube being withdrawn earlier than necessary.

Of course, if there are reasons that make it inadvisable to place a tube in the nose, esophagopathies, gastropathies or emetic processes that cannot be medically controlled, nasoesophageal tubes are not recommended.

Finally, very often these tubes are not chosen due to the small number of foods formulated for this administration. They are of very low caliber, which forces the use of fully liquid commercialized diets that are totally free of lumps and have ideal rheological properties.

The tubes used are usually 3 to 6 Fr in diameter. Whenever possible, the placement of a 6 Fr tube is highly recommended to make it easier for the food to enter and more difficult for the tube to bend irreparably, forcing it to be changed.

Polyurethane tubes are preferred over silicone ones, and silicon tubes are preferred over PVC (polyvinyl chloride) ones.

For the **placement of a nasoesophageal tube** (see video):

1. First, we must choose the diameter of the tube (3 to 6 Fr) and mark the length we want to insert. Normally, this entails measuring from the tip of the nose to the 7th or 8th intercostal space. However, the authors use a faster and more practical technique, which is to elevate the elbow in a caudal direction. This point usually marks the base of the heart in the vast majority of cats and is a good place for the tube tip to rest once it is in place. In any case, what must be avoided is for the tip of the tube to remain inside the stomach, which may cause reflux, stimulate the emetic reflex or provoke esophagitis.
2. Once the tube has been marked to the chosen depth, a drop of topical anesthetic is applied in the nostril to be used for tube placement. Allow about 30 seconds for the anesthetic to take effect. Most cats will allow this maneuver without struggling too much. The use of a towel restraint technique (e.g., burrito technique) is recommended for the protection of both the patient and the assistant. If there is excessive struggling, mild sedation may be applied.
3. The tip of the tube is lubricated with water-soluble gel (it can be a gel such as ultrasound gel or one with lidocaine or even chlorhexidine).
4. The cat's head is then held firmly with one hand and tilted so that the tip of the nose is raised. The tube is inserted with

TABLE 1. Comparison of feeding tubes

	Nasoesophageal tube	Esophagostomy tube	Gastrostomy tube	Enterostomy tube
Advantages	■ Ease of placement ■ Economical ■ Well tolerated, although it requires an Elizabethan collar ■ No anesthesia or sedation required	■ Ease of placement ■ Economical ■ Very well tolerated ■ Administration of a wide variety of available foods ■ Can be used long term	■ Very well tolerated ■ Administration of a wide variety of available foods ■ Useful in patients with esophagopathy	■ Can be used in patients with uncontrollable vomiting or at risk for pulmonary aspiration ■ Useful in patients with oral, pharyngeal, esophageal, gastroduodenal or pancreatic problems ■ Can be placed in the duodenum or jejunum
Disadvantages	■ Only useful for liquid diets ■ Not applicable if esophagopathies or vomiting are present ■ Allows only short-term feeding (up to 7 days, maximum 10 days) ■ Produces rhinitis	■ Requires anesthesia ■ Not applicable in the presence of vomiting or esophagopathies	■ More technically complicated ■ Requires anesthesia ■ Necessary to wait 24 h to start feeding ■ May cause peritonitis as a complication ■ Necessary to wait 14 days to withdraw it	■ The most technically complicated ■ Requires anesthesia ■ May cause peritonitis as a complication ■ Must be removed under anesthesia
Tube diameter	3–6 Fr	10–16 Fr	12–20 Fr	6–8 Fr
Observations	—	—	There are open techniques, semiopen techniques with semiblind kits and endoscopically guided techniques	There are open techniques and endoscopic techniques, in which the tube is introduced through the stomach and advanced to the duodenum or jejunum

the other hand and introduced little by little. The tube should be introduced in a ventromedial direction so that it passes through the ventral nasal meatus and reaches the nasopharynx without much difficulty. If it is suspected that the meatus through which the tube is passing is the dorsal or middle meatus, the tube must be withdrawn and reoriented.

> From experience, the authors recommend passing the first 2-3 cm of the tube slowly, as this is the most uncomfortable part for the patient.

5. Once the nasopharynx has been reached, continue little by little so that the patient is aware that they have a foreign body in their throat and help us by means of the swallowing reflex. At this time, the assistant allows the cat's head to return to its normal position, which also helps prevent tracheal intubation.
6. Once the esophagus is reached, the tube is advanced to the mark that was made in the first step.
7. An X-ray is performed to check for perfect placement of the tube. The authors do not recommend serum aspiration or instillation techniques to verify tube placement because they have found that these systems are not foolproof.
8. The tube is affixed to the patient's cheek or forehead by means of a butterfly of medical adhesive tape and a pair of stitches using nonabsorbable, flexible suture material.
9. An Elizabethan collar is placed, since the vast majority of patients try to remove the tube and succeed very easily thanks to the use they make of the nail of the first finger on the side of the tube (Fig. 3).

VIDEO

Placement of a nasoesophageal tube

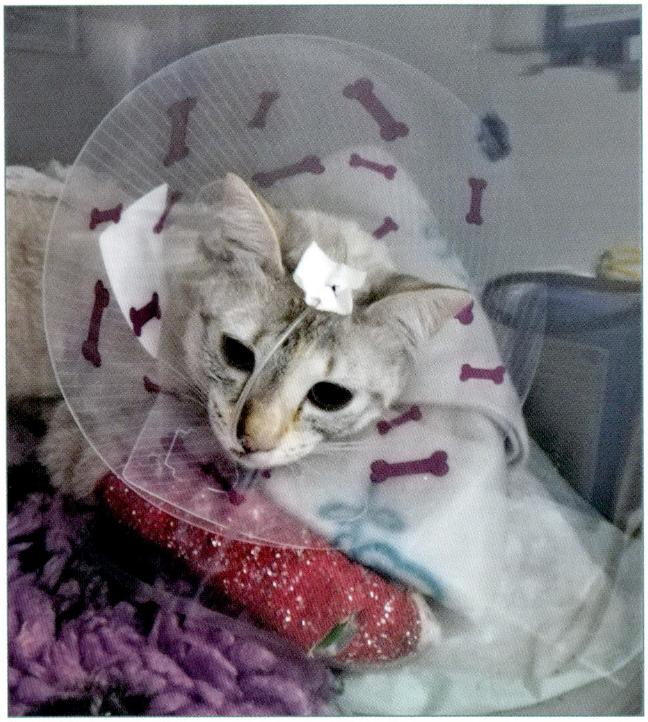

FIGURE 3. Patient after placement of a nasoesophageal tube.

Esophagostomy tubes

Currently, esophagostomy tubes are the most widely used and preferred by many clinicians. Their ease of placement, patient acceptance and minimal storage requirements make them even suitable for the guardian to feed their cat at home in a very simple and safe manner. In addition, they are suitable for administering almost any type of wet food that can be liquefied and their shelf life can range from one week to several months. The only two true contraindications are when the gastroesophageal area is not usable and when there are emetic syndromes that cannot be controlled with medication.

The materials from which these tubes are made include polyurethane, silicone, PVC and latex. The authors prefer polyurethane tubes because they are more resistant to bending and breaking, collapse less often and have sufficient stiffness to reduce leakage in the event of an emetic accident. Tube diameters ranging from 10 to 16 Fr (4.0–5.3 mm in diameter) are usually recommended. These diameters allow the use of almost any liquefied wet diet.

For the **placement of an esophagostomy tube** (see video):

1. The cat should be placed in lateral recumbency and the upper mid cervical region should be shaved and aseptically prepared (from the angle of the mandible to the cranial margin of the scapula and shoulder).

> Brief general anesthesia is required for this technique.

2. After the intratracheal intubation of the patient, curved Kocher forceps long enough to reach the esophagus are introduced. The forceps are oriented in a laterodorsal direction to identify both the esophagus in the mid cervical region and the jugular vein, which will be moved in a ventral direction to safeguard it.
3. Over the tip of the Kocher forceps, maintaining pressure at all times, the skin is incised directly with a scalpel blade. The tip of the forceps is pulled through the incision and the forceps is opened.
4. If not already done, the length of tube required should now be calculated. This is done by measuring the distance from the incision to the base of the heart, which can be easily calculated by moving the elbow caudally over the ribs or by using the 7th or 8th intercostal space as a reference.
5. The tip of the tube is held firmly with the forceps and gently pulled until it is extracted through the patient's oral cavity.
6. At this point, the tip of the tube is reintroduced into the esophagus. This can be done with the forceps again or with the hands. The tube is moved in the direction of the stomach. When the direction that the tube enters through the incision changes from cranial to caudal, the tube has been correctly positioned. The surgeon should ensure that the tube tip is in the correct position by checking the length of the inserted tube.
7. Next, a tobacco pouch suture is performed around the incision and, once completed and without cutting the ends, these are used to make a Chinese finger trap or Roman sandal suture (Fig. 4).
8. After this, and to finish, an antiseptic is applied again followed by a light bandage to protect the tube and at the same time allow it to exit, without bending, in a caudodorsal direction (Fig. 5). This bandage should be checked every 24–48 hours

to detect the presence of dermatitis or abscesses early. It is not necessary to use antibiotics with these tubes; in fact, aqueous solutions of chlorhexidine or hypochlorous acid or healing creams are now preferred to support the creation and care of the stoma.

This tube can be removed at any time after it has been placed, even the next day, without the need for sedation or anesthesia.

VIDEO

Placement of an esophagostomy tube

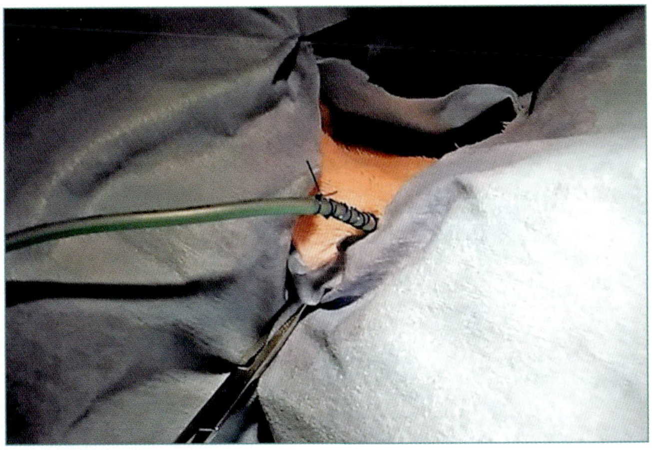

FIGURE 4. Detail of the Chinese finger trap suture.

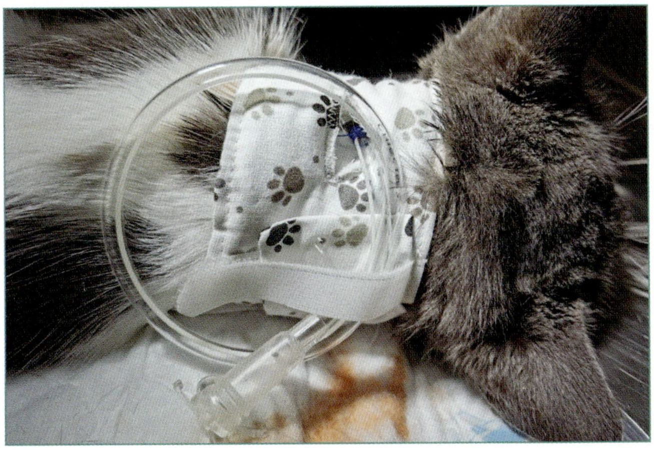

FIGURE 5. Bandage applied after esophageal tube placement.

Gastrostomy tubes

These tubes have practically fallen into disuse and are used in those patients that cannot tolerate an esophagostomy tube for whatever reason. They usually consist of mushroom-tip tubes with a diameter of up to 20 Fr. Placement of these tubes requires the use of endoscopy or laparotomy. The following is a brief explanation of how to perform the laparotomy technique.

For the **placement of a gastrostomy tube by laparotomy:**

1. The cat is placed in dorsal recumbency and the cranial abdominal surgical field is aseptically prepared for a linea alba celiotomy. This incision should be about 3–5 cm in length and made behind the xiphoid.
2. The scalpel blade is used to create a defect in the left abdominal wall to allow the gastrostomy tube to pass into the patient's stomach. The site of choice is usually just behind the last rib. To create this defect in the correct place, we will draw an imaginary line joining the spine with the midpoint of the celiotomy incision and make the defect at the level of the ventral third of this line. Using Kocher forceps, the end of the mushroom-tip tube is passed through the defect created.
3. Fixation sutures are then placed in the stomach wall in the area where the tube will enter.
4. A tobacco pouch suture is placed in the gastric body at the site where the tube will enter, before creating the incision with the scalpel.
5. The tube lumen must be clamped to avoid contamination of the surgical field.
6. After making the incision in the center of the tobacco pouch suture, the tip of the tube is inserted. To facilitate this step, the mushroom-shaped tip of the tube should be clamped with Kocher forceps.
7. Once the tube is inserted, it is withdrawn until the mushroom butts up against the gastric wall, and the tobacco pouch suture is knotted and well secured.
8. The stomach is attached to the abdominal wall using four horizontal mattress sutures between the stomach wall and the body wall, placed around the tube in sequence to create a box suture pattern.
9. The stoma is wrapped with some omentum, which should be placed around the tube and sutures.
10. The tube is secured externally with a Chinese finger trap or Roman sandal suture.
11. Finally, the exit point of the tube is bandaged before recovery from anesthesia to prevent accidental removal. This can be achieved by using a tubular mesh bandage.

Bibliography

Breheny CR, Boag A, Le Gal A et al. Esophageal feeding tube placement and the associated complications in 248 cats. *J Vet Intern Med*, 2019; 33(3):1306–1314.

Chan DL. The inappetent hospitalised cat: clinical approach to maximizing nutritional support. *J Feline Med Surg*, 2009; 11(11):925–933.

Chen X, Li Y, Cai X et al. Dose-effect of dietary L-arginine supplementation on burn wound healing in rats. *Chin Med J (Engl)*, 1999; 112(9):828–831.

Dhupa N. Hypothermia in dogs and cats. *Comp Cont Ed Pract Vet*, 1995; 17(1):61–68.

Fink L, Jennings M, Reiter AM. Esophagostomy feeding tube placement in the dog and cat. *J Vet Dent*, 2014; 31(2):133–138.

Formaggini L. Normograde, minimally invasive technique for oesophagostomy in cats. *J Feline Med Surg*, 2009; 11(6):481–486.

Glaus TM, Cornelius LM, Bartges JW, Reusch C. Complications with non-endoscopic percutaneous gastrostomy in 31 cats and 10 dogs: a retrospective study. *J Small Anim Pract*, 1998; 39(5):218–222.

Hale FA, Anthony JM. Prevention of hypothermia in cats during routine oral hygiene procedures. *Can Vet J*, 1997; 38(5):297–299.

Ireland LM, Hohenhaus AE, Broussard JD, Weissman BL. A comparison of owner management and complications in 67 cats with esophagostomy and percutaneous endoscopic gastrostomy feeding tubes. *J Am Anim Hosp Assoc*, 2003; 39(3):241–246.

Klaus JA, Rudloff E, Kirby R. Nasogastric tube feeding in cats with suspected acute pancreatitis: 55 cases (2001–2006). *J Vet Emerg Crit Care (San Antonio)*, 2009; 19(4):337–346.

Redondo JI, Suesta P, Gil L et al. Retrospective study of the prevalence of postanaesthetic hypothermia in cats. *Vet Rec*, 2012; 170(8):206.

Remillard RL. Nutritional support in critical care patients. *Vet Clin North Am Small Anim Pract*, 2002; 32(5):1145–1164.

Seaman R, Legendre AM. Owner experiences with home use of a gastrostomy tube in their dog or cat. *J Am Vet Med Assoc*, 1998; 212(10):1576–1578.

Sohail MA. The ingestive behaviour of the domestic cat: a review. *Nutrition Abstracts Rev*, 1983; 53:177–186.

Zaghini G, Biagi G. Nutritional peculiarities and diet palatability in the cat. *Vet Res Commun*, 2005; 29:39–44.

SUTURE TYPES AND TECHNIQUES 4

Salvador Cervantes

Introduction

All surgeries in which an incision is made require a system of closure. Although the most common method involves the use of sutures, nowadays other systems, such as surgical staples or biocompatible tissue adhesive, are used quite frequently in veterinary centers. Like any aspect of surgery, there are two clear dimensions when it comes to describing the use of sutures. There is a scientific dimension, in which choosing the type of needle and material, along with the suture pattern, basically are a function of scientific criteria; and there is also an "artistic" dimension, given that the choice of patterns and their placement can be called an art. If the reader is just beginning, or coming back after a while away, it would be worthwhile to use a silicone-based synthetic skin model in order to increase dexterity, speed and precision in the placement of stitches.

Types of sutures

There are many types of sutures, but for the sake of this chapter only those sutures that the clinician uses in 98% of surgeries will be described. In a first set of categories, we find absorbable and nonabsorbable sutures, both of which include monofilament and multifilament materials, as well as coated multifilament sutures, which aim to provide the advantages of both options.

> Note that, nowadays, a material is not considered reabsorbable if its mechanical resistance is maintained 60 days after its application, even if it may be eliminated later.

Absorbable sutures

Absorbable sutures are those that are dissolved by the patient's own body, whether they are made from natural materials, such as collagen, or artificial materials such as polyglycolic acid, polyglyconate and polydioxanone, to name a few with different rates of absorption. Natural materials are rarely used in cats, since the proteolytic process through which they are eliminated may easily produce inflammation and often rejection reactions in some cats. Due to their high available supply and reduced price, artificial sutures are currently indicated for almost any type of suture that will remain inside a feline patient. But the reason for their use is especially due to the lower inflammatory reaction produced when they are dissolved by hydrolytic processes.

Nonabsorbable sutures

Within this category of sutures, there is also a distinction between natural (e.g., silk, linen) and artificial; however, once again due to the higher rate of inflammation and complications in cats, natural materials are not often used and have been replaced by artificial sutures. The most commonly used artificial sutures are those made of polypropylene, polyamide (nylon) and polyester. In feline medicine, these products are usually used in skin sutures and in those situations that require tension for a long period of time, as can be the case in orthopedic surgery. Although the risk of reaction to these products is currently very low, the chance that a cat will have a foreign body reaction that may lead to a chronic inflammation process is not something that should be underestimated.

Selection of suture materials

The following characteristics should be kept in mind when selecting suture materials:

1. Duration of the useful resistance period
2. Degree of fixation and desired mobility
3. Risk of infection
4. Degree of reaction produced by the suture
5. Minimum caliber needed to provide sufficient resistance
6. Minimum caliber that can be used without producing tears

Table 1 shows recommendations and contraindications for different types of sutures, according to the tissue to which they will be applied.

Suture techniques

Much has been written about the number of wraps that each throw should have and the number of throws in each knot, and some manufacturers give recommendations. However, the clinician should know that this is dependent on:

- The material selected, since the friction coefficient and the memory, among other characteristics, vary.
- The tissue and the area that is being sutured. An area with high vascularity is not the same thing as an area without this vascularity, and a sterile area is not the same thing as an area with a high risk of infection.
- The chosen suture pattern, since a simple suture does not offer the same level of security as a continuous or continuous interlocking suture.
- The clinician's experience. As the surgeon acquires experience, they observe that the knot is either more secure or has a greater tendency to lose tension, depending on how the throws are tightened and the number of wraps they contain.

For these reasons, it is practically impossible to give fixed guidelines. Therefore, when switching to a new suture manufacturer, both beginner clinicians and experienced surgeons are advised to pay close attention to the condition of each stitch as it is being placed.

> Knotting techniques are also variable and depend on the tissue that is being sutured, the type of material and its caliber. Nevertheless, it seems to be accepted practice that a minimum of three throws is required for a secure knot. These throws can consist of single, double or triple wraps.

Common suture patterns in feline medicine

In general, suture patterns are divided into two groups: interrupted patterns and continuous patterns.

Interrupted patterns

These are sutures that close wounds through separate stitches:

- **Simple interrupted suture:** this is one of the most frequently used suture technique in feline medicine (Fig. 1a).

TABLE 1. Recommendations and contraindications of sutures as a function of the biological tissue

Type of tissue	Suture recommendation and contraindications
Skin	Nonabsorbable monofilament (polyamide, polypropylene)
Subcutaneous tissue	Absorbable (poliglecaprone, polyglactin 910, polyglytone)
Tendon	Nonabsorbable or delayed absorbable (polydioxanone, polypropylene, polyamide)
Abdominal, linea alba closure	Absorbable or nonabsorbable (polydioxanone, glycomer 631, polyamide)
Muscle	Absorbable (polyglactin 910, polyglycolic acid)
Parenchymal organs	Absorbable monofilament (poliglecaprone, glycomer 631)
Hollow organs (bladder)	■ Absorbable (poliglecaprone, polyglactin 910, glycomer 631) ■ Polyglycolic acid should not be used in the bladder since it dissolves quickly in urine
Infected or contaminated wounds	■ Absorbable (polyglactin, poliglecaprone) ■ Braided nonabsorbable sutures are not recommended since they may lead to fistula formation. Catgut is also not recommended since it absorbs rapidly
Blood vessels and vascular anastomoses	■ Ligatures: absorbable suture material ■ Vascular anastomoses: nonabsorbable monofilament (e.g., polypropylene) and with a needle:suture ratio of 1:1

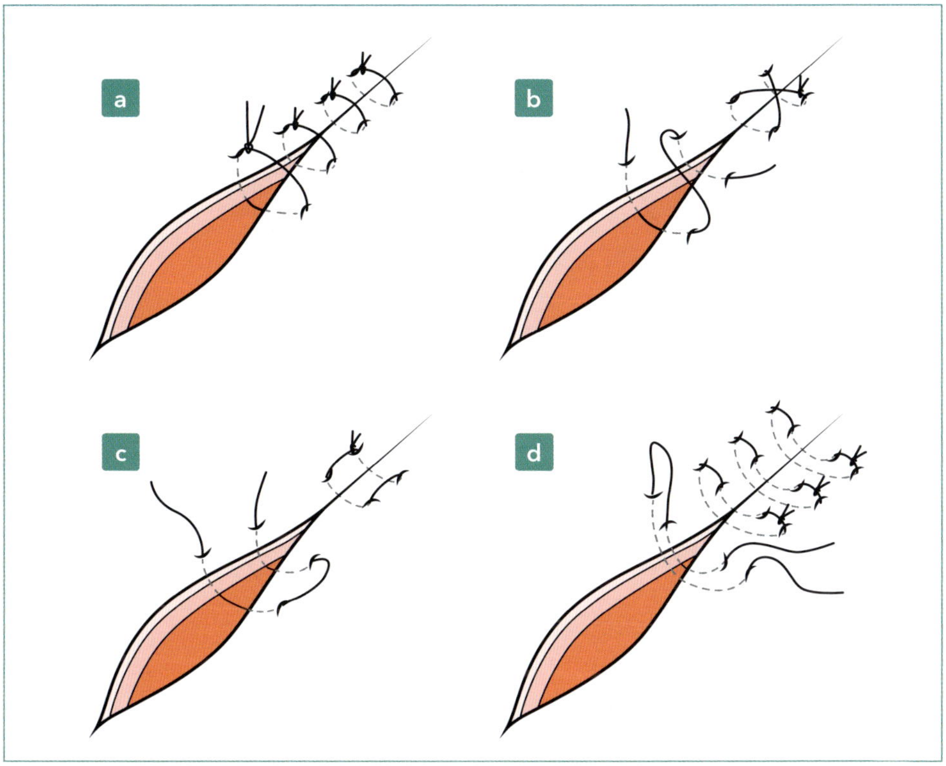

FIGURE 1. Interrupted suture patterns.
a) Simple interrupted suture.
b) Figure-of-X stitches or cruciate (cross mattress) suture.
c) Interrupted U-shaped suture.
d) Vertical mattress suture.

- **Figure-of-X stitches or cruciate (cross mattress) suture:** this provides added resistance (Fig. 1b).
- **Interrupted U-shaped suture:** this avoids passing strands over the wound (Fig. 1c).
- **Vertical mattress suture:** the main advantage is that it respects the vascularization of the area (Fig. 1d).

Continuous patterns

A major advantage of continuous suture patterns is that they cut down on the amount of time needed for surgery and anesthesia. However, a complication is that if they become loose or come undone, this increases, at least theoretically, the risk of dehiscence. Nevertheless, because they involve fewer stitches that the patient can pull at, these sutures are typically better tolerated. If this suture pattern is chosen, the use of shirts or bandages to protect the integrity of the suture may be recommended (see video).

VIDEO

How to make a homemade postoperative shirt for cats

The continuous patterns used most in feline medicine are:

- **Simple continuous suture pattern** (Fig. 2a).
- **Reverdin suture:** also known as Ford interlocking, this continuous suture pattern, if fairly tight, minimizes the risk of dehiscence if one of the stitches loses tension or comes undone. However, this extra security comes at the cost of weakening the suture material as it rubs excessively against the loop below the new stitch (Fig. 2b).
- **Continuous vertical mattress or U-shaped suture:** this pattern has all the advantages of continuous sutures, while minimizing the number of passes over the wound (Fig. 2c).
- **Schmieden suture:** this is an inverting suture in which the needle goes from inside the wound to the outside at every stitch. The rate of inversion is low, however, and this suture is indicated for nearly all tubular or vesical organs (Fig. 2d).
- **Intradermal suture with Aberdeen knot:** this suture has become popular in feline medicine because, if done correctly, it does not come out over the skin at any point. It starts with a simple intradermal stitch that is not cut. It then continues with simple intradermal stitches placed at short intervals from each other (Fig. 2e). Finally, an Aberdeen knot is made at the end of the suture pattern; this knot also remains buried (see video). This suture is very useful for wounds that

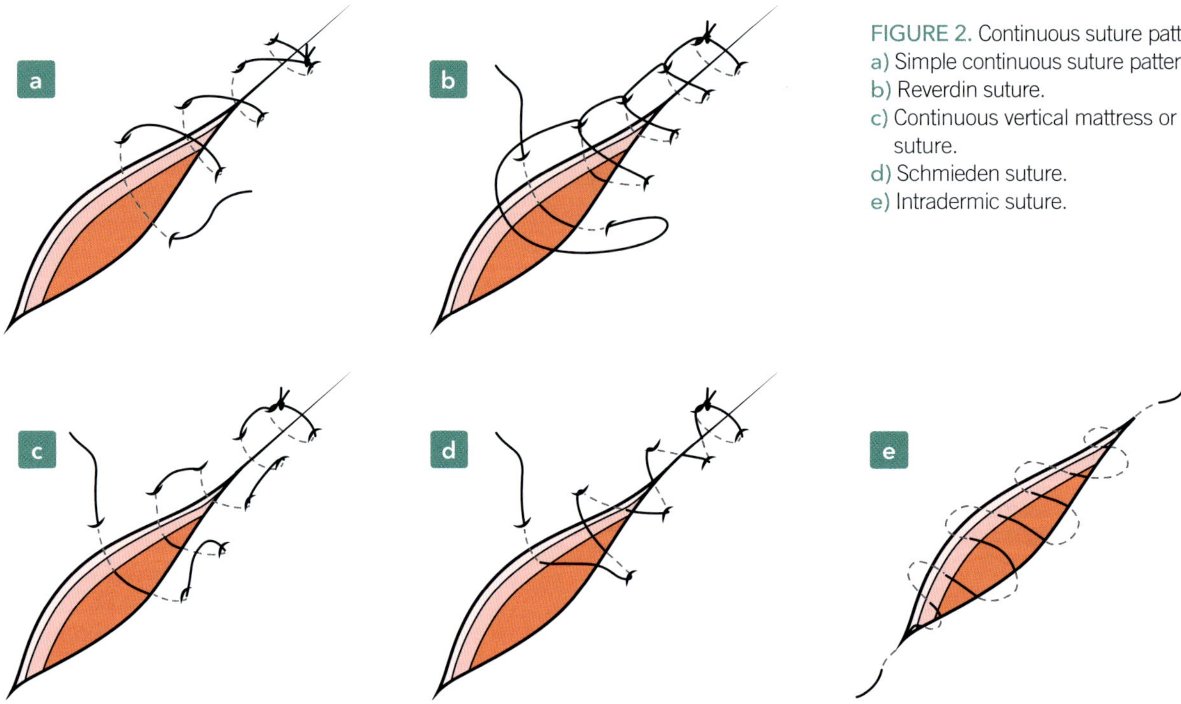

FIGURE 2. Continuous suture patterns.
a) Simple continuous suture pattern.
b) Reverdin suture.
c) Continuous vertical mattress or U-shaped suture.
d) Schmieden suture.
e) Intradermic suture.

are not very large, and in which there is little tension, such as in those made in small interventions like ovariectomies or ovariohysterectomies.

VIDEO

Intradermal suture with Aberdeen knot

Retention sutures

In addition to the traditional simple or continuous patterns, there is what is known as retention sutures. They provide extra security to the main suture, and are especially used to decrease the tension on the first sutures. These sutures, therefore, improve blood flow to the area of the closure by taking pressure off the stitches of the main suture (Fig. 3).

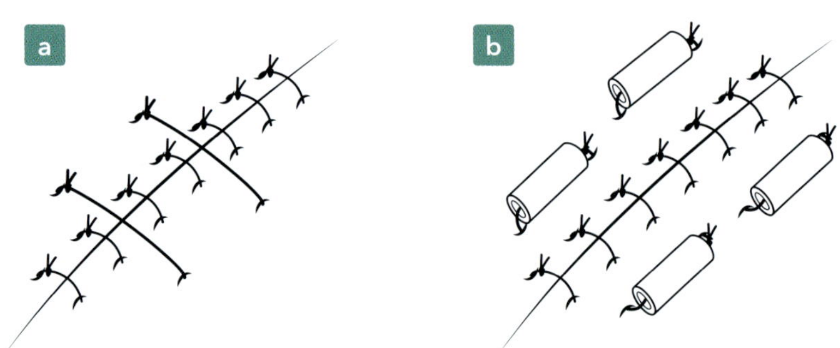

FIGURE 3. Retention sutures.
a) Suture with vertical retention stitches.
b) Suture with U-shaped retention stitches with rubber tubes.

Suture needles

Modern sutures use atraumatic needles, in which the material is attached to the eyeless needle. This makes threading the needle unnecessary, and moreover, the end of the suture is smaller than the body of the needle, allowing it to easily pass through the tissue.

In essence, there are three types of needles, classified according to the shape of their body:

- **Straight needles** are used in accessible surface areas where the needle can be directly handled with the fingers.
- **Curved needles** are used with a needle holder. Their curvature is in the shape of 1/4, 3/8, 1/2 or 5/8 of a circle. This allows the surgeon to access smaller areas with the needle.
- **Half-curved needles** are mainly used in ophthalmic surgery.

Needles are also available with various shaped tips and bodies (Table 2).

TABLE 2. Type of needle by tip and cross section of body, along with indications for use

Type of needle	Description	Indications
Round-bodied needles 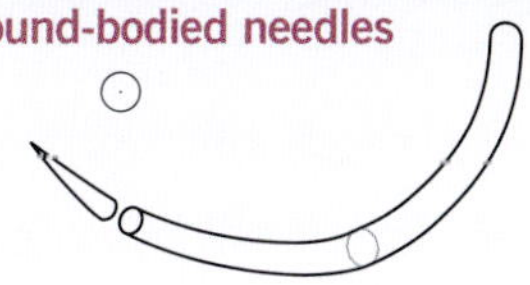	This needle is round-bodied and tapers gently towards the sharpened tip, which perforates and penetrates the tissue without cutting it.	Used in tissue that is easy to penetrate, such as intestine, subcutaneous tissue, loose fascia and blood vessels.
Cutting needles 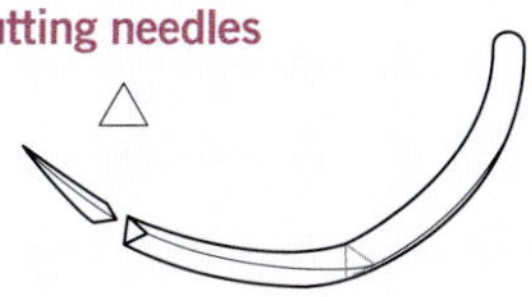	The body of the needle is triangular and has a sharp interior cutting edge (towards the wound).	Recommended for firmer tissues such as skin, fascia, tendons and ligaments.
Reverse cutting needles 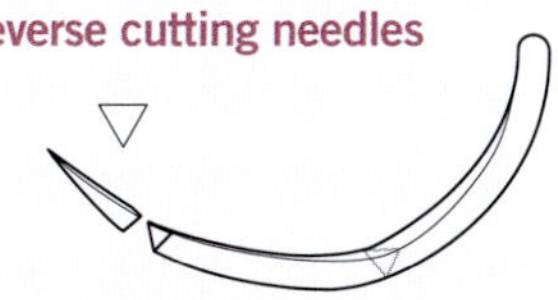	The body of the needle is triangular and has a sharp exterior cutting edge (away from the wound).	Recommended for firmer tissues such as skin, fascia, tendons and ligaments.
Tapercut needles 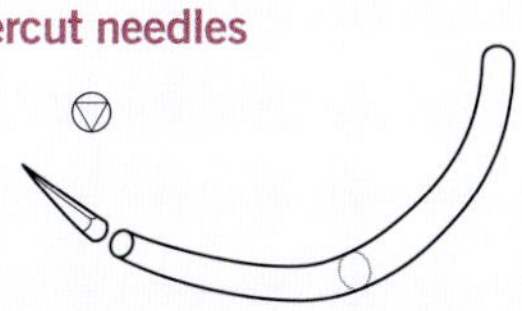	A combination of a reverse cutting needle tip and a round body.	Used to suture firm and dense tissue such as tendons or for vascular grafts.
Blunt-tipped needles 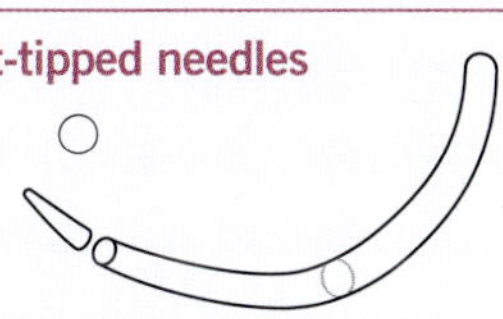	Has a rounded blunt tip that can dissect friable tissue without cutting it.	For suturing soft parenchymal organs such as the liver or kidney.
Spatulated needles 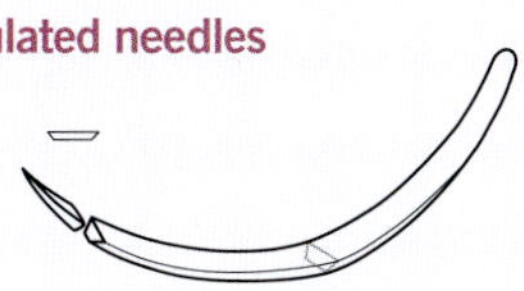	A flat needle on the top and bottom, with cutting edges along either side.	Used in ophthalmology.

Bibliography

Bellenger CR. Sutures part I. The purpose of sutures and available suture materials. *Comp Contin Educ Pract Vet*, 1982; 4(6):507–514.

Bellenger CR. Sutures part II. The use of sutures and alternative methods for closure. *Comp Contin Educ Pract Vet*, 1982; 4(6):587–600.

DeNardo GA, Brown NO, Trenka-Benthin S, Marretta SM. Comparison of seven different suture materials in the feline oral cavity. *J Am Anim Hosp Assoc*, 1996, 32(2):164–172.

Freeman LJ, Pettit GD, Robinette JD et al. Tissue reaction to suture material in the feline linea alba. A retrospective, prospective, and histologic study. *Vet Surg*, 1987; 16(6):440–445.

Runk A, Allen SW, Mahaffey EA. Tissue reactivity to poliglecaprone 25 in the feline linea alba. *Vet Surg*, 1999; 28(6):466–471.

Schiller TD, Stone EA, Gupta BS. In vitro loss of tensile strength and elasticity of five absorbable suture materials in sterile and infected canine urine. *Vet Surg*, 1993; 22(3):208–212.

Stashak TS, Yturraspe DJ. Considerations for selection of suture materials. *Vet Surg*, 1978; 7(2):48–52.

SURGICAL MATERIALS 5

Llibertat Real

As we have seen previously, feline surgery involves many peculiarities. The surgical instrument set (i.e., the ensemble of indispensable, specially designed surgical tools) required for correctly working with feline patients will be described in this chapter.

One part of the set is required for all surgeries performed, while other instruments are only needed for specific surgeries. We can organize it in various packages or bags. All the basic surgical material can be placed in some of these packages, while materials for each different type of surgery can be placed in separate, smaller packages. The surgical material packages should be color coded with tape, which makes it easy to identify the material belonging to each bag.

If we have a high volume of varied surgeries, we can also have bags prepared with different proportions of basic material components. This enables the operating room to be more efficiently used, optimizing the time and energy spent on maintenance and sterilization of the material.

It is also useful to keep lists of material required for different surgeries (along with the color-coded bags where they can be found). Not only does this allow us to quickly put the material in order, but it also makes it easy for any new member of the surgical team to adapt to their new environment.

Certain instruments have many different designs and differ from each other in small details. Each surgeon has their own preferences. Below the materials that the authors find to be most practical and most comfortable for use in feline patients will be described.

Materials required for all feline surgeries

This material is used in any surgery to suture, make incisions, perform hemostasis at points of bleeding, grasp tissues, etc. It comprises:

- **Hemostatic forceps:** Halstead mosquito, Spencer Wells, Rochester-Pean.
- **Scissors** for cutting and dissecting tissues, and for cutting sutures: baby Metzenbaum, Carless or other such scissors.
- **Dissecting forceps:** Adson with teeth and Adson with straight tip.
- **Forceps for grasping/traction** of tissues: baby Allis, Babcock.
- **Towel clamps**: Jones or Backhaus.
- **Scalpel blades and handles:** No. 3 or no. 7 handles, and no. 11 or no. 15 scalpel blades for fine handles.
- **Needle holders:** Mayo-Hegar, Olsen-Hegar.
- **Gauze.**
- **Surgical drapes:** we can use reusable cotton drapes, including two large ones to completely cover the operating table and the cat, or a fenestrated one to cover the table and the cat along with a small one over a Mayo table for the material. We can also use disposable (adhesive or nonadhesive) drapes that can be adapted to whatever surgery we will be performing. Because the patients are small, the material required for simple surgeries occupies little space.

Other materials that we may need and which must be prepared separately include:

- **Metal bowl or basin for saline solution:** the assistant will fill it with warm sterile saline for lavaging, moistening tissues, cleaning the surgical field, using saline for irrigation or for injecting into organs to check for leaks, etc. (Fig. 1).
- **Retractors:** these are needed in some surgeries in order gain access to the abdominal or thoracic cavity, or the surgical field (thyroidectomies, orthopedic surgery, etc.). They can be handheld or self-retaining:
  - Handheld retractors:
    - Langenbeck retractor: held by the assistant. It is used to retract soft tissues to gain access to other structures.
  - Self-retaining retractors for prolonged retraction of tissues in complex surgeries:
    - Gelpi retractor (Fig. 2): used for retraction of deep and superficial tissues. It is especially useful for retraction of thick tissues or for accessing difficult to reach

areas (e.g., in orthopedics to reach the neck of the femur) or for small, sensitive surgical fields (e.g., for a thyroidectomy).
- Gosset retractor: used for abdominal surgery in cats. Consists of two adjustable metal blades (solid or fenestrated) mounted on a bar. It is also indicated for rib retraction in thoracic surgery and for retraction of ventral cervical structures in neck surgery.
- Balfour retractor (Fig. 3): consists of three adjustable blades (curved outwards) and mounted on a bar. It may also be fenestrated. It is very useful in abdominal surgery, allowing the surgical field to be clearly exposed.

The box on the following page shows the contents of a basic surgical materials bag (Fig. 4). If there is a high volume of a particular surgery (e.g., sterilizations), packages with instruments and drapes required exclusively for these surgeries can be prepared in advance.

A **package for sterilization surgery** may contain:
- Surgical drapes (if disposable ones are not used): we can wrap them around the materials in such a way that everything is already in place when unfurled.
- Baby Allis tissue forceps (×1).
- Halstead mosquito forceps, 10 cm (×3).
- Rochester-Pean curved forceps, 14 cm (×1).
- Small Jones or Backhaus towel clamps (depending on the drapes that are used) (×4–10).
- No. 3 scalpel handle.
- Mayo-Hegar or Olsen-Hegar needle holder, 14 cm (×1).
- Baby Metzenbaum scissors (×1).
- Adson forceps with teeth (×1).
- Adson forceps with straight tip (×1).
- Spay hook (optional, for lateral access; Fig. 5) (×1).

Simpler packages can be prepared for short surgeries, for applying sutures, or for specific feline interventions such as for **esophagostomy tube placement**:
- Mayo-Hegar or Olsen-Hegar needle holder, 14 cm (×1).
- Adson forceps with teeth (×1).
- Adson forceps with straight tip (×1).
- Baby Metzenbaum scissors (×1).
- Rochester-Pean forceps or other forceps with a curved tip (×1).

Materials for biopsy collection

Depending on what area we wish to biopsy, we may need, in addition to basic materials:
- Tru-cut needles: automatic biopsy devices that extract a cylinder of tissue. Used for renal biopsies (Fig. 6).
- Punch: a punch is a circular scalpel with a plastic handle, available in different sizes. The diameter is measured in millimeters. Used for skin, intestine and liver biopsies.
- Stevens tenotomy scissors: for conjunctival and intestinal biopsies (Fig. 7).

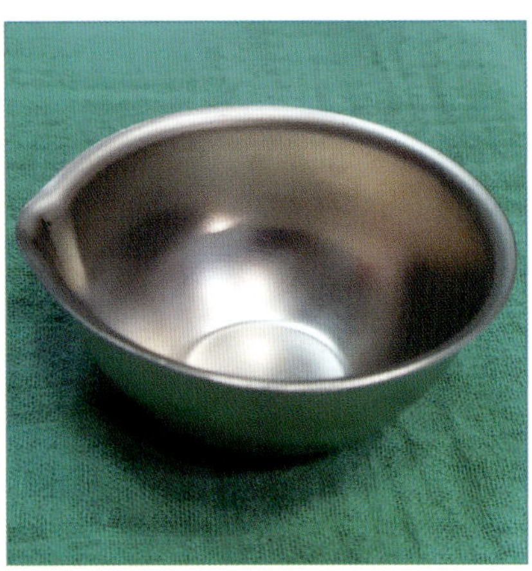

FIGURE 1. Metal bowl for saline.

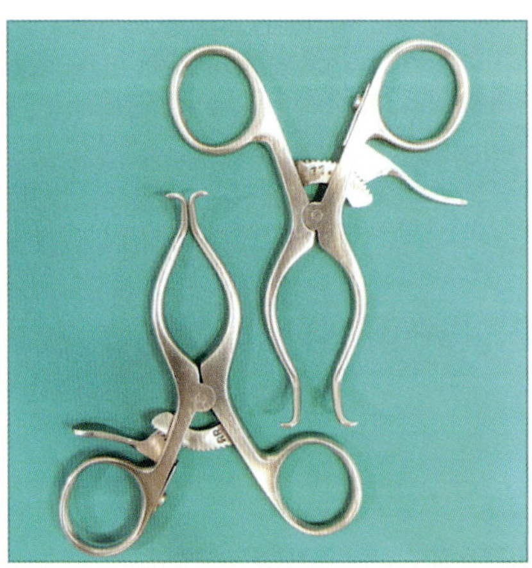

FIGURE 2. Small Gelpi self-retaining retractors.

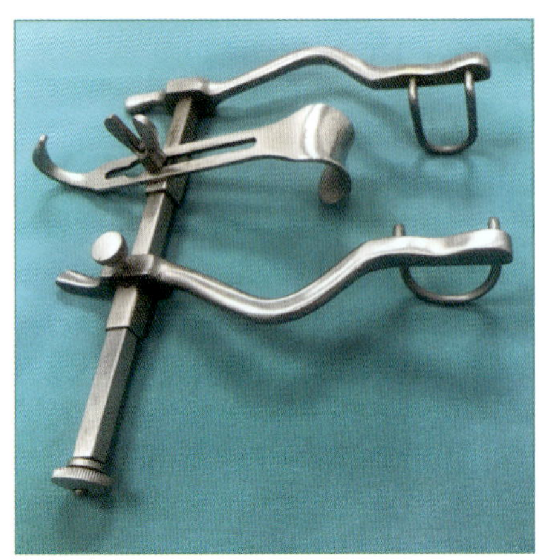

FIGURE 3. Balfour self-retaining retractor.

Contents of a basic surgery materials bag

1. Carless or standard scissors (or similar) for cutting sutures
2. Baby Metzenbaum scissors, straight or curved
3. Metzenbaum scissors, straight or curved
4. No. 3 scalpel handle
5. Rochester-Pean curved forceps, 14 cm (×2)
6. Small Jones or Backhaus towel clamps (×10–14)
7. Adson forceps with teeth
8. Adson forceps with straight tip
9. Tissue forceps: baby Allis forceps, 13 cm (×3)
10. Hemostatic forceps: Halstead mosquito forceps, straight and curved, 10–12.5 cm (×5)
11. Mayo-Hegar or Olsen-Hegar needle holder, 14 cm

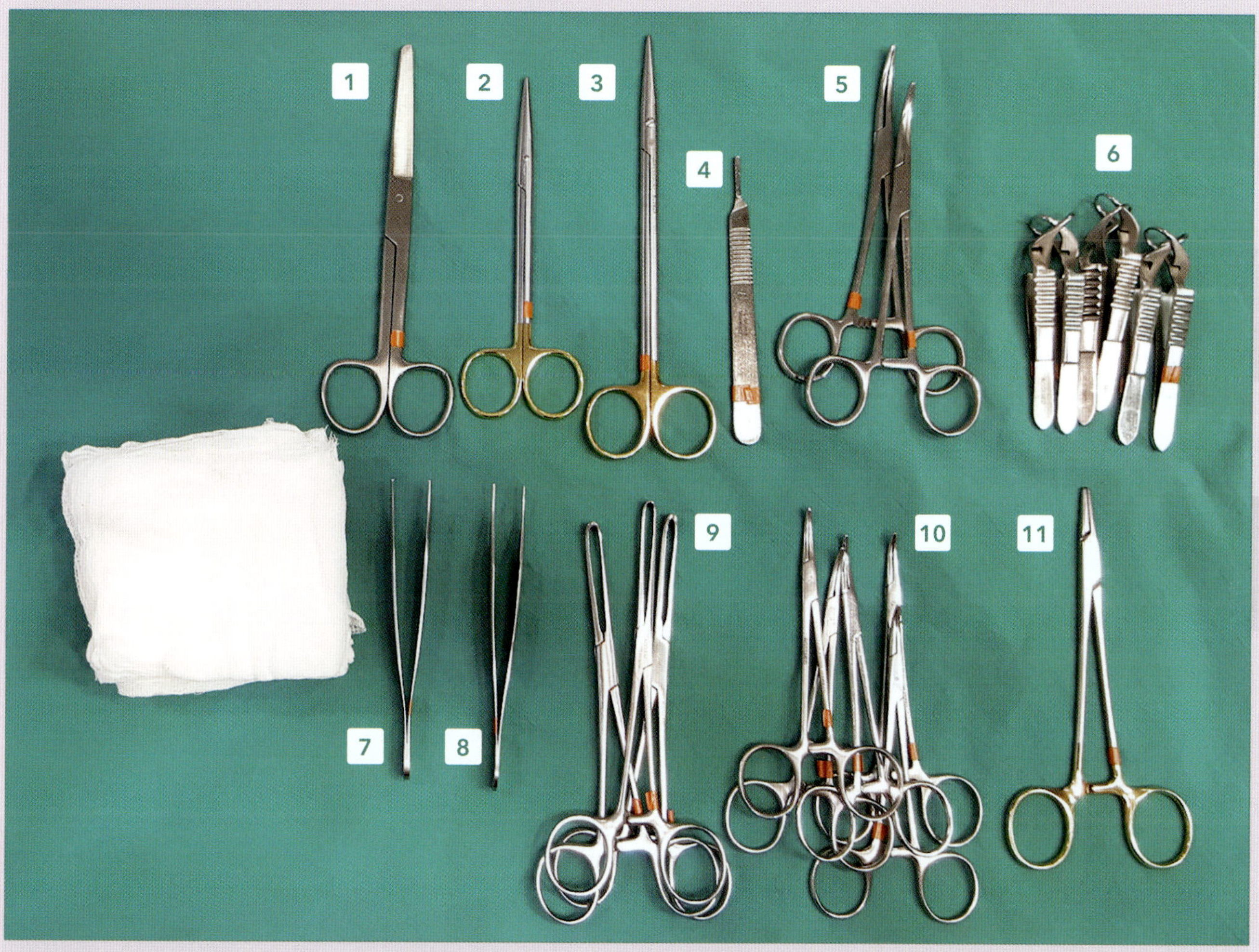

FIGURE 4. Basic surgical material.

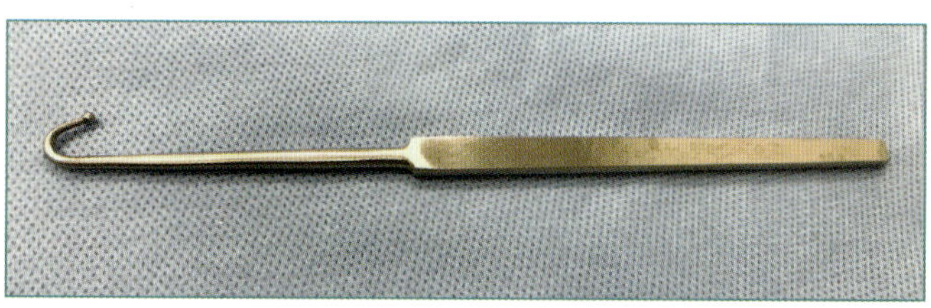

FIGURE 5. Spay hook.

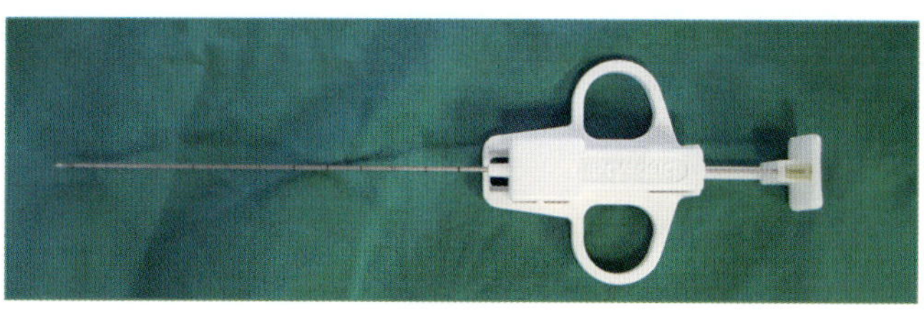

FIGURE 6. Tru-cut needle for renal biopsies.

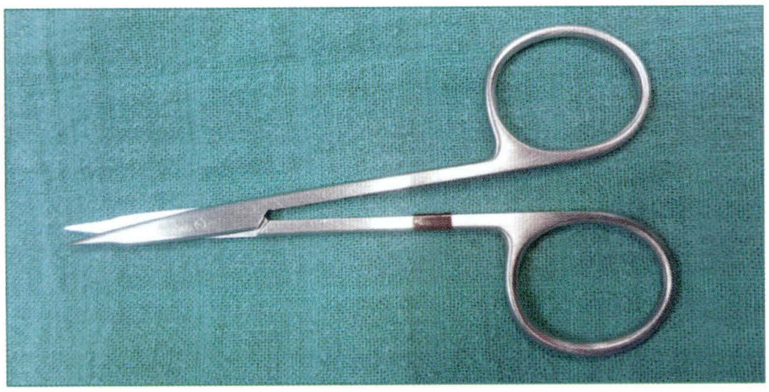

FIGURE 7. Stevens tenotomy scissors for use in corneal or intestinal biopsies.

Materials for dental extractions

To comfortably and safely perform dental extractions, we should always have the following sterile material available:

- Basic surgery and dental surgery kit (see below, Fig. 8).
- No. 11 scalpel blade.
- Lucas curette (Fig. 9): used in case of severe inflammation or infection of the alveolar process, to eliminate all necrotic or inflamed material and to promote clotting.
- Binocular headband magnifier (Fig. 10).
- Sharpening stone or mechanical sharpener: it is essential to keep luxators and elevators well sharpened.

Contents of a dental extraction materials bag

1. Small extraction forceps
2. Bone fragment forceps
3. Dental burs with round head, cross-cut fissure, and diamond burs, 16 mm (sizes between 1/4 and 4)
4. Curved baby mosquito forceps
5. No. 3 scalpel handle
6. (Superslim) straight elevator, 1 mm
7. Winged elevator, 1 mm
8. Winged elevator, 2 mm
9. Winged elevator, 4 mm
10. Luxator, 1 mm
11. Luxator, 2 mm
12. Freer periosteotome or elevator
13. Small periodontal curette
14. Dental probe and explorer
15. Dental mirror
16. Adson forceps with straight tip
17. Adson forceps with teeth
18. Mayo-Hegar needle holder, 14 cm
19. Baby Metzenbaum scissors

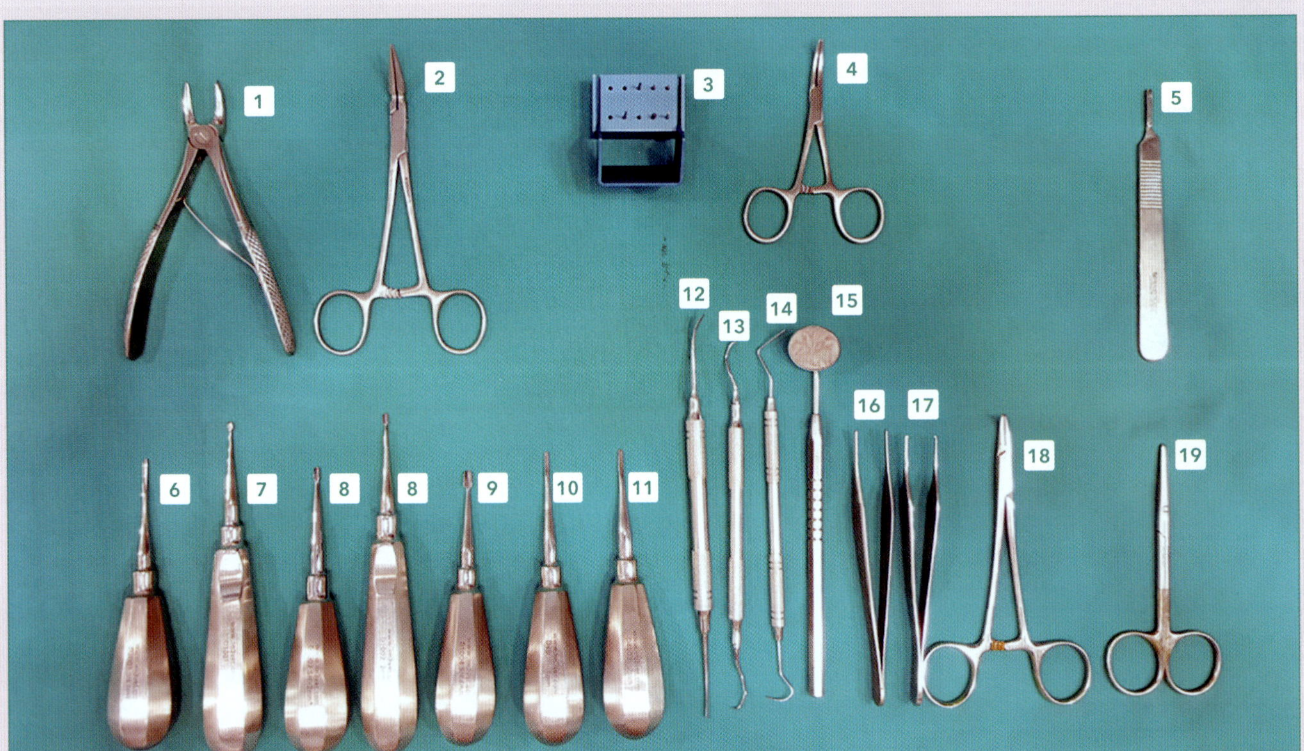

FIGURE 8. Material for dental extractions.

Materials for nasal surgery

To perform rhinotomies, we will need, along with basic surgical materials, a Freer elevator or periosteotome for removing periosteal tissue from the nasal bone.

Materials for trauma and orthopedic surgery

The following **basic material** is required:

- Forceps for grasping and bone reduction: used for holding and realigning bone fragments in fracture fixation.
- Point-to-point bone reduction forceps (Fig. 11): helps keep bone fragments in position before permanent fixation, especially in long and/or oblique bones.
- Bone-holding forceps with serrated jaws: with grooves on each opposing surface. Used in fractures of long bones. Maintains stability in the fracture area, so that the fracture can be fixed.
- Kern bone-holding forceps (Fig. 12): useful in fractures that require the use of wires, pins or other fixation methods. Allows bone fragments to be grasped in a firm and controlled manner to facilitate repositioning and reduction of the fracture.

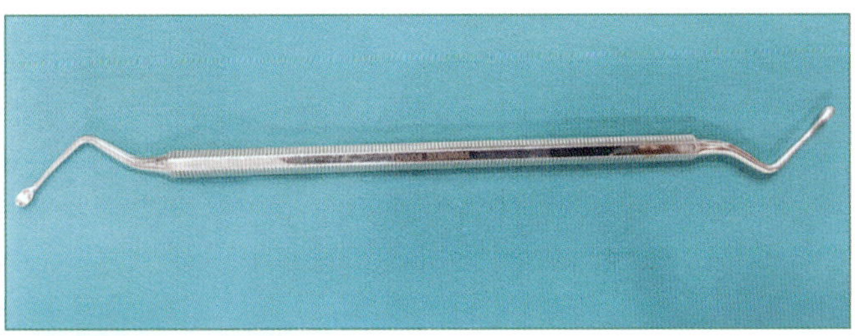

FIGURE 9. Lucas curette.

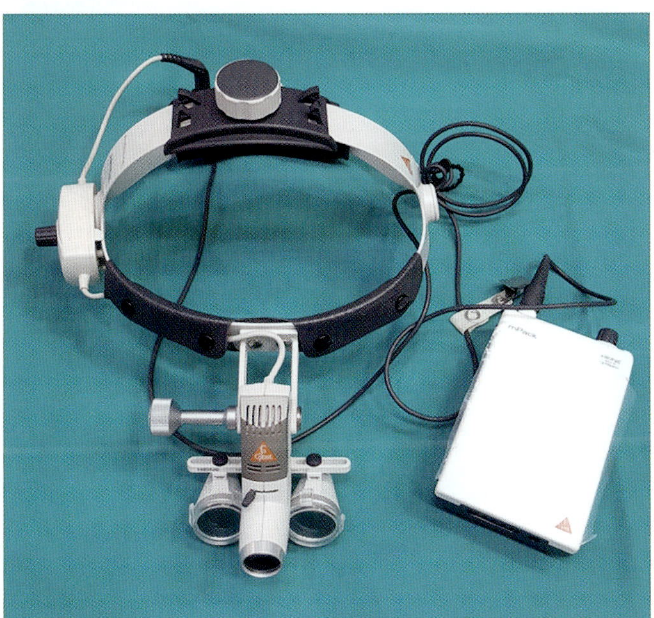

FIGURE 10. Binocular headband magnifier.

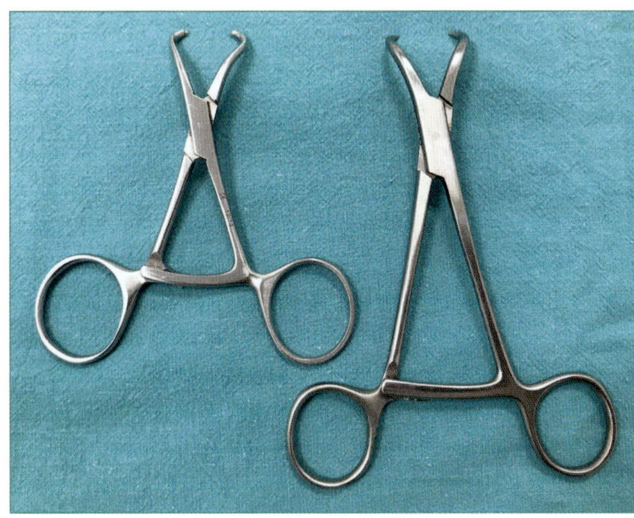

FIGURE 11. Point-to-point bone reduction forceps.

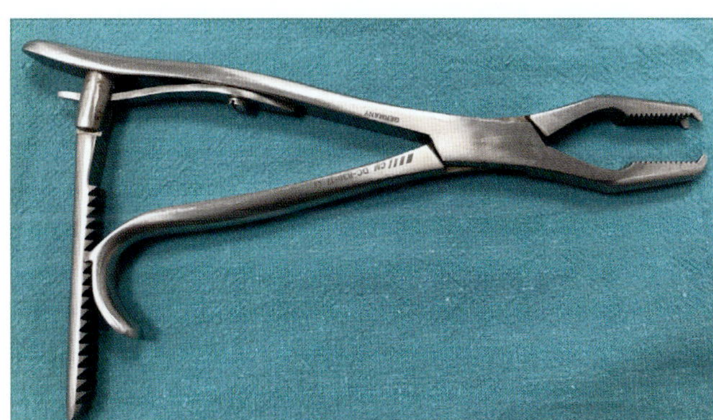

FIGURE 12. Kern bone-holding forceps.

- Rongeur forceps (Fig. 13): sharp-edged blades that touch each other when the handles are squeezed, cutting the bone. Also used in tympanic bulla surgery to break the bulla wall.
- Periosteotome (Fig. 14): to eliminate soft tissue on the surface of the bone. This makes it easier to work on the surface of bones and fix plates to them.
- Gelpi retractor (Fig. 15a).
- Weitlaner retractor with blunt tips (Fig. 15b): used to separate tissues and gain greater access to the surgical field.
- Senn-Miller retractor (Fig. 16): this is a double-ended retractor. One end consists of a hook with three curved tips and the other end is L-shaped.
- Hohmann retractor (Fig. 17): retracts and flattens soft tissue while elevating the bone and articular structures, improving visualization of the surgical field. Facilitates the fixation of fracture segments during alignment and in reconstruction of fractures of large bones.
- Volkmann bone curette (Fig. 18): with one end in the shape of a spoon to remove hard tissue and a grooved handle for improved grasping.

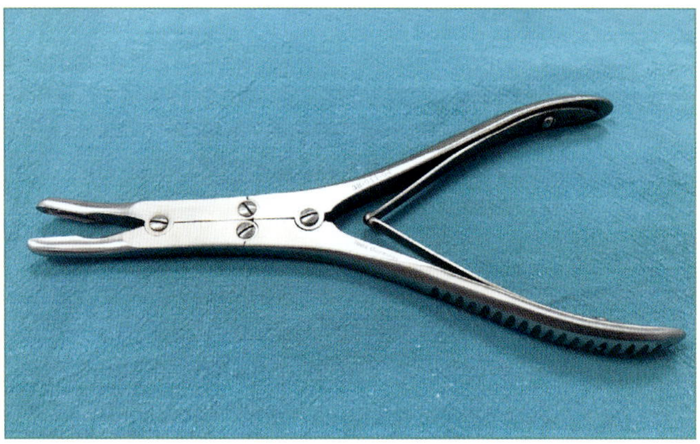

FIGURE 13. Rongeur forceps.

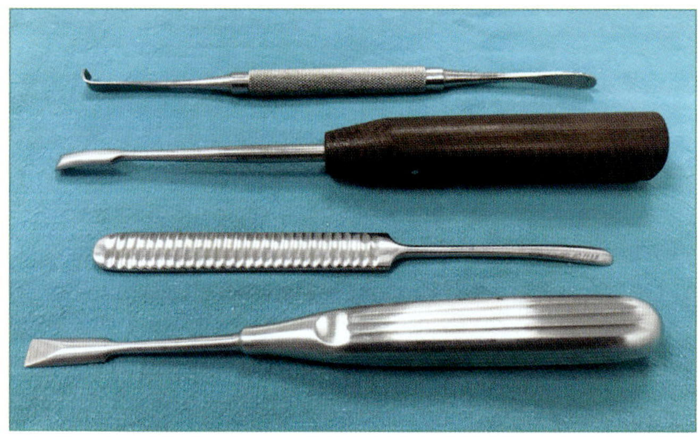

FIGURE 14. Periosteotomes.

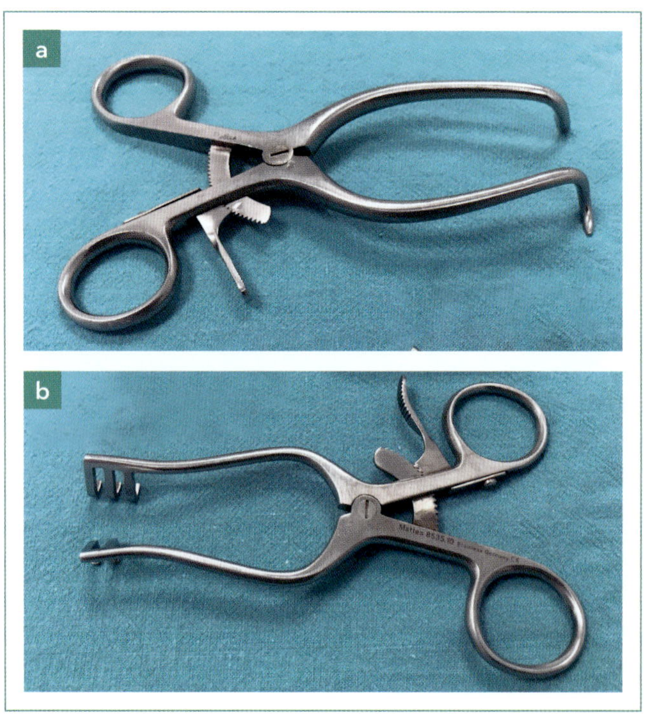

FIGURE 15. (a) Gelpi retractor. (b) Weitlaner retractor with blunt tips.

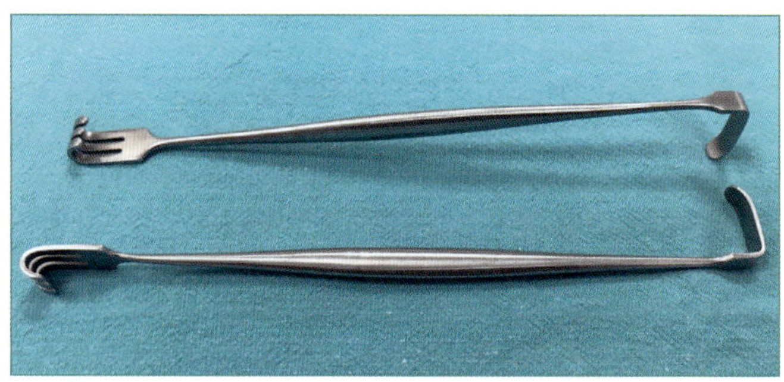

FIGURE 16. Senn-Miller retractors.

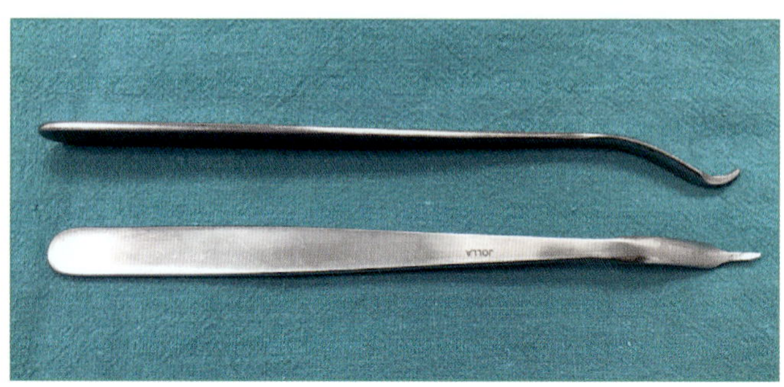

FIGURE 17. Hohmann retractors.

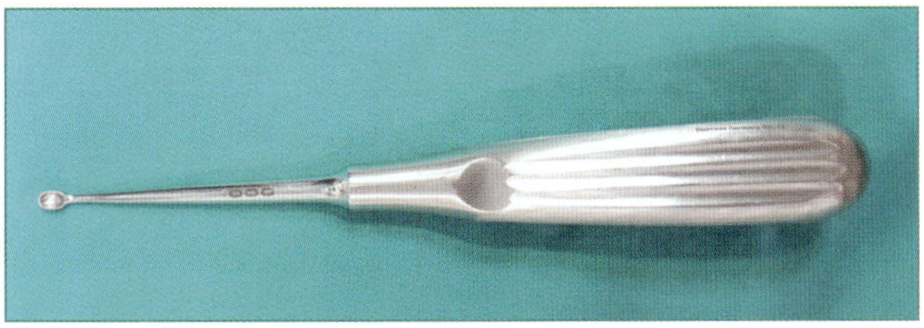

FIGURE 18. Volkmann bone curette.

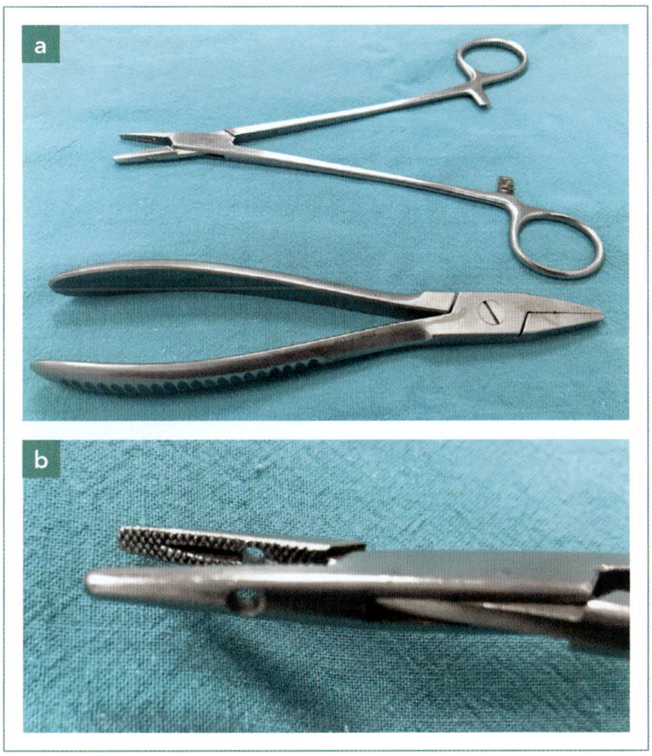

FIGURE 19. (a) Cerclage pliers and forceps. (b) Detail view of the tip of cerclage forceps.

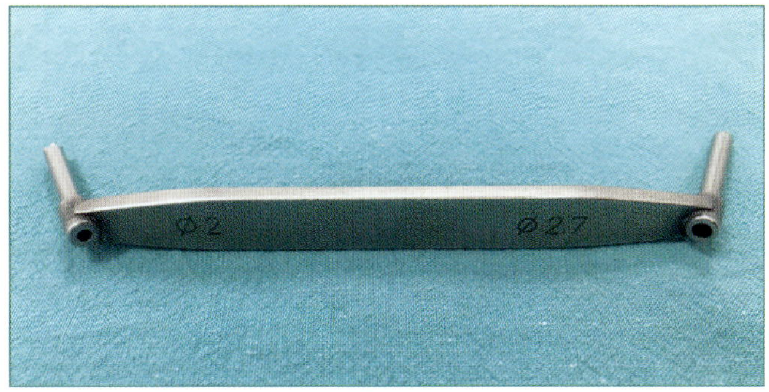

FIGURE 20. 2 and 2.7 mm drill sleeve.

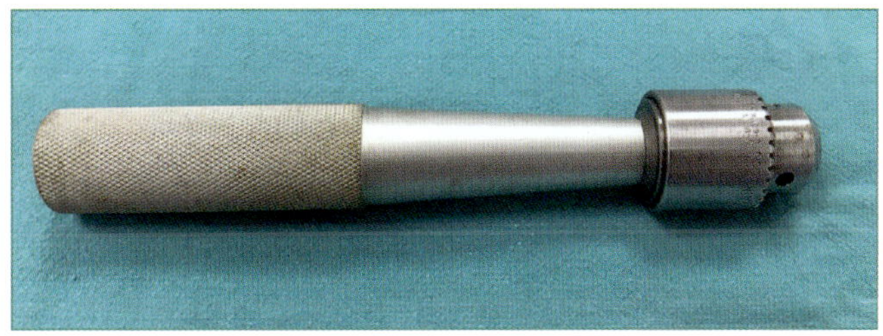

FIGURE 21. Jacobs mandrel.

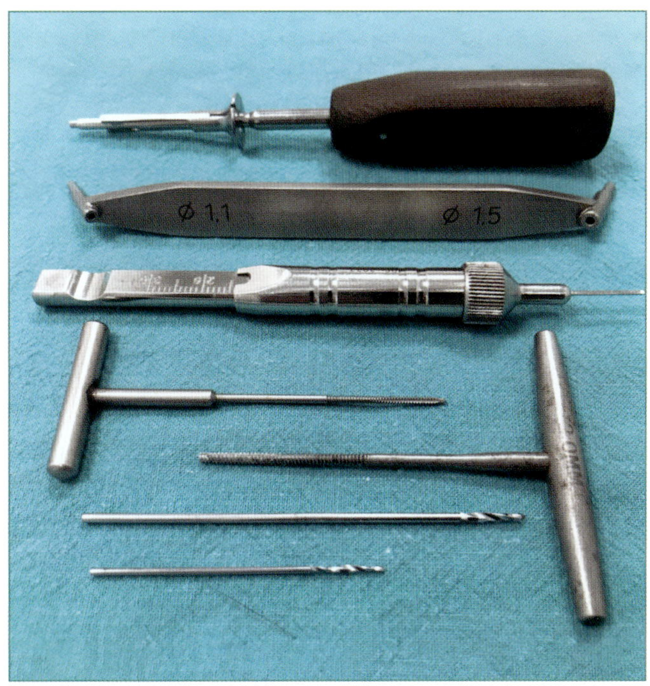

FIGURE 22. Material used for placement of screws.

- Cerclage pliers and forceps (Fig. 19a): these forceps have a slotted jaw that facilitates placement of cerclage wire (Fig. 19b).
- 2 and 2.7 mm drill sleeve (Fig. 20).
- Jacobs mandrel (Fig. 21): used to handle transfixing pins and to perforate the bone (manually or with a puncture pin).
- Material for placement of 1.5 and 2 mm screws (Fig. 22).
- Cerclage and pin cutters (Fig. 23).

The following is also needed for **hip surgery**:

- Oscillating saw and blades (Fig. 24).
- Hohmann retractor for the femoral head.

And for **stifle surgery**:

- Small stifle distractor (6 mm).
- Meniscus knife for meniscectomy: designed to remove damaged cartilage in the stifle.

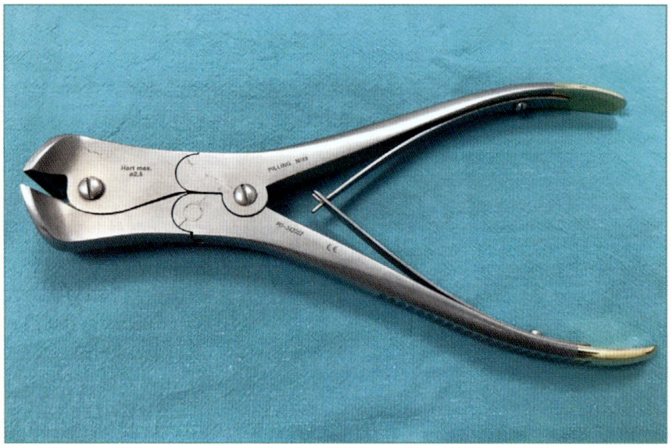

FIGURE 23. Cerclage and pin cutters.

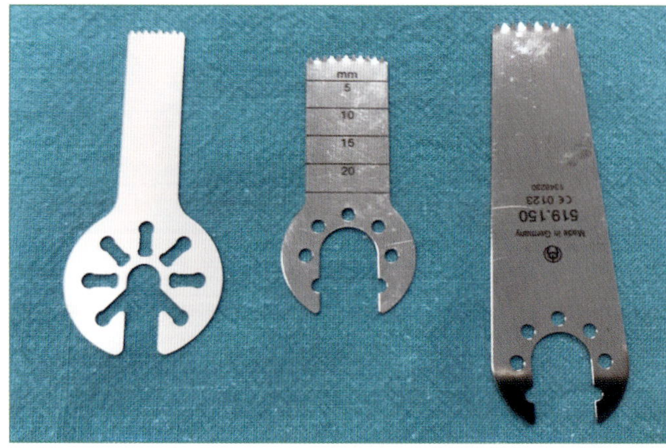

FIGURE 24. Oscillating saw blades.

Electrosurgery equipment

This is a system that converts low voltage electricity into heat.

Monopolar electrosurgery

Also known as electric scalpel or electroscalpel. The electric current passes through the cat between the electroscalpel and a metal plate that is in contact with the patient's body. Generated heat accumulates in the active electrode, which allows the surgeon to simultaneously cut and coagulate tissues and lesions. This method is not appropriate for large lesions since they are sectioned/coagulated slowly. It is not effective if the surgical field is wet (due to excessive bleeding). Incorrect use can cause tissue damage, burns and delayed scarring. While this method has been around for a long time, it is simple and economical.

Bipolar electrosurgery

The electric current does not pass through the cat (a metal plate in contact with the patient's body is not needed). Instead, it passes through the tips of a forceps, which acts as the active electrode. This forceps does not accumulate heat; rather it focuses electrical energy to a limited area. This allows tissue masses and blood vessels to be sealed. It produces less damage to tissues, uses less electrical current, and may be used in a wet surgical field. It may also be used in interventions involving highly vascularized organs such as the spleen or liver, as well as near nerves and in spinal surgeries, among others. Also known as bipolar sealing devices, these instruments come in a variety of forms. One of the most well-known of these devices uses a combination of manual pressure and thermal energy to melt the collagen and elastin in blood vessels, thereby sealing them permanently.

Ultrasonic coagulation equipment

Uses electrical energy to achieve high-frequency vibration of piezoelectric crystals in the treatment probe (Fig. 25). This enables the tip of the treatment probe to reach a temperature that denatures proteins, cutting and coagulating tissues at the same time. Minimal thermal damage is produced since the temperature of the surrounding tissues does not increase. It is especially useful in areas of the body that are sensitive to inflammation, such as the larynx, or in areas where heavy bleeding may occur, such as during liver biopsy. Blood vessels cannot be cauterized without cutting them. It does not produce smoke, and no muscular stimulation occurs.

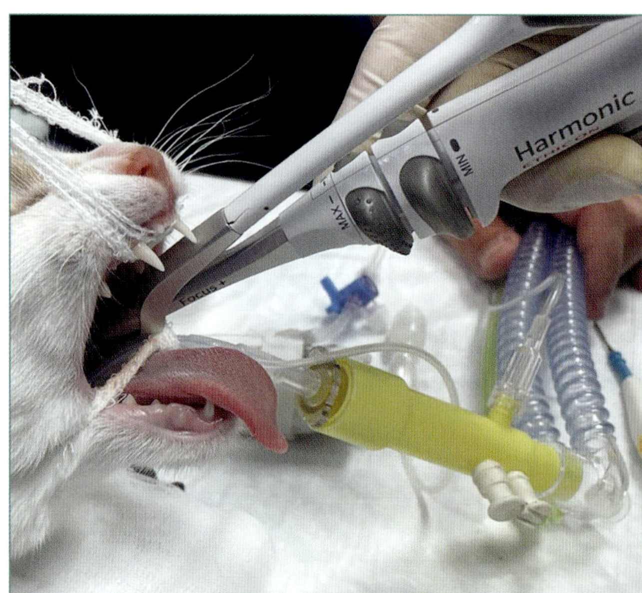

FIGURE 25. Ultrasonic coagulation device.

Maintenance and sterilization of the material

Proper handling of the material, rigorous washing and optimal sterilization will extend its lifetime. We should use the material only as it was designed to be used and avoid other uses (e.g., we should not cut gauze or other material with dissecting scissors in order to avoid damaging the cutting edge). We should also avoid letting the material fall on the floor or throwing it into the sink roughly when gathering up the surgical field to be washed. We should separate delicate instruments from other material to avoid damaging them with heavy weight (we should never place other materials on top of these instruments). We should carefully close mosquito forceps, Allis forceps, etc., so that their parts fit together properly.

After use, we should carefully wash the instrument set with surgical soap and cold water until all organic material has been eliminated (any material that is made up of multiple sections should be taken apart, and any fasteners or clasps should be opened, etc.). Enzymatic cleaners specifically designed for surgical material can also be used.

The material should not be left in water for long periods of time, since this can damage its surface.

If we need to use a brush, it should be soft in order to avoid abrasive damage. After this step, the material can be placed into an ultrasonic tank to eliminate residue from the most difficult-to-reach areas. Next, we should rinse the material thoroughly to eliminate any remaining cleaner or enzymatic solution, and dry it well.

One point we should pay special attention to after drying is the color-coded tapes or strips on the material, as these can become havens for bacteria if they are not replaced appropriately. Before putting the instruments into their bags or sterilization boxes, we should check that all the material is in pristine condition (including the cutting edges of the instruments). We should also review the checklist of materials to ensure that nothing is missing.

The packages or bags can be self-sealing, sterilizable, and disposable. This has the advantage of being convenient, but the cost of purchasing the material is higher and it generates more waste. An alternative is to use stainless steel sterilization boxes, which can be perforated or nonperforated, and may come with sterile membranes that must be replaced with each use. Any self-sealing materials should be double wrapped.

The material is placed inside an autoclave that is suitable for surgical sterilization. That usually means a temperature of around 273°F (134°C) for a 30-minute cycle. The time may vary according to the material to be sterilized and the machine. We should always confirm that the sterilization was completed correctly before putting the material in its storage place. We should also check to make sure that the bag has no tears or cracks and that the boxes are tightly closed.

Bibliography

Cowperthwaite L, Holm RL. Guideline implementation: surgical instrument cleaning. *AORN J*, 2015; 101(5):542–549.

Langley-Hobbs SJ, Voss K, Lapish JP, Montavon PM. Orthopedic implants. In: Montavon PM, Voss K, Langley-Hobbs SJ (eds.). *Feline Orthopedic Surgery and Musculoskeletal Disease*, 1st ed. Edinburgh, UK: Saunders Elsevier, 2009; pp. 259–282.

Lapish JP, Langley-Hobbs SJ. Instruments. In: Langley-Hobbs SJ, Demetriou JL, Ladlow JF (eds.). *Feline Soft Tissue and General Surgery*, 1st ed. Oxford, UK: Saunders Elsevier, 2014; pp. 133–138.

Lapish JP. Orthopedic instrumentation. In: Montavon PM, Voss K, Langley-Hobbs SJ (eds.). *Feline Orthopedic Surgery and Musculoskeletal Disease*, 1st ed. Edinburgh, UK: Saunders Elsevier, 2009; pp. 249–257.

MacPhail C, Fossum TW. Instrumental quirúrgico. In: Fossum TW (ed.). *Cirugía en pequeños animales*, 5th ed. Barcelona, Spain: Elsevier, 2019; pp. 50–59.

Parker RB. Técnicas electroquirúrgicas. In: Bojrab MJ (ed.). *Técnicas actuales en cirugía de pequeños animales*, 4th ed. Buenos Aires, Argentina: Intermédica, 2000; pp. 37–40.

Siemon H. Use of a bipolar vessel-sealing device for splenic parenchymal resection in three dogs and one cat. *J Am Anim Hosp Assoc*, 2021; 57(1):32–36.

The College of Animal Welfare. *Instrumentos quirúrgicos veterinarios*. Zaragoza, Spain: Acribia, 2000.

DIAGNOSTIC IMAGING 6

Alberto Barneto

Several different diagnostic imaging methods are used in modern feline veterinary medicine, with all the concomitant benefits that this entails when it comes to the diagnostic protocol. From the 1970s, when conventional radiology was the norm, until today, in which modern computed tomography is standard practice, diagnostic imaging techniques constitute a fundamental aid to an accurate diagnosis and for supporting the treatment of multiple pathologies.

Radiology

X-rays continue to be a basic pillar in the diagnosis of pathologies of the thorax and abdominal cavity. In most cases, they reveal pathologies that we can then follow up with additional testing. Furthermore, the use of contrast media inside cavities or hollow organs provides more choices and sensitivity in diagnoses (Fig. 1).

At present, **digital radiology** equipment has lowered the cost of radiographic studies while optimizing the storage capability of radiographic images. The quality of the images has also improved, with the additional advantage that digital radiology equipment comes with software that can edit images. In this process, a single radiographic image can give us not only morphological information, but also information on changes in texture of different tissues. Finally, digital radiology does not require a darkroom to develop film.

The only disadvantage of digital radiology is that the ease and speed of imaging has multiplied its use. Therefore, we should pay attention to the patient's risk of overexposure to radiation, and make sure not to relax protection protocols for technicians.

Ultrasound

In veterinary medicine, the use of high-frequency sound waves (ultrasounds) to obtain images of the anatomy and liquid flow dates to the 1980s. The waves are sent through a transducer (**probe**) into the organs, bounce back (form echoes = echography) and are captured and processed to generate moving 3D images with different textures. Its use is limited in anatomical areas that are protected by bone tissue and in organs with too

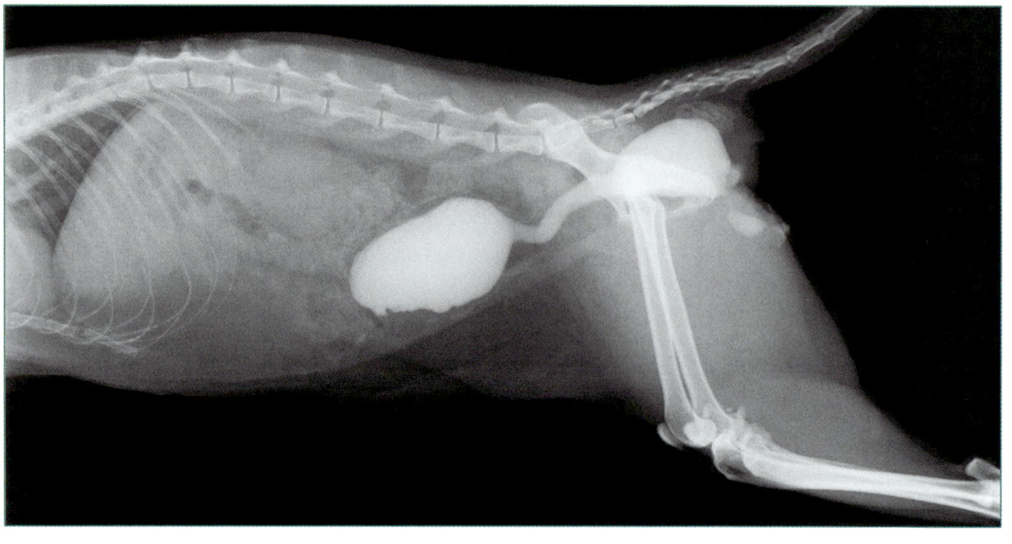

FIGURE 1. Radiographic image of a bladder with positive-contrast technique. Although usually done by retrograde route (the contrast enters via a urethral catheter), in this case, the contrast agent was injected into the bladder, which was gently squeezed to confirm a urethral disruption at the pelvis (white stains underneath the rectum and in the prepuce).

much air inside them (in both cases, the transmission of ultrasound waves is obstructed).

Nevertheless, ultrasound is very useful when it comes to examining soft tissues of the neck, the mediastinum (Fig. 2) and especially the abdomen. In addition, these images enable us to take very precise **ultrasound-guided biopsies** in different organs.

Computed tomography (CT)

In this technique a series of transversal radiological images are obtained as the patient advances on a moving table. This provides two major advantages:

- Greater image contrast; the different textures of each tissue are fully visible.
- As multiple cross sections of the body are obtained, each tissue is visible **without overlaps** (tomographically).

Furthermore, CT equipment has become more and more economical and has achieved better spatial resolution (finer slices). As a result, since the end of the twentieth century, it has increasingly gained traction in every veterinary center. The majority of modern CT equipment enables us, through advanced software, to reconstruct 3D images of each area of the body or a specific pathological structure (Fig. 3). If combined with the use of contrast agents, this improves the diagnosis of neoplasia (Fig. 4), as well as the functionality of certain organs, and specific vascular pathologies (e.g., portosystemic shunt).

The disadvantages are that the patient requires sedation (sometimes anesthesia) with all the concomitant risks associated in case of certain diseases. Moreover, it continues to be an expensive test that is centralized at referral centers, given that advanced interpretation expertise is required (technicians with a degree in diagnostic imaging).

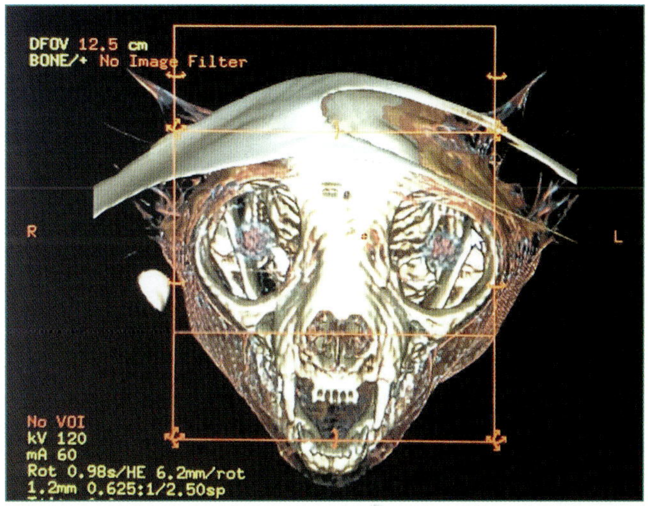

FIGURE 3. 3D reconstruction from a computed tomography scan of a cat's skull. Image courtesy of Diagnosfera.

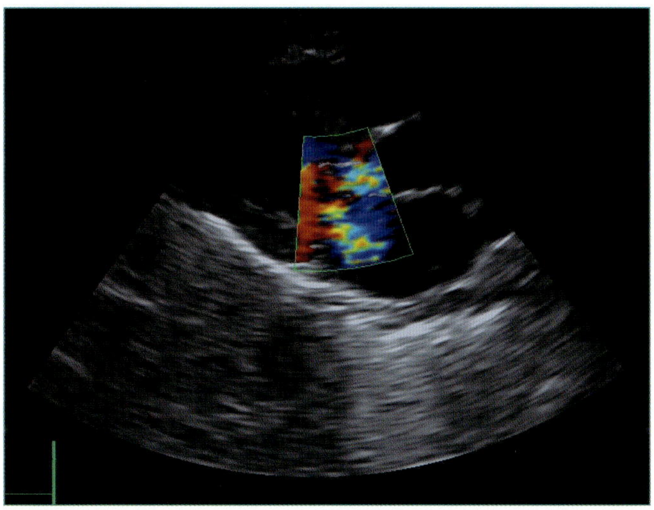

FIGURE 2. Doppler echocardiogram of a cat with severe concentric hypertrophic cardiomyopathy, with preserved systolic function and a restrictive diastolic pattern. Severe mitral valve regurgitation is seen, along with marked aortic stenosis with a velocity of 6 m/s (different from the mitral regurgitation). Image courtesy of Diagnosfera.

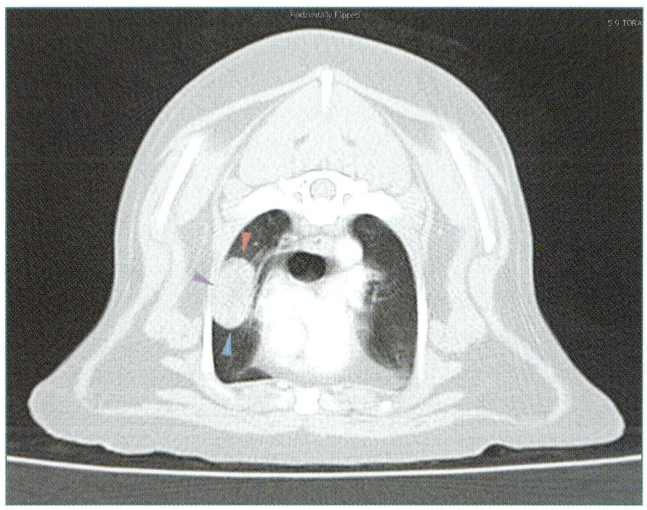

FIGURE 4. Thoracic computed tomography (CT) scan of a cat with a bronchogenic tumor. The combination of contrast angiography with CT is the best way to diagnose neoplasias in tissues that are hard to access with other methods.

Magnetic resonance (MR)

This is probably the most modern diagnostic imaging technique used in veterinary clinics (adopted in the early 2000s). A non-ionizing imaging technique, it can be used for evaluating both osseous structures and soft tissues with high precision. As is the case with CT, the images are not overlaid on each other. In contrast to CT, however, the image is directly digitalized in 3D, and the two-dimensional cross sections are obtained later through the use of software.

This technique has traditionally been preferred by neurologists due to the detail and precision in the localization of lesions, making it an invaluable tool when it comes to **planning surgeries**. It is now increasingly being used in the diagnosis of both soft tissue and bone pathologies, with the advantage of providing higher contrast between tissues than other techniques that use X-rays.

Unfortunately, this test still requires the use of equipment that is expensive to purchase and maintain. It also requires the patient to be sedated or anesthetized. Another limitation specific to feline medicine is that due to the size of the patients, the images have less precision.

Scintigraphy

Scintigraphy consists of creating images with special cameras that detect emissions of radioactive isotopes that circulate in organs as radiotracers. Since the 1940s, this technique has been used in nuclear medicine for the diagnosis and treatment of different tumors. In feline medicine, it is used in the diagnosis and treatment of thyroid disease and in the evaluation of renal function.

The most commonly used radioactive isotopes are technetium-99m (^{99m}Tc) for diagnosis and iodine-131 (^{131}I) for treatment. Generally speaking, ^{99m}Tc is taken up by the thyroid gland and is metabolized in approximately 6 hours. This allows morphologic diagnostic images (thyroid) or functional diagnostic images (kidney) to be taken. Later ^{131}I is used for the treatment of hyperthyroidism, since it takes 8 days to metabolize and, therefore, to eliminate tumor cells from the thyroid gland.

Endoscopy

This is an advanced diagnostic imaging method in which we insert a device into an opening (either natural or surgically created) in a bodily cavity or a hollow organ. This allows us to confirm a diagnosis after a previous examination of the condition. At the same time, this method is also used on occasion as a treatment (e.g., extraction of foreign bodies, gallstones) and often for taking biopsies. There are two modalities according to the type of endoscope:

- **Rigid endoscope:** in feline medicine, its use is limited to anterograde rhinoscopy, tracheoscopy, and otoscopy.
- **Flexible endoscope:** due to its mobility and increasingly fine caliber of optics, this instrument is much more versatile. It is very well suited to evaluate the digestive tract and respiratory tree (Fig. 5). A limitation of the finest flexible endoscopes (1.9 mm) is that in many cases they do not have a working channel in which to insert a biopsy forceps.

Each of the above diagnostic imaging methods has its pros and cons according to the anatomical area involved and the findings we wish to see. Table 1 shows anatomical areas and most frequent uses in feline medicine.

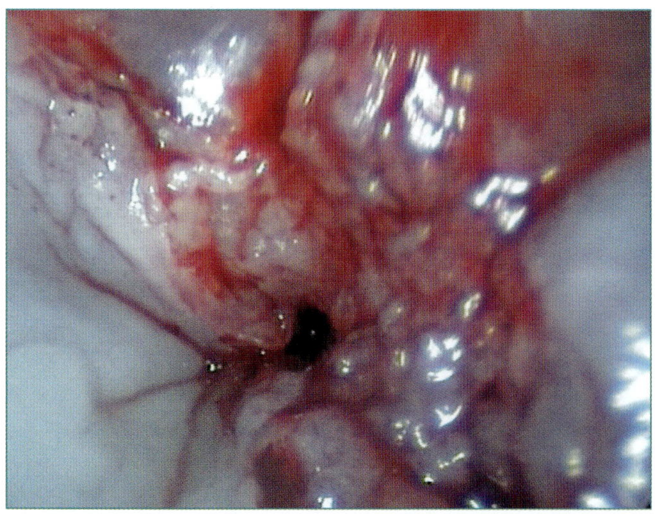

FIGURE 5. Endoscopic image of an adenocarcinoma in the esophageal lumen of a cat with chronic regurgitation.

TABLE 1. Uses of various common diagnostic imaging methods in feline medicine in different anatomical areas (green background: very useful; yellow background: moderately useful; gray background: not very useful)

Anatomical area	Radiology	Ultrasound	Computed tomography	Magnetic resonance	Scintigraphy	Endoscopy
Thorax	■ Requires good technique and good use of radiological projections ■ Cardiac silhouette ■ Pulmonary patterns ■ Pleural fluid ■ Diaphragm defects	■ Advanced diagnostics of heart disease ■ Mediastinum ■ Can detect pleural effusion ■ Pleural fluid ■ Ultrasound-guided cystocentesis	■ Same uses as in radiology ■ Very useful for detecting tumors	Not at all useful	Very useful for detecting ectopic thyroid tissue and thyroid diseases	■ Evaluation of the tracheal and bronchial lumen, and biopsies ■ Evaluation of the esophageal lumen
Abdomen	■ Provides much information with good technique ■ At least two projections are required (LL and DV) ■ Very useful in lithiasis and calcifications ■ Preferred technique for urethral stones	■ Essential for wall and contents of the digestive system ■ Renal diseases ■ Parenchymal organs, thick tissues and ultrasound-guided cytologies ■ Pregnancy ■ Effusions and sampling ■ Evaluation and aspiration of lymph nodes	■ Same uses as in radiology, but preferable for detecting tumors ■ With the use of angiography, enables functional evaluation and detection of vascular pathologies (portosystemic shunt) ■ Evaluation of pneumoperitoneum	May have some applications in the liver and parenchymal organs	Renal function (glomerular filtration rate)	■ Evaluation of the digestive system, including lumen, contents and sample collection (stomach, duodenum, ileum, colon and rectum) ■ Cystoscopy is increasingly useful ■ Laparoscopic interventions
Musculoskeletal system	Preferred technique for bone lesions	Not very useful, if at all, in muscular diseases	Same uses as in radiology, with the advantage of avoiding overlapping images in complex areas (skull, vertebrae, pelvis, mandible)	Not usually used	Not usually used	Not usually used

TABLE 1. Uses of various common diagnostic imaging methods in feline medicine in different anatomical areas (green background: very useful; yellow background: moderately useful; gray background: not very useful)

Anatomical area	Radiology	Ultrasound	Computed tomography	Magnetic resonance	Scintigraphy	Endoscopy
Head and neck	▪ Although it is used, difficult to interpret ▪ Several projections should always be obtained	▪ Not usually used in the head, except rarely in ophthalmology ▪ Diseases of the neck (thyroid gland, lymph nodes)	▪ Preferred technique for avoiding overlaid images of structures ▪ Very useful in the upper respiratory tract	▪ Not usually used in the head, except for the central nervous system ▪ Evaluation of the cervical spinal cord	Preferred technique for thyroid gland disease	Rigid and flexible rhinoscopy, for visualization and sample collection
Central nervous system	Only in case of associated bone disease	Not usually used	Although not as sensitive as MR, the most modern CT devices can aid in neurological diagnosis	Preferred diagnostic method	Not usually used	Not usually used

Bibliography

Holland M, Hudson J (eds.). *Feline Diagnostic Imaging*. NJ, USA: Wiley Blackwell, 2020.

Ohlerth S, Kircher P, Posch B. Diagnostic imaging. In: Langley-Hobbs SJ, Demetriou JL, Ladlow JF (eds.). *Feline Soft Tissue and General Surgery*, 1st ed. London, UK: Saunders Elsevier, 2014; pp. 75–90.

Ohlerth S, Voss K, Steffen F. Further diagnostic procedures. In: Montavon PM, Voss K, Langley-Hobbs SJ (eds.). *Feline Orthopedic Surgery and Musculoskeletal Disease*, 1st ed. London, UK: Saunders Elsevier, 2009; pp. 21–38.

Willard MD, Schulz KS, Hayashi K, Fossum TW. Principios de la cirugía minimamente invasiva y diagnóstico por imagen del paciente quirúrgico. In: Fossum TW (ed.). *Cirugía en pequeños animales*, 5th ed. Barcelona, Spain: Elsevier, 2019; pp. 158–178.

BIOPSY TECHNIQUES AND MOST COMMON USES IN FELINE MEDICINE 7

Llibertat Real

Biopsy is the extraction and examination of a tissue sample taken from a living being for diagnostic purposes.

There are many situations in feline medicine where we might need this technique to diagnose a cat and administer the proper treatment.

We can take an **incisional** biopsy (a sample of a small part of a lesion taken for purposes of diagnosis and administration of the proper medical or surgical treatment) or an **excisional** biopsy (complete removal of a lesion and subsequent analysis thereof). In the case of skin and skin appendages, excisional biopsies can be performed on small or medium-sized nodules that are not adhered to subcutaneous tissue. In other organs, they can be performed on small noninfiltrative nodules. If the presence of a neoplasm is confirmed, and if it is found that the margins are not tumor-free, we will be required to reintervene. On the other hand, if the lesion has been fully removed, performing a second surgery will not be necessary. An incisional biopsy is performed when a diagnosis is needed to plan treatment for lesions that are multifocal, extensive, deep, or adhered to subcutaneous tissue. On most occasions, we will be performing incisional biopsies.

> An excisional biopsy should never be performed if a fibrosarcoma or other infiltrative subcutaneous tumor is suspected.

Gastrointestinal biopsy

Gastrointestinal biopsies are indicated when:

- The patient's medical history and imaging tests lead us to suspect the presence of a diffuse neoplasm or if we detect masses.
- We encounter a case of gastric/gastrointestinal atony for which we have no explanation and which does not respond to treatment.
- There is gastrointestinal ulceration or necrosis for which we have no explanation.
- We see chronic weight loss with a gastrointestinal cause, and it is not improved by dietary changes (especially if this is paired with cobalamin levels that are below the normal range).
- An ultrasound detects changes in the thickness of any layers of the gastrointestinal tract.
- An exploratory laparotomy shows highly infiltrative lesions that we cannot remove. In this case, we would take a biopsy to plan the best treatment, if treatment is at all possible.
- After an exhaustive medical history and diagnosis process, therapeutic tests and a nutritional assessment, we are unable to control the cat's condition, and we suspect enteropathy or chronic gastritis. In some cases, if the clinical, laboratory or ultrasound abnormalities of these patients are severe, biopsies are performed during the initial phases of the diagnostic process.

Biopsies can be taken with a **scalpel**, with **Stevens tenotomy scissors** or with a **punch** during an **exploratory laparotomy**, or even during an **endoscopy** (when we only need samples of the stomach, duodenum, ileum or colon).

Biopsies taken during an exploratory laparotomy enable direct visualization of the serosa and mucosa of the affected parts. They also enable us to take a larger sample that is the full thickness of the gastric or intestinal wall, thus increasing the likelihood of correctly diagnosing a high- or low-grade lymphoma. Finally, they also allow us to perform excisional biopsies of masses that are small and well defined. Endoscopic biopsies do not include the muscular layer, and some parts of the small intestine cannot be reached. However, this technique is less invasive.

The most severe **complication** of a biopsy taken by laparotomy is the dehiscence of sutures, which can lead to septic peritonitis. This occurs infrequently (in 1%–3% of cases) and is associated with abnormally low levels of albumin as well as with sampling of neoplastic tissues. It also occurs more frequently in colon biopsies (at a much higher rate, up to 10% of cases).

Stomach biopsy

To take gastric tissue samples, we must first identify the stomach and isolate it from the other organs. If we have detected an abnormal area in a prior ultrasound, we must locate that area and take the sample from it. If a defined lesion has not been observed, we should extract a sample from the gastric fundus, which is the part of the stomach with the least vascularity. To do this, we place two stay sutures at each end of the area that will be biopsied and make a 1 cm long incision in the shape of a rhombus or spindle. The biopsy should include all layers of the stomach, until reaching the lumen. Once the first incision is made, we can take a sample with a scalpel or baby Metzenbaum scissors. After the biopsy is taken, the incision is sutured in two layers (as explained in Ch. 21 "Gastric foreign bodies and tumors"). Before putting the sample in formol, we must always check to make sure it contains all the layers, including the mucosa.

Small intestine biopsy

When biopsy of the small intestine is performed, the samples should be taken from the duodenum, the jejunum and the ileum, even if their macroscopic and ultrasound appearance is normal. Often the lesions with the most diagnostic significance are found in the ileum (especially in the case of alimentary lymphoma). This is especially evident in cats with cobalamin levels that are below normal or at the low end of the reference range. Samples taken during laparotomy (in contrast to endoscopic samples) enable the pathologist to better visualize the area, and furthermore, they involve all layers of the intestine. They can be taken with a scalpel or a punch after an exploratory laparotomy.

For this procedure, we isolate a segment of the intestine from the other organs. We cover the surrounding area with gauze moistened with lukewarm sterile saline solution. If the lesions were detected by ultrasound, we pinpoint their location, and if not, we thoroughly examine the section of intestine to choose the biopsy site. The assistant should gently massage the biopsy area to displace any ingested material, pressing each side with their index finger and thumb to clear the section where the incision will be made (Fig. 1). The fingers will not always be placed at the same distance apart with respect to the cutting area. This distance should be large enough so that the surgeon can work comfortably, but not so large that the gripped section is loose. Too much mobility will complicate the surgeon's work. This pressure can also be effectuated with Doyen intestinal forceps or a Penrose drain. Using a no. 15 scalpel, an incision is made through the entirety of the wall on the antimesenteric side, until reaching the intestinal lumen. A 4–5 mm long and 1–2 mm wide sample is then taken with the scalpel or tenotomy scissors. An alternative is to place a stay suture, apply traction to it, and, using tenotomy scissors, cut the portion of the intestine that rises with the stay suture (Fig. 2). Another possibility is to use a punch. This requires heavy pressure in order to be able to make a good cut; therefore, the direction of the pressure and the amount of force applied should be carefully controlled to avoid taking a sample incorrectly or causing a iatrogenic injury. We place a 4 mm punch on the antimesenteric border of the intestinal loop we wish to biopsy and rotate it forward until reaching the intestinal lumen. After withdrawing the punch the sample is collected from its cylindrical core.

Biopsies taken with a scalpel or tenotomy scissors can be sutured lengthwise, but the circular wound made by a punch is sutured transversally to avoid causing stenosis.

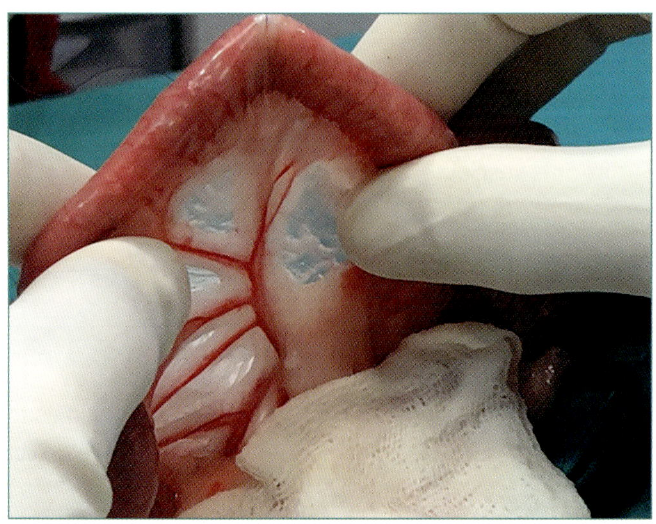

FIGURE 1. Pressure applied by the assistant with their index fingers and thumbs on each side of the section where we make the incision prevents intestinal contents from coming into the area.

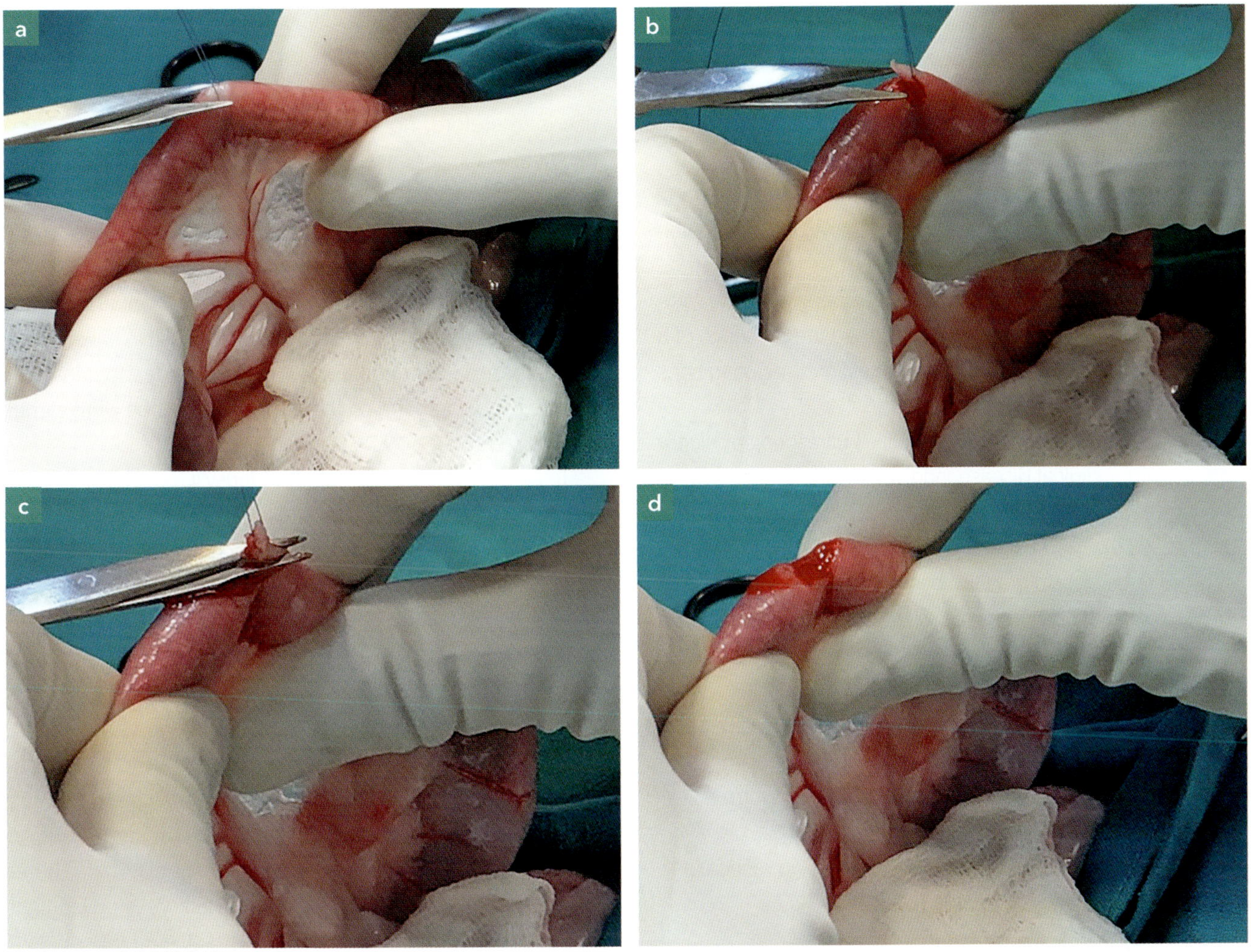

FIGURE 2. Intestinal sample taking with tenotomy scissors. (a) After placing a stay suture, (b) it is pulled up (c) and the portion of the intestine that rises with the stay suture is cut with tenotomy scissors. (d) The resulting wound.

Before closure, we should check to make sure that the sample contains mucosa. The sample should be handled in such a way as to cause minimal trauma, to avoid damaging it to the point that it has no diagnostic value. The incision, including the submucosa, is then closed with simple 5-0 absorbable monofilament sutures. Omentum can be wrapped around the area and tacked with sutures, especially in patients that have an elevated risk of dehiscence.

Large intestine biopsy

The large intestine is biopsied if nodular lesions are found, if structural abnormalities are detected ultrasonographically, or if the patient has colitis that has not responded to any dietary or medical treatment and all the most common infectious causes have been discarded. To minimize complications, it is usually performed by endoscopy, but this method entails long preparation and does not allow us to take samples that are the full thickness of the wall. When this is required, an exploratory laparotomy is performed, and the sample is collected with a no. 15 scalpel blade, using the same technique as described for the small intestine. Due to the higher risk of suture dehiscence (around 10% of colon surgeries in general, including biopsies) and contamination with colon flora, we should close the incision with a double suture (the risk of stenosis is lower): the first suture is simple continuous and the second is inverting, with an absorbable 4-0 size. This is followed with routine postoperative management for a gastrointestinal surgery. The cat is closely monitored for 48–72 hours to detect as soon as possible any dehiscence of sutures or other complication that may arise.

Liver biopsy

In the liver, biopsies can be taken of nodules, masses, multifocal lesions or diffuse lesions that affect the whole organ. A liver biopsy is performed when:

- We suspect the presence of a neoplasm after detecting abnormalities ultrasonographically or analytically, and cytology is not indicated.
- Hepatic enzyme or bile acid levels are persistently or progressively elevated and we have discarded the presence of a portosystemic shunt, endocrine diseases, or other conditions associated with hepatic alteration.
- We have detected hepatic abnormalities ultrasonographically in cats with a clinical disease, and we find no other explanation for the disease or there is no response to treatment for the disease that we suspected.
- In order to be able to plan the best medical or surgical treatment, we also biopsy liver masses that cannot effectively be resected in their totality.

We should keep in mind that persistently or progressively elevated hepatic enzymes does not mean that the levels need to be extremely high before making the decision to perform a liver biopsy. If any levels are persistently elevated without explanation for a sufficiently long period of time and there is no response to treatment, a biopsy may be indicated.

> A liver biopsy should never be performed in a cat without first testing for thyroid disease.

Given the possibility of excessive bleeding due to vitamin K deficiency (possibly associated with an abnormal enterohepatic circulation of bile acids), we should do tests for clotting and administer 0.5–1.5 mg/kg of subcutaneous vitamin K every 12 hours, beginning 36–48 hours before the intervention.

As we have described previously, different types of lesions or pathologies may require a biopsy; therefore different techniques are used in the liver. We do not use the same technique for lesions that affect the entire parenchyma, in which a biopsy of the edge is sufficient, as for lesions found in the center of the organ. An excisional biopsy can be performed on a single medium or large lesion through lobectomy, as long as the location of the mass allows it. We should also keep in mind that some pathologies can increase the friability of liver tissue. Therefore, it should always be handled with care to avoid tears.

The most frequent complication is postoperative bleeding. The use of tru-cut automatic needles carries an increased risk of death due to shock associated with severe vagotonia. Their use is, therefore, not advised. If we deem this technique to be suitable for our case, the use of a semiautomatic needle is recommended.

At least 12–15 complete portal triads (portal spaces) are needed to be able to correctly interpret the sample, and 40 g of tissue are needed to be able to quantify copper. Biopsying at least two hepatic lobules is advised, if possible. If we suspect a certain disease in particular, it is a good idea to contact the pathologist beforehand so that they can describe what samples they will need.

To perform a **marginal hepatic biopsy** we will use the **guillotine technique**. It is done on diffuse lesions that affect the whole organ or when we ultrasonographically detect an abnormal area that comprises the entire lobe or its margin. Excisional biopsies can be performed on small noninfiltrative nodules (nevertheless, ultrasonic coagulation is preferred; see Ch. 5, "Surgical materials").

To carry out the guillotine technique, we gain access to the abdominal cavity and examine the organ to confirm that the lesion is diffuse. A lobe of the liver whose margin is easily accessible is isolated (Fig. 3). Using a 3-0 absorbable monofilament suture, we make a loop with a simple knot. The end of the lobe is circled by the loop, and the knot is pulled tightly. As the knot is tightened, the blood vessels and bile ducts are ligated (Fig. 4). We make two or three more knots to secure the suture in place. Using baby Metzenbaum scissors, we cut the portion of liver isolated by the suture (Fig. 5). We

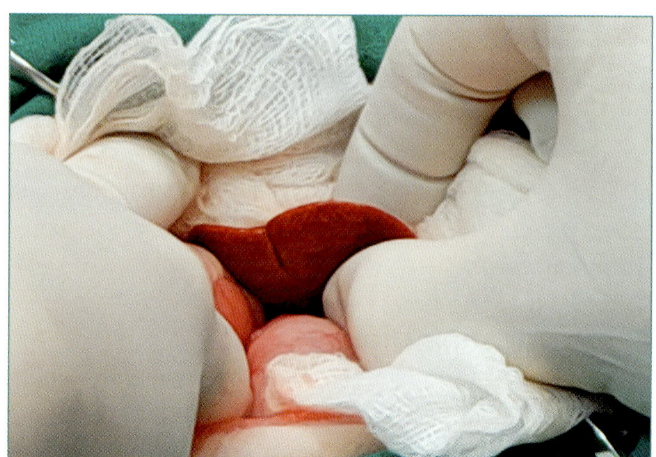

FIGURE 3. Isolation of the hepatic lobe selected for biopsy using the guillotine technique.

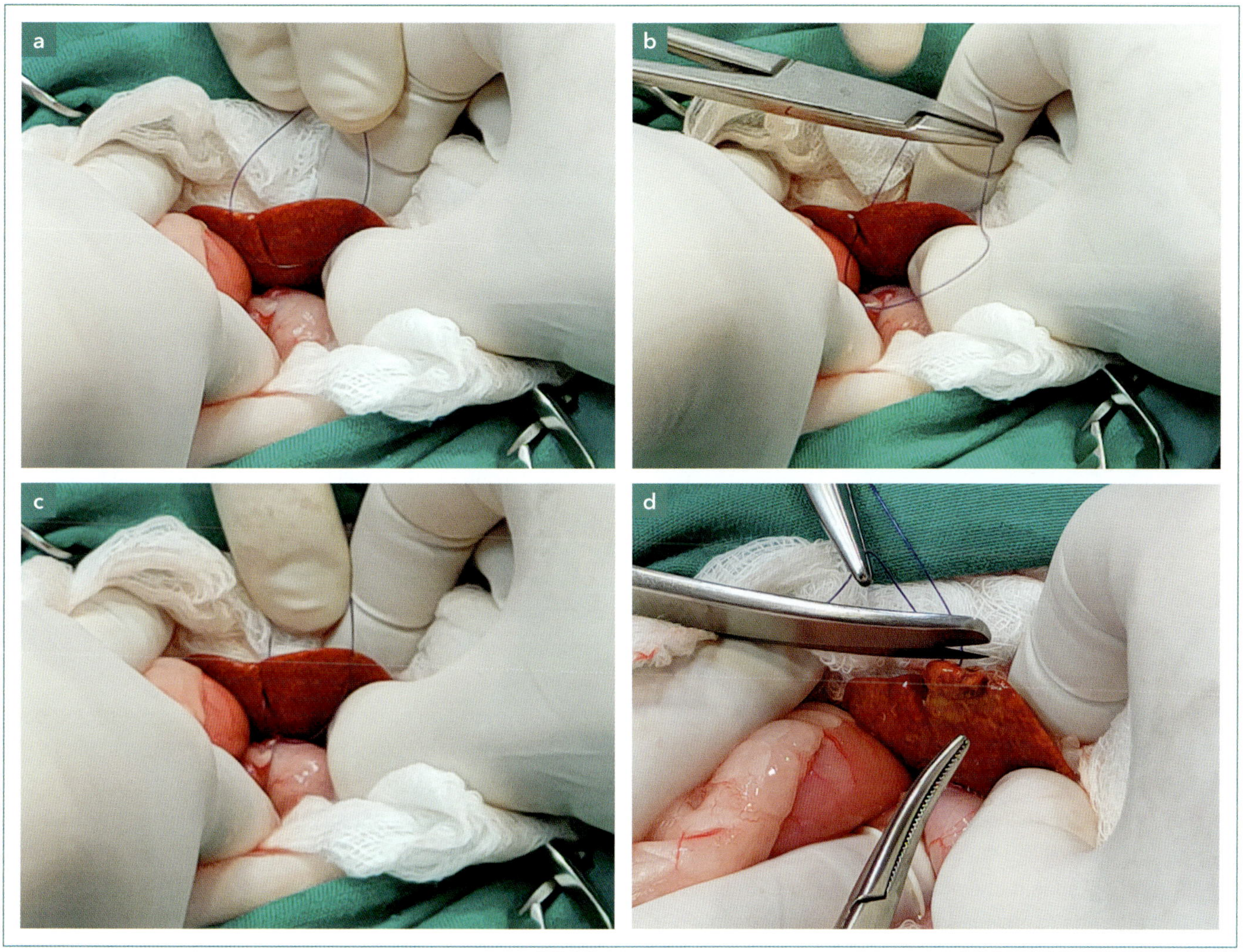

FIGURE 4. Taking a liver sample with the guillotine technique. (a) A suture loop is formed with a simple knot, (b,c) with which the end of the lobe is circled, and it is moved forward while squeezing the knot tightly. (d) The knot ligates the blood vessels and bile ducts.

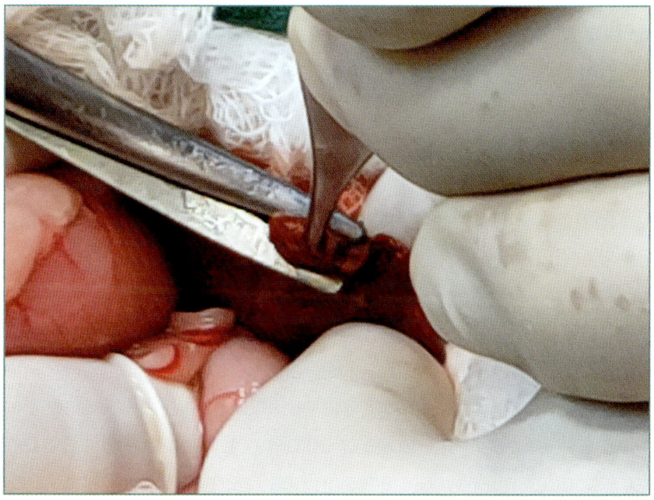

FIGURE 5. Cutting a hepatic fragment. We should make sure there is no bleeding after withdrawing the sample.

should take care not to cut the suture and handle the sample with the minimal trauma possible before placing it in formol. Imprints can be made before the sample is placed in the container. If we also wish to make a culture, using the liver tissue is not advised; instead we should retrieve a sample of bile at the same time by performing a cholecystocentesis. This will increase the chance of obtaining a positive result in the culture. Cholecystocentesis is done by puncturing the gallbladder through a lobe of the liver (the quadrate lobe in most cases, if done during a laparotomy) with a 23-gauge needle attached to a syringe (2 or 5 ml, depending on the size of the gallbladder) (Fig. 6). Emptying the gallbladder completely is advised in order to minimize the risk of biliary peritonitis. A marginal biopsy can also be collected using ultrasonic coagulation equipment. In this case, we simply cut the section with

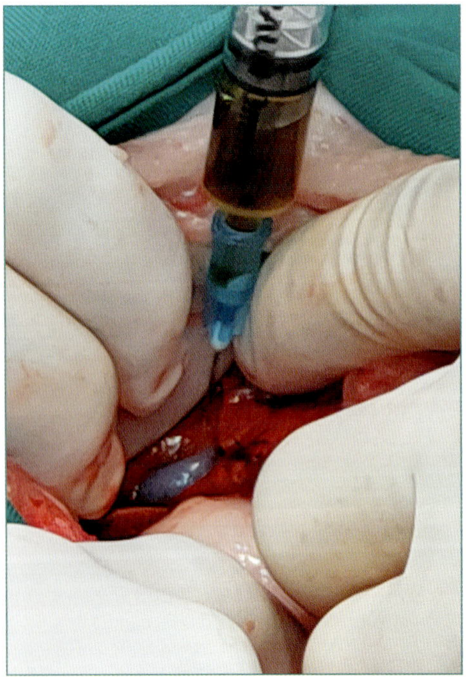

FIGURE 6. In cholecystocentesis, we should try to extract as much biliary content as possible within a margin of safety.

the scalpel. There are special forceps for taking biopsies, such as the clamshell type. Another option is to obtain the biopsy through laparoscopic surgery. For diffuse lesions, a tru-cut needle is not recommended, since the samples are smaller and have a lower diagnostic value. Regardless of the technique used, we should check to make sure that there is no bleeding after the sample is taken. Once the intervention is over, we should keep the patient at the clinic for a sufficient amount of time to ensure that there is no postoperative bleeding. The patient is administered opioid pain medication and antibiotics. The cat may begin to ingest food as per the usual guidelines for any surgery.

If we want to biopsy a **nodule** or other **lesion or lesions located at a distance from the margin of the liver,** we can use a **tru-cut** needle, a **punch** or **ultrasonic coagulation** equipment. If we use a punch, it will be 4 mm. Once the pressure and rotation has been applied, we cut the base with baby Metzenbaum scissors, pressing with our fingers for 3–5 minutes to control the bleeding. If it does not stop, we should use hemostatic colloid to seal it. If a tru-cut needle is used, bleeding should be controlled in the same way. In any case, using ultrasonic coagulation equipment if we can is highly recommended, since it minimizes the risk of hemorrhaging and produces minimal trauma in the tissue. As with biopsies done when we suspect a diffuse condition, the diagnostic value of samples obtained by needle is much lower than samples obtained with a scalpel or a punch.

Pancreatic biopsy

The pancreas is not biopsied as commonly as other organs because of the possible negative aftereffects caused by handling (postoperative pancreatitis). Today, taking pancreatic biopsies in cases where it is indicated is considered safe if it is done with proper technique and minimal trauma to the tissues.

Pancreatic biopsies are taken when:

- We detect masses in an ultrasound, computed tomography (CT) or magnetic resonance (MR). If they are small, these masses may be located in areas where we can even perform an excisional biopsy. In other cases, their size or location means only an incisional biopsy can be performed.
- We are faced with patients with clinical signs, laboratory tests and imaging tests compatible with chronic pancreatitis (with or without clinical signs in other digestive organs), and we may not be able to control the condition with the established treatment.

A disadvantage of biopsies in these cases of chronic pancreatitis is that the biopsied area may not show signs of the lesion that is producing the clinical condition. This can happen because while all of the tissue may have a similar macroscopic appearance, some areas could be more affected than others. Another reason is that there may be a higher level of fibrosis in areas that show greater ultrasonographic or macroscopic alteration.

We should never euthanize a cat because of the macroscopic appearance of its pancreas when a biopsy is taken or in an ultrasound image. Chronic pancreatitis can cause the organ to enlarge considerably, sometimes in a heterogeneous and infiltrative way and with an appearance similar to carcinoma. However, the prognosis is completely different. Although not very common, we may encounter postoperative pancreatitis as a complication.

To minimize the risk of injuring the cranial and caudal pancreaticoduodenal blood vessels, the common bile duct (CBD), and the pancreatic duct, we should always take a sample of the **left lobe** if we can. For diffuse lesions we should use the **guillotine technique**, as with a liver biopsy. To do this, we isolate the pancreas by separating the omentum. We then select the biopsy site, usually the edge or border of the left lobe if it is a diffuse condition, or where a lesion has been detected. The mesentery should be separated through blunt dissection if possible, although sharp dissection may be required at some points. We then make a simple knot with a 4-0 absorbable monofilament, placing a loop around the pancreatic area we wish to biopsy (a small area), and tie the knot to ligate the pancreatic tissue. The end that is circumscribed within the loop is cut with baby Metzenbaum scissors.

An alternative to this technique is to place two stitches in the shape of a V to demarcate the area we wish to cut. We can also take the sample with ultrasonic coagulation equipment.

After the intervention, an antiemetic is administered (maropitant: 2 mg/kg), along with an analgesic. Arterial pressure is monitored, and we continue fluid therapy until the patient has woken up and is in stable condition to ensure that there is constant blood flow to the pancreas.

Renal biopsy

In contrast to other organs, renal biopsies are rarely performed when we suspect the presence of a neoplasm. This diagnosis is obtained much more frequently in a post nephrectomy pathology report on the removed kidney or by cytology when we suspect renal lymphoma. A biopsy should be performed to obtain a definitive diagnosis of the cause of chronic kidney disease when:

- Kidney disease is coupled with severe proteinuria.
- The disease progresses with unusual rapidity and we are unable to determine the cause.
- We suspect renal amyloidosis (or another hereditary or congenital disease) or when we may be dealing with reactive amyloidosis.
- We suspect glomerulonephritis even in the absence of severe proteinuria.

There are different renal biopsy techniques. It can be **ultrasound guided with a tru-cut** needle, a **wedge biopsy through abdominal laparotomy** or with laparoscopy through an **incision in the flank of the abdomen**. It can also be performed by laparoscopy with a tru-cut needle (Fig. 7).

> If possible, we should always take wedge samples via laparotomy, since their diagnostic value is much higher than other techniques. It is also easier to detect and control postoperative bleeding.

The most frequent complication is microscopic hematuria, followed by macroscopic hematuria, and postoperative bleeding. We may encounter subcapsular bleeding up to 2 days after the biopsy. It is important to biopsy only in the renal cortex (Fig. 7b). If we reach the medulla or the pelvis, this can cause severe iatrogenic injury, which can cause hydronephrosis or even death of the cat. Clotting tests should be performed before the biopsy.

After gaining access to the abdominal cavity, the left kidney is located (this kidney is more accessible). The assistant immobilizes the kidney and uses their fingers to squeeze the renal vessels for a few brief moments while the sample is being taken. We access the convex lateral aspect. A 4-0 absorbable monofilament suture is used to place a U-stitch across the renal cortex and parenchyma, without closing it, around the area that will be biopsied. An incision is made with a no. 15 scalpel blade in the capsule to take an approximately 0.5 cm wedge-shaped sample of the renal parenchyma. We can use a hemostatic colloid to stop the bleeding. Next, the capsular incision is closed. Alternatively, the suture can be placed after making the incision and tightened immediately. It is important to make sure that there is no bleeding before closing the abdominal cavity.

The cat should remain under observation for a minimum of 4–6 hours after extubation to confirm that there is no bleeding. Body temperature, heart rate and blood pressure is monitored. In case of doubt, a complete blood count and a follow-up ultrasound can be performed.

Lymph node biopsy

Lymph node biopsies are performed relatively often in the following situations:

- Sometimes during an exploratory laparotomy, while performing biopsies of other organs, an abdominal lymph node is detected with a significant alteration of its characteristics (size, shape, color) or else after having detected a lymphadenopathy on a preoperative abdominal ultrasound.
- We may also have to biopsy peripheral lymph nodes (prescapular, popliteal, etc.) if they are notably swollen in size without explanation, if cytology does not provide a diagnosis or information on the cause, or if there is no response to treatment administered after a cytological diagnosis. We should keep in mind that we may fail to diagnose a neoplasm of the lymph nodes if we only carry out cytology.
- If we have diagnosed a neoplasm and we would like to determine if it has spread to regional lymph nodes.

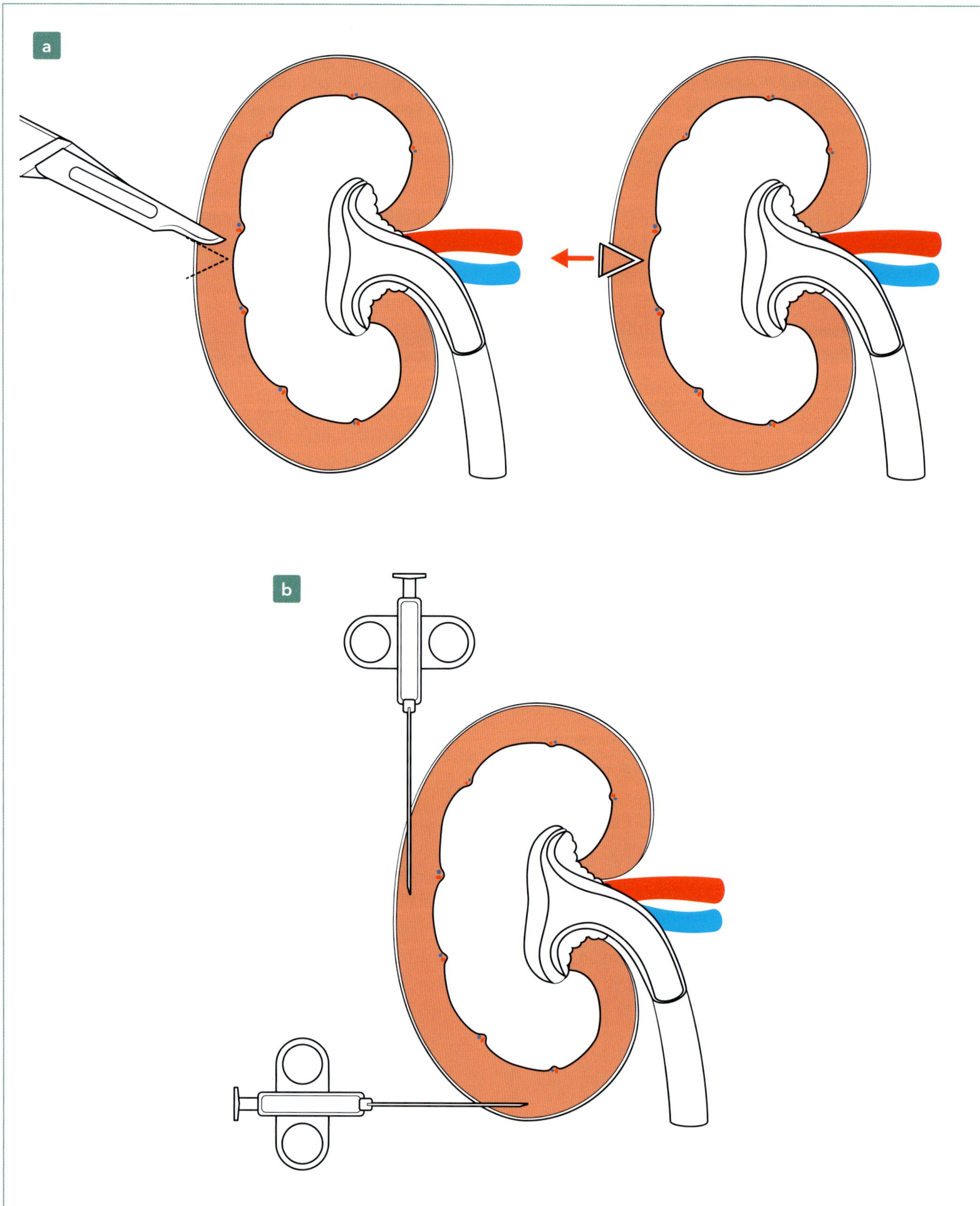

FIGURE 7. (a) Renal wedge biopsy. (b) Renal biopsy with a tru-cut needle. A biopsy of the kidney should be done exclusively within the renal cortex; it should not reach the renal medulla or pelvis.

We can take a **wedge biopsy** with a scalpel or with a punch. Less frequently, we may fully excise the node, depending on the sample required or the condition that we suspect. On occasion, pathologists may require the full node after having ordered a wedge biopsy to confirm a diagnosis. PARR, or PCR for antigen receptor rearrangements, is a very helpful complementary test when there is doubt whether a lymphoma is present. Before performing a biopsy, we should remember that many regional blood vessels are close to the lymph nodes, and we should be careful when dissecting them to avoid bleeding.

For this technique, the lymph node we wish to biopsy is located and accessed. A wedge fragment is obtained through the capsule. Subsequently, the area is closed with a 3-0 absorbable monofilament suture, using a U-stitch (Fig. 8). In some cases the lymph node tissue is very friable, and it is difficult to obtain such a fragment. In this case, full excision of the lymph node is better so that the pathologist can correctly evaluate the lymph node architecture. This is only done in those nodes that are easily accessed. To do this, after accessing the lymph node, it is isolated by performing a blunt dissection of the surrounding tissue. The blood vessels are ligated and it is extracted. After making several imprints, it is preserved in formol. A portion of it can be kept frozen, or several fine needle aspirates can be frozen in case a specific technique is required. Before performing the biopsy, it is highly advisable to contact the pathologist and the laboratory to find out how we should preserve the samples, so that the surgery is as diagnostically useful as possible.

Splenic biopsy

Biopsies of the spleen are not taken frequently. Rather, splenectomy is usually indicated in the various pathologies that affect this organ (severe splenomegaly, masses). If a biopsy is required, we should use the **guillotine technique** (similarly to the liver biopsy) for the head and the tail. Or, if lesions affect the body of the spleen, we should perform a partial resection. To do this, we ligate the vessels of the portion to be resected, apply an atraumatic clamp forceps, and after cutting the fragment of spleen, the capsule is sutured. In the latter situation, ultrasonic coagulation equipment should be used whenever possible.

Conjunctival biopsy

This is a simple and quick technique that can be very useful in the diagnosis of certain ocular pathologies. It is performed when:

- A moderate or severe abnormality of the conjunctiva is present for which we have no explanation, which does not respond to the usual empiric therapies for feline herpesvirus type 1, and for which the cytology did not provide diagnostic information.
- Neoplastic disease is suspected.

The biopsy is obtained under sedation or general anesthesia, and after administering local anesthesia. Anesthetic eye drops are applied with a swab for 10 seconds, taking effect within a

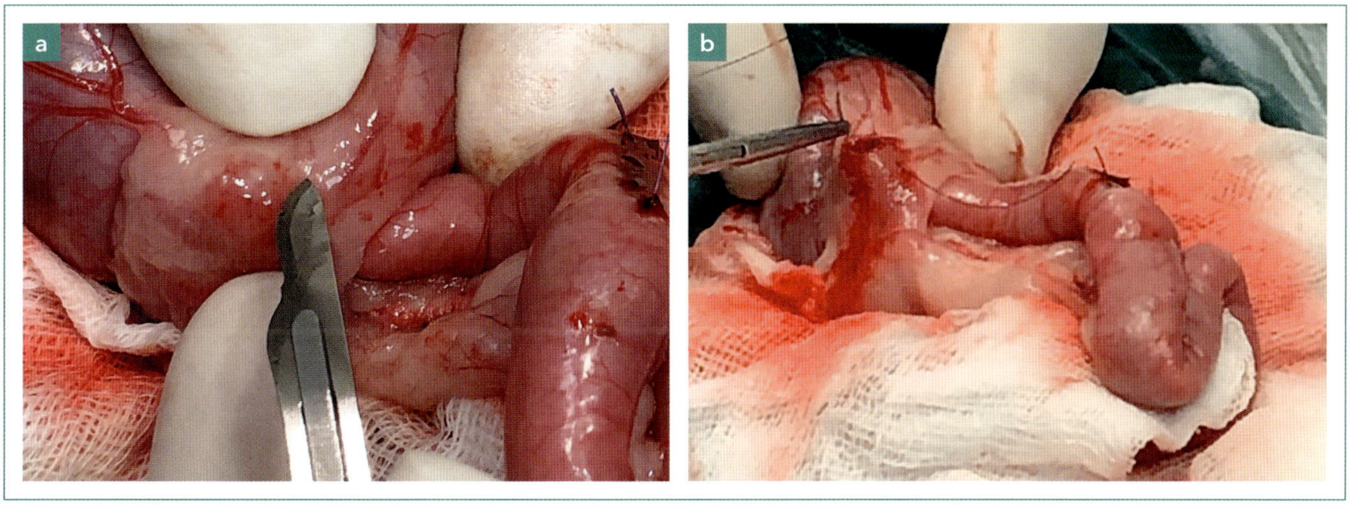

FIGURE 8. (a) Taking a sample of a mesenteric lymph node during an exploratory laparotomy, (b) in which intestinal samples have also been taken.

minute of application and lasting approximately 25 minutes. Next, the conjunctival sac is washed with a 1:50 dilution of povidone-iodine. We take a pinch of conjunctiva with Adson non-toothed forceps or with Bishop-Harmon forceps (with small teeth), we lift it similarly to a tent, and section the part furthest from the eye with tenotomy scissors (Fig. 9). The sample should be handled with utmost care to avoid damaging it. We place it on a heavy-paper or cardboard surface to aid with orientation and to avoid producing folds or contraction of the tissue. The conjunctiva does not require a suture unless the defect created is greater than 1 cm. Bleeding is controlled by applying pressure for 2–3 minutes. If the bleeding does not stop, we can apply a 1:10,000 dilution of local adrenaline. Antibiotic eye drops are administered for a few days after taking the sample.

Biopsy of skin and subcutaneous tissue

A biopsy of the skin and subcutaneous tissue is performed to:

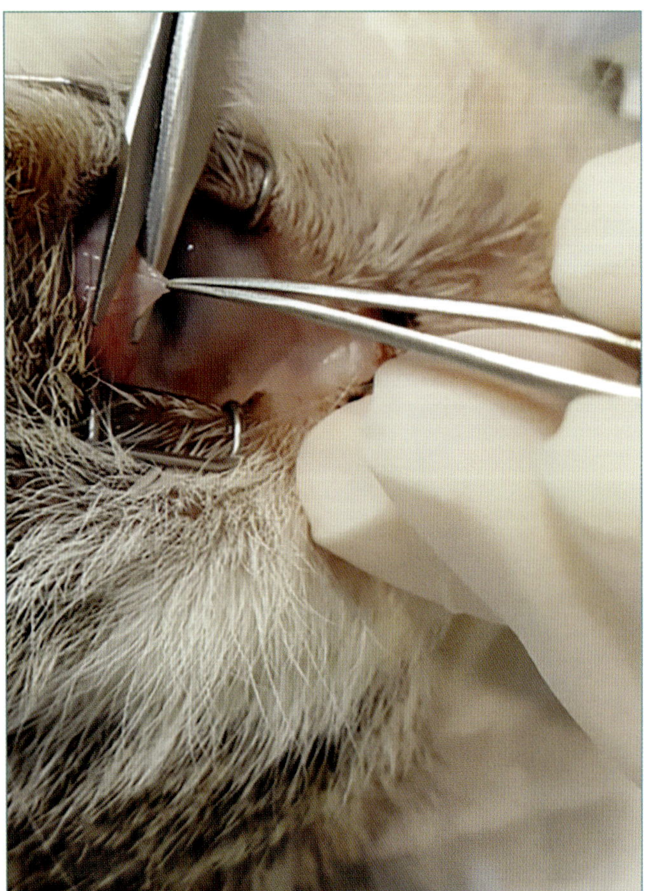

FIGURE 9. Conjunctival sample taken with tenotomy scissors.

- Obtain or confirm a precise diagnosis in the presence of specific skin lesions (mainly immune-mediated and neoplastic diseases, unusual infections, or endocrine diseases).
- Discard certain conditions or confirm a diagnosis that has been established on the basis of medical history or other tests such as cytologies, skin scrapes, adhesive tape tests, or cultures, among others, and there has not been adequate response to treatment (hypersensitivity, parasitic and fungal conditions).

No strict criteria exist concerning when (at which point in the diagnostic process) we should take a skin biopsy in a feline patient. In many cases, it depends on:

- The medical history.
- Whether or not the patient has received previous treatment (and their response to that treatment).
- The cat's overall condition (normal appearance or with signs of systemic infection).
- The amount of time since the lesion or lesions manifested.
- Geographic origin or current place of residence.
- Retroviral status.
- Age of onset and current age of the cat.
- If the cat lives with other cats or alone.
- If the cat goes outdoors or has contact with other cats.
- Color of the skin and fur.

As a general rule (but with some exceptions) chronic conditions in which lesions have existed for very long durations give us little information, since changes that the skin undergoes, such as fibrosis or infiltration of inflammatory cells, can hinder a diagnostic pathology report.

The key to obtaining the best possible information from a skin biopsy is in the technique, the careful handling of the sample, and in very carefully choosing of the area or lesion that will be biopsied. We should make sure we have controlled all the secondary conditions that can affect the results of the biopsy. Some authors recommend the use of antibiotics a week before the biopsy if we have confirmed the presence of a secondary infection (after a culture and antibiogram) so that it does not complicate the interpretation of the pathology report. If corticosteroid treatment is being administered, it should be discontinued, if possible, 2–3 weeks before the biopsy in the case of oral medication, and 6–8 weeks in advance if using long-lasting injectable corticosteroids.

As a general rule, we should try to take samples of primary lesions: papules, pustules, vesicles, macules, or nodules in their fully developed state, if possible, or in several stages of development. It is best to send pustules in an early phase of development. We should be careful in the presence of crusts and try to preserve them in the sample. Biopsies are also indicated in some locations such as at mucocutaneous junctions or the nail bed. Sometimes only secondary lesions such as alopecia, ulcers, erosions, etc., are observed. If that is the case, we should keep in mind that the diagnostic value is much more limited. We should avoid biopsies in areas where there is self-inflicted trauma. Biopsies are obtained of lesions that increase in size quickly and do not respond to treatment. A biopsy is also obtained whenever we suspect a skin tumor; subcutaneous masses with fistulous tracts, samples of which yielded a negative result on a bacterial culture; or when we suspect diseases for which treatment may entail aggressive surgery. We should explain to the animal's owner that we are not always able to obtain a diagnostic result and that it may sometimes be possible that we will have to take another biopsy during another phase of the diagnostic process.

Cutaneous biopsies can be performed with a 3, 4 or 6 mm **punch** or by taking a **wedge fragment** with a **scalpel** (if masses have adhered to subcutaneous tissue). In the case of a large skin lesion, a fragile lesion (pustule, vesicle) or a deep lesion (when we suspect panniculitis), a scalpel is used to take **an ellipsoid sample**. This may include a section of healthy skin along with a part of the lesion.

This technique can be carried out with the cat deeply sedated or anesthetized, or we can administer local anesthesia and mild sedation. We should prepare the area by lightly removing fur from the area (if possible, with scissors), taking care not to damage the skin. If this is difficult due to the nature of the lesion, it is best not to do it until after the samples are taken. The area should not be washed or disinfected. We should always try to take a sample that contains the entire lesion. For solitary ulcers, the central area should be avoided and there is no need to include adjacent skin. For progressive multifocal ulcerative lesions, however, the biopsy should comprise the ulcer and the area adjacent to the lesion. If the lesion is very large, we should consider whether to send several samples from different areas of the lesion or whether to take one ellipsoid sample. If the sample is needed for immunohistochemical staining, it should include the lesion (new lesions or well developed lesions) and areas immediately adjacent to it. If we believe it is important to send healthy skin, it is better to take another sample separately.

When using a punch, 3–5 samples should be obtained, if possible from different areas. We should always take biopsies from areas that look different. The process consists of selecting an area to which we apply pressure with the punch while rotating it (Fig. 10). In order to obtain a correct sample, it should contain the full thickness of the skin, up to the subcutaneous fat, where we cut the sample with iris or baby Metzenbaum scissors. Adson nontoothed forceps are used to hold the hypodermis during handling. A very important point is that we should avoid handling it from any other area, since we can damage the sample and obtain results that are not diagnostic. The sample should be placed on a flat surface (e.g., a piece of cardboard or a tongue depressor). This ensures that the sample will not fold in on itself, and helps the pathologist understand the orientation of the sample (Fig. 11). We then place it into a properly marked container with 10% formaldehyde solution. The biopsy area is sutured with a simple suture or a cross suture with 3-0 or 4-0 nonabsorbable monofilament material.

If possible, we should always send the sample to a dermatopathologist with a medical history that explains the most relevant clinical and laboratory data.

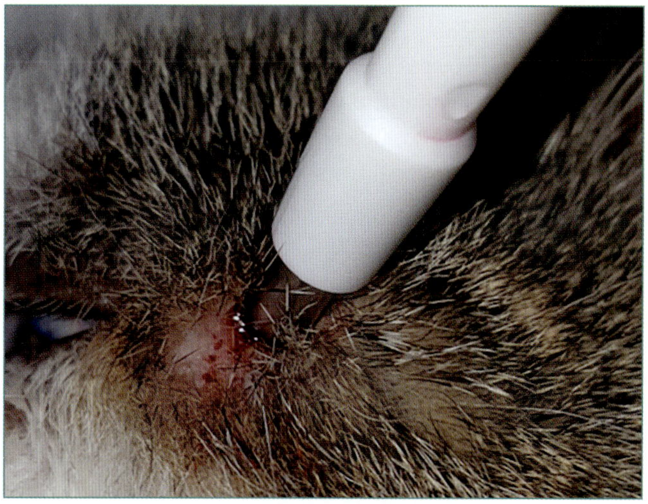

FIGURE 10. Rotation and pressure with a punch to obtain a skin sample.

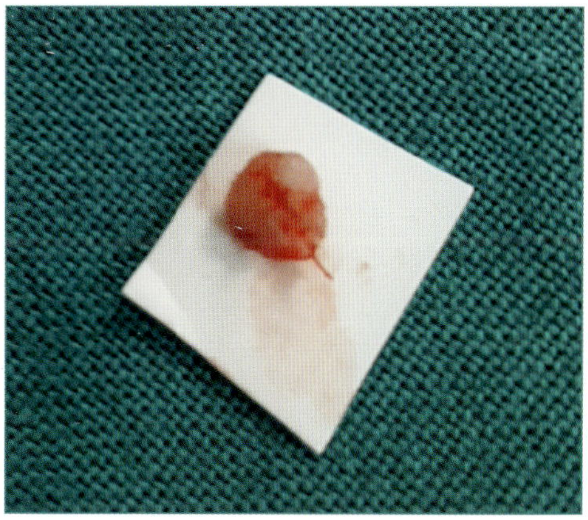

FIGURE 11. Placing the sample on a piece of cardboard to prevent it from deforming before placing it into formol.

Bibliography

Aronson LR. Kidney and ureter. In: Langley-Hobbs SJ, Demetriou JL, Ladlow JF (eds.). *Feline Soft Tissue and General Surgery*, 1st ed. Oxford, UK: Saunders Elsevier, 2014; pp. 401–422.

Cole TL, Center SA, Flood SN et al. Diagnostic comparison of needle and wedge biopsy specimens of the liver in dogs and cats. *J Am Vet Med Assoc*, 2002; 220(10):1483–1490.

Corrêa LM, Demetriou JL. Retrospective assessment of the clinical relevance of surgical biopsies of abdominal lymph nodes in cats: 51 cases (2014–2018). *J Feline Med Surg*, 2020; 22(12):1168–1175.

Evans SE, Bonczynski JJ, Broussard JD et al. Comparison of endoscopic and full-thickness biopsy specimens for diagnosis of inflammatory bowel disease and alimentary tract lymphoma in cats. *J Am Vet Med Assoc*, 2006; 229(9):1447–1450.

Guttin T, Walsh A, Durham AC et al. Ability of ultrasonography to predict the presence and location of histologic lesions in the small intestine of cats. *J Vet Intern Med*, 2019; 33(3):1278–1285.

Kleinschmidt S, Harder J, Nolte I et al. Chronic inflammatory and non-inflammatory diseases of the gastrointestinal tract in cats: diagnostic advantages of full-thickness intestinal and extraintestinal biopsies. *J Feline Med Surg*, 2010; 12(2):97–103.

Lidbury JA. Getting the most out of liver biopsy. *Vet Clin North Am Small Anim Pract*, 2017; 47(3):569–583.

Linder KE. Skin biopsy site selection in small animal dermatology with an introduction to histologic pattern-analysis of inflammatory skin lesions. *Clin Tech Small Anim Pract*, 2001; 16(4):207–213.

Mitchell N, Oliver J. The conjunctiva. In: *Feline Ophtalmology*, 1st ed. Zaragoza, Spain: Servet, 2015; pp. 99–100.

Murgia D. Investigation of parenchymal abdominal organ disease in cats: aiming for the ideal biopsy. *J Feline Med Surg*, 2014; 16(3):216–230.

Odenweller PH, Smith MM, Taney KG. Validation of regional lymph node excisional biopsy for staging oral and maxillofacial malignant neoplasms in 97 dogs and 10 cats (2006–2016). *J Vet Dent*, 2019; 36(2):97–103.

Pratschke KM, Ryan J, McAlinden A, McLauchlan G. Pancreatic surgical biopsy in 24 dogs and 19 cats: postoperative complications and clinical relevance of histological findings. *J Small Anim Pract*, 2015; 56(1):60–66.

Proot SJM, Rothuizen J. High complication rate of an automatic Tru-Cut biopsy gun device for liver biopsy in cats. *J Vet Intern Med*, 2006; 20(6):1327–1333.

Scott KD, Zoran DL, Mansell J et al. Utility of endoscopic biopsies of the duodenum and ileum for diagnosis of inflammatory bowel disease and small cell lymphoma in cats. *J Vet Intern Med*, 2011; 25(6):1253–1257.

Shales C. Celiotomy. In: Langley-Hobbs SJ, Demetriou JL, Ladlow JF (eds.). *Feline Soft Tissue and General Surgery*, 1st ed. Oxford, UK: Saunders Elsevier, 2014; pp. 245–252.

Swinbourne F, Jeffery N, Tivers MS et al. The incidence of surgical site dehiscence following full-thickness gastrointestinal biopsy in dogs and cats and associated risk factors. *J Small Anim Pract*, 2017; 58(9):495–503.

Vaden SL, Levine JF, Lees GE et al. Renal biopsy: a retrospective study of methods and complications in 283 dogs and 65 cats. *J Vet Intern Med*, 2005; 19(6):794–801.

Vaden SL. Renal biopsy of dogs and cats. *Clin Tech Small Anim Pract*, 2005; 20(1):11–22.

Yager JA, Wilcock BP. Skin biopsy: Revelations and limitations. *Can Vet J*, 1988; 29(12):969–975.

WOUND MANAGEMENT 8

Anna Calvet

Characteristics of wounds in cats

The wound healing process begins immediately after a wound has occurred and involves a series of overlapping events or stages. These phases include a synchronized molecular and biochemical process in the cells that culminates in healing.

The wound healing process in cats has unique characteristics that will influence the process itself and how we should approach it:

- Compared to dogs, cats' epidermis, dermis and hypodermis are thinner.
- Cats' skin is more elastic.
- The blood supply is more limited, with fewer perforating arteries and a lower density of cutaneous angiosomes, especially in the trunk area, which are defined as the block of tissue comprising the skin, subcutaneous tissue, fascia, muscle and bone that receives blood supply from a specific artery and is drained by a specific vein.
- With regard to the wound healing phases (discussed below), the progression of the proliferative phase is slower.
- In wounds closed by first intention, there is lower collagen production (always compared to dogs) and the tensile strength at 7 days is 50% lower.
- In wounds treated by secondary closure, the inflammatory phase is longer.
- Cats take twice as long as dogs to "fill" a wound with granulation tissue. This is because while in the dog granulation tissue originates from the entire hypodermis, in cats it starts at the edges of the wound and progresses towards the center.

The relationship between wound healing and the nature of cats deserves a small section:

- Cats generally tolerate bandages and immobilizations poorly.
- Repeated sedation may be required for dressing changes.
- In order to change dressings as often as needed, it may be necessary to keep the cat hospitalized. The downside is that hospitalization causes stress and patients tend to eat less, which is detrimental to the healing process. We should never underestimate the importance of adequate caloric intake in a recovering cat. We must calculate their daily energy needs and ensure that our patient meets them, either by eating on their own or through a feeding tube.
- Cats wearing bandages sometimes stop using the litter box, and the bandages may become soiled or wet.

Phases of wound healing

Wound healing involves several stages:

1. **Hemostasis:** vasoconstriction and the formation of fibrin clots occur to stop bleeding. Platelets and growth factors such as platelet-derived growth factor (PDGF) and transforming growth factor beta (TGF-β) are involved. This phase lasts 0 hours to 1 day.
2. **Inflammation:** vasodilatation, increased capillary permeability and the chemotaxis of inflammatory cells (macrophages) occur. PDGF triggers the release of growth factors (vascular endothelial growth factor —VEGF— and TGF-β) and cytokines (interleukin 1 —IL-1— and tumor necrosis factor alpha —TNF-α—) by macrophages. This phase lasts 3 hours–5 days.
3. **Proliferation:** tissues reepithelialize, new blood vessels are generated and collagen production by fibroblasts increases. This phase lasts 3 days–5 weeks.
4. **Remodeling:** old collagen is resorbed by the action of matrix metalloproteinases and newly synthesized collagen is reorganized and cross-linked. This phase lasts 3 weeks–2 years.

Wound management

It is important to perform a rigorous clinical examination and round out that information with imaging tests, which may include thoracic and abdominal X-rays, with or without abdominal ultrasound, and minimal blood tests.

> The first step is to assess the cat's general condition, the presence of comorbidities and to not focus solely on the wound.

Once we have a general idea of the patient's health condition, we will assess the wound or wounds (Fig. 1).

Wound closure options

Depending on the type of wound and the characteristics present at the time of evaluation, different closure options can be considered:

- **Primary closure:** it is performed by tissue apposition and suturing; it is basically used to close surgical wounds.
- **Delayed or deferred primary closure:** in this case, the wound must be cleaned before closure. Many feline injuries have an unknown cause, but trauma and fights are common. An injury such as this will be treated as an open wound for a period ranging from 2 to 4 days and then closed by suturing.
- **Secondary closure:** suturing the wound is delayed until wound infection has been controlled. Heavily contaminated wounds or wounds with extensive tissue loss require a few days for the appropriate wound bed to form in order to attempt closure. The formation of granulation tissue will be the indicator that it is time for closure.
- **Management or closure by secondary intention:** the wound is remodeled by the emergence of new tissue, the aim is to accelerate the process by applying the appropriate dressings. The main stumbling block to overcome in the management of extensive wounds is time (the slow nature of tissue recovery in cats has already been mentioned). The number of dressing changes necessary requires that the owners be well informed and cooperative, and also that the patient cooperate. Although it is a long and difficult road, it can also be very rewarding. In these cases it is almost always necessary to perform surgical closure at some point (see Ch. 9 "Most common flaps and plasties in feline surgery").

Reconstructions should be performed, as already mentioned, when the wound bed and the donor skin in the case of plasties are in good enough condition to carry out all the cellular processes involved in the healing process.

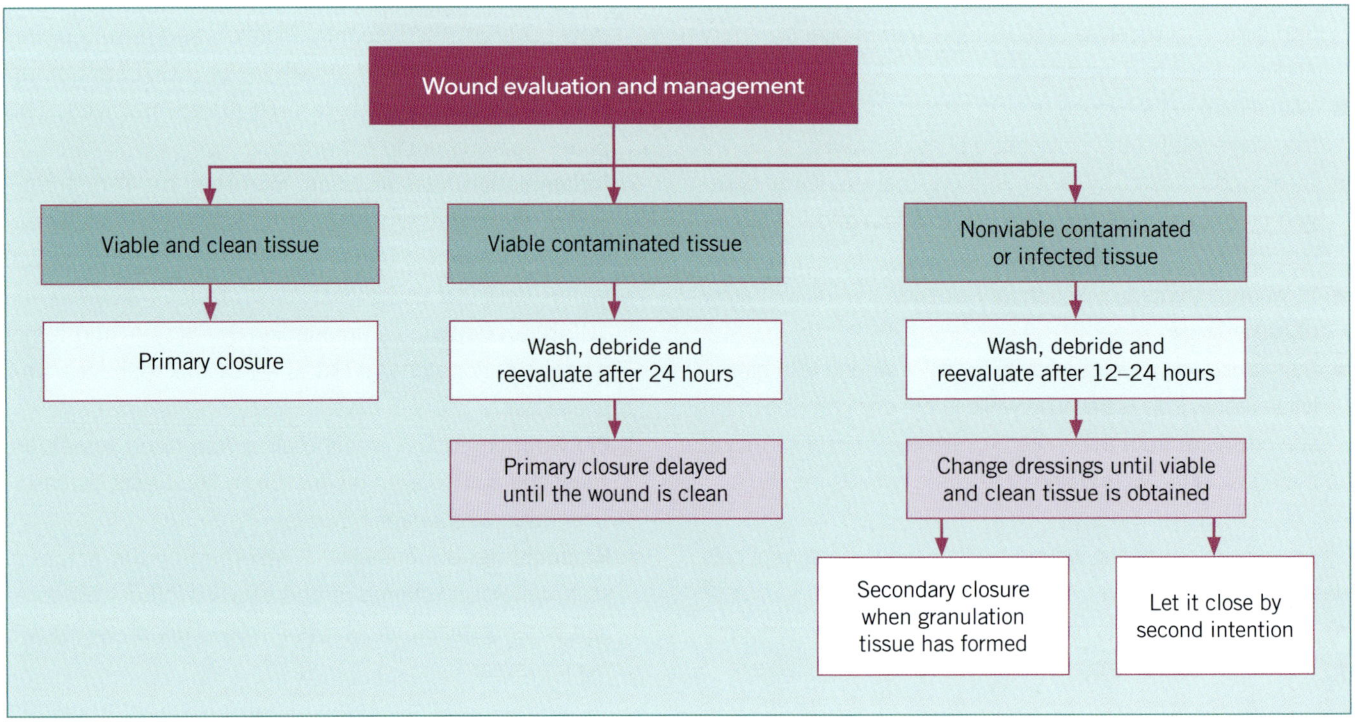

FIGURE 1. Protocol for evaluating and managing wounds.

Sometimes healing becomes chronic or scarring is abnormal or pathological. Concomitance with diseases that can affect the immune system's response capacity, such as diabetes mellitus, liver or kidney problems, neoplasms and neurological problems, or diseases such as feline immunodeficiency or viral leukemia can hinder healing. In these cases it is advisable to proceed with primary wound closure.

Initial treatment of the wounded cat

Assessing the patient's clinical status is crucial in extensive wounds and especially in traumatic wounds, as the cat may be suffering from shock. Before addressing the wound (except in case of heavy bleeding, which must be stopped as soon as possible), we should correct any abnormalities that may be present:

- **Hypothermia:** by means of appropriately positioned heaters in large cages, blankets that accumulate heat, warm saline solution (fluid heater), etc. It is important not to raise the patient's temperature too quickly (recommended: 34°F or 1°C per hour).
- **Hypovolemia:** the necessary fluid therapy must be administered to restore volemia.
- **Dyspnea:** during the stabilization period, even when it is unknown whether it is due to stress/pain or chest injury, an oxygen-supplemented environment must be provided.
- **Pain:** it is very important in all cases to establish an appropriate analgesic treatment to improve the patient's condition and to prevent excessive stimulation of the pain pathway neurons (known as the wind-up phenomenon) prior to the start of treatment.

Initial care

Open wounds should be considered contaminated, whether by endogenous, environmental or nosocomial (from the hospital environment) bacteria, so we should treat them as such and always handle them using gloves, while employing procedures that prevent cross-contamination.

While we stabilize the patient, we can cover wounds with a soft waterproof bandage, which can be left on for 1 or 2 hours.

Definitive wound treatment

To apply the appropriate treatment, it is necessary to:

- Establish what type of wound the patient has (Table 1).
- Record its initial extent.
- Evaluate the quality of the vascular supply. In this case, the gold standard would be an angiography, but this is not recommended because it is a procedure that may require lengthy anesthesia and the use of contrast agents, which is contraindicated in patients with vascular compromise. Conversely, Doppler ultrasound or color Doppler can be used with relative ease to look for the arterial beat.

Daily care

Initially, the wound should be washed with warm saline or even with water if it is very dirty, the hair at the edges of the wound should be cut with scissors and then shaved around a wide enough area to allow us to clean and disinfect properly and assess the viability of the tissue.

Washing must be performed correctly, otherwise it can damage tissue, delay healing and increase the risk of infection. The key is:

- Pressure: to maximize the removal of debris and bacteria while minimizing tissue damage, the pressure should be 48–55 kN/m^2 (kilonewtons/square meter). This means that it is not correct to irrigate with a syringe, spray with an aerosol or put the wound under the tap.
- Volume: the more volume, the better. We can start with a crude wash with tap water, but later we should use a washing solution.
- Composition of the washing solution: we should use solutions prepared for washing, not products with the same active ingredients but intended for presurgical cleaning of the skin, as the detergents they usually contain damage the subcutaneous tissue.

As for **antiseptics**, these are the most common:

- **Povidone-iodine:** antimicrobial effect, eliminates bacteria, viruses, fungi and protozoa. It is inactivated in the presence of organic matter. It is cytotoxic at all concentrations. It has a residual effect of 3 hours (the appropriate dilution is 1%, i.e., 100 ml at 10% in 900 ml of diluent).
- **Chlorhexidine:** is also broad-spectrum, has a residual effect of approximately 6 hours and is active even in the presence of organic matter. It is cytotoxic at commercial concentrations (the appropriate dilution is 0.05%, which would be 25 ml of 2% chlorhexidine in 975 ml of diluent).
- **Hypochlorous acid:** bactericidal effect; does not appear to be cytotoxic at concentrations of 0.02%. It is considered, compared to the two previous antiseptics, to be better tolerated in conscious feline patients due to its odor.

TABLE 1. Wound types and etiologies		
Type	**Etiology**	**Characteristics and observations**
Traumatic wounds	Cut	In addition to lost skin, there is also a loss of underlying tissue. They usually present extremely contaminated.
	Avulsion	There is little loss of underlying tissue, but an initially invisible loss of vascularization may cause us to underestimate the extent.
	Gash/tear (degloving)	The loss of the entire skin circumference of an area of a limb or the tail. These are really problematic wounds because they occur in areas where skin is normally already lacking and strangulation may occur due to fibrous stenosis. Nevertheless, they should be allowed to heal by secondary intention. If circulatory problems appear, plasties or grafts will be necessary.
	Laceration	They cause little involvement, usually only the skin and underlying tissue are affected.
	Puncture wound	In cats these are usually bite wounds and are always very infected. We must observe whether they penetrate a cavity, since the case may become very complicated if combined with pyothorax or peritonitis.
	Projectile	Besides the wound in the skin, the damage caused to the internal organs is more related to the power and distance reached by the projectile.
	Abrasion	Abrasions are superficial and heal well, but if they are extensive they produce significant fluid loss.
	Crushing	Crush injuries can be difficult to assess at first, as the visible damage to the skin will be minor, but the underlying organs and especially the musculature can be severely damaged.
Skin loss	Thermal or chemical burns	Burns from electric mats during surgery or from the extravasation of intravenous medications. In this case it can take days (on average: 1 week–10 days) to see the extent of the problem.
	Detachment due to vasculitis or necrosis	Produced by immune-mediated vasculitis, drug reactions, extensive/poisonous stings, vasculitis secondary to coagulopathies, hypotension or pyrexia, or necrosis secondary to thromboembolism. In all these cases, the focus is on the treatment of the primary cause and on complications that appear in other organs and systems.
	Chronic wounds	Chronic wounds occur because the cat does not stop licking the affected area, because the wound becomes infected, because of its location or because some comorbidity hinders the healing process.
	Fistulas secondary to foreign bodies	These are uncommon in cats but occur more often in young cats or in cats with access to the outdoors. Fistulous tracts may be caused by plant material, bone sequestrations or contaminated implants. Fistulas may also be observed due to bites in the perineal area leading to perforation of the rectum.
Injuries due to physical causes	Pressure ulcers	Feline patients are usually not heavy enough for these wounds to occur, but, in rare cases of hyperadrenocorticism, thinning of the skin and loss of regenerative capacity can result in their appearance on the extremities.
	Cold or heat (sunburn)	Cats are usually well protected from temperature, but if in extreme weather they are unable to shelter properly, they may lose distal areas of their limbs and the tips of their pinnae. House cats can also suffer burns from stepping on a hot glass-ceramic cooktop or accidentally touching boiling water in the kitchen; in these cases the pads are affected.

TABLE 1. Wound types and etiologies		
Type	**Etiology**	**Characteristics and observations**
Iatrogenic wounds	Surgical wound dehiscence	The causes are varied; too much tension, poor technique, infection, poor circulation to the wound edges or self-injury.
	By tourniquets	Usually from applying too much pressure to a bandage on the extremities, which can cause necrosis.
	Esophagostomy tube stoma infection	Due to poor management of the stoma. Cleaning every 48 hours with chlorhexidine and checking for inflammation or redness is recommended. Occasionally, the primary disease that led to the need for this tube to be placed is the complicating factor that facilitates infection despite all care.
	Intravenous catheter infection/ phlebitis	This is an ongoing problem, but now more important because of the increased number of multidrug-resistant bacteria we are facing. Catheter placement should be done aseptically and should be checked periodically in hospitalized animals.

Enzymatic ointments are extremely helpful in initial wound care. These contain proteolytic enzymes whose purpose is enzymatic debridement, a chemical process selective for necrotic material. The topical application of these enzymes allows them to act on the necrotic area, destroying it without damaging healthy tissue. In other words, these exogenous enzymes eliminate eschar or slough (inflammatory and necrotic tissue debris), thus promoting wound cleansing.

> Enzymatic ointment is administered daily without the simultaneous use of other products and the residue from the previous day is removed before the next dressing is applied, and so on until viable tissue is obtained.

Initially, treatment will be daily, then spaced out over time depending on the evolution of the healing process and the degree of contamination present (Figs. 2–6).

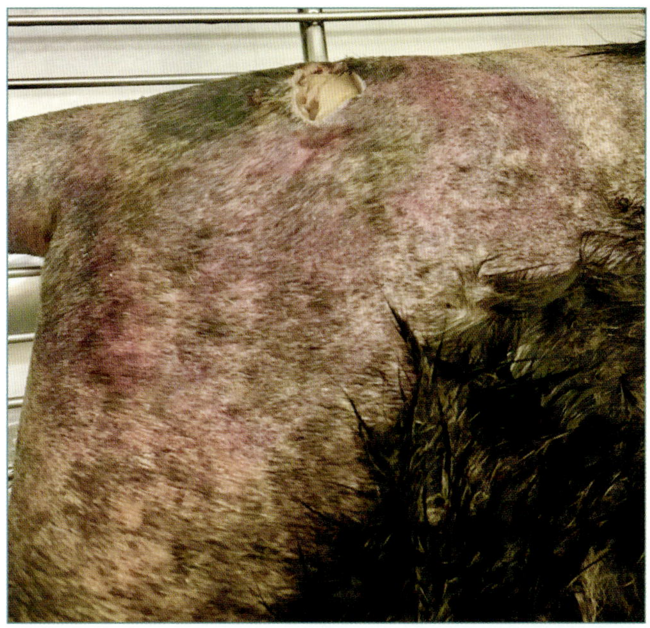

FIGURE 2. Cat that had been missing for 72 hours showing a deep bite wound. The bluish discoloration that defines the extent of the affected skin can be seen around the wound orifice.

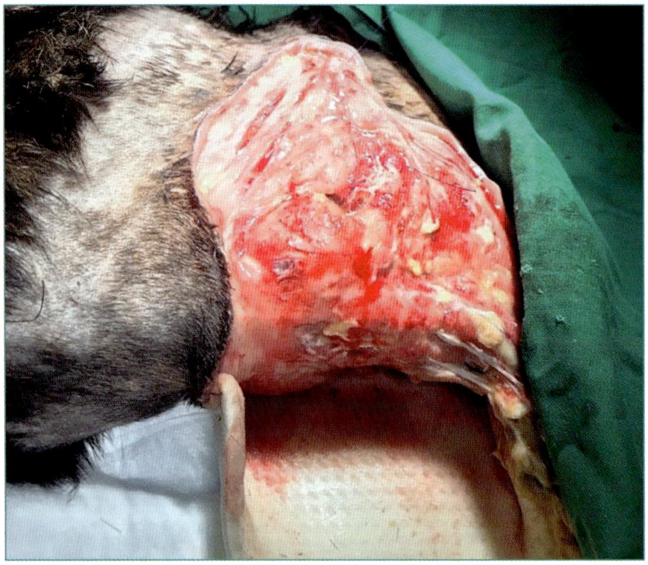

FIGURE 3. Patient from the previous figure after initial care. Nonviable skin and subcutaneous tissue has been removed and a highly absorbable polyurethane foam has been applied to promote granulation tissue formation.

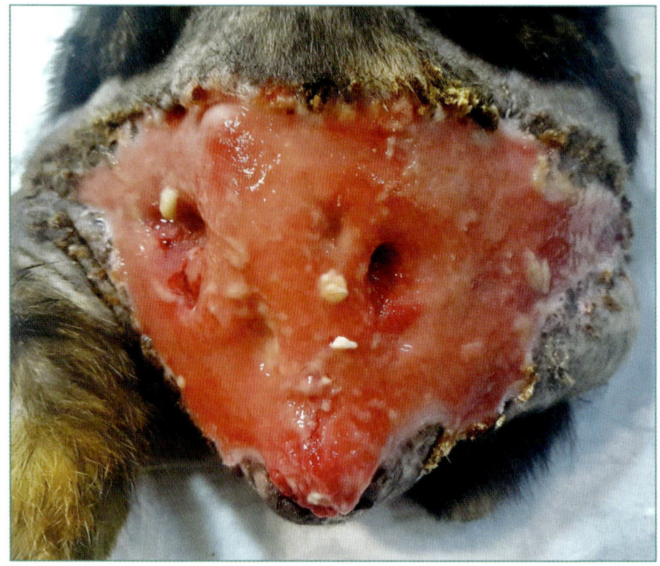

FIGURE 4. Wound appearance after one month of wound care and tail amputation.

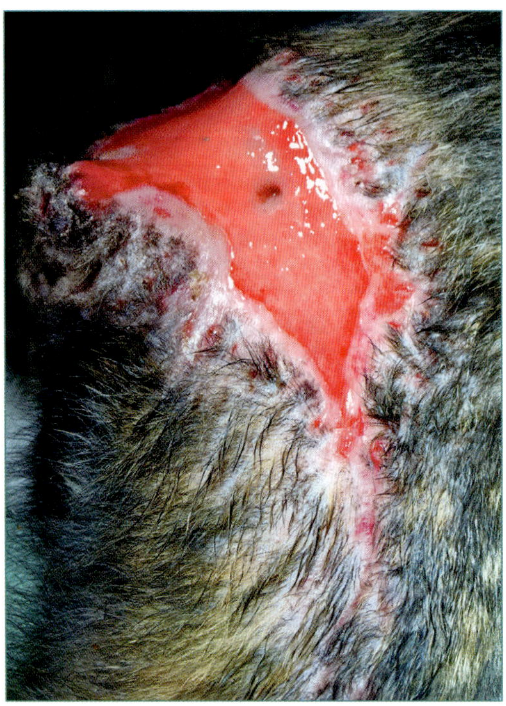

FIGURE 5. Scar formation and retraction of the patient's wound.

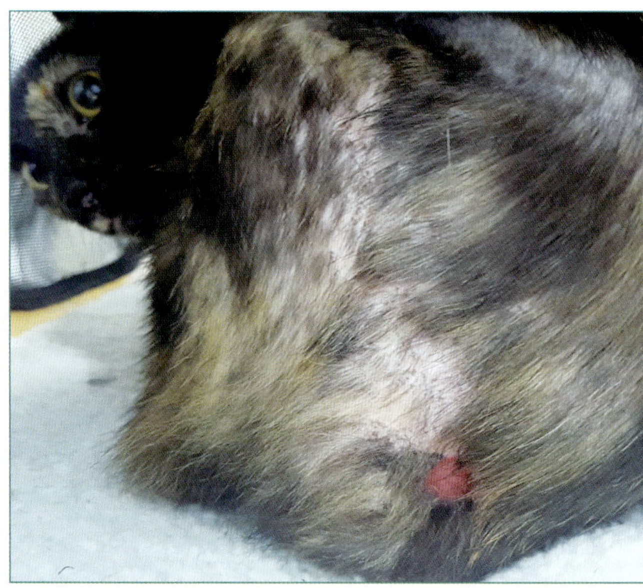

FIGURE 6. Patient 5 months after starting treatment, almost completely recovered. The first month and a half was spent in the hospital, after which dressings were changed first weekly, then every 2 weeks and then the rest of the time at home.

Supplementary care

It is extremely important to ensure that the patient receives an adequate caloric intake and to add food supplements when necessary. Esophagostomy tubes, as already mentioned, are a great ally. Weight loss should be monitored. For this purpose, all cats should be weighed daily and their water and calorie intake should be calculated, in addition to assessing their losses through urine and stool, as well as through the wound itself.

Bandages

Cats, admittedly, tolerate bandages poorly, but in the experience of the authors, with good pain management and close monitoring of the patient, it is possible to treat these wounds, making our patient relatively comfortable. As mentioned at the beginning of the chapter, bandage changes are also very stressful for cats and should be performed under conditions involving minimal stress for the patient and staff, thus sedation should typically be used.

In order to follow a wound management protocol, the Wound Bed Advisory Board (international advisory board on wound bed preparation) has designed a mnemonic rule to control the evolution between dressing changes with the acronym TIME.

Initial bandage layer

Almost all the products on the market come from human medicine and there is no single choice among the many options available, which makes it difficult to establish recommendations for some products over others. The indications in Table 2 can be followed.

Mnemonic rule TIME proposed by the Wound Bed Advisory Board

- **T** for **tissue**: referring to its condition, since necrotic tissue must be removed, dry tissue must be moistened or rehydrated and avascular tissue must be revascularized or trimmed.
- **I** for **inflammation and infection**: should be treated correctly.
- **M** for **moisture**, referring to the tissue moisture level: just the right amount is needed, wounds with dehydrated tissue will require dressings that provide water such as those incorporating gels or hydrocolloids, while very suppurative wounds will need absorbent products that prevent the "inflammatory broth" from remaining on the wound for too long and also prevent the wound from macerating.
- **E** for **epithelialization**: leading to wound healing. Bandages should protect this fragile new tissue from abrasion or desiccation.

TABLE 2. Products most commonly used in the initial layer of the dressing

Product	Exudate level	Properties	Indications	Contraindications
Calcium alginate	High	Looks like felt and when it absorbs liquid from the wound it turns into a gel.	Hemostatic. Stimulates granulation. Good for autolytic debridement of contaminated wounds.	Insufficient exudate can dehydrate the wound.
Polyurethane foam	Moderate–high	Soft foam.	Versatile, since it can be used dry for oozing wounds and moistened for dry wounds. Stimulates granulation and epithelialization.	Too soft to protect bony protrusions.
Hydrocolloids	Moderate–low	Supplied in sheet, paste or powder form, they have an occlusive backing and an adhesive perimeter. They also turn to gel on contact with wound fluids.	Good for autolytic debridement in wounds with moderate suppuration.	Adhesive edges may delay wound contraction and the fact that there is an occlusive layer may favor the proliferation of anaerobic bacteria in infected wounds.
Hydrogels	Low	Composed of 90%–95% water, they require the application of an occlusive layer on top.	Add moisture to dry wounds and can improve contraction in wounds affecting the extremities.	Can inhibit contraction in trunk wounds.

Depending on the effect sought with this initial bandage layer, these products include:

- **Debridement:** at the beginning of treatment, adequate debridement should always be performed to eliminate foreign material and purulent exudates. It is most effective in infected wounds. The enzymatic ointments mentioned above are supplemented by other options. The most commonly used in the past is gauze moistened with Ringer's lactate/Hartmann's solution to create a wet-to-dry dressing, but it is painful to change, can damage the forming granulation tissue and must be redone within 12–24 hours. The best current option is hydrogels that rehydrate the necrotic material and trap these products of the autolytic process by separating them from the underlying layer.
- **Drying dressings:** not widely used in cats in which desiccation is the most frequent problem and whose wounds produce little fluid. Absorbent human medicine dressings with a semipermeable membrane allow water vapor to be present on the wound surface, which creates a better environment for healing (Figs. 7–9).
- **Moisture-retaining dressings:** their dual behavior, providing hydration through hydrocolloids or hydrogels while absorbing the fluid produced by the wound, keeps inflammatory mediators away from the surface and allows exudates to move only in one direction (outward), keeping the wound clean and hydrated.

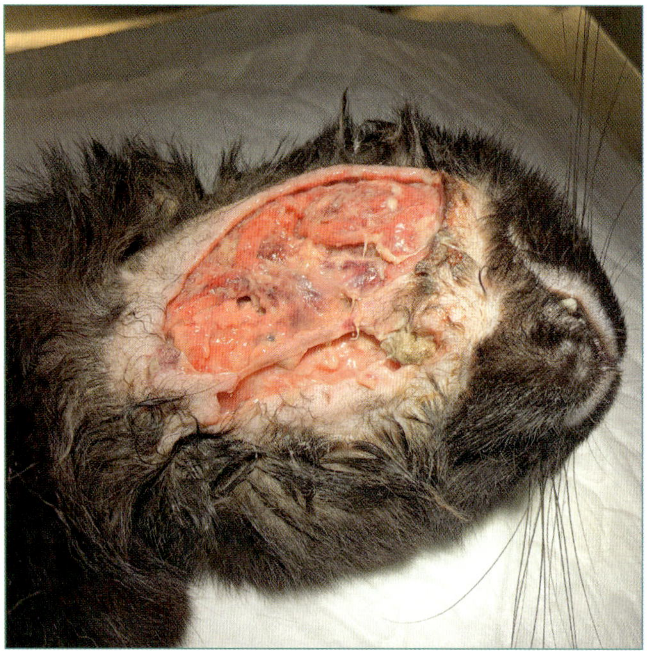

FIGURE 7. Feline patient with a wound on the skin of the mandible and neck after the debridement phase.

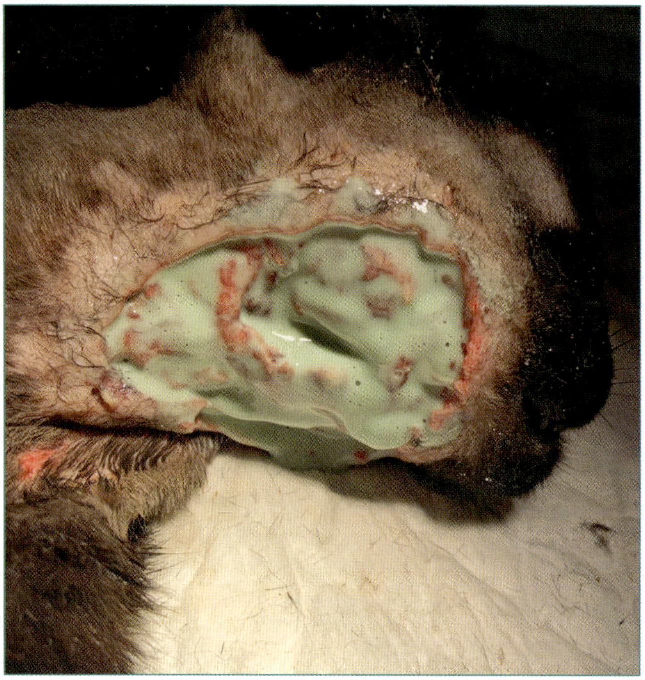

FIGURE 8. Application of a healing product on the wound.

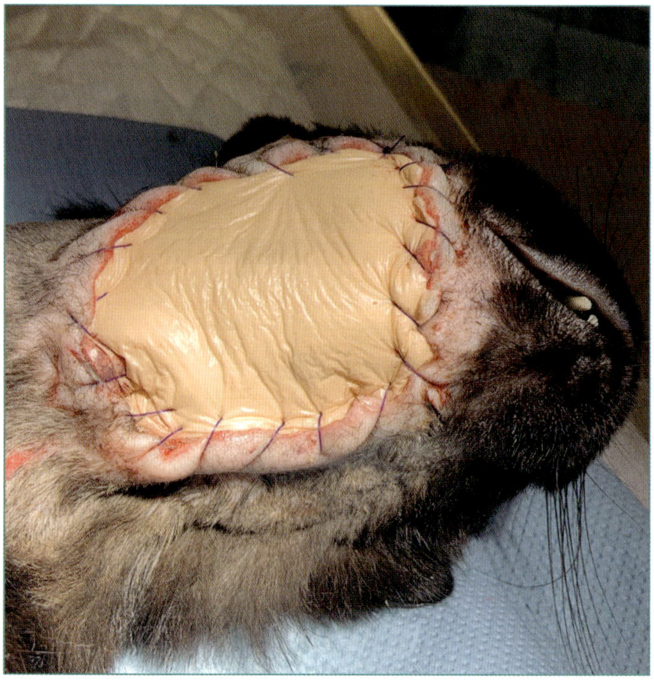

FIGURE 9. Placement of an absorbent bandage to stimulate and improve healing.

There are numerous products on the market that can be used, but there are no extensive veterinary studies available, so their use is not supported by scientific evidence, but rather by a number of published cases and personal experience. These are some of them:

- **Honey:** has an osmotic effect that reduces the capacity for bacterial growth, and it also contains antibacterial and anti-inflammatory substances. Medical-grade honey should always be used.
- **Microcrystalline silver:** is eliminated slowly on the wound (unlike the sulfadiazine silver ointment widely used in the treatment of wounds, especially burns). It has bactericidal effects and allows the time between dressing changes to be extended. Unfortunately, cases of drug-resistant bacteria have already been described and in cats an accumulation in serum and distant organs has been reported, resulting in toxicity.
- **Negative pressure:** eliminates suppuration and accelerates the formation of granulation tissue, although it delays contraction and epithelialization. Closed active drains also obliterate dead space and decrease the risk of infection.
- **Photobiomodulation:** also inherited from human medicine. It consists of an LED lamp and a chromophore gel that fights bacterial infection, improves tissue oxygenation and promotes vascularization and healing.
- **Ozone:** among the beneficial effects of ozone, noteworthy are its powerful antimicrobial activity and the increased tissue oxygenation that accelerates healing.

Subsequent layers of the bandage

The chosen dressings or adjuvant treatments are covered with a layer of gauze bandage, followed by a thicker absorbent layer of gauze or wadding and, finally, with an outer supporting layer, for which a cohesive bandage may be used, although it tends to exert excessive pressure. The authors use hypoallergenic non-woven tape with synthetic rubber adhesive, which is very soft and adaptable, elastic and has high air and vapor permeability. Or wide silk adhesive tape.

When the patient's wound is ready, we can consider closure by plasty. On other occasions, repeating these steps, we will have to wait for the wound to finally heal.

Bibliography

Bohling MW, Henderson RA, Swaim SF et al. Cutaneous wound healing in the cat: a macroscopic description and comparison with cutaneous wound healing in the dog. *Vet Surg*, 2004; 33(6):579–587.

Crisi PE, De Santis F, Aste G et al. Inflammatory, mechanical and infectious complications associated with peripheral intravenous catheters in dogs and cats: a risk factor analysis. *Vet Sci*, 2022; 9(3):118.

Davidson JR. Current concepts in wound management and wound healing products. *Vet Clin North Am Small Anim Pract*, 2015; 45(3):537–564.

Lascelles BD, Davison L, Dunning M et al. Use of omental pedicle grafts in the management of non-healing axillary wounds in 10 cats. *J Small Anim Pract*, 1998; 39(10):475–480.

Orlandin JR, Machado LC, Ambrósio CE, Travagli V. Ozone and its derivatives in veterinary medicine: A careful appraisal. *Vet Anim Sci*, 2021; 13:100191.

Scapagnini G, Marchegiani A, Rossi G et al. Management of all three phases of wound healing through the induction of fluorescence biomodulation using fluorescence light energy. Photonic Diagnosis and Treatment of Infections and Inflammatory Diseases II. Vol. 10863. International Society for Optics and Photonics, 2019.

Schultz SG, Sibbald RG, Falanga V et al. Wound bed preparation: systematic approach to wound management. *Wound Repair Regen*, 2003; 11 Suppl 1:S1–S28.

Wang XQ, Kempf M, Mott J et al. Silver absorption on burns after the application of Acticoat: data from pediatric patients and a porcine burn model. *J Burn Care Res*, 2009; 30(2):341–348.

2

SKIN SURGERY

MOST COMMON FLAPS AND PLASTIES IN FELINE SURGERY

9

Alberto Barneto

In recent years, skin reconstruction techniques have been developed for wounds with extensive tissue loss or those resulting from oncological surgeries. In feline medicine there are several common techniques, some of them specifically for this species. We will cover them in this chapter.

Surgical anatomy

The skin is the largest organ of the body. In the cat it is very loose, which contributes to a better wound healing capacity. Its layered anatomical structure is distributed as follows (Fig. 1):

- **Epidermis (external):** composed of stratified squamous epithelium. The cat's epidermis is thinner than that of dogs or humans.
- **Dermis (internal):** consists of dense connective tissue and is also thinner than in other species. In the cat, the dermis is loosely attached to the hypodermis.
- **Hypodermis:** innermost layer that supports the main vasculature. This vascular network is distributed parallel to the cutaneous surface and originates from arterial branches that supply the skeletal musculature.

Another significant difference in the feline species is their cutaneous vascularization. The major cutaneous vessels of the cat have a lower relative density than in other species, especially those in their trunk. However, the loose nature of the skin and the elasticity of the cutaneous vessels in this species allow their blood supply to be distributed very efficiently, resulting in efficient recovery and healing. The cutaneous vascular system is structured in three interconnected layers:

- **Subdermal plexus (deep):** is the primary blood supply to the skin. It is distributed from main vessels that irrigate very large cutaneous areas (**angiosome**). Together with fat and a layer of loose connective tissue, they constitute the **panniculus carnosus**.
- **Cutaneous plexus (middle):** fine secondary vessels that penetrate the dermis.
- **Subpapillary plexus (superficial):** tertiary vessels from the cutaneous plexus in the same dermal thickness.

Skin flaps

In wound repair surgery, the loss of skin and surrounding tissue surface area often forces us to use adjacent or distant portions

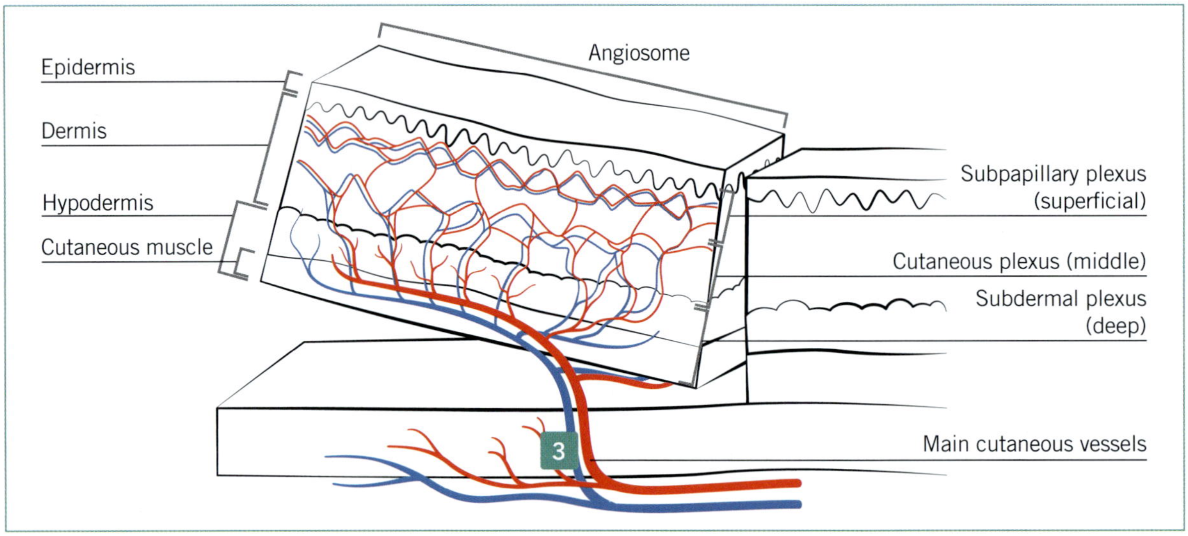

FIGURE 1. Structure and vascularization of the skin.

of skin tissue for adequate treatment. **Skin flaps** are areas of skin that maintain their vascular supply and can be moved from a donor area to aid in the healing of a wound or defect.

> The high elastic capacity of the cat's skin makes reconstructive techniques an important tool for treating complicated cases of skin defects.

Uses of skin flaps

- Covering defects with poor vascularization
- Improving circulation in an area
- Covering areas that are difficult to immobilize for proper healing
- Covering orifices over body cavities

According to their location in relation to the defect to be covered, these flaps are divided into:

1. **Local skin flaps (random):** due to the elasticity of the subdermal plexus. As they require a larger surface area to anchor to the skin that nourishes them, the amount of displacement achieved with them is less. Depending on the type of displacement, there are advancement, transposition and rotation flaps.
2. **Distant skin flaps:** the skin graft we use for repair is located far away from the wound. There are three types:
   - **Bipedicle distant flaps (pockets):** mainly used in major defects of distal parts of the extremities. The limb is flexed over the trunk where a full-thickness pocket flap is made and sutured over the limb and left for days or weeks until the flap integrates into the wound bed.
   - **Free skin flaps**: a full-thickness patch of skin is excised, used to prepare a covering that is loosely fitted to the defect and then sutured in place.
   - **Axial pattern flaps:** portions of pedicled skin with a wide surface area (angiosome) that preserve their direct cutaneous arteries and veins and are used to cover large defects at a certain distance.

For a skin flap to be successful there are a series of general principles that must be respected.

In the **donor area** we have to evaluate whether the skin is sufficiently elastic to cover the defect and to allow suturing with simple stitches and without tension on the wound area. Avoid donor areas with excess mobility (e.g., axillary and inguinal folds in the cat). Width and length are not important factors if the vascularity of the flap is well preserved (see below in flap types). Dissection of the flap bed must be done carefully, maintaining the full thickness of the hypodermis, and even the cutaneous muscle where it exists.

The graft **recipient bed** must be clean of dead tissue and infection. To achieve this, it is sometimes necessary to perform surgery beforehand to remove tumor tissue, necrotic tissue or tissue infected with a bacterial biofilm. Flap grafting can be performed in the same procedure as long as the donor tissue is well vascularized (e.g., random or distant axial pattern flaps). For free skin flaps, the recipient bed will need to be repaired days beforehand to obtain vascularized and healthy granulation tissue that accepts the implant.

Most common local skin flaps

Their general use is for the synthesis of small to moderate sized skin defects. To make these, a portion of elastic skin adjacent to the defect is needed. Healing occurs thanks to the blood supply from the subdermal plexus. In general, these are small flaps with moderate displacement (Fig. 2).

There are two types of **advancement flaps**:

- **Simple pedicled advancement flap:** after removing the defect, the skin is incised with two parallel lines the same distance apart as the length of the defect. The flap created will be approximately twice as wide as the defect. The flap bed is debrided, respecting the layers up to the hypodermis and the cutaneous muscle if present. The flap is advanced until the defect is covered, avoiding excessive tension. The initial sutures will be at the vertices of the graft, joining it to the corners of the defect. The preferred material is monofilament suture, in a simple interrupted pattern (Fig. 2a).
- **Bipedicled advancement flap:** this technique is identical to the previous one, except the defect is repaired with two simple pedicled advancement flaps facing each other and displaced one in front of the other (after suture, the final wound is H-shaped) (Fig. 2b). Another technique consists of preparing the area of the primary defect and dissecting the skin thickness down to the hypodermis on one side. At a distance somewhat greater than the thickness of the primary defect, an unloading incision is made on the dissected skin (secondary defect), so as to allow suturing of the initial defect without tension. Finally, the secondary defect is closed (Fig. 2c).

Rotation flaps can be rectangular or fan-shaped and cover defects by rotating on their base up to a maximum of 90°. Typically, one of the edges of the defect becomes one of the edges of the flap. The width of the defect is equal to the width of the flap. The more rotation, the more tension, and creases will form that need to be repaired. It is the technique most commonly used to close small skin defects (Figs. 3 and 4).

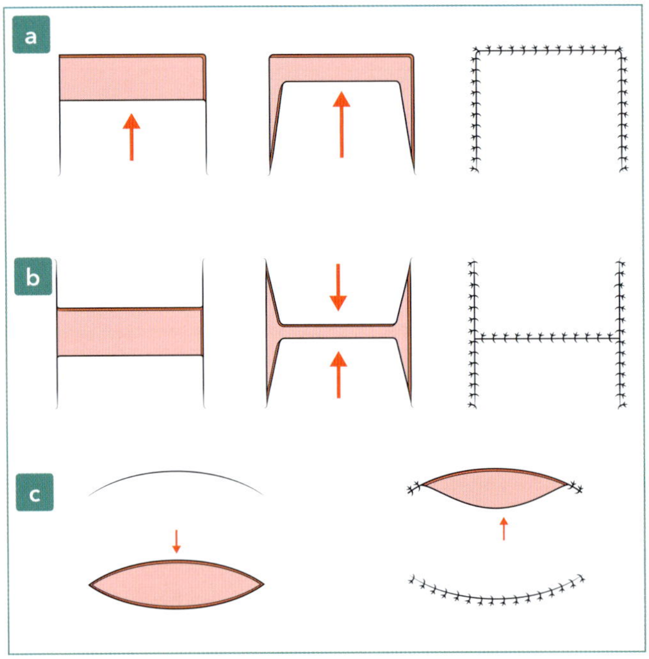

FIGURE 2. (a) Simple pedicled advancement flap. (b) Bipedicled H-shaped advancement flap. (c) Bipedicled advancement flap.

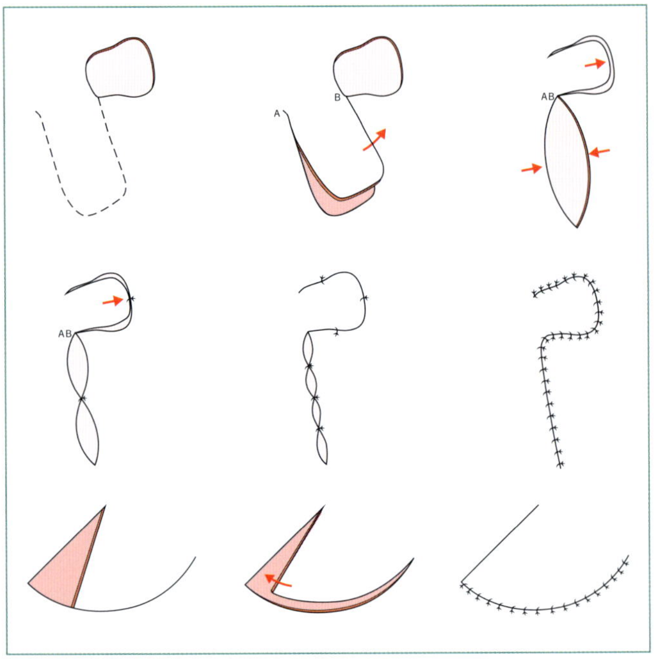

FIGURE 3. Rotation flaps.

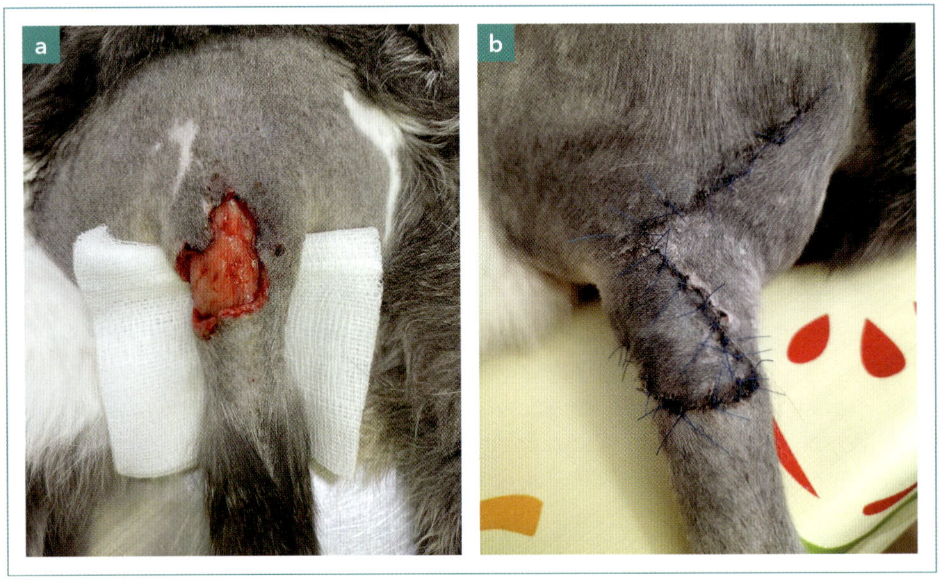

FIGURE 4. (a) Defect at the base of the tail of a cat after a bite that needed a rotation flap, as it was an area with little integument elasticity. (b) Appearance of the plasty after 14 days of healing.

Preoperative considerations

- Before selecting a repair technique, we should study the area to be treated. Regarding the wound type, if it is recent, it will be thoroughly cleaned and we will repair it immediately. If, on the other hand, the wound is an old and infected open wound, it will have to be treated beforehand to create a healthy bed that can accept the donor tissue.
- As part of this preparation, we will also study the characteristics and extent of the wound area and the possibility of using distant flaps, depending on the presence of major cutaneous vascular branches nearby. We will design the flap according to the size of the defect. It is helpful to use a template made of sterile paper and draw the defect (or even on the donor skin itself with a sterile marker pen).
- Avoid designing flaps with too small a surface area. If the base length is understood to be the measurement of the distance from the base of the flap to the defect, this should be increased by 10%–20% in size to avoid excessive tension during both suturing and subsequent healing.
- The flap must be handled very carefully during dissection and transfer so as not to damage its vascularization. If the surgery time is long and the defects are large, the tissues should be rehydrated with warm saline. A Penrose drain or an omental flap could also be added to the technique when possible (defects close to the trunk).
- Following extension of the flap and coverage of the defect, with rotation or displacement as appropriate in each case, we secure the flap to the bed with absorbable monofilament stitches. Once the flap is secured and dead spaces have been minimized, we will begin placing simple skin stitches with nylon thread, starting from the most distal ends and respecting the correct apposition and symmetry of the edges of the tissues.

Halsted's principles for the correct handling of tissues in surgery

At the end of the 19th century, William Stewart Halsted, cofounder of Johns Hopkins Hospital (Baltimore, USA), developed his basic principles for the correct handling of tissues in surgery. To this day, they remain the foundation for reconstructive surgery:

- Gentle tissue handling
- Meticulous hemostasis
- Preservation of blood supply
- Strict aseptic technique
- Minimal tissue tension
- Accurate tissue apposition
- Elimination of dead space

Elbow skin fold (axillary skin fold) reconstruction

The elbow fold is a skin structure typical of the feline species. It is composed of two opposing triangular layers of skin (lateral and medial) separated by loose connective tissue. Each triangular layer of the elbow has two anchor points:

- **Outer layer**: lateral attachment to the arm and dorsal attachment to the trunk (lateral thorax) (Fig. 5a).
- **Inner layer:** medial attachment to the arm and dorsal attachment to the trunk (ventral thorax) (Fig. 5b).

The ventrocaudal edges of each layer are joined together. The vascularization of the fold originates from the lateral thoracic artery.

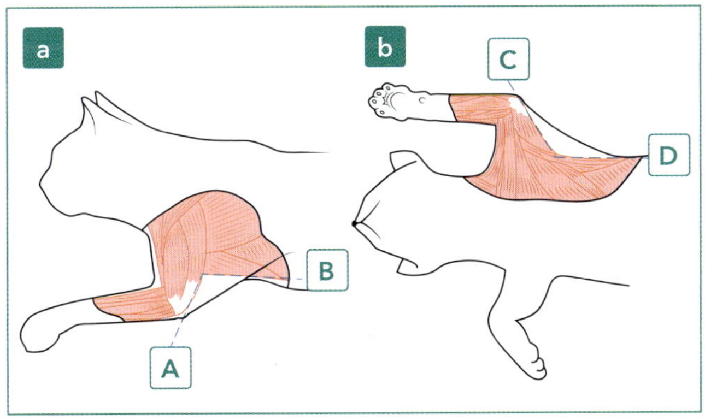

FIGURE 5. (a) Lateral and (b) medial elbow skin fold. In the outer layer, the lateral attachment is to the arm (A) and the dorsal attachment is to the trunk (B). In the inner layer, the medial attachment is to the arm (C) and the dorsal attachment is to the trunk (D).

The elbow fold has two key features:

- Extreme elasticity.
- No skin of the fold is attached to the arm. Rather the arm "floats" within the loose connective tissue.

> When a cat flexes its forelimb, the entire elbow and part of the arm move into the pocket formed by the two layers of the elbow skin fold.

The clinical presentation of axillary wounds in the cat involves a loss of the elbow skin fold due to chronic strangulation by the cat's collar, which traps and embraces the elbow producing a cut and necrosis. If the animal has been trapped for a long time, the elbow fold disappears and is replaced by granulation tissue. The granulation tissue itself does not heal because it is in a space that is too mobile, thus becoming a chronic wound, which means that the elbow does not have the anatomical pocket where it is protected.

Several unsuccessful techniques for debriding and suturing the wound bed of these wounds have been described. Some repairs with an axial pattern flap coupled with omental flap techniques have been successful. Here we will explain a technique for reconstructing the elbow skin fold that is simpler and more effective than those previously described (Fig. 6):

- **Patient positioning:** once the collar or rope strangling the elbow fold has been released, the area with necrotic tissue and hair is washed and debrided. Antibiotic therapy is started with amoxicillin–clavulanic acid. The animal is placed in lateral recumbency with the affected axilla facing upwards. The skin of the thorax, arm, forearm and neck is thoroughly shaved. The affected granulation tissue is covered with water-soluble gel while the entire area is disinfected with chlorhexidine and irrigated with pressurized Ringer's lactate solution to remove all residue. It is important to avoid any contamination of the surgical field. Once the area is thoroughly disinfected, the sterile surgical field is assembled in a square configuration with the unshaved part of the forearm and the rest of the extremity protected with a sterile bandage.
- **Approach:** the granulation tissue is resected, taking extreme care to remove all of it. The resulting defect will expose the caudomedial aspect of the arm, axilla and ventrolateral thorax. Wide blunt dissection of the entire edge of the skin of the wound is performed, in order to thoroughly free all the attachments of the underlying tissues (this dissection encompasses the skin of the arm and the ventrolateral skin of the thorax, including the hypodermis and the cutaneous muscle in this thickness).

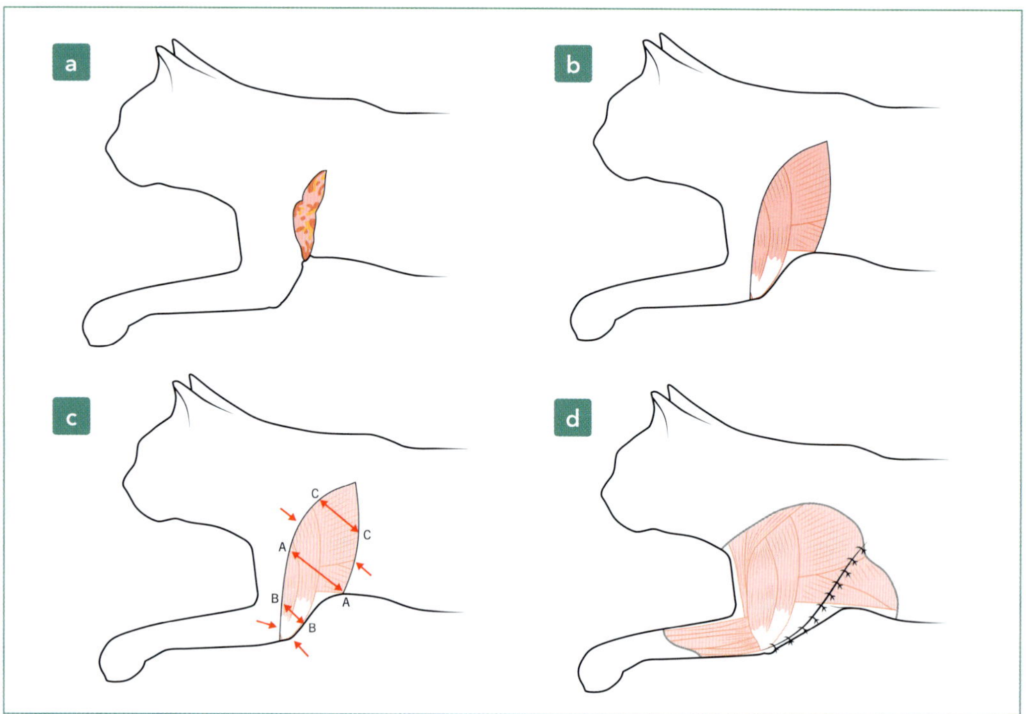

FIGURE 6. (a) Diagram of the resolution of a nonhealing wound with loss of the axillary fold. (b) After debriding the abnormal tissue, the defect will expose the caudomedial aspect of the arm, axilla and ventrolateral thorax. (c) Wound closure should begin from the skin of the arm adjacent to the elbow to its opposite symmetrical point on the skin of the lateral thorax. (d) This and subsequent subdermal stitches will create a wound line that reconstructs the new axillary fold. No stitches should be anchored to the wound bed to allow the elbow to flex properly within the skin pocket.

- **Reconstruction:** once the dissection of the adjacent skin allows us to redo the elbow fold, an initial subdermal suture stitch using 3-0 gauge polyglactin 910 is placed from the skin of the arm adjacent to the elbow to its symmetrical point on the skin of the lateral thorax. This and subsequent subdermal stitches will create a wound line that reconstructs the new axillary fold, which should allow the elbow to tuck in when flexing. During reconstruction we should never anchor stitches in the wound bed. To decrease the risk of seroma accumulation, we should place a Penrose drain in the axillary pocket once reconstructed. Interrupted skin stitches are used, with 3-0 nylon (Figs. 7–9).

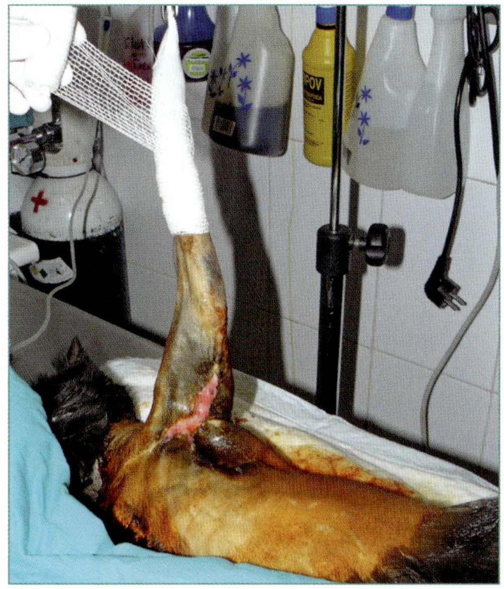

FIGURE 7. Typical axillary fold wound in a cat that got caught in its own collar prepared for surgery. Note the scar that has eliminated the elbow fold.

VIDEO

Testing the elasticity of the elbow fold in a cat that underwent an axillary fold plasty several years ago. Note how the elbow hides in the fold.

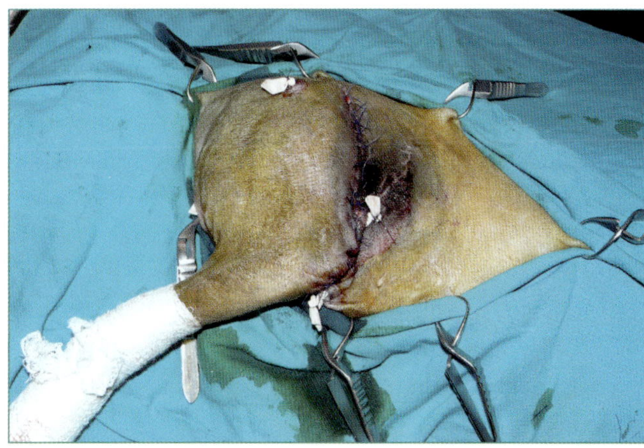

FIGURE 8. Reconstruction of the elbow fold after surgery. In this case, a Penrose drain was kept in place for 5 days to avoid seromas.

Distant flaps: axial pattern flaps

These flaps are pedunculated skin grafts whose only vascularization comes from a cutaneous artery and vein, whose branches supply blood to the subdermal plexus of the entire surface of the graft. This technique provides large and long surface areas of skin that we can transpose at a distance and with an excellent blood supply ideal for healing. Given the elasticity of cat skin, these types of flaps are very useful for covering very extensive defects in areas close to regions where major cutaneous vessels are located (Fig. 10). By grafting a different type of skin, the characteristics of the glands, as well as the color and length of hair, may be altered in the recipient area.

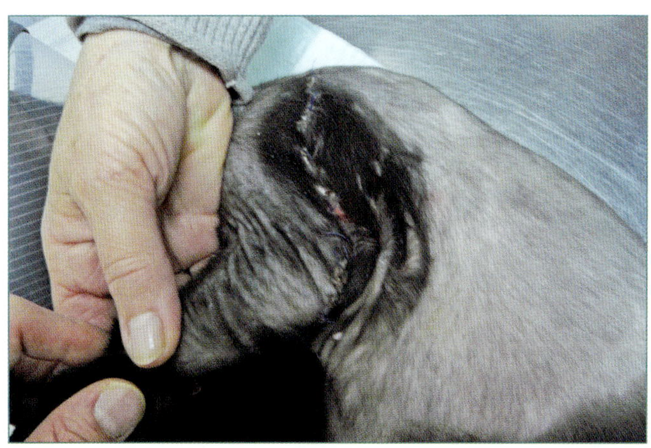

FIGURE 9. Follow-up on the elasticity of the new skin fold one week after surgery. The elbow should tuck under the new fold with ease when flexing the shoulder joint.

In feline medicine, the most commonly used axial pattern flaps are:

- Angularis oris axial pattern buccal flap
- Thoracodorsal axial pattern flap
- Caudal superficial epigastric axial pattern flap

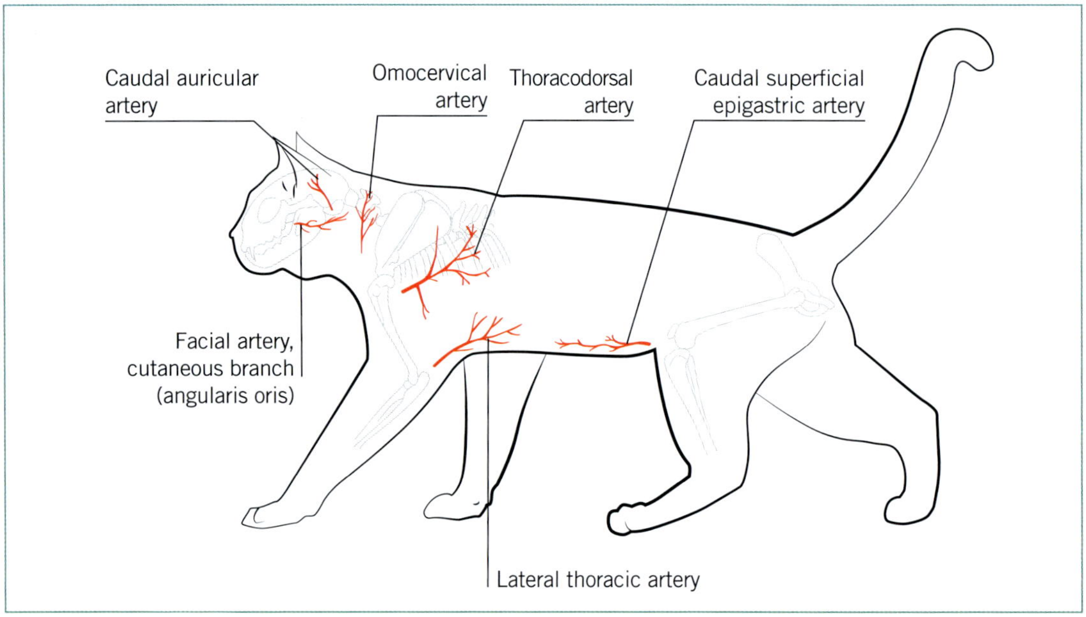

FIGURE 10. Distribution of cutaneous vessels used as the basis for axial pattern flaps in cats.

Angularis oris axial pattern buccal flap

Reconstructive or oncologic surgery on the face is usually limited by the lack of skin and very little elasticity. Closures by apposition or with subdermal advancement flaps are used when defects are small. When the size of the defect is larger, there is necrosis or dehiscence of the previous techniques or the wound is very rostral, axial pattern flaps are preferred.

Four axial pattern flaps have been described to repair major defects in a cat's head:

- **Caudal auricular flap:** from the caudal auricular artery, which originates at the base of the auricular cartilage, in its posterior aspect, distributed towards the skin of the neck in a caudal direction. It is a flap that can rotate up to 180° to cover defects in the temporomaxillary region.
- **Superficial temporal flap:** uses the blood supply from the superficial temporal artery, a superficial branch of the carotid artery that runs cranially from the posterior part of the zygomatic arch. Rotating 90° allows for the closure of defects in the temporal and maxillofacial region. It is more limited in its size than the previous one.
- **Omocervical flap:** in this case, the flap uses the blood supply from the cutaneous branch of the omocervical artery. It originates from the cervical artery, which starts near the shoulder joint and runs dorsally through the neck. The resulting angiosome allows for the treatment of defects on the neck and the caudal portion of the face and skull within a rotation of less than 90°. Its use in defects that are more cranial is limited.
- **Angularis oris flap:** although limited to rotations of between 90° and 180°, it is a very versatile flap that can reach almost any area of the face, skull and jaw in cats. Its blood supply comes from the angularis oris artery, a cutaneous branch of the facial artery, more cranially located than all the previous ones. It starts at the commissures of both lips and extends to the atlas. With this portion of tissue, defects of the nasal plane, face, skull, mandible and maxillary region can be repaired with shorter flap lengths.

Classically, in feline medicine, facial defects were repaired using the omocervical axial pattern flap or more specifically the caudal auricular flap. In recent years, the angularis oris axial pattern flap has been described with very promising results in the reconstruction of all skin defects of the face and neck in cats. Its use has been broadened to include the removal of facial tumors of all sizes, chronic infections with large skin defects, resections of the nasal plane, enucleation, otectomy or the total ablation of the ear canal. For defects in the temporomaxillary region, the most commonly used technique is currently the superficial temporal axial pattern flap, which, although showing good results in this region, allows for less distance displacement than the angularis oris flap. The latter also requires little surgical time.

- **Patient positioning:** in lateral recumbency, the entire lateral area of the head up to the middle of the neck should be thoroughly shaved. It is useful to place a soft towel roll under the neck.
- **Surgical field:** once the field has been shaved and disinfected, we will design the extension (width and length) of the flap according to the size and location of the defect to be treated. As a general rule, we will add 0.5 to 1 cm to each measurement we take of the defect to achieve a wider flap and avoid subsequent tension. The flap can even be drawn on the skin of the prepared field with a sterile surgical marker.
- **Technique**
  1. The dorsal edge of the flap should start at a point dorsal to the lip commissure, 1.5 cm away from it, in a direction coinciding with the ventral edge of the zygomatic arch and extending to the wing of the atlas. At a distance of 3 cm ventrally (and 1.5 cm from the commissure) the ventral edge of the flap starts out parallel (slightly divergent). Thus, the end of the flap will be approximately 1 cm wider than its base. Both lines will be of equal length, joined caudally with another vertical line. We can get an idea of the measurements of the flap using the following rule:
     - The distance from the dorsal origin of the flap to the **most cranial apex** of the defect will be the **length of the dorsal edge of the flap (+1 cm)**.
     - The distance from the ventral origin of the flap to the **most caudal apex** of the defect will be the **length of the ventral edge of the flap (+1 cm)**.
     - The **width of the dorsal edge of the defect (+1 cm)** will be the width of the caudal portion of the flap (Figs. 11–17).
  2. Careful dissection of the flap is performed in a caudal to rostral direction, including the panniculus muscle, taking care not to damage the jugular, maxillary and linguofacial veins or the vascular pedicle of the flap. The flap should be rotated as necessary to cover the defect. If the defect is remote and there is a portion of skin between the defect and the flap, we must make an incision in the skin to directly connect the rotated flap to the defect. The lips of the wound must be sutured to the flap.
  3. The suture should be performed in two planes; first a 4-0 or 5-0 absorbable subdermal suture (e.g., poliglecaprone), and afterwards the lips are sutured with 4-0 or 3-0 gauge non-absorbable interrupted stitches. The donor flap bed is then sutured using a simple appositional pattern. Drains may or may not be used, depending on the disease being treated.

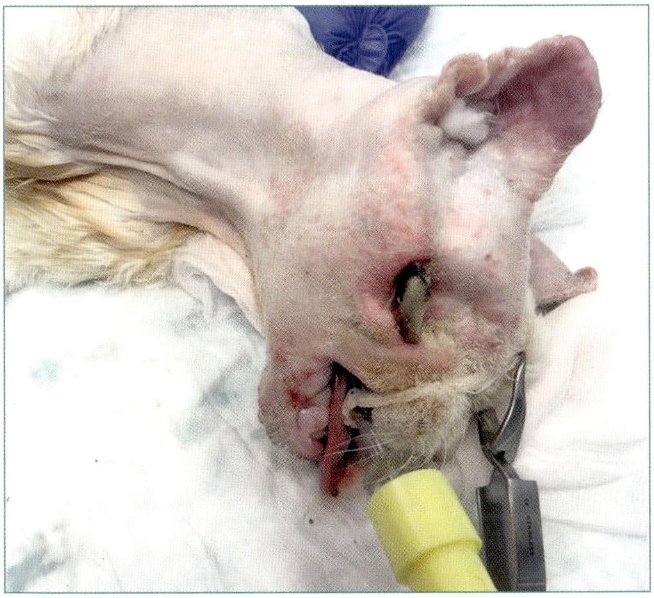

FIGURE 11. Patient with an old abscess affecting the orbit and exposing a portion of the zygomatic arch with osteomyelitis. Defect reconstruction was planned using an angularis oris axial pattern flap.

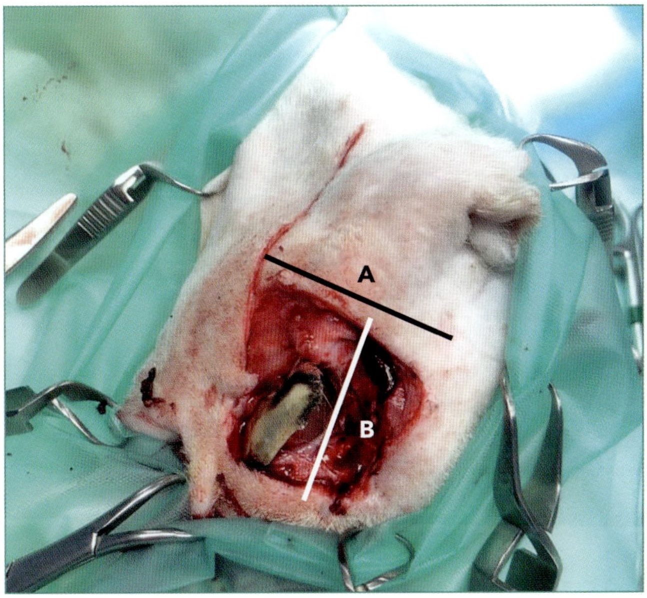

FIGURE 12. The entire orbital bed is prepared and debrided in order to delimit the defect and to be able to measure the size of the flap based on the width (A) and length of the defect (B).

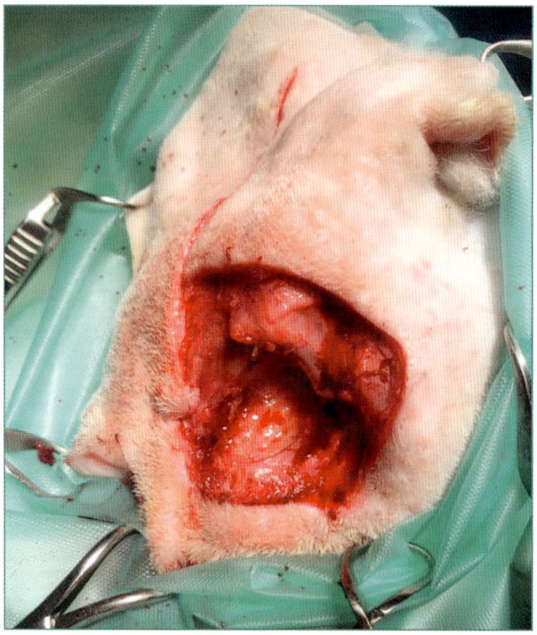

FIGURE 13. Appearance of the defect after removal of the necrotic zygomatic arch. Marking of the longitudinal line of the flap has begun.

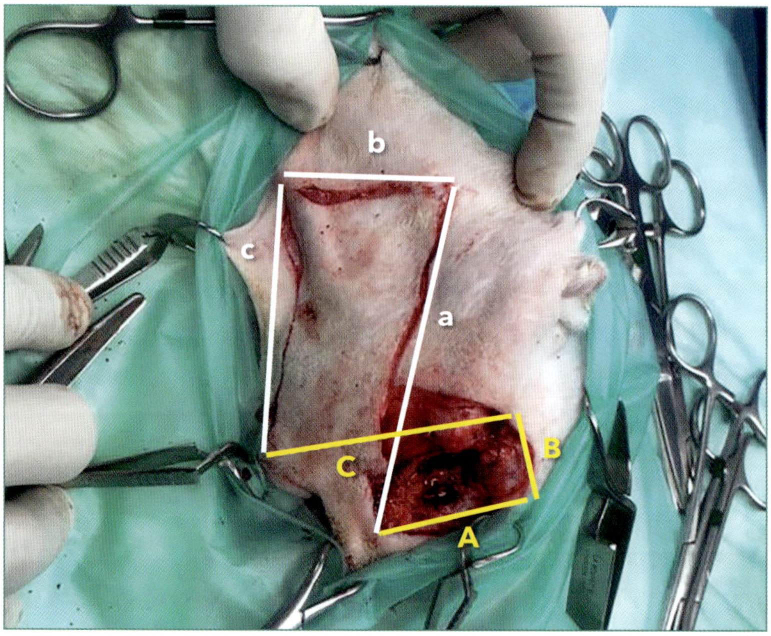

FIGURE 14. Flap marked along its entire length. The dorsal edge of the flap extends from the beginning of the defect to the end of the dorsal incision (length a) and should cover the distance between the starting point of the flap (start of a) to the dorsocranial apex of the defect (distance A). In this case, the length of the flap (a) is much longer than that of the defect (A), as the defect is very deep and the flap will lose length as it adapts to its bed. As for the ventral edge of the flap (length c), it will correspond to the caudal edge of the defect (distance C). In this case, the length of c will be approximately C + 1 cm. Finally, the width of the flap at its caudal end (length b) will be somewhat greater than the width of the defect (distance B; b = B + 1 cm).

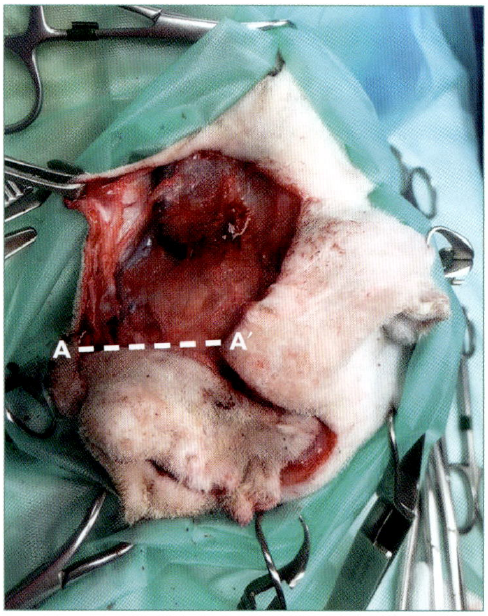

FIGURE 15. Once the thickness of the flap has been dissected to its full length, the flap is rotated over the defect and suturing is started. The first stitch is the most important to avoid creasing and puckering the skin: point A at the beginning of the flap is joined to point A′ at the apex of the defect (dotted line).

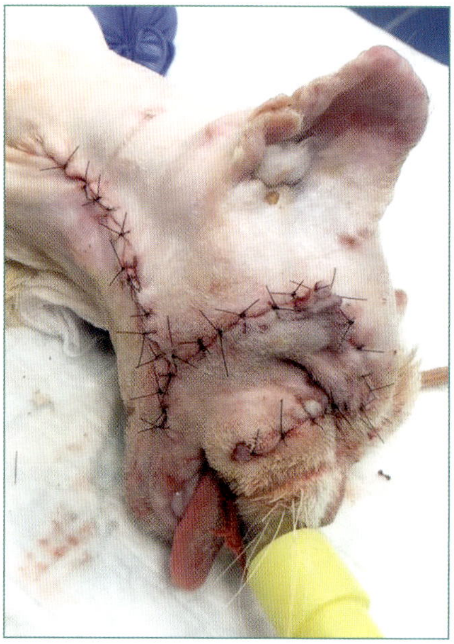

FIGURE 16. Final appearance. When the defect is deep, stitches should be placed between the inner layer of the flap and the wound bed.

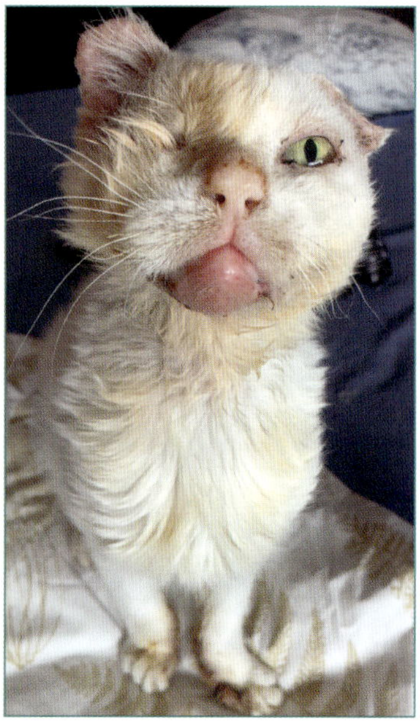

FIGURE 17. Check-up of the patient 3 months after surgery.

Thoracodorsal axial pattern flap

This flap technique is among the longest used in reconstructive surgery. It is used for reconstructions of surgical defects in the thorax, axilla, elbow, shoulder, arm or forearm (in its most dorsal portion). Even some carpal lesions in cats can be treated thanks to the elasticity of their skin.

A slightly more ventral alternative is the **lateral thoracic axial pattern flap**, associated with the lateral thoracic artery, just behind the elbow. Dissection of the flap is in a caudodorsal direction to the last ribs, which provides a pedicle long enough to cover defects of the entire forearm and even the carpus. In recent years, this technique has been complemented by the use of **omental flaps** to take advantage of the vascularization of this structure in the reconstruction of large defects with necrotic tissue and compromised irrigation near the trunk.

To perform this technique:

- **Patient positioning:** in lateral recumbency with the forelimb unrestrained, shave the entire neck, arm and scapula (beyond the midline of the thoracic spinal column), thorax and forelimb up to the carpus, depending on the location of the defect to be treated.
- **Surgical field:** the **cutaneous branch of the thoracodorsal artery** and its vein originate between the intermuscular fascia behind the caudal border of the shoulder joint, at the level of the acromion. From there it runs parallel to the caudal border of the scapula, at a distance of approximately 1–2 cm, and branches in a dorsocaudal direction approaching the dorsal thorax.
- **Technique**
  1. The cranial edge of the flap is parallel and slightly caudal to the spine of the scapula. Its origin is immediately caudoventral to the acromion. The caudal edge is parallel to the cranial edge in a dorsocaudal direction, starting halfway between the acromion and the caudal shoulder depression. The dorsal edge will join the cranial and caudal edges near the midline of the thoracic spine.
  2. We carefully dissect the skin starting from the dorsal edge of the flap, including the cutaneous muscle of the trunk until we reach the base of the flap. We will be extremely careful not to damage the thoracodorsal artery and vein, so we may leave some subcutaneous fatty tissue around them.
  3. Once dissected, the flap can be pivoted to bring it over the defect. As always, we will incise the island of skin remaining between the flap and the defect to give the flap continuity. This surgical wound will be integrated into the repair suture. The suture should be performed in two planes: subcutaneous with absorbable monofilament and cutaneous with nylon in a simple interrupted pattern.
  4. If an **omental flap** is included in the procedure, a mid-cranial laparotomy is performed prior to the aforementioned technique. The sheet of the greater omentum is removed starting from its connection to the greater curvature of the stomach and one-third of its width is dissected to increase the length of the pedicle. The omental flap is removed through the laparotomy opening and tunneled under the subcutaneous tissue through a saline-moistened Penrose drain to the axillary area where the thoracodorsal flap will be made. The omental pedicle is sutured over the defect before the thoracodorsal flap is applied (Figs. 18–22).

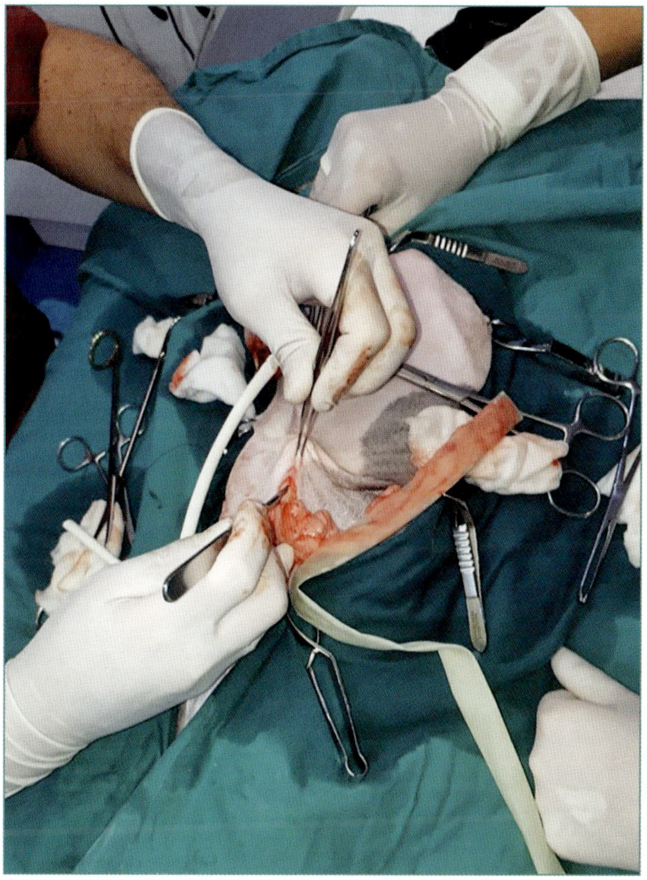

FIGURE 18. Start of a surgery using a thoracodorsal axial pattern flap with an omental flap to cover and resurface a severe elbow defect in a cat with osteomyelitis associated with bone implants. A portion of the greater omentum has been harvested by laparotomy and is prepared for tunneling through a Penrose drain. The cutaneous tunnel is made from the exit point of the omentum through the laparotomy to the axilla.

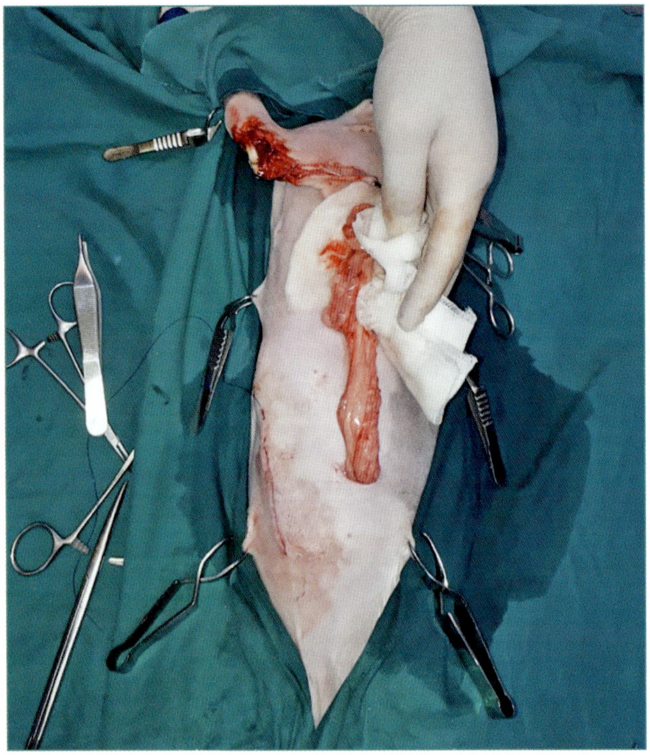

FIGURE 19. Exit of the omental flap through the axillary wound; it is ready to be applied over the defect.

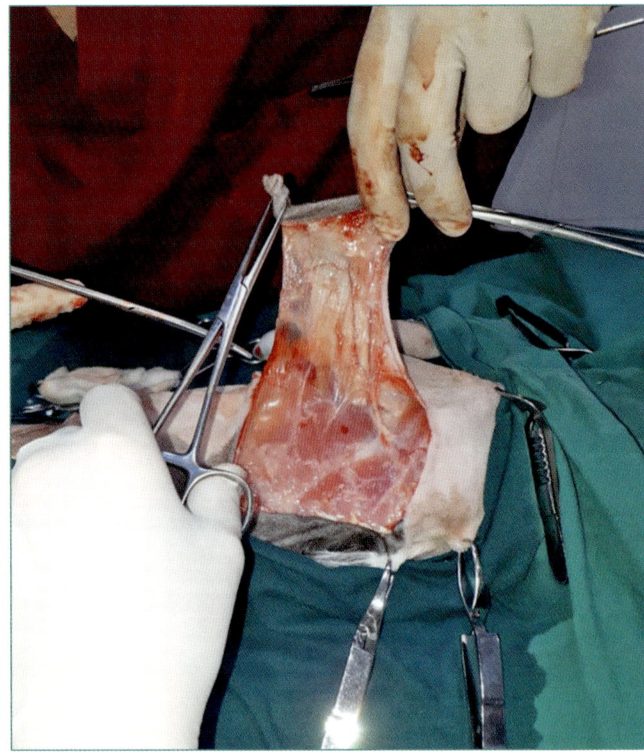

FIGURE 20. Dissection of the thoracodorsal flap with sufficient thickness and width to cover the defect. The thoracodorsal artery and vein are visible.

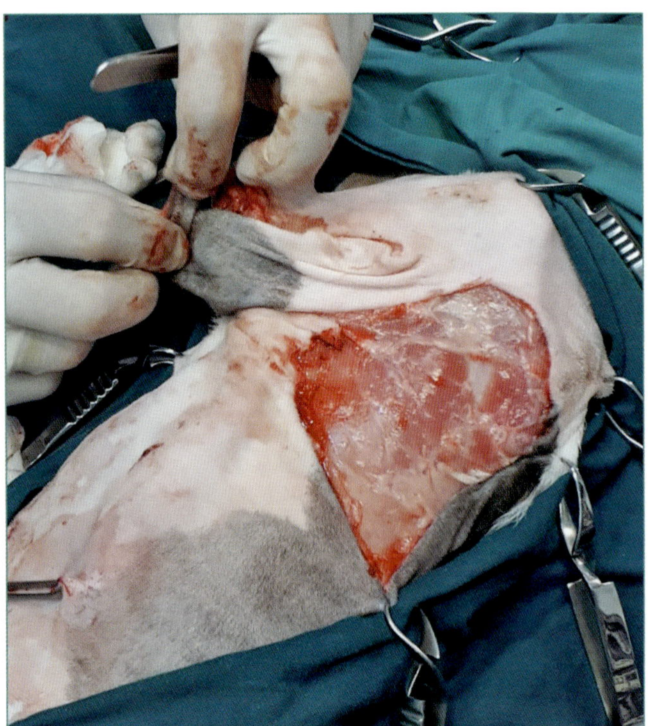

FIGURE 21. Rotation of the axial pattern flap over the defect to be covered. In this case, the omental flap layer will have already been sutured.

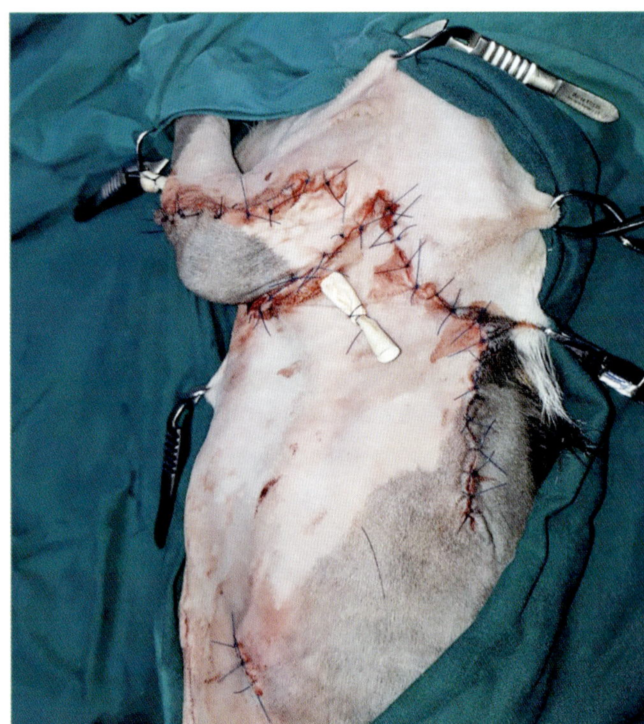

FIGURE 22. Appearance of the finished suture. In this case, a Penrose drain was kept in place for 7 days to eliminate any secretions that may occur during healing.

Caudal superficial epigastric axial pattern flap

This is the axial pattern flap most commonly used to correct large tissue defects in the ventrocaudal portion of the body in cats. A flap of considerable length with good vascularization is obtained, which can repair the abdomen, flanks, inguinal region (uni- or bilateral), perineum, thigh and hind limb, all the way to the tarsus:

- **Patient positioning:** in dorsal recumbency with the extremities extended and supported to achieve good fixation. If the defect is in a hind limb, that extremity will be left free. The entire abdomen should be shaved from the perineal area to both axillae to obtain the flap, and the flap recipient area should be prepared in the same manner.
- **Surgical field:** the **caudal superficial epigastric artery** is a branch of the external pudendal artery that passes through the inguinal ring and supplies the mammary tissue of the 2nd, 3rd and 4th glands in a cranial direction.
- **Technique**
  1. The beginning of the flap should be centered on the area of the inguinal ring. From this location, we will outline two parallel incisions on both sides of the nipples that can reach up to the 2nd mammary gland, depending on the length of the flap we need. The medial incision of the flap should coincide with the ventral midline of the abdomen (above the linea alba). The lateral incision should be parallel in a cranial direction and twice the distance from the abdominal midline to the nipple. The cranial edge of the flap will join both lines (Fig. 23.1).
  2. Once the surface of the flap has been outlined, dissection begins starting at the cranial edge. The flap should include mammary tissue and the full depth of the supramammary muscle, so that once the flap is dissected, only the clean surface of the fascia of the external abdominal oblique muscle will remain.
  3. We should handle the flap carefully and rotate it to place it over the defect, taking care not to excessively kink or stretch the vascular pedicle. If there is an island of skin between the flap and the defect, it is incised to include it in the suture of the plasty (Fig. 23.2). As always, a double layer of stitches is placed: absorbable monofilament for the subcutaneous tissue and nylon for the skin (Fig. 23.3).

Postoperative management and complications

Reconstructive surgery requires careful postoperative care, especially in feline medicine:

- The use of drains may be considered for the first 2–4 days after surgery if there is risk of seroma formation.
- Protective padded bandages can be used and should be changed every 48 hours following the first 3 days after surgery. They not only protect the wound but also help reduce the dead space between the tissues.
- An Elizabethan collar will protect the patient from self-injury.
- Antibiotic therapy may be administered based on antibiogram results. Cephalosporins are a good prophylactic option.
- The application of multimodal analgesia (opioids, NSAIDs, local anesthesia) is recommended.

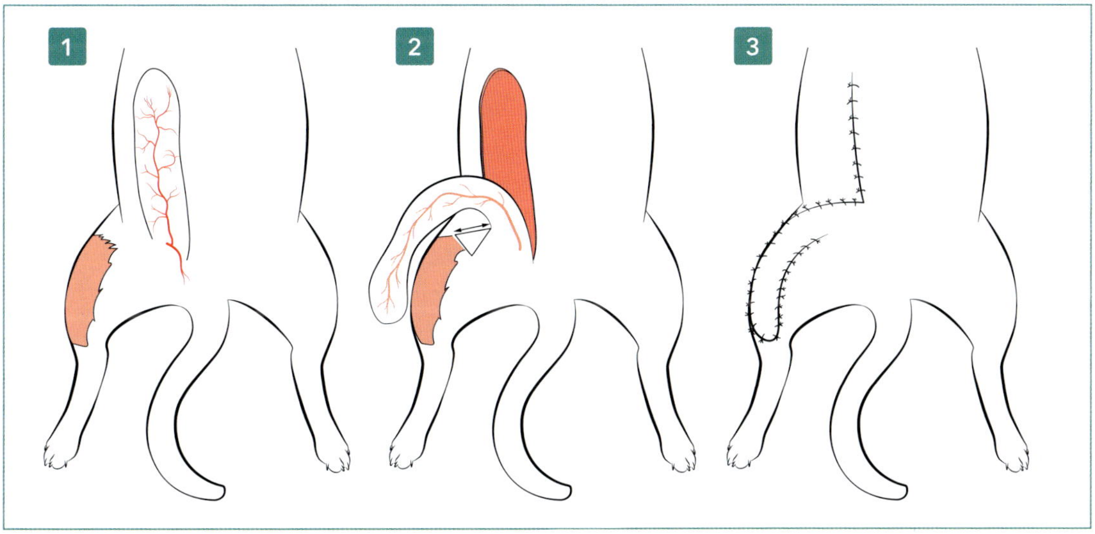

FIGURE 23. Caudal superficial epigastric axial pattern flap.
1. The flap, including the caudal superficial epigastric artery and vein, is harvested by means of two parallel incisions and their cranial junction.
2. Flap rotation and removal of the skin isthmus between the flap and the defect.
3. Double-layered (subcutaneous tissue and skin) suture of the flap.

The most common complications of reconstructive skin surgery are edema, suture dehiscence and infection. Edema is common in the first few days, especially if the flap has been rotated or displaced too much without sufficient size. Soft bandages may lessen this effect.

The causes of suture dehiscence can vary: too much tension on the flap, suture knotted too close to the edge, poor circulation in the donor tissue due to improper handling, uncontrolled infection or poor healing due to an underlying metabolic disease. Hydrocolloid bandage dressings and good antibiotic prophylaxis will help combat these complications. If the surgery is performed well, healing will be delayed, but it will usually occur correctly.

Bibliography

Albernaz VGP, Oblak ML, Quitzan JG. Angularis oris axial pattern flap as a reliable and versatile option for rostral facial reconstruction in cats. *Vet Surg*, 2021; 50(8):1688–1695.

Amsellem P. Complications of reconstructive surgery in companion animals. *Vet Clin North Am Small Anim Pract*, 2011; 41(5):995–1006.

Benzioni H, Shahar R, Yudelevich S et al. Lateral thoracic artery axial pattern flap in cats. *Vet Surg*, 2009; 38(1):112–116.

Bradford M, Degner DA, Bhandal J. Use of the angularis oris cutaneous flap for repair of a rostral mandibular skin defect in a cat. *Vet Comp Orthop Traumatol*, 2011; 24(4):303–306.

Brinkley CH. Successful closure of feline axillary wounds by reconstruction of the elbow skin fold. *J Small Anim Pract*, 2007; 48(2):111–115.

Bryant KJ, Moore K, McAnulty JF. Angularis oris axial pattern buccal flap for reconstruction of recurrent fistulae of the palate. *Vet Surg*, 2003; 32(2):113–119.

Buick SC, Haar GT. Reconstructive techniques of the facial area and head. In: Kirpensteijn J, Ter Haar G (eds.). *Reconstructive Surgery and Wound Management of the Dog and Cat.* London, UK: Manson, 2013; pp. 95–115.

Clarke BC, Findji L. Bilateral caudal superficial epigastric skin flap and perineal urethrostomy for wound reconstruction secondary to traumatic urethral rupture in a cat. *Vet Comp Orthop Traumatol*, 2011; 24(2):142–145.

De la Puerta B, Buracco P, Ladlow J et al. Superficial temporal axial pattern flap for facial reconstruction of skin defects in dogs and cats. *J Small Anim Pract*, 2021; 62(11):984–991.

Defoor J, Bosmans T, Doom M et al. The use of islandized angularis oris axial pattern buccal flap for the reconstruction of a recurrent cleft palate in a cat. *Vlaams Diergeneeskd Tijdschr*, 2013; 82:350–355.

Gray MJ. Chronic axillary wound repair in a cat with omentalisation and omocervical skin flap. *J Small Anim Pract*, 2005; 46(10):499–503.

Lascelles BDX, White RAS. Combined omental pedicle grafts and thoracodorsal axial pattern flaps for the reconstruction of chronic, nonhealing axillary wounds in cats. *Vet Surg*, 2001; 30(4):380–385.

Lester S, Pratschke K. Central hemimaxillectomy and reconstruction using a superficial temporal artery axial pattern flap in a domestic short hair cat. *J Feline Med Surg*, 2003; 5(4):241–244.

Losinski SL, Stanley BJ, Schallberger SP et al. Versatility of the angularis oris axial pattern flap for facial reconstruction. *Vet Surg*, 2015; 44(8):930–938.

Milgram J, Weiser M, Kelmer E, Benzioni H. Axial pattern flap based on a cutaneous branch of the facial artery in cats. *Vet Surg*, 2011; 40(3):347–351.

Osborne MP. William Stewart Halsted: his life and contributions to surgery. *Lancet Oncol*, 2007; 8(3):256–265.

Remedios AM, Bauer MS, Bowen CV. Thoracodorsal and caudal superficial epigastric axial pattern skin flaps in cats. *Vet Surg*, 1989; 18(5):380–385.

Stiles J, Townsend W, Willis M et al. Use of a caudal auricular axial pattern flap in three cats and one dog following orbital exenteration. *Vet Ophtalmol*, 2003; 6(2):121–126.

Woods S, de C Marques AI, Yool DA. Simultaneous bilateral caudal superficial epigastric flaps in a cat. *Vet Rec*, 2009; 164(14):435–435.

MOST COMMON SKIN TUMORS IN THE CAT 10

Anna Calvet

Introduction

The **skin** is the most extensive **organ** in the body, extending entirely over its surface. Together with its accessory structures, that is, the **hair follicles**, **glands** and **nails**, they comprise the integumentary system.

As noted in Chapter 9 "Most common flaps and plasties in feline surgery" (see Fig. 1, p. 66), the skin is organized in overlapping layers, beginning with the most external layer, the epidermis, followed by the dermis, then the hypodermis, in which the adipose tissue connects the skin to the underlying musculature or periosteum through a fascia.

The nerves and the sensory nerve endings reach into the three layers of the skin, while blood vessels are found only in the two deepest layers. In addition to the different types of skin that comprise the abovementioned accessory structures, the skin undergoes significant modifications to create special structures, such as the skin covering the ear canal, nasal planum or paw pads.

Keeping in mind the epidermis and dermis, the thickness of the skin is variable in cats. Although it varies according to the region of the body, this thickness ranges between 0.4 and 2 mm, being thickest on the dorsal side of the body and the more proximal parts of the limbs, and thinnest on the ventral side of the body, as well as the more distal parts of the limbs, and the ears. The hypodermis varies greatly in thickness, depending on the quantity of the patient's fat tissue and the anatomical region. This layer is thickest in the belly, and it may essentially be absent from the limbs.

Of all the skin conditions observed in the feline clinic, those that require surgical treatment are principally of neoplastic origin.

Because this organ is visible to the naked eye, it is easy for the patients' guardians to observe changes in the skin. Therefore, the appearance of cutaneous tumors is detected easily. On the other hand, the skin's function as protective barrier means it is exposed to a large variety of environmental carcinogens. Keeping this in mind, along with other possible causes, the etiology of skin tumors can be broken down as follows:

- Mechanical processes or trauma: origin of granulomas and lesions that have a tumor-like appearance.
- Chronic inflammation: as can occur in injection-site sarcomas.
- Sun, ultraviolet (UV) light: as occurs in squamous cell carcinomas or hemangiosarcomas.
- Genetics: Siamese cats are predisposed to developing mast cell tumors.
- Virus induced:
  - Papillomavirus: papillomas, carcinoid lesions, squamous cell carcinoma.
  - Feline leukemia virus (FeLV): cutaneous lymphoma.
  - Feline sarcoma virus and FeLV: multiple sarcomas in young cats.

The frequency of certain skin tumors is a function of what latitude the patient lives at or the color of their fur (carcinoma in cats with white fur). Others such as injection-site sarcomas are equally spread out across the globe (a chapter is devoted to this due to its clinical significance and the difficulty of surgical treatment).

When we plan to surgically remove a cutaneous tumor, especially when we have to remove a large amount of skin, we should consider the particularities of cutaneous irrigation, which is discussed extensively in Chapter 9 (see Fig. 10, p. 72).

Classification of skin tumors

Cutaneous tumors affect the skin or the subcutaneous tissue and can be classified according to their cellular origin (Table 1).

TABLE 1. Classification of skin tumors according to their cellular origin

Cellular origin	Type of tumor
Epithelial	■ Basal cell tumor ■ Basal cell carcinoma ■ Papilloma ■ Squamous cell carcinoma ■ Nail bed tumors
Skin adnexal	■ Adenoma or adenocarcinoma of sebaceous glands ■ Ceruminous adenoma ■ Apocrine gland anal sac adenocarcinoma ■ Sweat gland tumors ■ Trichoepithelioma ■ Pilomatrixoma ■ Meibomian gland adenoma
Mesenchymal	■ Soft tissue sarcomas ■ Myxomatous tumor ■ Nerve tumor
Round cell	■ Mast cell tumors ■ Histiocytomas ■ Melanocytic nevi ■ Plasmocytomas ■ Lymphomas
Melanocytic	■ Benign cutaneous melanocytic nevi ■ Malignant melanoma

General diagnostic approach and staging of skin tumors

When dealing with any cutaneous or subcutaneous mass, we should always perform a fine needle aspiration (FNA) cytology (Figs. 1 and 2). We should also consider:

- The time of appearance.
- Its evolution, changes in size and color, and the appearance of the surrounding tissue.
- The presence of clinical signs or other masses to determine if any concomitant pathologies exist or if we are dealing with a paraneoplastic syndrome, observations that could impact the prognosis.
- If there is a solitary lesion or multiple lesions.
- The anatomical location and the size of the mass, information that is recorded in the medical history.
- The consistency of the mass upon palpation, as well as adhesion to tissues.

> Before preparing the surgical plan, the tumor should be staged, and its type and histological grade determined.

Preoperative tests

For benign tumors that are easy to diagnose via cytology, it is not necessary to run the whole battery of tests, but it is always better to have as much information as possible:

- **Blood tests:** especially for tumors that may be associated with paraneoplastic syndromes or that may directly affect the hematology.
- **Diagnostic imaging:** it is usually not necessary to image the area of a cutaneous lesion, with the exception of tumors that are adherent or very close to bone. In general, thoracic

Aspects to keep in mind

- In contrast to dogs, mast cell tumors and basal cell tumors usually behave benignly in cats.
- Hair matrix tumors are rare, although Persian cats are predisposed to them.
- Papillomas are usually virus induced.
- Lipomas may present in any part of the body, and Siamese cats are predisposed to them.
- Complete excision of benign tumors usually has a curative effect, but a sample should always be sent out for histopathology.

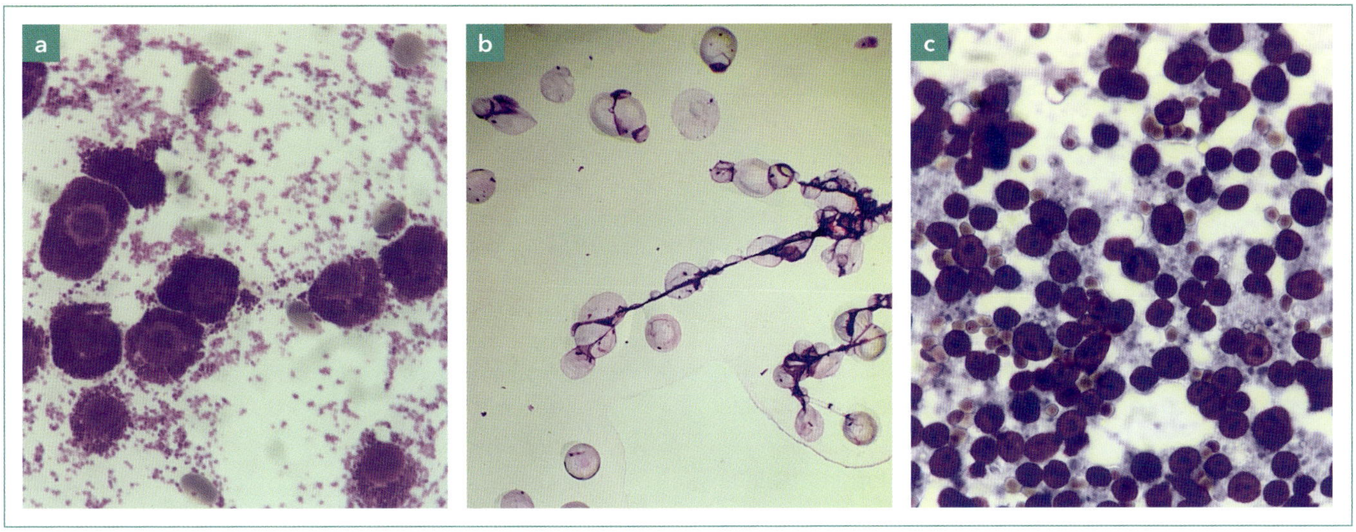

FIGURE 1. Fine needle aspiration and subsequent cytology can sometimes orient us perfectly toward a diagnosis. (a) Mast cell tumor. (b) Lipoma. (c) Carcinoma.

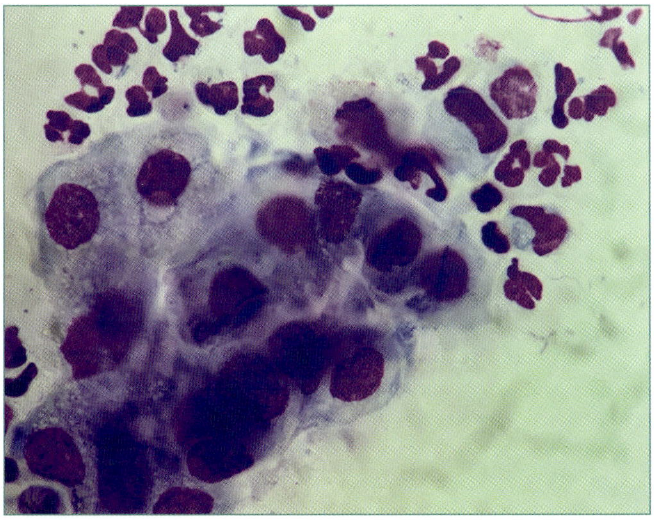

FIGURE 2. In other cytological samples, the presence of concurrent inflammation/infection means that either the infection should be treated first or a sample of tissue should be obtained by incisional biopsy to plan the surgical approach.

radiographs in four positions (right and left lateral, ventrodorsal and dorsoventral) and an abdominal ultrasound enable us to stage a malignant tumor. If advanced imaging techniques are available, it is reasonable to conduct magnetic resonance or computed tomography scans with or without contrast.

- **FNA/biopsy:** some skin tumors such as mast cell tumors or lymphoma can be diagnosed by cytology. In other cases, an incisional biopsy is required. Ulcerated or necrotic areas should be avoided in such a biopsy, given that a diagnosis cannot be made without a representative tissue sample to enable an evaluation of the histological pattern. An excisional biopsy is only recommended when multiple lesions are present.
- **FNA of regional lymph nodes:** to check for metastasis.

As with all tumors, staging is based on the size, location and infiltration of the tumor in adjoining tissues (T), the presence or absence of metastasis in regional lymph nodes (N) and the presence or absence of distant metastasis (M).

Characteristics of primary tumors (T)

Determination of T for canine and feline tumors of dermal or epidermal origin (excluding lymphomas and mast cell tumors):

- **Tis:** preinvasive carcinoma or carcinoma in situ
- **T0:** no evidence of tumor
- **T1:** tumor is less than 2 cm, superficial or exophytic
- **T2:** tumor is 2–5 cm, or any size but minimally invasive
- **T3:** tumor is over 5 cm or has invaded the hypodermis
- **T4:** tumor has invaded other structures such as fascia, muscle, bone or cartilage

Diagnosis and treatment of the most common skin tumors

Basal cell tumor

Some of its characteristics are:

- Represents approximately 20% of skin tumors and 34% of epithelial tumors.
- Usually affects middle-aged and older cats.
- Typically solitary, firm to the touch (although cystic ones also exist), well defined, and located in the dermis and epidermis of the head and neck, though they may also appear in other locations (Fig. 3).
- They are usually relatively small, 0.5–2 cm in diameter, although they can sometimes be over 10 cm.
- The surface skin may be ulcerated.
- They are often highly pigmented, and can therefore be confused with melanomas at first glance.
- They can be benign or malignant. The latter are invasive and not pigmented, with metastasis in regional lymph nodes (although not very frequent).

They can be diagnosed by cytology, although the cells do not always have the same appearance. These tumors usually have slow, noninvasive growth, and respond well to full excision, which usually has a curative effect.

In the case of malignant basal cell tumors, needle biopsy of regional lymph nodes must be considered to check for metastasis, and in the case of incomplete excision, radiation therapy can be applied. If there is metastasis, administration of carboplatin or doxorubicin is indicated.

Example of biopsy results

- **Macroscopic examination:** dissected skin fragment with wart-like appearance, 1×0.7 cm.
- **Microscopic examination:** cutaneous tissue with circumscribed dermal proliferation, prominent, composed of small epithelial cells arranged in solid plaques and nest structures separated by fine bands of connective tissue. The cell contains little cytoplasm, basophilic, with round or oval-shaped nucleus, hyperchromatic, with low-grade anisokaryosis. Mitotic activity is not visible. Presence of abundant melanophages and intercellular melanin clusters. Evaluation of surgical margins: absence of marginal neoplastic cells. Complete excision.
- **Diagnosis:** Basal cell tumor.
- **Comments:** benign neoplasm with origin in the follicular or epidermal basal layer, with a very good prognosis after complete surgical removal. Recurrence and metastasis are not reported.

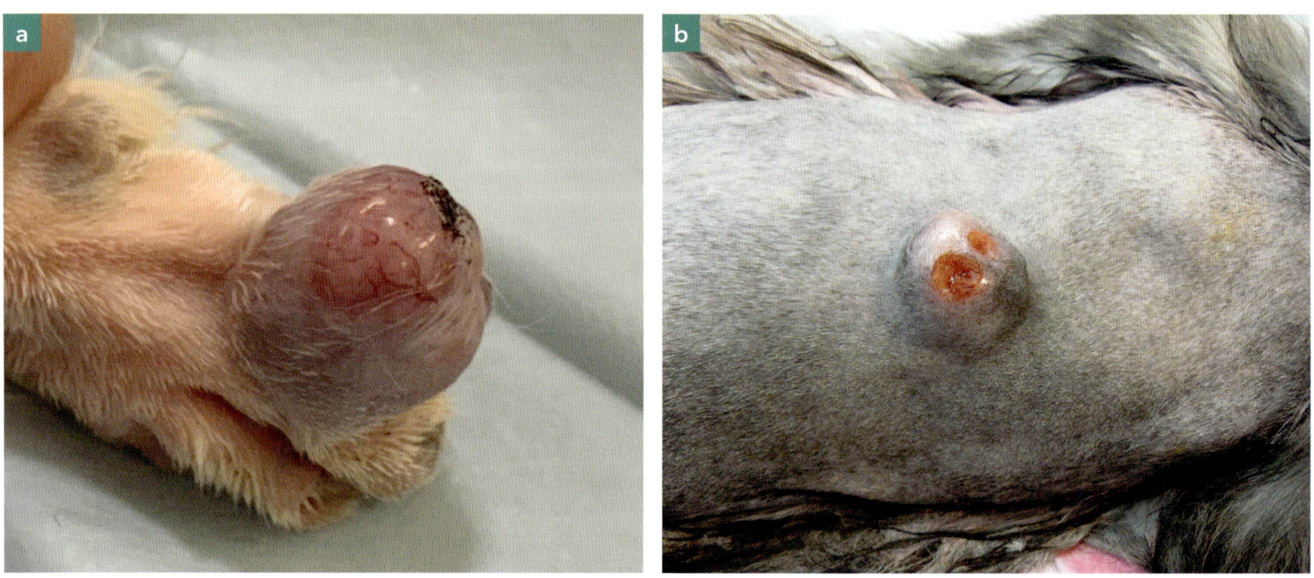

FIGURE 3. Examples of basal cell tumors, (a) in a finger and (b) on the dorsum.

Fibrosarcoma

As noted previously, fibrosarcomas are sufficiently significant and complex to have a separate section devoted to them (see Ch. 12 "Feline injection-site sarcoma"). They represent 17% of skin tumors.

Squamous cell carcinoma

Some of its characteristics are:

- They represent 11% of cutaneous tumors. They are the leading malignant skin epidermal tumor.
- They are locally aggressive, but tend not to metastasize.
- This tumor is induced by sunlight and is most common in older cats with white fur or, in general, little pigmentation (cats with white fur are up to 5 times more likely to develop it).
- A precancerous lesion, **actinic dermatitis**, appears similar to an ulcerative lesion due to excessive licking or scratching and can have a long duration.
- Its distribution:
  - 72% in the ear pinnae (Fig. 4)
  - 15% in the nose (Fig. 5)
  - 8% in the eyelids
  - 5% in other places such as the chin, the palate or the lips (Fig. 6)
- The size is highly relevant to the prognosis. It is important to act quickly.
- It may be associated with feline immunodeficiency virus (FIV).

It is diagnosed by cytology, and the surgical plan for its removal is based on the location, extension and depth of the lesions.

> Surgery in patients with squamous cell carcinoma generally yields good results without recurrence, but in the most severe cases, radiation therapy, cryotherapy, electrochemical therapy or medication can be used.

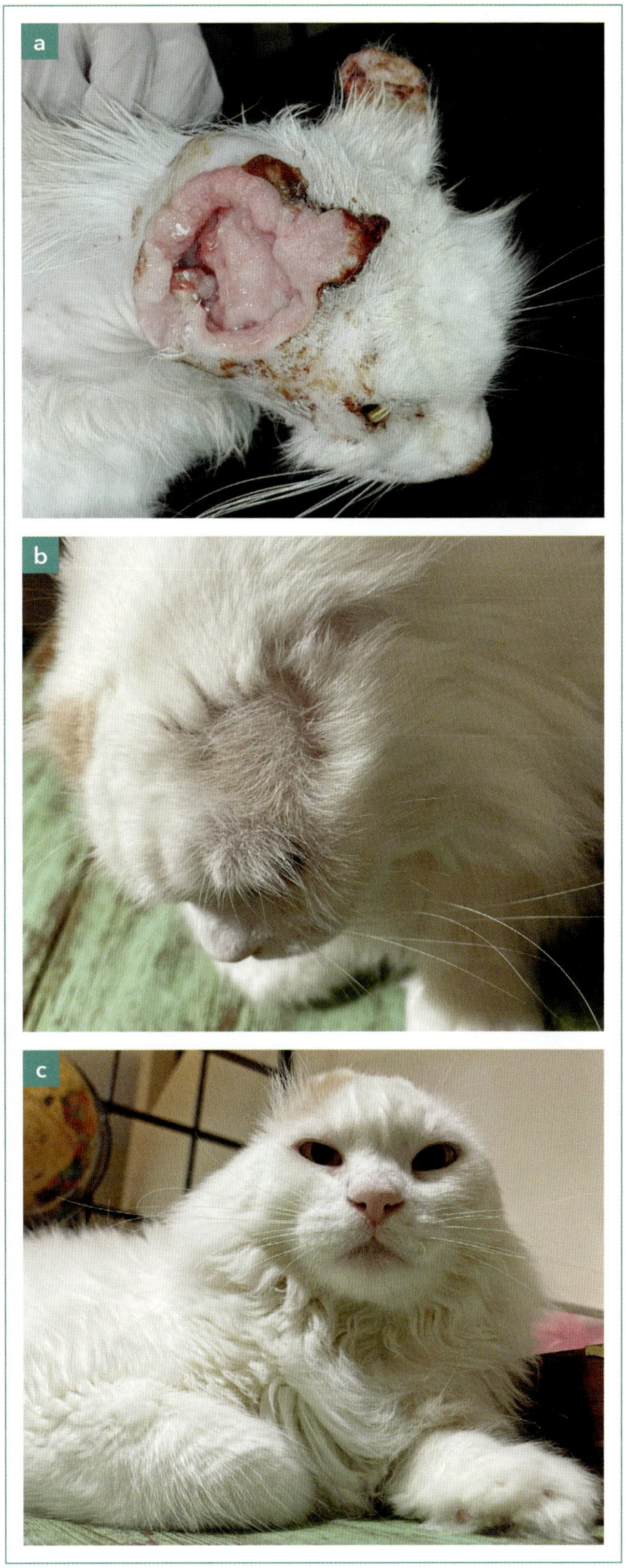

FIGURE 4. (a) Squamous cell carcinoma in both pinnae. (b,c) Current appearance of the patient.

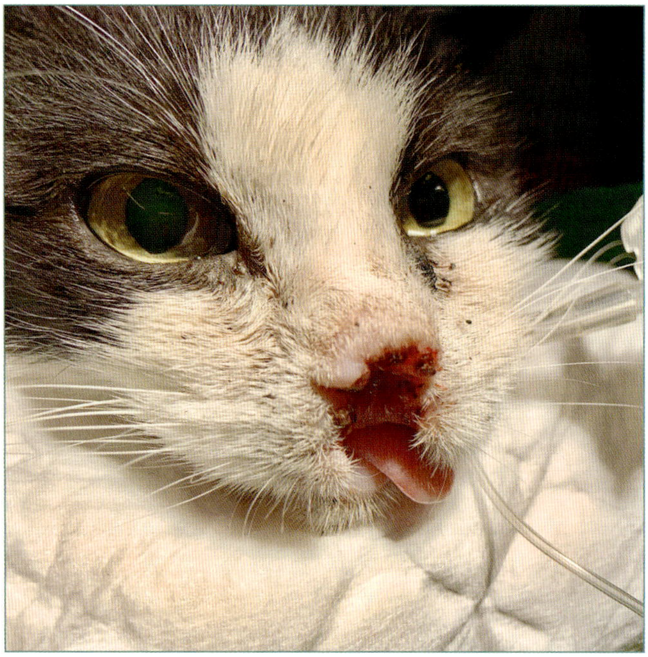

FIGURE 5. Patient with carcinoma in the nasal planum before surgical intervention.

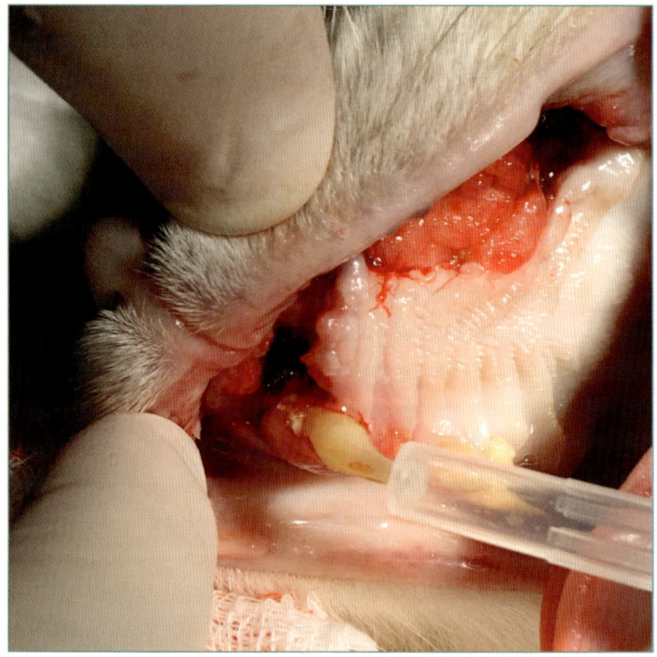

FIGURE 6. Squamous cell carcinoma in a cat's palate.

Multicentric squamous cell carcinoma (in situ)

In terms of histology, this premalignant lesion is biologically similar to Bowen's disease in humans. It usually affects middle-aged and older cats, and the lesions present in pigmented areas. They can be located in the trunk, limbs, head or neck (Fig. 7). As with Bowen's disease, the papillomavirus is implicated in its etiology, and the lesions can evolve into invasive squamous cell carcinoma with aggressive behavior and higher metastatic capacity.

Full removal of the lesions is initially indicated if there are only a few of them, but new ones may appear. We can use 5% imiquimod cream on the lesions 3 times per week. It does not always work, and is more useful in the initial stages. Interferon has also been used.

Sphynx and Devon Rex breeds are predisposed. The prognosis is worse for hairless cats.

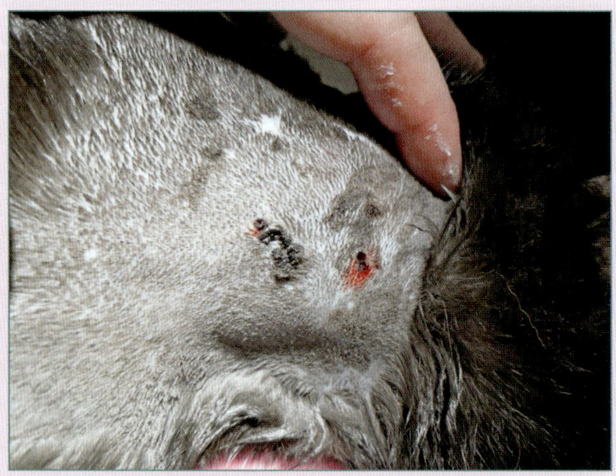

FIGURE 7. Multicentric squamous cell carcinoma in the neck area in a 4-year-old domestic shorthair cat.

Mast cell tumor

Some of its characteristics are:

- They represent approximately 7% of skin tumors.
- Feline mast cell tumors are less frequent and pose less of an issue than in dogs.
- There are two types of mast cell tumors: cutaneous and visceral.
- Cutaneous mast cell tumors have a benign behavior, are scaly and easily diagnosed with cytology.
- The most common areas where they occur are the trunk and the head.
- The majority are solitary (Fig. 8).
- Tumors that are not extracted with sufficient margins or those that are unresectable can be treated with radiation therapy or lomustine.

Cutaneous mast cell tumors that cannot be extracted with sufficient surgical margins or those that are unresectable can be treated with radiation therapy or chemotherapy (lomustine).

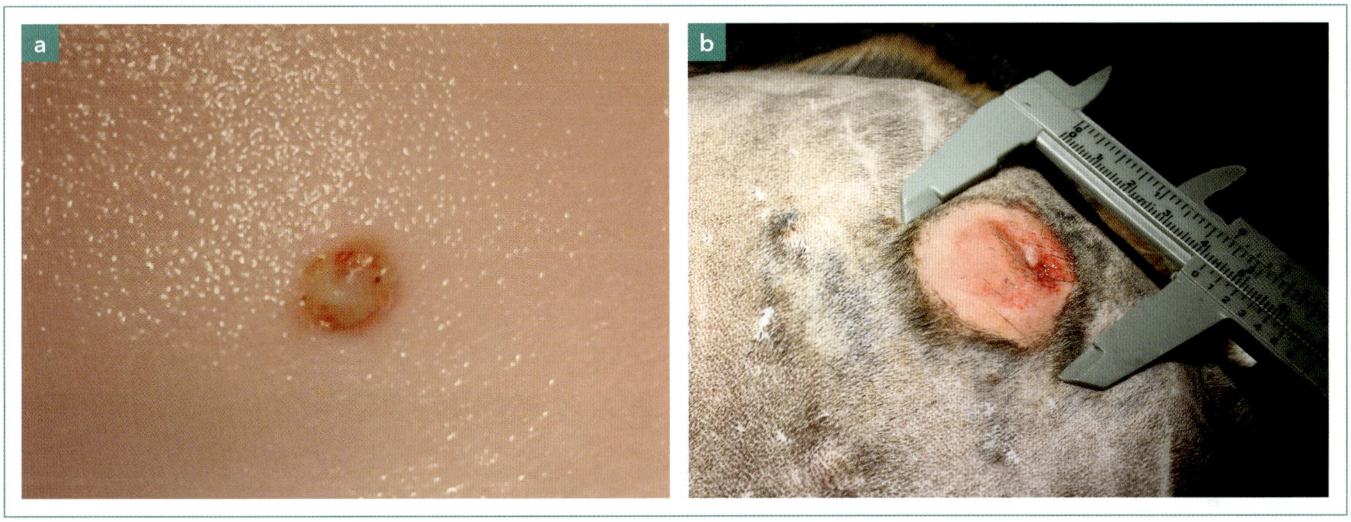

FIGURE 8. Examples of cutaneous mast cell tumors. (a) Single nodule. With proper excision, no further complications are expected, and the surgery may have a curative effect. (b) Large mast cell tumor invading the underlying structures. The prognosis is guarded due to the high risk of recurrence.

Noncutaneous mast cell tumors

Visceral and systemic mast cell tumors

The primary tumor is found in the spleen, and the treatment is splenectomy. Cats usually present with nausea and anorexia, with mastocytosis and bone marrow involvement. In addition, mediastinal involvement with pleural effusion may be observed. The presence of mast cell tumors / skin lesions may incorrectly be thought to have a dermal origin with subsequent organ involvement.

Intestinal mast cell tumor

This pathology is distinct from visceral mast cell tumors (which do not affect the intestine). It is a severe, malignant disease with high metastatic capacity and a poor prognosis.

In contrast to other conditions in which mastocytes are involved, sclerosing intestinal mast cell tumors present cells with little cytoplasmic granulation. Metastasis occurs in 66% of cases (especially in lymph nodes and the liver) and according to one study, the life expectancy is 2 months from the time of diagnosis.

Melanoma

Some of its characteristics are:

- It affects mostly older cats.
- Usually they are pigmented lesions that tend to be located on the head and pinnae, at the edge or tips or at the base.
- Amelanotic melanomas have a worse prognosis.
- Multiple melanoma is rare.
- They may exhibit rapid growth and ulcerate.
- They are more frequent in cats with black or gray fur.
- In general, all feline melanomas should be considered potentially malignant, even if they behave benignly. In this type of tumor, criteria such as growth rate, histological picture, or mitosis rate do not always correlate with behavior, so it is more difficult to establish a prognosis. In general, however, we can consider intratumoral necrosis or the presence of more than 4 mitoses per field to be negative prognostic factors.
- Ocular and oral melanomas have a more malignant behavior.

The treatment of choice is excision with wide margins. Recurrence may occur, and there are currently no good adjuvant therapies available for those that have malignant behavior, since they are not sensitive to chemotherapy. Radiation therapy can be used. The reaction to immunotherapy is not yet clear, although the efficacy of the canine melanoma vaccine is being tested (current studies aim to evaluate its tolerance in cats).

Diffuse or multifocal cutaneous neoplasms

Although not considered surgical pathologies once a biopsy is performed, they are described below.

Cutaneous lymphoma

Lesions in the form of plaques are most frequent. However, nodules or crusted, exfoliative lesions accompanied by pruritus may also present, and such lesions may be confused with other skin diseases (Figs. 9 and 10).

On occasion, what begins as a single lesion quickly evolves, increasing in number as the condition progresses.

Affected cats usually test negative for feline leukemia virus (FeLV).

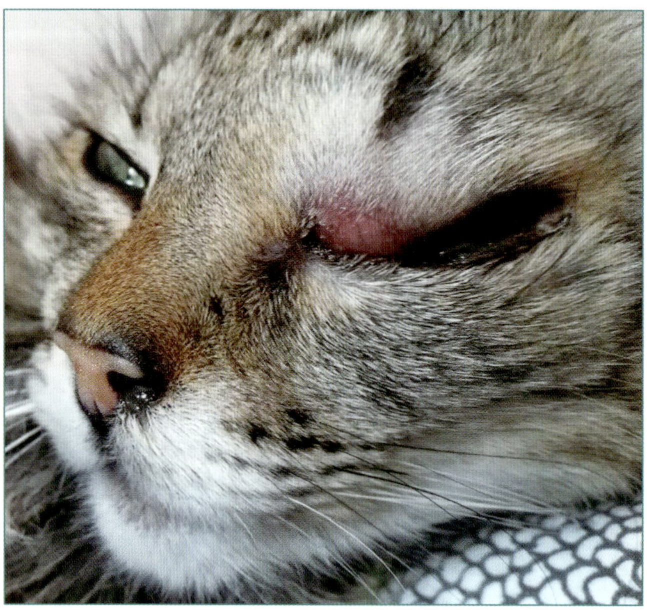

FIGURE 9. Lymphoma in the eyelid of a 12-year-old long hair domestic cat; single nodule.

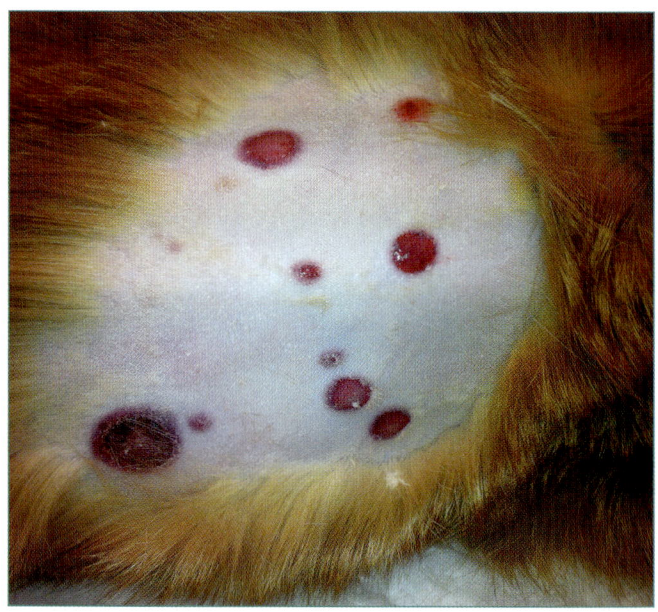

FIGURE 10. Another cutaneous lymphoma.

It is often associated with systemic lymphoma. Epitheliotropic lymphoma usually has its origin in T cells.

In rare cases, early on in the condition, surgery can have a curative effect if there is a single lesion that has not yet spread. But in the remaining cases, it should be treated as a systemic condition. The treatment protocol includes a combination of chemotherapy drugs.

Feline progressive histiocytosis

This can present in the form of a single lesion or as multiple nodules, firm/hard papules, or nonpruritic plaques, especially exhibiting tropism for the feet, limbs and head.

A neoplasm that originates in dendritic cells, it progresses over time: indolent in its initial phases (during which it remains in the cutaneous area, with long periods of latency, up to 3 years), it becomes more aggressive as it progresses (lesions exhibit greater cellular atypia and involve lymph nodes or other internal organs). The etiology of these lesions is unknown.

It does not respond well to treatment; usually immunosuppressants, immunomodulators or chemotherapy is used.

In all cases, crusted lesions and ulcerated areas may appear.

In contrast to pathologies associated with lymphocytes, which are more aggressive but may respond to chemotherapy treatment, histiocytosis evolves more slowly, but its response to treatment is also worse (Fig. 11).

Surgical procedures associated with skin tumors

The surgical procedures for the removal of skin tumors are described in other chapters of this atlas:

- Incisional and excisional biopsies (see Ch. 7) (Fig. 12)
- Nasal planum surgery/rhinotomy (see Ch. 15)
- Eyelid plasties (see Ch. 17)
- Excision of the pinna/otectomy (see Ch. 18)
- Total ablation of the ear canal (see Ch. 18)

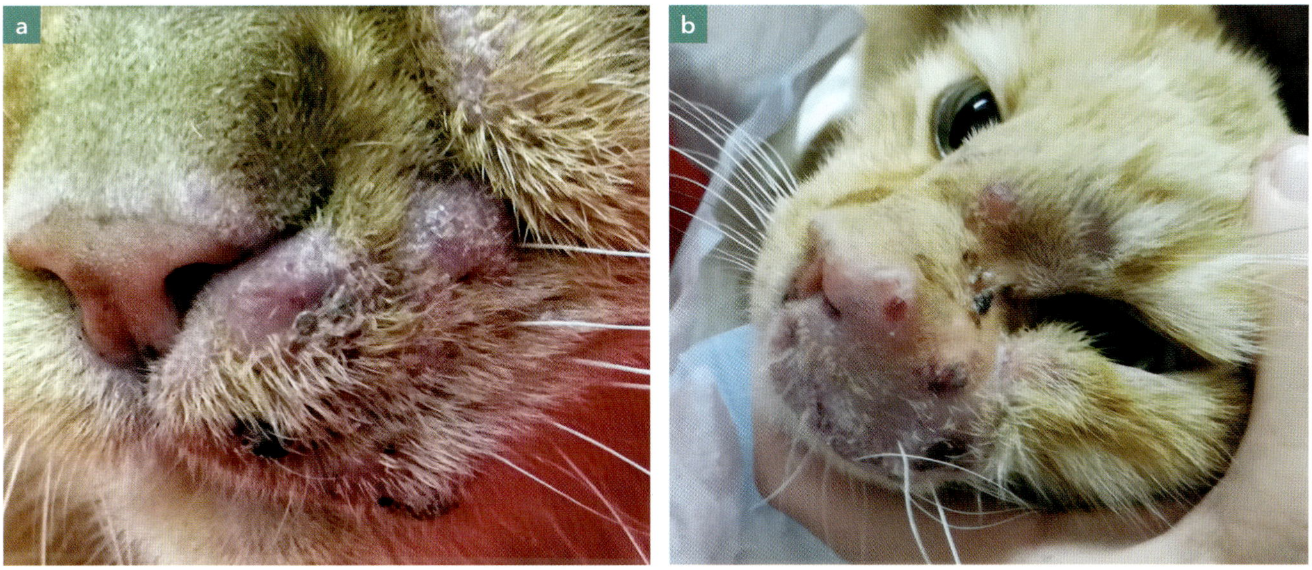

FIGURE 11. Progressive cutaneous histiocytosis. (a) Day of the diagnostic biopsy (02/14/18). (b) Evolution of the patient despite treatment (10/16/19).

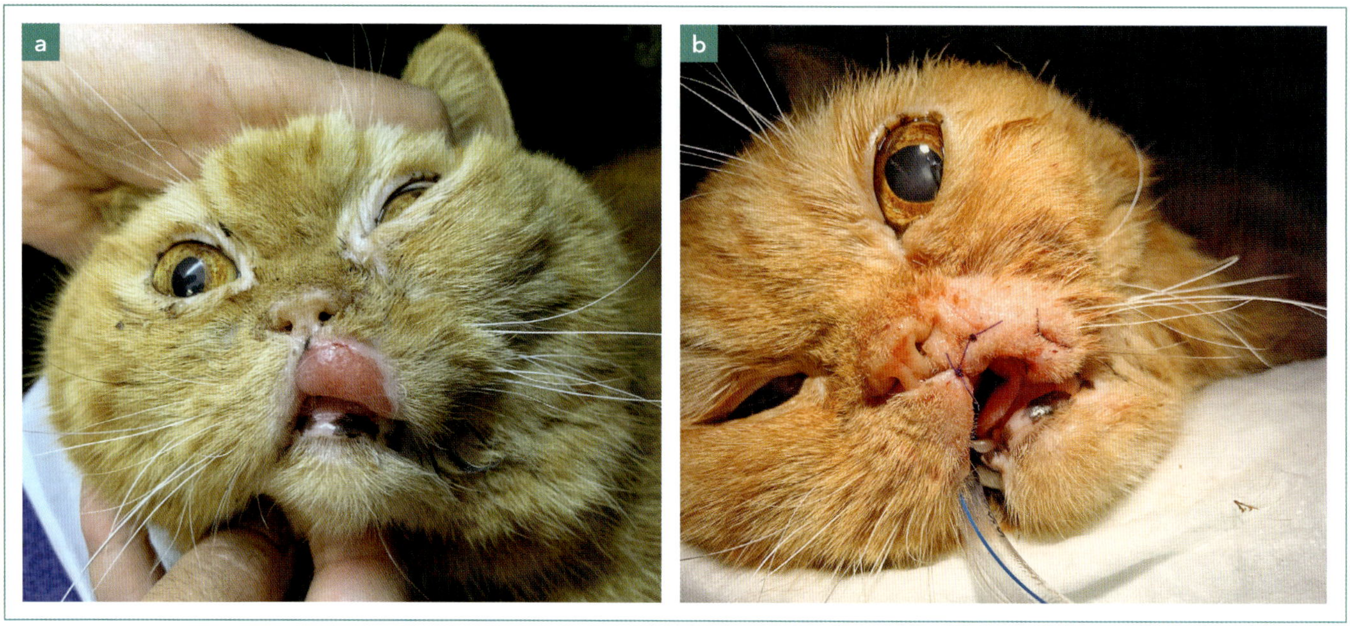

FIGURE 12. (a) Cat with a tumor on the lip. (b) Result after tumor biopsy.

Bibliography

Affolter VK, Moore PF. Feline progresive histiocytosis. *Vet Pathol*, 2006; 43(5):646–655.

Diters RW, Walsh KM. Feline basal cell tumours: a review of 124 cases. *Vet Pathol*, 1984; 21(1):51–56.

Goldschmit MH, Shofer PS. *Skin Tumours of the Dog and Cat*. Pergamon Press, 1992; pp. 2–3.

Halsey CH, Powers BE, Kamstock DA. Feline intestinal sclerosing mast cell tumour: 50 cases (1997–2008). *Vet Comp Oncol*, 2010; 8(1):72–79.

Liska WD, MacEwen EG, Zaki FA, Garvey M. Feline systemic mastocytosis: a review and results of splenectomy in seven cases. *J Am Anim Hosp Assoc*, 1979; 15:587–597.

Miller MA, Nelson SL, Turk JR et al. Cutaneous neoplasia in 340 cats. *Vet Pathol*, 1991; 28(5):389–395.

Sarbu L, Kitchell BE, Bergman PJ. Safety of administering the canine melanoma DNA vaccine (Oncept) to cats with malignant melanoma - a retrospective study. *J Feline Med Surg*, 2017; 19(2):224–230.

Spugnini EP, Vinzenzi B, Citro G et al. Electrochemotherapy for treatment of squamous cell carcinoma in cats: A preliminary report. *Vet J*, 2009; 179(1):117–120.

MAMMARY SURGERY 11

Anna Calvet

Surgical anatomy

Mammary glands are formed from epithelial buds on the mammary crests in the embryo. Female cats usually have four pairs of **mammary glands**, lying on either side of the ventral midline. Thus, there are two pairs of thoracic mammary glands and two pairs of abdominal mammary glands. On occasion, however, more buds emerge during development that may persist into adulthood, giving rise to supernumerary mammary glands.

Different terminology is used to orient us, but we will always number from cranial to caudal.

To understand the metastasis pattern that we might find in malignant feline mammary tumors (FMTs), it is very important to learn the particularities of vascularization and lymphatic drainage.

Vascularization

Principal vascular supply is provided by the **cranial and caudal epigastric arteries**, which anastomose in the umbilical region (Fig. 1). In some cases branches exist connecting the arteries on either side of the abdomen.

The venous pattern mirrors the arterial, but we should note that these vessels cross the midline most often through accessory branches.

In the thoracic region, there are also **perforating branches of internal thoracic arteries** as well as **vertebral veins**.

The abdominal region contains **cutaneous branches** of the **phrenicoabdominal and deep circumflex iliac arteries**, and cranially cutaneous branches of the most caudal **intercostal arteries**.

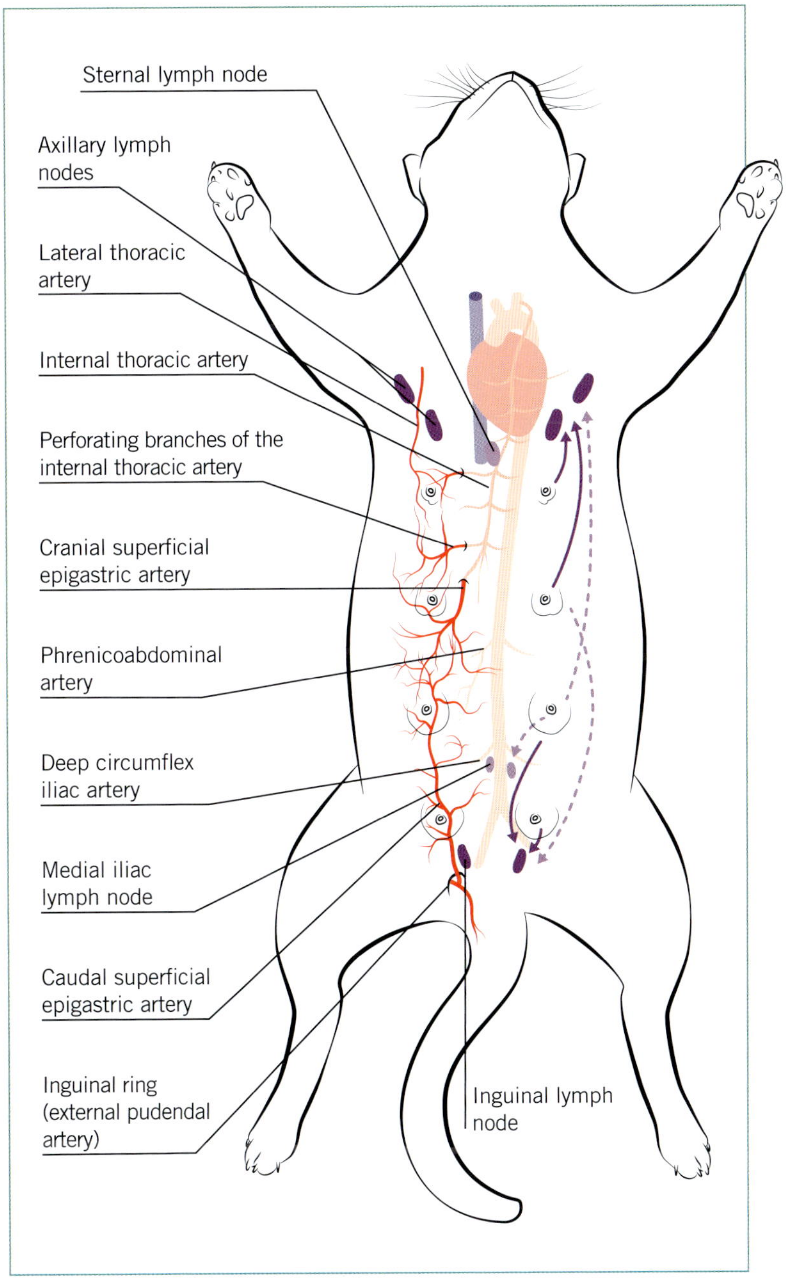

FIGURE 1. Vascularity and lymphatic drainage of feline mammary glands.

Lymphatic drainage

In normal conditions, the thoracic mammary glands are drained by the **axillary lymph nodes** and the abdominal mammary glands are drained by the inguinal nodes (Fig. 1). Nevertheless, numerous exceptions exist, and thus, on occasion, the second thoracic gland can also be drained by the **inguinal lymph node** and the first abdominal gland can be drained by the axillary and inguinal lymph nodes.

It has also been observed that the third mammary gland (first abdominal) can be drained by the **medial iliac lymph node**; however, drainage by the sternal lymph node has not been confirmed.

It has also been observed that when a tumor exists, the first three mammary glands (two thoracic and the first abdominal) can be drained by the same mammary glands of the contralateral mammary chain, a situation not observed in healthy cats.

> Local metastasis has a higher chance of occurring through the venous system than through the lymphatic system.

Diseases of the mammary glands

Feline mammary glands can have benign, nontumoral lesions, both inflammatory and noninflammatory, as well as benign and malignant tumoral lesions. It is vitally important to be meticulous when diagnosing due to their different prognosis and possible treatment.

Nonneoplastic lesions

Inflammatory: mastitis

Usually infection is produced in one or more glands during lactation. Therefore, our diagnosis is based on the medical history. In most cases, clinical signs include fever, anorexia, pain on palpation of the mammary glands and purulent discharge, while subclinical presentation includes only galactostasis in the affected mammary glands.

The diagnosis is made via the medical history, a cytology and a culture of mammary secretions. A complete blood count may also show leukocytosis with neutrophilia. Treatment consists of proper antibiotic therapy based on the culture and subsequent antibiogram, keeping in mind that the environment of the mammary glands is highly lipophilic, which reduces the concentration of hydrophilic antibiotics (e.g., penicillins and cephalosporins).

Noninflammatory: fibroadenomatoid hyperplasia

Caused by a rapid and abnormal, but benign, proliferation of mammary tissue due to hormonal stimulation. This pathology is most often diagnosed in young females in estrus (usually after a silent estrus), but it can also be diagnosed in gestating females or even in males that have been exposed to progestogens.

It can affect one or more mammary glands, and occasionally all of them are severely affected. In these cases, ulceration is not rare (Fig. 2). The diagnosis can be established on the basis of the history and clinical signs, but a pathology report provides definitive confirmation.

Treatment is centered on controlling the pain and blocking progesterone receptors with aglepristone (10–15 mg/kg subcutaneously on days 1, 2 and 7). In addition, we should perform an ovariohysterectomy (OHE) on any females that have not been sterilized. Remission sometimes occurs spontaneously. This condition can take weeks to months to resolve, even with treatment.

> If we observe inflammation in one or more mammary glands, we should consider the possibility of mastitis or fibroadenomatoid hyperplasia as a differential diagnosis, keeping in mind that both conditions may present simultaneously.

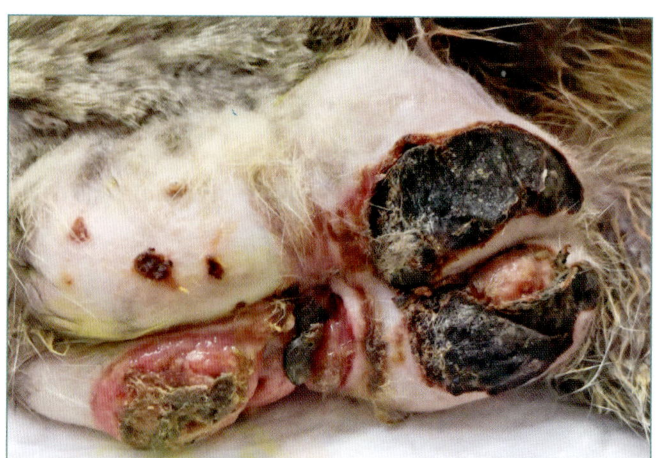

FIGURE 2. Patient with ulcerated fibroadenomatous hyperplasia with necrotic areas.

Neoplastic lesions

Feline mammary tumors are the third most frequent neoplasm in female domestic cats, after skin and lymphohematopoietic tumors. As the majority of them are malignant (80%), early detection and intensive, radical therapy will greatly influence how long our patients' survival time and quality of life.

Benign tumors

Between 10% and 20% of mammary neoplasms are benign. The age of presentation can vary widely, ranging between 1 and 9.5 years. The most frequent benign tumors are:

- Ductal papilloma
- Simple adenoma
- Complex adenoma
- Benign mixed tumor

Malignant tumors

There are three cell lines in the mammary glands (epithelial, myoepithelial, and mesenchymal), but malignant tumors arise most commonly from epithelial cells. Therefore, carcinomas and adenocarcinomas are observed most frequently, although other types of tumors also exist (Fig. 3).

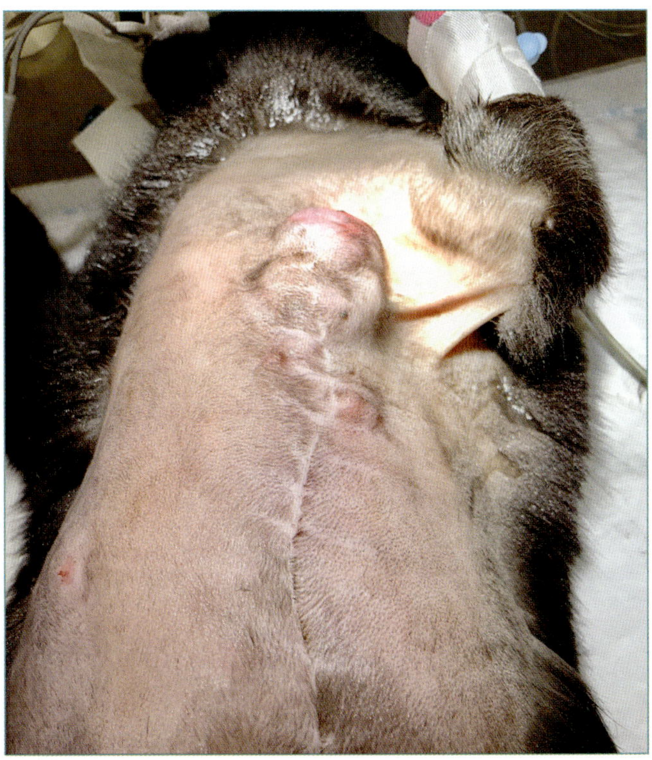

FIGURE 3. Recurrence of a malignant mammary tumor.

Risk factors identified for these conditions are, among others:

- Age (10–12 years old).
- Breed: the incidence in Siamese cats is much higher. They have a 2 times greater chance of developing these conditions and have a lower median age of presentation (9.5 years old).
- Hormonal status: early sterilization has a protective effect. Unspayed female cats have a 7 times higher risk of developing a malignant mammary tumor as compared to spayed female cats (Box 1).

BOX 1. Decreased tumor risk as a function of the time of sterilization

- Before 6 months: 91% decrease
- 6–13 months: 86% decrease
- After 24 months: 11% decrease

Estrogen and progestogen receptors have been detected in benign FMTs, but not in malignant or metastatic ones. Therefore, after diagnosis of a malignant FMT, OHEs are usually performed to prevent complications such as pyometra, rather than for its protective effect.

Diagnosis

Malignant FMTs behave aggressively. The majority of them are high-grade carcinomas, and in 60% of cases, the cat has more than one tumor at the time of diagnosis. The main cause of death is metastasis, and the most common metastatic sites for these tumors are:

- Regional lymph nodes
- Lungs
- Pleura
- Liver

The diagnostic protocol that we have to design should enable us to correctly stage the patient before planning our surgical approach.

Diagnostic protocol for patients with mammary tumors

1. Routine blood testing including T_4 and retroviral status.
2. Cytology of the mass or masses: cytology can be very helpful when establishing differential diagnoses of lesions that affect a cat's mammary glands. FMTs are usually composed of homogeneous populations, which facilitates their cytological diagnosis.
3. Urinalysis.
4. Systematic palpation of all regional lymph nodes and cytology to confirm the presence or absence of suspicious cells.
5. X-rays to detect pulmonary masses, ideally four projections: right and left lateral, dorsoventral and ventrodorsal.
6. Abdominal ultrasound, paying special attention to the liver and subiliac lymph nodes.

Preoperative considerations

The general consensus is that when dealing with a **malignant FMT**, the best course of action with the highest chance for success is **early detection and total mastectomy**.

Unilateral, or preferably bilateral, mastectomy is the best option. The bilateral option can be performed in a single intervention. Otherwise, one mammary chain can be removed first and the second one removed 4–8 weeks later.

In these cases, the issue that the clinician usually faces is that the diagnosis is rarely done early enough, and therefore, surgery must be considered in combination with other therapeutic options. Numerous studies have been done on the use of chemotherapy, whether more intensive or low-dose (metronomic). The goal, when choosing one of these options, is to improve life expectancy and the quality of life of our patients, even though we currently lack sufficient scientific evidence thereon.

A staging system has been established (Table 1) that will inform the prognosis once we have considered the histopathology results in combination with all the information obtained in the proposed diagnostic protocol.

Aspects to keep in mind

- Always remove the inguinal lymph node together with the abdominal mammary gland.
- Prophylactic removal of the axillary lymph node has not been shown to be useful if it is not enlarged, if it does not have a different texture upon palpation, or if cytology does not indicate a possible metastasis. Therefore, a supplementary cranial incision may be unnecessary.
- The sample should be prepared correctly before sending it to the laboratory, marking cranial and caudal, and sending the entire sample together for proper evaluation of the surgical margins, since this is a significant factor in the prognosis.
- If there is no prior infection as a result of an ulcerated tumor, good aseptic and surgical techniques enables us to avoid the use of antibiotic therapy.

TABLE 1. Staging system of malignant tumors, modified for cats (Mc Neill et al., 2009)

Stage	Size (T)	Lymph node (N)	Metastasis (M)
I	T1	N0	M0
II	T2	N0	M0
III	T1, T2, T3	N1	M0
	T3	N0	M0
IV	T1, T2, T3	N0/N1	M1

T1: >2 cm; T2: 2–3 cm; T3: >3 cm.
N0: no presence of metastasis in regional lymph nodes; N1: with metastasis in regional lymph nodes.
M0: no metastasis to other parts of the body; M1: with metastasis to other parts of the body.

Surgical techniques

Unilateral mastectomy

A simple mastectomy can be performed for small benign lesions, making an elliptical incision around the affected mammary gland. However, unilateral mastectomy is the surgery of choice as part of a bilateral mastectomy performed on two different occasions, or as a single surgery for solitary malignant tumors if they are detected early and in stage I (Fig. 4).

Technique

1. We place the patient in dorsal recumbency and prepare a large extension of the abdominal area by shaving and antiseptic cleaning. The area clipped should extend cranially towards the axilla if our intention is to remove the axillary lymph node.
2. With a skin incision, we mark the entire area that will be removed, keeping in mind that we should create a 2 cm margin of macroscopically healthy tissue around the neoplasm(s).
3. The fascia of the abdominal musculature should also be excised with the scalpel if the neoplasm appears fixed.
4. With Metzenbaum scissors, we then separate and cut all of the tissue we willl remove, in a cranial to caudal direction.
5. During this entire process, we carefully and accurately perform hemostasis, ligating all vessels we come across with a simple suture, using 3-0 or 4-0 caliber absorbable material and minimizing the use of electrocautery, since it can result in a delay in healing and, furthermore, complicate the subsequent histopathological evaluation of the surgical margins.
6. One of the important points in this surgery is the accurate ligation of blood vessels. First the cranial epigastric vessels, followed by the caudal epigastric vessels (we will find them in the inguinal region, usually surrounded by a significant amount of fat, and use scissors to dissect them delicately, although it is also useful to use our fingers or sterile cotton swabs). Once identified, it is worthwhile to ligate the veins first and then the arteries. It is very important to accompany the single or double ligature of these vessels with the distal application of hemostatic forceps because if they are cut accidentally before being ligated, they can retract towards the abdomen through the inguinal canal, causing heavy bleeding, which will then force us to perform a caudal laparotomy.
7. A large amount of tissue will be exposed during the intervention. This will essentially cause tissue desiccation and increase the risk of hypothermia (one of the principal surgical complications in cats). For this reason, during the surgery, we should cover the exposed tissue with gauze moistened with lukewarm saline solution.
8. Once all the mammary tissue is removed, the area is washed with lukewarm saline solution. We also change our gloves and surgical material before proceeding to close each layer, thus preventing the spread of tumor cells.
9. To close the wound, we approximate the subcutaneous edges first using a simple continuous suture (3-0 absorbable material). We should include small "bites" of muscle fascia from the center of the wound in order to minimize the presence of dead spaces that can predispose the formation of seromas. If a continuous suture is not possible, we can approximate the edges with a simple interrupted suture or an interrupted X suture, which should likewise include parts of the muscle fascia; subsequently, we join these stitches together in the subcutaneous suture.
10. Subcutaneous closure is performed with a different continuous suture to avoid too much tension.
11. With respect to the closure of the skin, although intradermal suturing has been described, the tension in the wound means that other cutaneous suture patterns are preferable. This includes simple interrupted stitches, X sutures, or a mattress suture, using nonabsorbable material such as 3-0 surgical nylon.

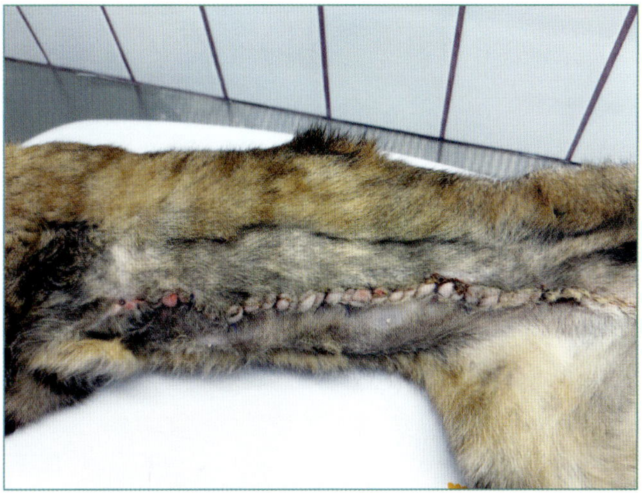

FIGURE 4. Unilateral mastectomy.

Bilateral mastectomy

This technique is indicated when tumors are detected in both mammary chains during diagnosis. One of the most significant difficulties of bilateral mastectomy is the tension created at the wound. For this reason, it is highly recommended that skin elasticity be evaluated prior to surgery, along with the chances of obtaining surgical margins with minimal tension. It is also important to note that it will be even more difficult to obtain the desired 2 cm margins.

Preparation will be the same as for unilateral mastectomies, although extending preparation of the cutaneous area to the entire abdomen.

The surgery is performed in exactly the same fashion, except that we must keep in mind a couple key points:

1. Preserving a triangular area of skin between the two mammary chains, both cranially and caudally to the incision, in order to facilitate closure (Fig. 5).
2. We have already discussed tumors that appear adhered to muscle fascia and how to resolve this, but we should also keep in mind that in the case of larger malignant tumors, we may have to remove the affected area en bloc (extracting all the abdominal musculature). In this case, the closure of this surgical wound should be done with a muscle flap or with a surgical polypropylene mesh.

Complications

Tension

Tension, especially at the cranial end of the surgical wound, is one of the most frequent complications we might come across, especially in our most obese patients.

Tension produces discomfort during the first few days after surgery, but this can be reduced with good perioperative and postoperative analgesia. It can also cause dehiscence of sutures, ulceration in the area, necrosis and inflammation of the limbs caused by edema.

Seroma

Closure in layers and the consequent elimination of dead spaces is essential to avoiding this complication.

If the seroma is minor, it is best not to intervene. In that case, we should monitor and observe until it reabsorbs on its own.

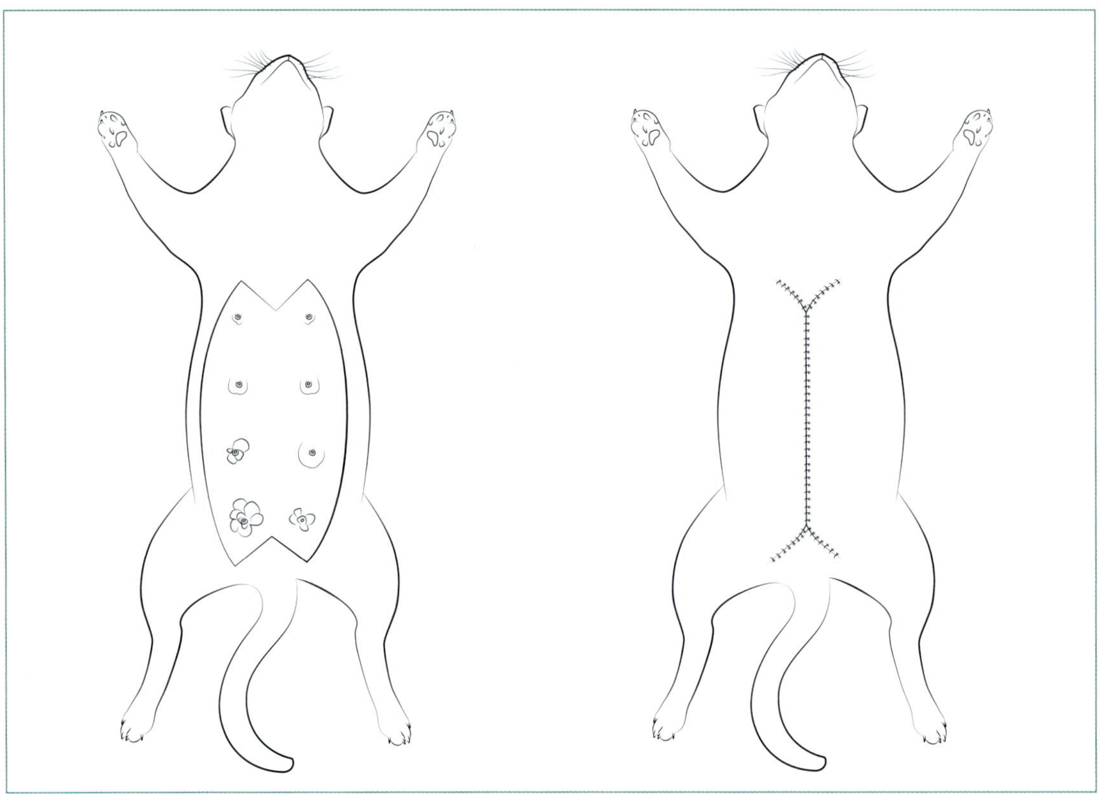

FIGURE 5. Bilateral mastectomy. It is recommended to preserve a triangular area of skin between the two mammary chains, both cranially and caudally to the incision, in order to facilitate closure.

With more significant seromas, it is not advisable to empty them with a needle and syringe. Not only does this carry a risk of infection, but it will not fundamentally resolve the issue, and as such, the seroma may refill. We have various options to resolve seromas:

- Remove the sutures, allowing the space to drain and heal by secondary intention.
- Use either a closed or open drainage system, but which we should always accompany with an abdominal compression bandage.

In either case, the procedure is accompanied by anti-inflammatory medication (NSAIDs) and analgesics.

Other complications

Although more rare, another complication could be herniation of the abdominal contents due to dehiscence of the abdominal sutures or due to loss of containment of the surgical mesh. This can only be resolved through corrective surgery.

Prognosis

The mean survival time after detection of a FMT is 10–12 months. Even so, we should keep in mind:

- **The breed:** not only do Siamese cats have a higher chance of developing malignant FMTs, but they also tend to develop them at an earlier age and have a worse prognosis.
- **The size:** the size of FMTs is one of the most important prognostic factors, since it determines the risk of developing metastasis and is associated with the recommendation to use chemotherapy as an adjuvant therapy. The survival time of patients with solitary tumors that are less than 2 cm can be over 24 months; with a size of 2–3 cm, the mean survival time is 12–24 months; and if the tumor measures over 3 cm, the survival time falls to 4–12 months.
- **The type of surgery:** it is very important to keep in mind that complete mastectomies result in a notable increase in the amount of time free of disease.
- **Histologic malignancy grade (HMG):** only valid for carcinomas.
- **COX-2 expression:** the expression of this isoenzyme may be associated with the prognosis for FMTs. Specifically, higher levels of expression have been linked with a poor prognosis, most likely because it influences the tumor's metastasic capacity, and therefore, the patient's survival. Admittedly, the results of these studies should encourage us to use long-term administration of NSAIDs as an antiangiogenic therapy for patients with FMTs, although at present, their effectiveness has not been sufficiently demonstrated.

Table 2 summarizes the factors that influence the prognosis for FMTs.

Adjuvant treatments: chemotherapy

There is not enough data to recommend the use of chemotherapy for malignant FMTs, but studies show some efficacy of cytostatic drugs such as doxorubicin, methotrexate, cyclophosphamide or vincristine (Fig. 6). Adding the use of doxorubicin and cyclophosphamide for inoperable or stage-IV FMTs, a response can be obtained in half of cases. Therefore, we believe that given the lack of more conclusive studies, making use of these protocols may be beneficial depending on the case.

TABLE 2. Prognostic factors in feline mammary tumors

Prognostic factor	Description
Size (diameter)	■ <3 cm; MST: 21–24 months ■ >3 cm; MST: 4–12 months
Clinical stage	■ I; MST: 29 months ■ II; MST: 12.5 months ■ III; MST: 9 months ■ IV; MST: 1 month
Type of surgery	If it is radical, recurrence is reduced
Mitotic index	<2 mitoses per field, better prognosis
Histologic malignancy grade (HMG)	■ Well differentiated: 100% survival 1 year after surgery ■ Poorly differentiated: 0% survival 1 year after surgery

MST: median survival time.

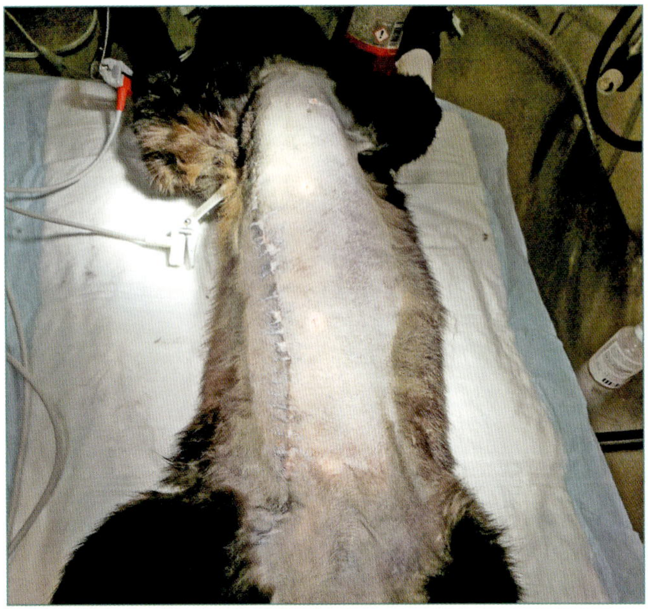

FIGURE 6. Female cat with mastectomy previously performed in the operating room for surgery of the other mammary chain. Surgical treatment is complemented with chemotherapy 15 days after the operation.

Available chemotherapy protocols

- Stage III or IV: **doxorubicin** (20–30 mg/m² or 1 mg/kg every 3 weeks IV) **+ cyclophosphamide** (100 mg/m² for 3 days every 3 weeks PO). The reported response rate is more than 50%.
- Stage III or IV: **doxorubicin** (25 mg/m² or 1 mg/kg IV) **+ cyclophosphamide** (50 mg/m² for 4 days every 3 weeks PO).
- **Surgery + carboplatin** (200 mg/m² every 3 weeks IV, 4 doses): median survival time of 428 days.
- **Surgery + doxorubicin** for tumors <2 cm: median survival time of 450 days.
- **Surgery + doxorubicin + meloxicam** (0.2 mg/kg SC at surgery, followed by 0.1 mg/kg/day for 5 days and 0.025 mg/kg/day for the rest of treatment): survival time of 460 days.
- **Surgery + mitoxantrone** (6 mg/m² every 3 weeks IV, 4 doses): survival time of 450 days.

Bibliography

Görlinger S, Kooistra HS, van den Broek A, Okkens AC. Treatment of fibroadenomatous hyperplasia in cats with aglepristone. *J Vet Intern Med*, 2002; 16(6):710–713.

Hayes AA, Mooney S. Feline mammary tumors. *Vet Clin North Am Small Anim Pract*, 1985; 15(3):513–520.

MacEwen EG, Hayes AA, Harvey HJ et al. Prognostic factors for feline mammary tumors. *J Am Vet Med Assoc*, 1984; 185(2):201–204.

McNeill CJ, Sorenmo KU, Shofer FS et al. Evaluation of adjuvant doxorubicin-based chemotherapy for the treatment of feline mammary carcinoma. *J Vet Intern Med*, 2009; 23(1):123–129.

Morris J. Mammary tumours in the cat: size matters, so early intervention saves lives. *J Feline Med Surg*, 2013; 15(5):391–400.

Ogilvie GK. Feline mammary neoplasia. *Compend Contin Educ Pract Vet*, 1983; 5:384–391.

FELINE INJECTION-SITE SARCOMA 12

Alberto Barneto and Salvador Cervantes

Introduction

In 1991, Pennsylvania saw an increase in the number of diagnoses in cats of subcutaneous tissue sarcomas located in places where vaccines were often applied. It was found to be statistically related with the increase in rabies vaccination in this state in previous years. Although it was later shown that any type of vaccine, and even other types of injections, could cause sarcomas in cats, the resulting controversy was significant in the United States and other countries. In 1996, a group of experts was appointed to scientifically study the causes, prevent them, and give the best treatment guidelines. Thus was born, in partnership with pharmaceutical laboratories, the **Vaccine-Associated Feline Sarcoma Task Force (VAFSTF)**, a working group on feline injection-site sarcoma, which continues to update its recommendations on this pathology to this day (Fig. 1).

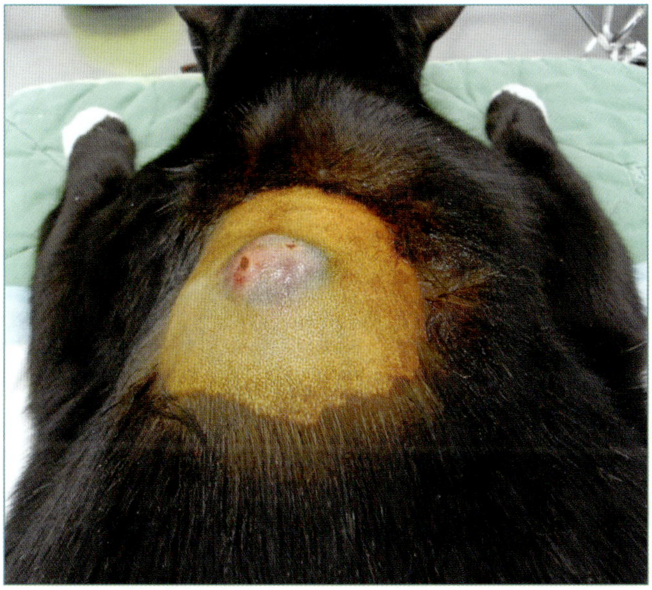

FIGURE 1. Feline injection-site sarcoma (FISS) in a standard location, the withers. This area is the most difficult to operate on, and has the most recurrence caused by surgery.

These tumors are highly invasive and have a tendency to recur locally. Although the name references sarcomas, different types thereof have been described: fibrosarcoma (the most common), liposarcoma, malignant fibrous histiocytoma, extraskeletal osteosarcoma, rhabdomyosarcoma, myofibrosarcoma and chondrosarcoma.

Epidemiology and risk factors

According to the literature, the prevalence varies from 1–3.6 cases per 10,000 vaccines administered, up to 1 out of every 400. Initially it was linked to feline leukemia vaccines, rabies vaccines, and adjuvants like aluminum hydroxide. Today we believe a mix of several factors is involved, and that the patient's genetic disposition plays a large role, along with the number of injections in the same area. Sarcomas of this type have been described after all types of injections and even implants like microchips. It has not been demonstrated that any specific manufacturer or type of vaccine causes more such sarcomas than others. It has also not been demonstrated that any specific practice (using a certain caliber of needle, mixing vaccines in one syringe, or shaking the vials more vigorously) promotes or protects from this condition. It was discovered in 2006, however, that populations of cats affected by this disease had a genetic alteration in the *p53* gene, which protects against tumors. This would explain the irregular distribution of FISS diagnoses in different countries over the past 30 years.

> In general, it is believed that any type of chronic or repeated inflammation in genetically predisposed cats can give rise to injection-site sarcomas.

In terms of predisposition by age, there are two peaks of presentation in cats, one at 6–7 years of age and a later peak at 10–11 years of age.

Clinical course and signs

These sarcomas develop between 4 weeks and 10 years after vaccination. The clinician should be aware of the speed of onset in some cases and advise cat owners to watch for the first signs of postinjection inflammation.

This type of sarcoma grows faster than other sarcomas that appear in older or geriatric cats.

It usually begins with firm inflammation of the subcutaneous tissues in an area that was previously injected with any substance. Shortly thereafter, a painless mass with undefined borders may appear. This mass may or may not be fixed to the underlying structures. Sometimes necrosis is observed, along with the consequent accumulation of fluid in the center of the mass, caused by rapid growth of the tumoral mass. This causes an even greater increase in volume of the sarcoma (Fig. 2).

Diagnosis

As with any mass that exhibits abnormal growth, the primary diagnostic test is biopsy. Cytologies using fine needle aspiration are not advised for this type of tumor for two reasons: sarcomas do not shed easily, so it is easy to get an insufficient sample that the pathology laboratory will reject. Secondly, since the presence of necrosis-associated seromas is frequent, a sample of the existing inflammatory process may be obtained, resulting in a false negative diagnosis (low sensitivity of the test). Therefore, the test with the highest sensitivity and specificity for FISS is **incisional biopsy**. Clinicians are advised to take a sample that is sufficiently representative (the ideal is in the shape of an orange wedge in its depth). In addition, in contrast to the usual recommendation to obtain margins of healthy tissue during incisional biopsies, if FISS is suspected, the sample should not include the periphery in order to avoid increasing inflammation and causing tumors to appear in new areas (Fig. 3).

Once inflammation is identified (or a mass if transformation has already occurred), the patient should be referred to an advanced imaging test, usually computed tomography (CT), although magnetic resonance (MR) may also be useful. These techniques are especially helpful in the second part of the diagnosis/treatment process, which is surgery, and they enable the surgeon to plan the depth that they should reach in order to leave the margins of the wound clean (Fig. 4).

These tumors have a low distant metastatic capacity, with the prevalence of metastasis being 0%–26%. The most common place where metastasis may appear is in the lungs. Therefore, a plain X-ray can be very helpful in ruling out this complication (Fig. 5).

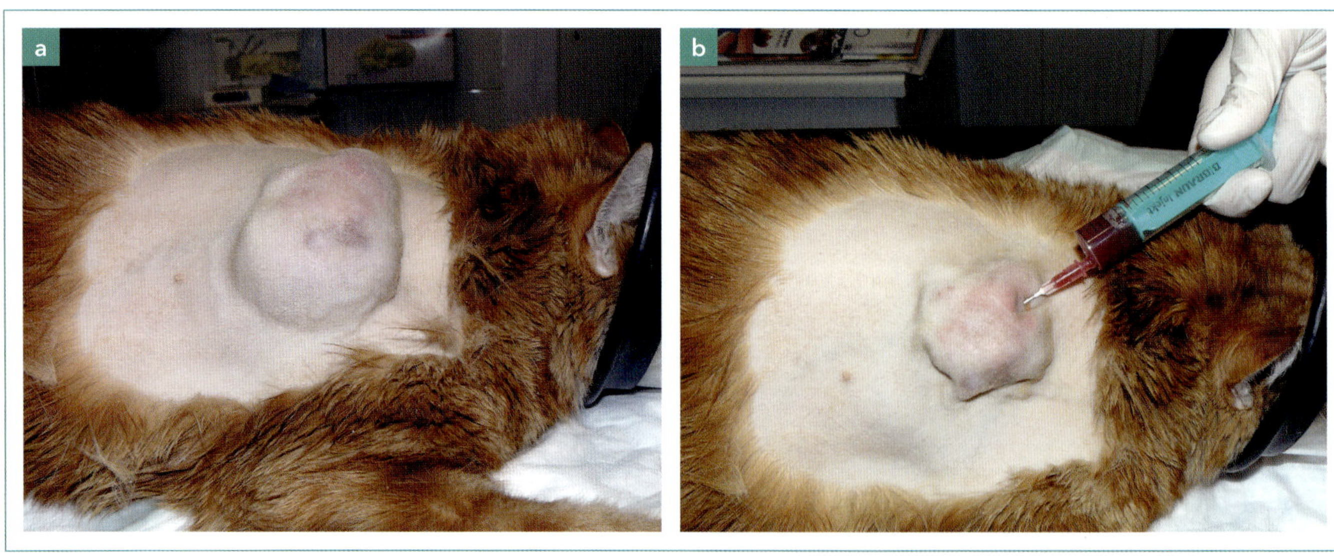

FIGURE 2. Large feline injection-site sarcoma (FISS) with serohemorrhagic fluid originating from interior necrosis. This fluid should not be used for cytological diagnosis because the likelihood that it contains sarcoma cells is low. Once emptied, an incisional biopsy should be performed.

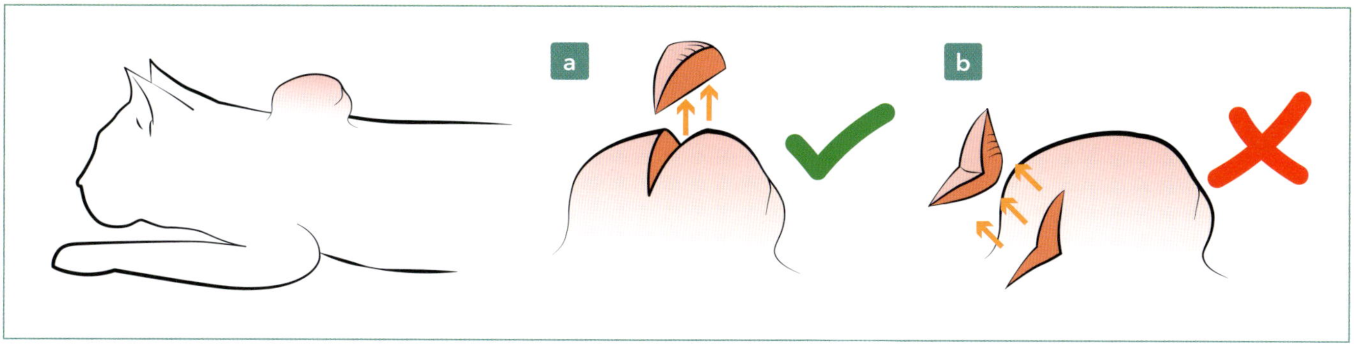

FIGURE 3. Incisional biopsy of sarcoma performed (a) correctly and (b) incorrectly.

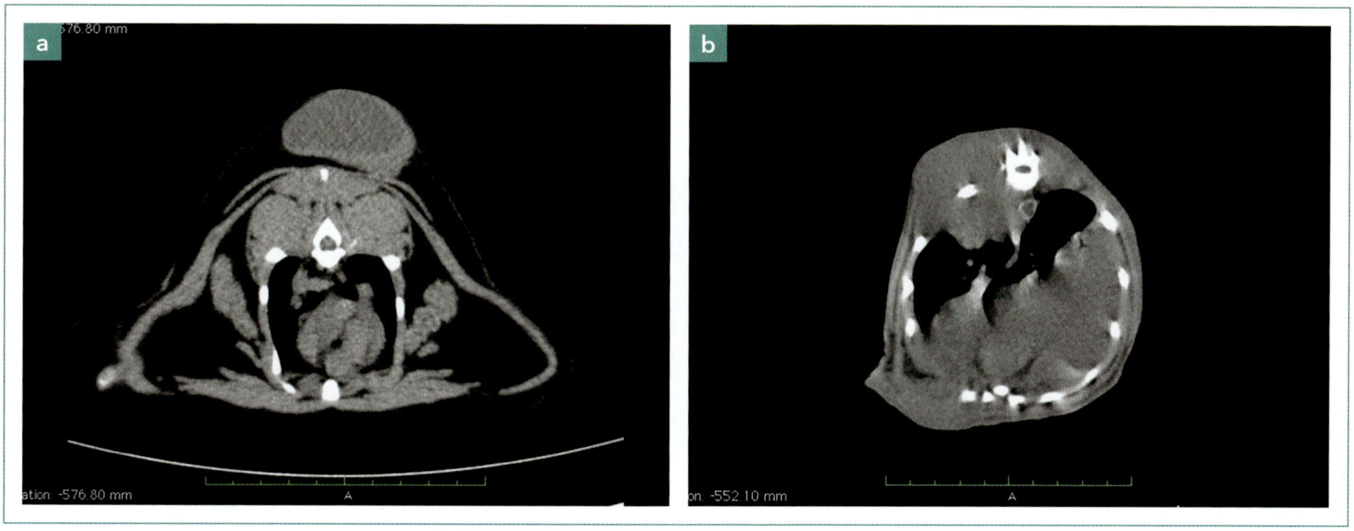

FIGURE 4. (a) Computed tomography of a well-defined case of feline injection-site sarcoma (FISS) located on a small piece of muscular tissue. Wide surgical removal had a curative effect in this case. (b) Computed tomography of a complex case of FISS. Infiltration in deep dorsal planes, up to the pleural cavity, is seen. The sarcoma recurred because it had not been removed correctly. Previous therapy and a second surgery were not sufficient to control the disease. Images courtesy of Diagnosfera.

VIDEO

Computed tomography of the case from Figure 4a, where it is confirmed that the tumor does not go beyond the muscle fascia, with good prognosis after wide oncological surgery (video courtesy of Diagnosfera)

VIDEO

Computed tomography of the case from Figure 4b, where infiltration in deep dorsal planes, up to the pleural cavity, is seen, with poor prognosis (video courtesy of Diagnosfera)

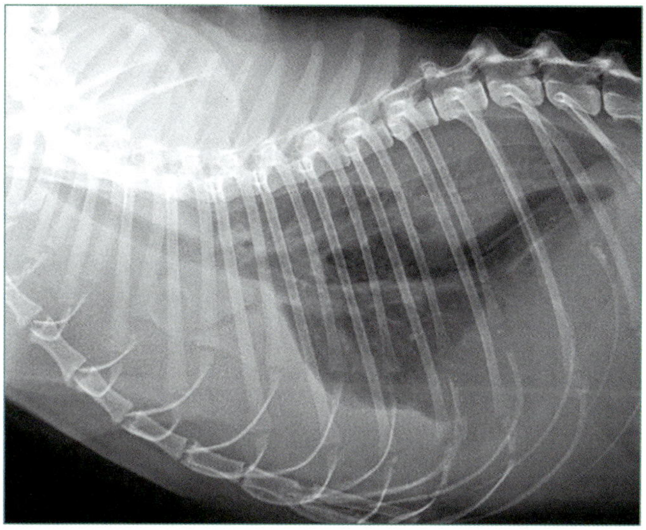

FIGURE 5. Pulmonary metastasis of the sarcoma shown in Figure 4b.

3-2-1 rule to alert veterinarians and pet owners of a possible FISS

In 1999, the conclusions of the VAFSTF (the American group of experts known as the Vaccine-Associated Feline Sarcoma Task Force) led to the publication of a large number of recommendations for the early detection and prevention of this disease. One of them was the 3-2-1 rule for owners to understand when to see a veterinarian if they suspect this type of tumor:

- If a mass persists at an injection site for more than 3 months* after the injection.
- If a mass is present and it is larger than 2 cm, regardless of the amount of time since the injection.
- If a mass continues increasing in size 1 month after the injection.

* In some of the authors' clinics, the recommendation is not to wait more than 2 months, since their experience has led them to think that if postinjection inflammation or a mass persists more than 2 months, it should be removed before transformation occurs.

Treatment

The most successful treatment is centered around radical surgery, including clean margins of 3–5 cm at the periphery and 1–2 planes of fascia in depth. If it occurs in a limb, total amputation is advised. Unfortunately, these tumors grow very rapidly. Therefore, in many cases, removal of the tumor as the sole modality of treatment is not feasible.

Surgery for this disease is designed on the basis of advanced imaging of the affected area (CT or MR). Safety margins are essential in FISS surgery: several studies noted that the tumor margins exhibited healthy tissue macroscopically, while histologically, the accumulation of lymphoid cells and active macrophages conferred characteristics of malignancy to the tumor. Therefore, from the perspective of practice, there are two types of surgical removals for this disease:

1. **Wide surgical removal:** surgical margins of 2–3 cm on each side, and removal of one fascia (one muscle) in depth. This approach is usually applied in early-stage tumors located in areas that are easily resectable in depth.
2. **Radical surgical removal:** surgical margins of 5 cm on each side, and at least 2 fascias (2 muscles) in depth. If signs of malignancy are observed or if the tumor is located in areas that are difficult to operate, this modality is usually chosen. Radical removal includes amputation of the limb in cases with appendicular sarcoma.

The location of FISS varies (Figs. 6 and 7). Of course, since it is associated with injection sites, statistically they are located in certain regions more frequently:

- **Interscapular area:** the use of this area is on the decline, since more and more veterinarians are following the recommendations of the VAFSTF for vaccination in cats (see below). Radical removal requires the elimination of certain vertebral spinous processes and sometimes a partial scapulectomy.
- **Hind limbs:** depending on how distal the location of the tumor is, coxofemoral disarticulation or some level of hemipelvectomy is performed.
- **Forelimbs:** partial scapulectomy is done frequently if the tumor appears on the surface of this bone.

Surgical technique

Once a wide surgical field is shaved and disinfected, we make an oval-shaped incision around the tumor, at a distance of 3 or 5 cm, depending on the chosen modality of removal (Fig. 8). After incising the skin and subcutaneous tissue on one end, we deepen the dissection without moving towards the tumor, going down through the number of muscles that will be included in the removal (Fig. 9). At the same time as the muscle is dissected, it may be necessary, depending on the area, to perform osteotomies (spinous processes, scapula, pelvis) or disarticulations in full limb amputations. Hemostasis is carried out carefully through electrocautery, hemostatic clips or sutures.

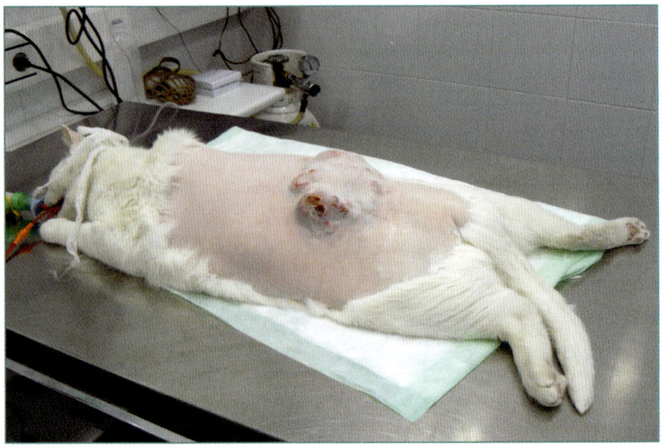

FIGURE 6. Feline injection-site sarcoma (FISS) located in the dorsolumbar region, standard location of subcutaneous injections. The more caudal the tumor is to the withers, the easier it is to remove.

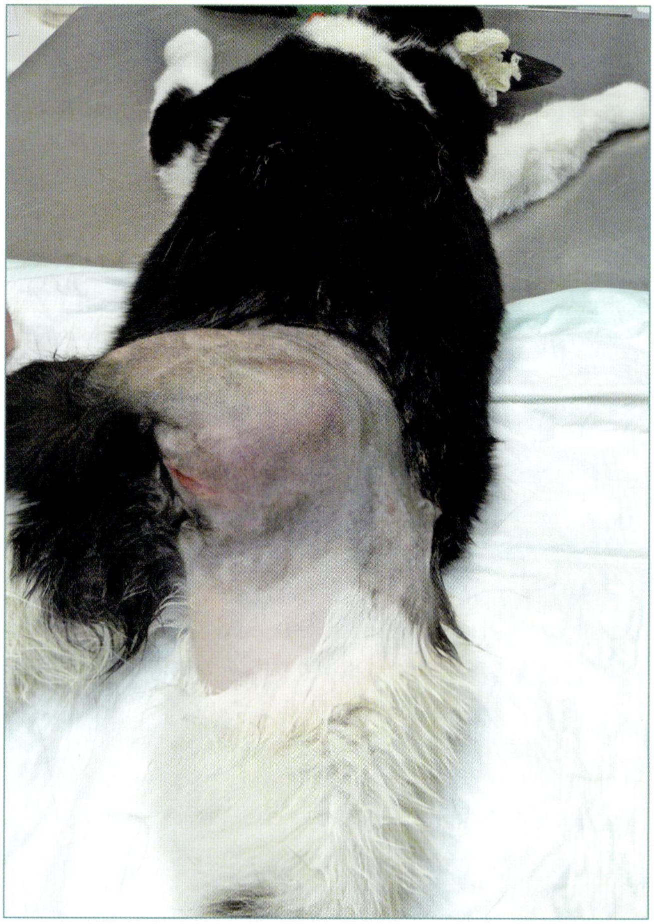

FIGURE 7. Liposarcoma located in the region of the coxofemoral joint. Radical surgical removal is mandatory, with amputation of the hind limb, including some level of hemipelvectomy.

It is essential to understand that this is an oncological surgery: **the goal is not to touch or come close to the tumor.**

Absorbable sutures are preferred in order to decrease the risk of new tumors resulting from chronic inflammation associated with the suture material. Reconstruction of the defect is done via approximation of the muscles and connective tissue. Sometimes muscle advancement flaps and often skin flaps are required. Before closing, it is highly recommended to apply a fenestrated catheter system through which irrigation with local anesthesia can be administered postoperatively (Fig. 10).

The entire specimen is sent to the pathology laboratory en bloc, identifying each edge with sutures (different stitches in each area, with explanations notated in the report). Sometimes the edge of the tumor is the same as the edge of the removed tissue. If that is the case, repetition of the surgery is advised, widening the surgical margins to the location indicated by the laboratory.

If the surgery was not sufficiently effective, several adjuvant treatments have been described that can improve the effectiveness of the therapy and lengthen the survival time. Based on their experience, the authors prefer to use these treatments **before surgery** to reduce the size and edges of the FISS, thus improving the chance of recovery.

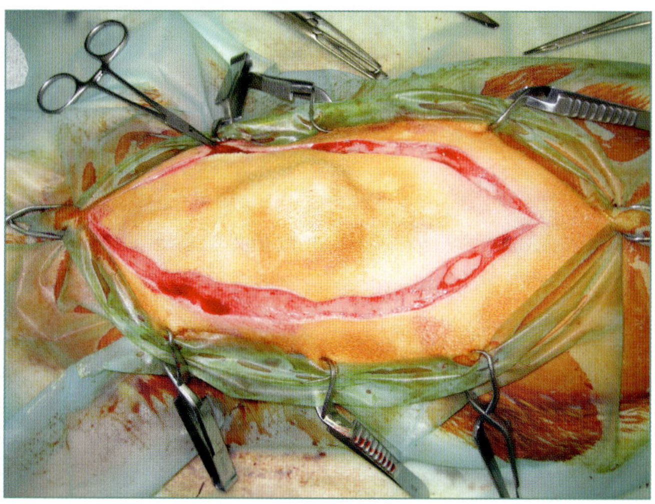

FIGURE 8. Initial planning of radical surgical technique for a dorsolumbar sarcoma.

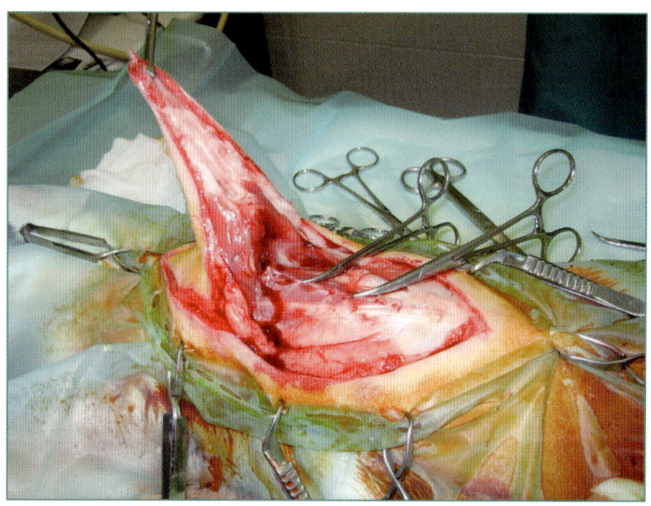

FIGURE 9. Resection of the sarcoma in the previous figure. Two deep muscular planes were removed, along with ostectomy of the local dorsal and lumbar spinous processes. All of this was done at the beginning of the incision, so that the surgeon could stay several centimeters away from the tumor during the entire intervention.

Reasons for treatment failure

The most important factors leading to surgical treatment failure are:

1. Large tumors (>5 cm)
2. Patients that have undergone several surgeries in the area
3. Histological type: malignant fibrous histiocytomas have a worse prognosis than fibrosarcomas
4. Incomplete surgical margins
5. Presence of metastasis before surgery

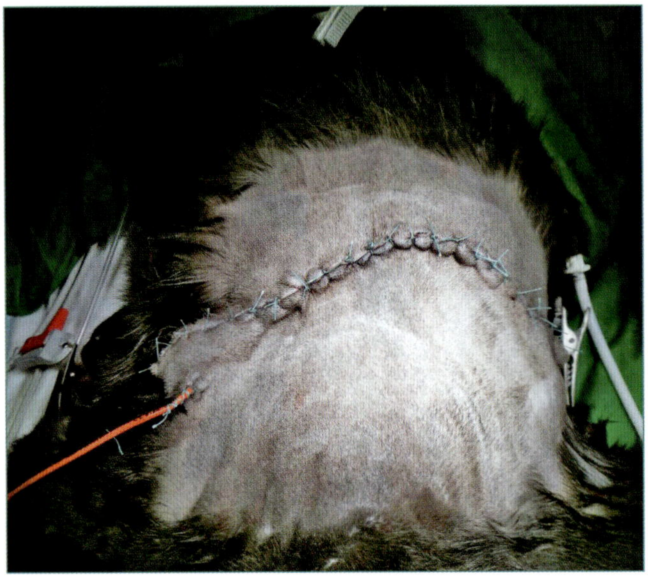

FIGURE 10. Fenestrated catheter system for the application of postoperative local anesthesia.

Radiation therapy

This can be applied preoperatively or postoperatively. The objective of preoperative radiation therapy is to reduce the quantity of viable tumor, thus reducing the length and depth of the incision with clear margins. Postoperative application is used as an adjuvant treatment when the surgical excision is not complete.

Chemotherapy

As in the above case, this can be used before or after surgery to attempt to reduce the amount of affected tissue, or as an adjuvant therapy in the case of incomplete removal. Usually, drugs such as doxorubicin (or, if available, epirubicin) or mitoxantrone are administered (Table 1).

Electrochemotherapy

Cases of treatment with electrochemotherapy have begun to be published in the last few years. In these cases, electricity is applied to tumor cells so that they become more permeable to chemotherapy drugs. Protocols with intratumoral bleomycin and/or cisplatin have been used with good results. In cats, cisplatin should not be administered via systemic injection due to the severe risk of potentially deadly pulmonary disease associated with the dose.

Immunotherapy

It has been shown that interleukin-2, induced by injection of the recombinant canarypox virus expressing feline interleukin-2, combined with surgery and/or brachytherapy significantly reduces the frequency of relapse.

TABLE 1. Chemotherapy drugs that have shown some activity against injection-site sarcomas

Chemotherapy drug	Dose
Doxorubicin (anthracycline)	1 mg/kg IV every 3 weeks (not to exceed 20–25 mg/m² per dose or 240 mg/m² of total dose), 3 cycles
Mitoxantrone (anthracycline)	5.5–6.5 mg/m² IV every 3 weeks, 3 cycles
Epirubicin (anthracycline)	25 mg/m²
Toceranib (tyrosine kinase inhibitor)	1.5–3.5 mg/kg, 2–3 times per week

AAFP/AAHA recommendations for feline vaccination with respect to FISS prevention (2020)

- Avoid administering multiple injections in the same spot or area.
- Warm vaccines to room temperature before inoculation.
- Use new needles with the lowest caliber possible.
- There is an international convention that offers guidelines on where to vaccinate cats (Fig. 11):
  - Never inject in the interscapular area.
  - Inject limbs and as distally as possible.
  - Consider the tail as an injection site (in the author's experience it is a painful area due to the small amount of loose connective tissue).
  - An alternative is subcutaneous injection in the abdomen.
- Keep a record of the injection sites, along with information on the vaccine that was administered.

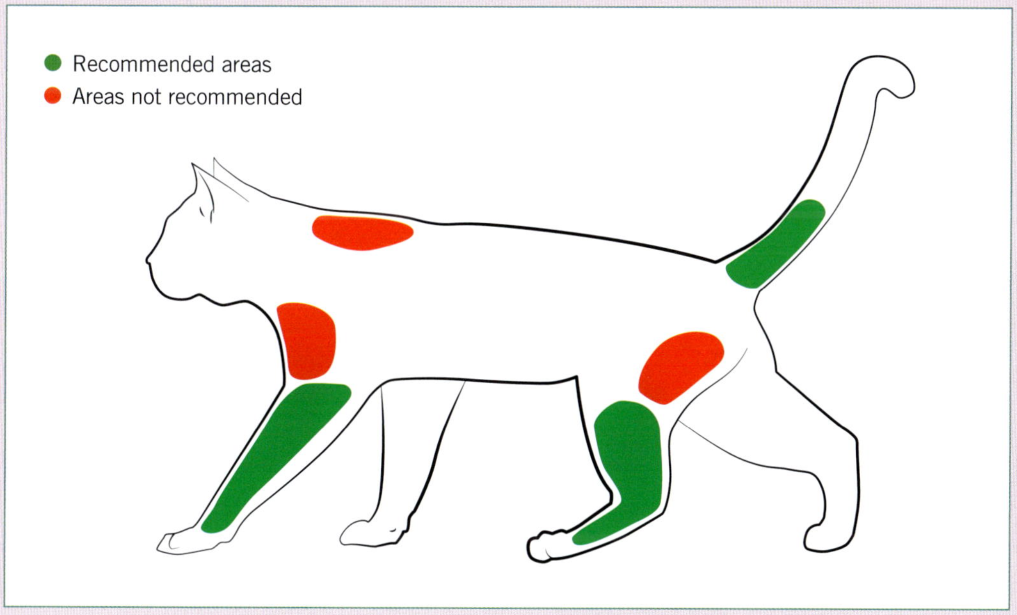

FIGURE 11. Areas that are recommended or not recommended for feline vaccination by the AAFP/AAHA, with the goal of prevention and effective treatment of injection-site sarcoma.

Prevention

Feline vaccination guides published by the AAFP/AAHA (American Association of Feline Practitioners/American Animal Hospital Association, latest edition from 2020) include some recommendations related to FISS prevention.

The goal of these recommendations is to minimize the occurrence of FISS, but when it does occur, the goal is that its location would enable safe removal with wide margins, leading to the patient being cured.

Prognosis

The prognosis is always guarded given the high recurrence rate of FISS. Early detection and effective surgical treatment has been shown to be the most effective protocol to cure this disease.

Bibliography

Banerji N, Kanjilal S. Somatic alterations of the *p53* tumor suppressor gene in vaccine-associated feline sarcoma. *Am J Vet Res*, 2006; 67(10):1766–1772.

Bray J, Polton G. Neoadjuvant and adjuvant chemotherapy combined with anatomical resection of feline injection-site sarcoma: results in 21 cats. *Vet Comp Oncol*, 2016; 14(2):147–160.

Esplin DG, Campbell R. Widespread metastasis of a fibrosarcoma associated with vaccination site in a cat. *Feline Pract*, 1995; 23(1):13–16.

Gobar GM, Kass PH. World Wide Web-based survey of vaccination practices, postvaccinal reactions, and vaccine site-associated sarcomas in cats. *J Am Vet Med Assoc*, 2002; 220(10):1477–1482.

Hartmann K, Day MJ, Thiry E et al., European Advisory Board on Cat Diseases. Feline injection-site sarcoma: ABCD guidelines on prevention and management. *J Feline Med Surg*, 2015; 17(7):606–613.

Hendrick MJ, Goldschmidt MH, Shofer FS et al. Postvaccinal sarcomas in the cat: epidemiology and electron probe microanalytical identification of aluminum. *Cancer Res*, 1992; 52(19):5391–5394.

Hendrick MJ, Goldschmidt MH. Do injection site reactions induce fibrosarcomas in cats? *J Am Vet Med Assoc*, 1991; 199(8):968.

Kass PH, Barnes WG Jr, Spangler WL et al. Epidemiologic evidence for a causal relation between vaccination and fibrosarcoma tumorigenesis in cats. *J Am Vet Med Assoc*, 1993; 203(3):396–405.

Knapp DW, Richardson RC, DeNicola DB et al. Cisplatin toxicity in cats. *J Vet Intern Med*, 1987; 1(1):29–35.

Ladlow J. Injection site-associated sarcoma in the cat: treatment recommendations and results to date. *J Feline Med Surg*, 2013; 15(5):409–418.

Martano M, Morello E, Buracco P. Feline injection-site sarcoma: past, present and future perspectives. *Vet J*, 2011; 188(2):136–141.

Phelps HA, Kuntz CA, Milner RJ et al. Radical excision with five-centimeter margins for treatment of feline injection-site sarcomas: 91 cases (1998–2002). *J Am Vet Med Assoc*, 2011; 239(1):97–106.

Spugnini EP, Vincenzi B, Carocci F et al. Combination of bleomycin and cisplatin as adjuvant electrochemotherapy protocol for the treatment of incompletely excised feline injection-site sarcomas: A retrospective study. *Open Vet J*, 2020; 10(3):267–271.

Stone AE, Brummet GO, Carozza EM et al. 2020 AAHA/AAFP Feline Vaccination Guidelines. *J Am Anim Hosp Assoc*, 2020; 56:249–265.

Vaccine-Associated Feline Sarcoma Task Force guidelines. Diagnosis and treatment of suspected sarcomas. *J Am Vet Med Assoc*, 1999; 214(12):1745.

Vaccine-Associated Feline Sarcoma Task Force: Roundtable Discussion. The current understanding and management of vaccine-associated sarcomas in cats. *J Am Vet Med Assoc*, 2005; 226(11):1821–1842.

Woodward KN. Origins of injection-site sarcomas in cats: the possible role of chronic inflammation-a review. *ISRN Vet Sci*, 2011; 2011:210982.

3

HEAD AND NECK SURGERY

RECONSTRUCTIVE SURGERY OF THE HARD AND SOFT PALATE 13

Alberto Barneto

Surgical anatomy

The palate of the cat is a bony and soft tissue structure that separates the oral and nasal cavities. It constitutes the roof of the oral cavity and is divided into an anterior part (**hard palate**) and a posterior part (**soft palate**). Based on their embryological origin, these are differentiated into a primary and a secondary palate. The **primary palate** extends from the lip to the caudal portion of the premaxilla (incisive bone). The **secondary palate** (which we will deal with in this chapter) includes the rest of the hard palate and the soft palate.

The hard palate is formed by the confluence of the **incisive, maxillary and palatine bones**. All are joined by suture joints. The mucosa of the hard palate forms cornified grooves of squamous epithelium and has no muscles. The soft palate, however, has a mucosa full of mucoid glands and several muscles that give it firmness and mobility. The soft palate joins caudally to both sides of the pharyngeal and mandibular mucosa, forming the **folds of the fauces** or caudal oral mucosa. On each side of the palatine bones, medial to each 4th premolar, are the **greater palatine foramina**, through which the two **greater palatine arteries** arise, which run cranially and are responsible for irrigating all the structures of the hard palate. The **lesser palatine arteries** also originate from the **maxillary artery** and are responsible for irrigating the soft palate, together with branches of the ascending pharyngeal artery and the greater palatine artery. They exit the skull through the two **lesser palatine foramina**, one on each side, immediately caudal to the greater palatine foramina.

The sensory innervation of the palate arises from the maxillary division of the **trigeminal nerve**, giving rise to the **greater and lesser palatine nerves**, which exit the skull alongside the homonymous arteries. The musculature of the soft palate is innervated by branches of the glossopharyngeal and vagus nerves.

Surgical diseases of the feline palate

Cleft palate

A congenital malformation with a recessive genetic cause of transmission, although intrauterine factors such as exposure to toxins or some infections also play a role in its occurrence. Classically, it affects the midline of the secondary palate (soft portion only or both). Its presentation, upon clinical examination, is a longitudinal defect in the center of the organ with a lack of tissue and rounded edges, which leaves the oral and nasal cavities in direct contact with each other. Kittens present with sucking difficulties when suckling, excrete milk through their nostrils and exhibit growth failure. A simple visual examination of the palate is sufficient to diagnose it, although the presence of other congenital defects should be evaluated (Fig. 1). Surgical correction too early (before 8 weeks) may carry an increased risk of dehiscence during healing. Until the kitten can be operated on,

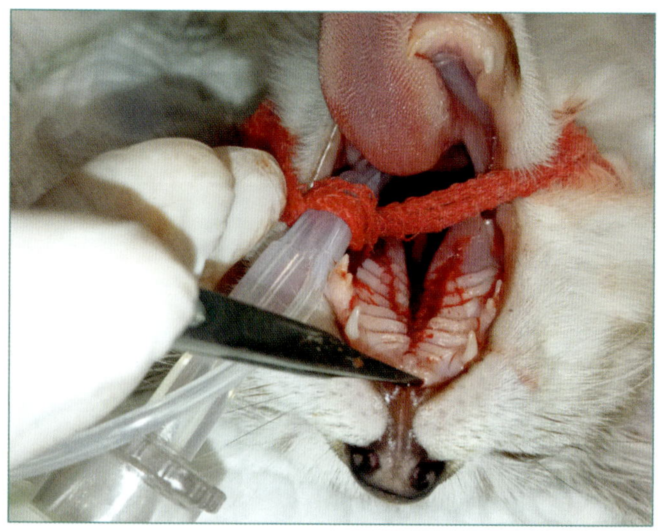

FIGURE 1. Kitten with cleft palate affecting both the hard and soft palate. Its caregiver fed it with an oral tube and syringe. When the kitten reached 1 kg in weight, the cleft palate was resolved in two phases: first the hard palate and then the soft palate.

it should be fed fluids through a tube or syringe, preferably in an upright position.

Palate fracture

The most classic traumatic causes are falls from high buildings (higher incidence of fractures in falls from a height of more than two floors). Due to the cat's instinct to place itself in the extended paw and standing position when falling (cat-righting reflex —CRR—), when they touch the ground the head hits the jaw, frequently resulting in a fracture of the mandibular symphysis (see Ch. 30, Fig. 8) and the palate (Fig. 2).

Oronasal fistulas

These defects are usually caused by necrosis of the palatal tissue. The causes in feline medicine are usually infectious (calicivirus complicated with chronic bacterial superinfections) or traumatic (burns from biting wires, caustic substances, unconsolidated fractures, etc.). When oronasal fistulas affect one or several dental alveoli, they are associated with periapical infections that generate osteomyelitis and a loss of considerable bone tissue in the maxilla. Palatal wounds of any origin tend to be complicated in cats, especially young cats, by bacterial infections. Treatment should always be based on the results of an antibiogram, knowledge of the patient's retroviral status and a sufficiently long course of therapy.

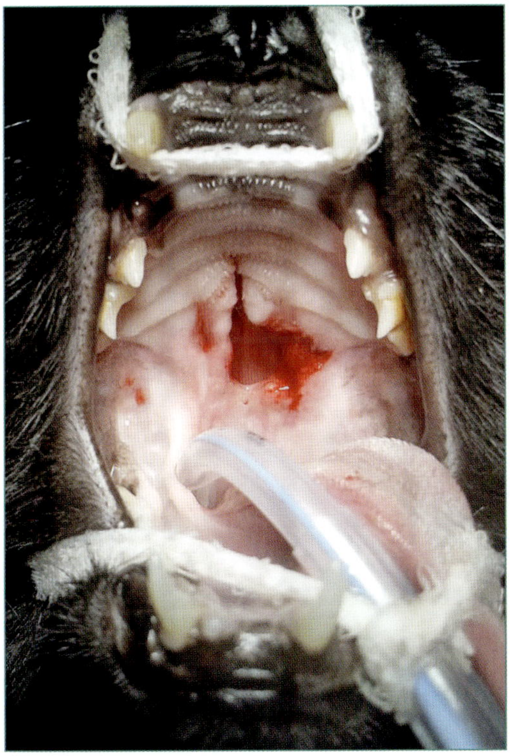

FIGURE 2. Defect of the soft and hard palates following a fall from a great height. The patient had been suffering from the wound for some time and it was complicated by chronic rhinitis, which lengthened the healing process.

Neoplasms of the palate

More common in older cats. The most frequent are squamous cell carcinomas, but fibrosarcomas, melanomas and eosinophilic plaques affecting the palate have also been described.

Diagnosis

The diagnosis of defects and other pathologies of the palate is clearly established from a clinical perspective: cats move their tongues excessively when eating, make noises when swallowing and sneeze after eating and especially when drinking.

> Whenever a cat presents with chronic rhinitis, the palate should be thoroughly explored for oronasal communications.

Even if the opening in the palate is not painful, the authors recommend sedating the patient in order to be able to perform a complete exploration, including the hard and soft palate, searching for deformities or abnormal tissues, gums and periodontal spaces.

> Many times very deteriorated teeth hide communications between alveoli and the nasal cavity.

The only imaging technique that can help in unclear cases is a CT scan, although its use is limited in the palate. It is recommended when we want to evaluate the extent of a lesion or the possibility of metastasis in cases of neoplasia.

Congenital palate defects should be diagnosed as early as possible (ideally screened in newborns), treated clinically with the necessary nutritional supplements and the surgical intervention scheduled as late as possible so that growth does not affect surgical success.

Preoperative and postoperative considerations

Aspects to be considered:

- Complicated or extensive palate defects will very often require several interventions and a long healing time, as well as the combination of various reconstructive techniques. This point should be made clear to the animal's caretaker and their cooperation should be sought in order to successfully resolve the case.
- The surgical field is cleaned with a swab moistened with an antiseptic solution (1% chlorhexidine or povidone iodine). Even so, these surgeries are considered clean-contaminated.
- Prior antibiotic therapy should be based on the results of the culture and antibiogram, especially in cases associated with chronic rhinitis.
- The use of an Elizabethan collar should be considered after surgery to avoid self-injury.
- Some complicated cases may require the use of feeding tubes to minimize trauma to the sutures.
- Feeding a soft diet during the first postoperative week is preferred.

Guidelines for a successful oral mucosal flap

- Always dissect flaps larger than the defect to be covered.
- Carefully study the anatomy in order to choose the most appropriate technique and preserve vascularization during the procedure (especially the greater palatine artery).
- Always incise tissues using a scalpel blade, which is less traumatic for the edges.
- Avoid placing sutures directly over the defect. It is preferable to always suture in two nonoverlapping layers (nasal and oral).
- The stitches should be placed using a good amount of tissue in order to preserve the vascularization of the wound edge. They should be placed without excessive tension, as this may induce retraction.
- When possible, choose 4-0 or 5-0 monofilament absorbable sutures and a continuous suture pattern. The fewer the number of knots, the less stimulus for trauma from the cat's abrasive tongue.

Surgical techniques

Double mucoperiosteal flap (hinged flap + bipedicled flap) for closure of a congenital cleft palate

The most commonly used techniques for the resolution of a cleft palate are double flap techniques, which are more effective because they provide a double reconstruction: the nasal mucosa on the one hand, and the oral mucosa on the other. The procedure can be done in two steps (hard palate and then soft palate) or both in the same surgical procedure. If it is done in two steps, the authors usually recommend leaving a one-month interval between the two surgeries.

Technique

1. The technique is started by incising one of the edges of the defect with a scalpel blade until the end of the hard palate is reached. A small strip 1–2 mm thick is removed along the entire length of the edge of the cleft palate. On the other edge of the defect, a longitudinal incision is made with the scalpel blade, leaving a band of palatal mucosa wide enough to cover the defect once the hinge flap is made (the measurement should be approximately 2.5 times the width of the palate defect). This second incision (and its resulting flap) has a **partial thickness** (Fig. 3.1).
2. Both sides of the defect are bluntly dissected using Stevens tenotomy scissors or with the aid of a Freer periosteal elevator. Dissection of the first lateral side along the entire length of the defect will serve to allow for a sufficiently wide bed to receive the sutures of the flap of the other side. On the second side, dissection is performed carefully to leave the entire length of the flap free until it can be rotated 180° and the free edge is apposed to the edge of the other side of the defect. Care must be taken to preserve arterial vascularization and not to perforate the palatal mucosa right at the angle of the hinge (Fig. 3.2).
3. The nasal **hinge flap** suture is placed with an atraumatic needle, 4-0 or 5-0 absorbable monofilament material (depending on the size of the kitten) and simple interrupted stitches, following the guidelines for oral reconstructive surgery (Fig. 3.3).
4. Once the defect is closed, with the reconstruction of the nasal part of the mucosa, we prepare to reconstruct the oral mucosa. Two bilateral incisions are made, parallel and adjacent to the maxillary dental arch, to create a **double bipedicled flap**. The flaps maintain their insertions rostral and

caudal to the palatal mucosa. Dissection of the bed should be complete **except in the area medial to the 4th premolar**, where the major palatine artery exits through the palatine foramen. If we dissect the tissues with sufficient width, the mobility of both flaps will be sufficient to suture them at the midline (Fig. 3.4).

5. To reconstruct the oral mucosal layer, we suture the entire length of both flaps at the midline of the palate, handling the tissues carefully. We will use 4-0 or 5-0 absorbable or non-absorbable material with an atraumatic needle. The authors prefer a continuous mattress suture to reduce the number of knots, which could lead to the kitten causing trauma with the spicules of its tongue (Fig. 3.5).
6. After the technique, there will be defects on each side of the hard palate, parallel to the dental arch. They will close by secondary intention without issue (by means of granulation tissue) in a few days (Fig. 3.6).

> Another technique for defects that are not too large is to make a bilateral double hinge flap with both smaller lips, which would be sutured in the center with interrupted stitches for closure and reconstruction of the nasal mucosa.

7. Once the hard palate defect is closed, we will do the same with the soft palate. The scalpel blade incision will be longitudinal, full thickness, trimming approximately 1–2 mm along both edges of the defect to the end of the soft palate. Thus, in the midline, we will obtain a double layer of tissue to make the double suture. If the defect is large, we may need partial thickness dissection to give elasticity to both sides of the soft palate. Sometimes, we may even need to make two parallel unloading incisions, at a certain distance from the midline, to improve the elasticity of the suture (similar to the double bipedicled flap).
8. We will first reconstruct the part of the nasal mucosa, with a continuous or interrupted suture pattern, starting at the end of the soft palate and proceeding in a rostral direction. We will use 4-0 or 5-0 absorbable monofilament material and an atraumatic needle. The second layer is performed the same way to close the defect in the oral cavity. In this second layer the authors prefer a continuous mattress suture. If the defect is very large or there is significant atrophy of the soft palate, we may need to make two partial-thickness unloading incisions parallel to the central incision and adjacent to the fauces, which will remain open after the repair and will heal in a few days by secondary intention.

Figures 4–9 show the application of this technique in the patient in Figure 1.

Split palatal U-flap

This technique was described in 1991 for the closure of very caudal defects of the hard palate or even those affecting the cranial part of the soft palate in dogs and cats. The origin of these defects is usually the formation of oronasal fistulas due to necrosis of the palatal tissue.

Technique

1. The mucosa is incised about 2 mm adjacent to the dental arch on both sides, starting at the level of the 4th premolar, and is joined by the cranial portion of the hard palate, forming a U. A second smaller U-shaped incision is made, following the cranial edge of the defect. We join both incisions with a third one at the midline of the hard palate, thus drawing the double split palatal U-flap. The length of this third incision should be slightly longer than the defect to be covered (Fig. 10.1).
2. The full thickness of both flaps is dissected, taking care to respect the greater palatine arteries. We must also finish dissecting the entire edge of the defect, or rather trim the entire thickness with a scalpel blade (Fig. 10.2).
3. One of the flaps is transposed first, rotating it towards the midline and covering the most caudal part of the defect. It is sutured in two layers (nasal and oral) with monofilament material in a simple interrupted pattern. In cats this is sometimes difficult, so a single-layer suture is acceptable (Fig. 10.3).
4. Finally, the flap on the other side is rotated in the opposite direction as the first flap and sutured to the first rotated flap and to the opposite side of the dental arch. A bony portion of the cranial part of the hard palate will be exposed and will heal by secondary intention in a few days (Figs. 10.4 and 11).

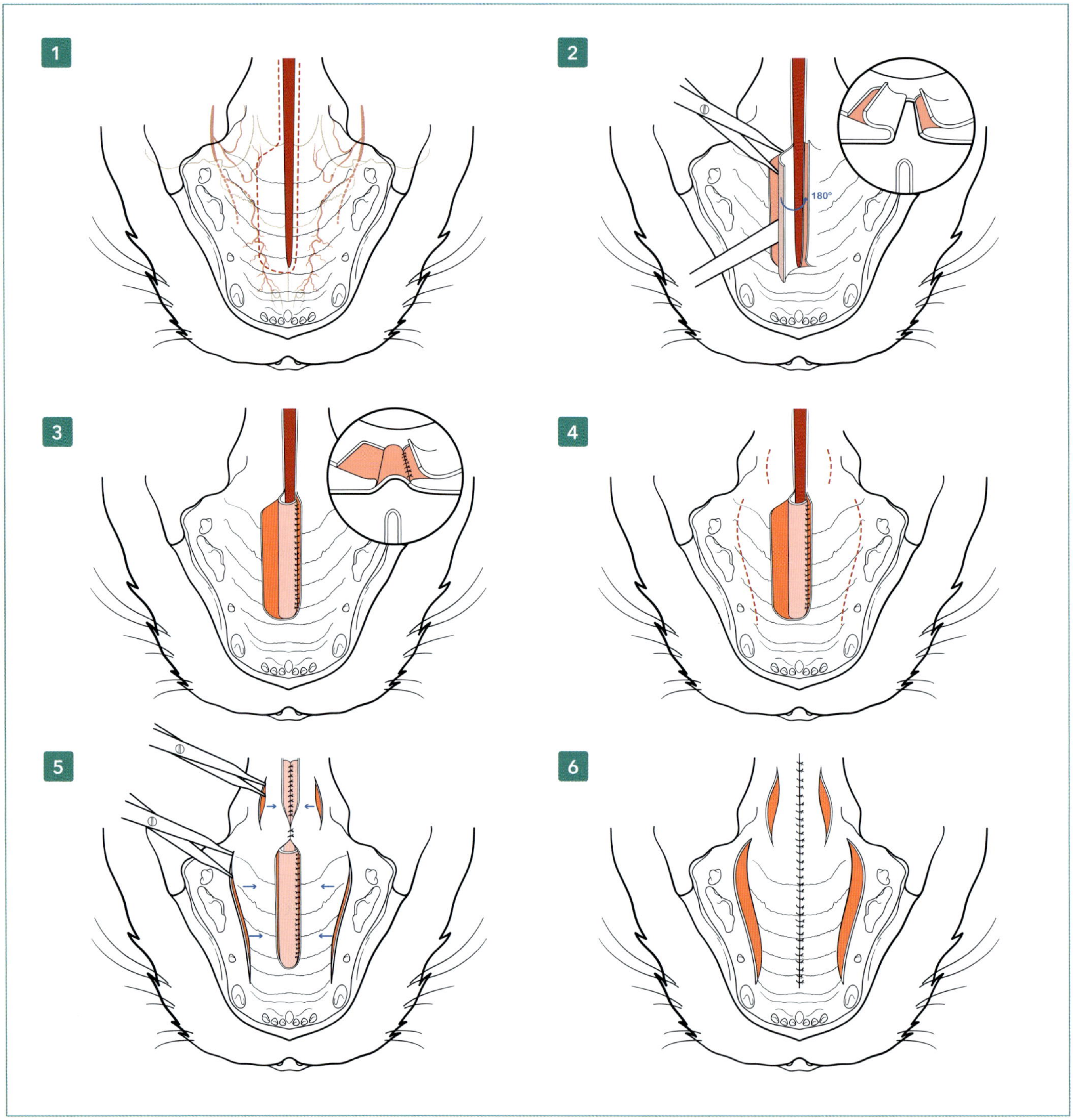

FIGURE 3. Steps of the double mucoperiosteal flap (hinged flap + bipedicled flap) for closure of a congenital cleft palate.

1. One of the edges of the defect is incised with a scalpel blade and a 1–2 mm thick strip is removed. A partial-thickness mucosal band is left on the other edge to cover the defect with the hinged flap (2.5 times the width of the palate defect).
2. Blunt dissection of both sides of the defect with Stevens tenotomy scissors or a Freer periosteal elevator, preserving the arterial vascularization. A nasal hinge flap is created, rotated 180° and sutured over the bed created on the other side of the defect.
3. The nasal hinge flap suture is placed with an atraumatic needle and 4-0 or 5-0 absorbable monofilament material in a simple interrupted pattern.
4. To reconstruct the oral mucosa, incisions are made adjacent to the maxillary dental arch to create a double bipedicled flap. Dissection of the bed should be complete except in the area medial to the 4th premolar, where the major palatine artery exits through the palatine foramen.
5. Ample dissection of the tissues in order to suture them on the midline with 4-0 or 5-0 absorbable or nonabsorbable material with an atraumatic needle in a continuous mattress pattern.
6. The defects created on each side of the hard palate will close by secondary intention in a few days.

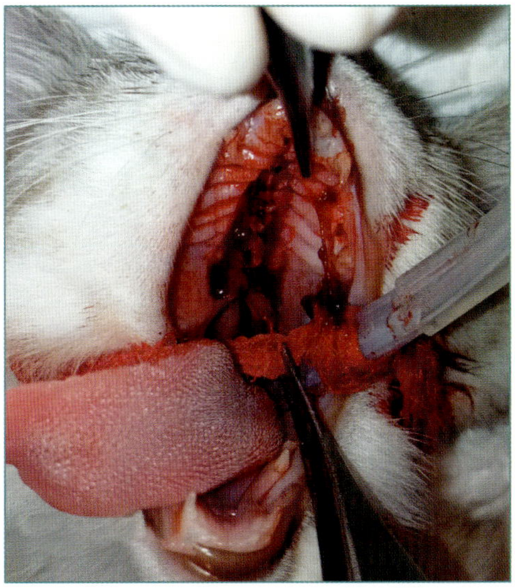

FIGURE 4. First step in the resolution of the cleft palate of the patient in Figure 1 using the double mucoperiosteal flap technique, in this case the hinged part of the flap.

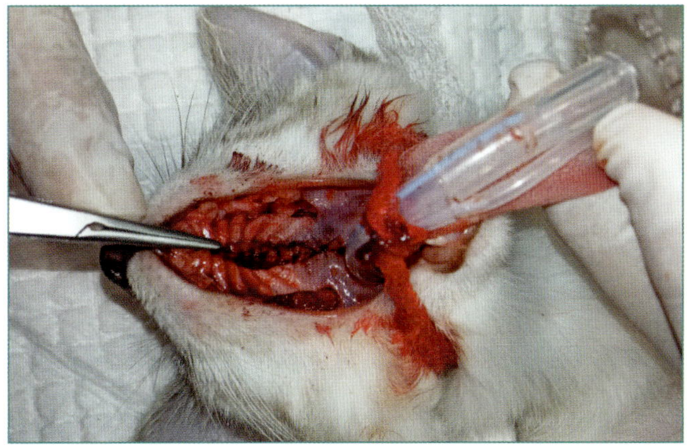

FIGURE 5. Beginning of the second phase of the technique, the double bipedicled flap. Careful periosteal elevation of both sides of the hard palate mucosa was performed with care to preserve the bilateral vascularization of the major palatine artery.

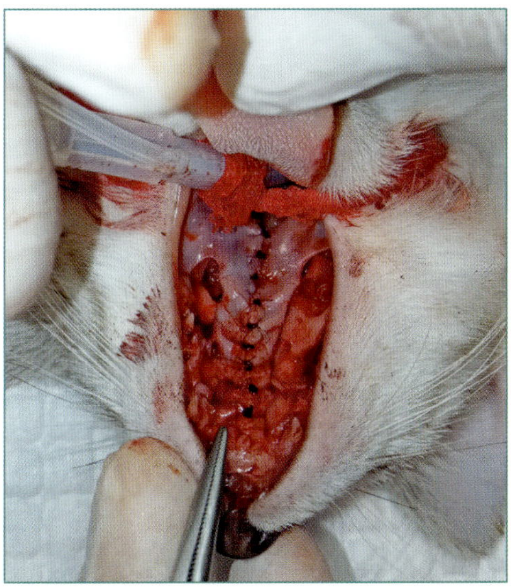

FIGURE 6. Both flaps are sutured in the center, avoiding the suture line of the hinged flap. In this case, a single interrupted suture pattern was used since the kitten was very small and its tissues were very delicate, so the authors preferred not to traumatize them any further.

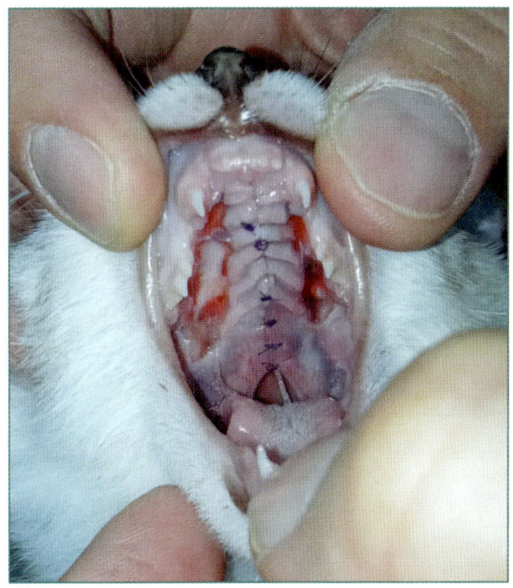

FIGURE 7. Patient 5 days after surgery. Note the suture is healing well, as are both sides of the hard palate (this area is filled with granulation tissue). After 2 weeks, the resolution of the most caudal part of the cleft palate was planned.

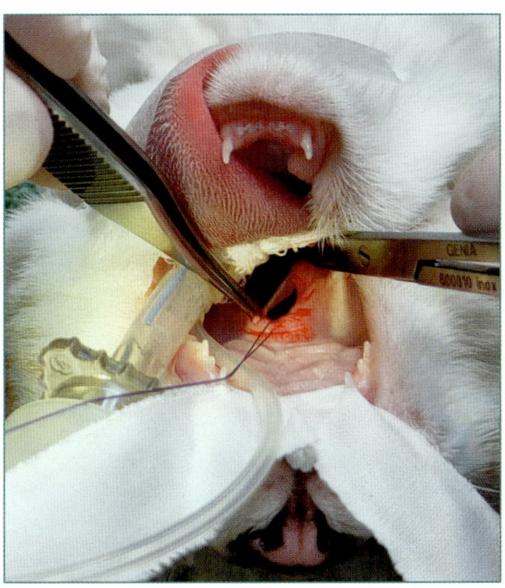

FIGURE 8. Incision and resurfacing of both sides of the soft palate defect. The suture will be placed first in the layer corresponding to the oral mucosa. A guiding point is used to pull the soft palate towards us and facilitate handling.

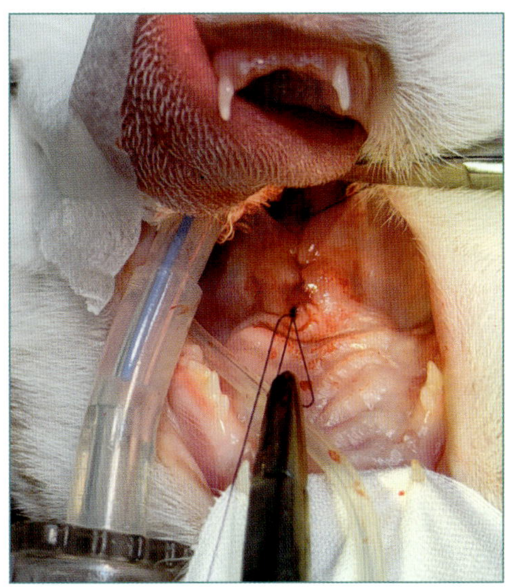

FIGURE 9. Completed continuous suture of the oral mucosa.

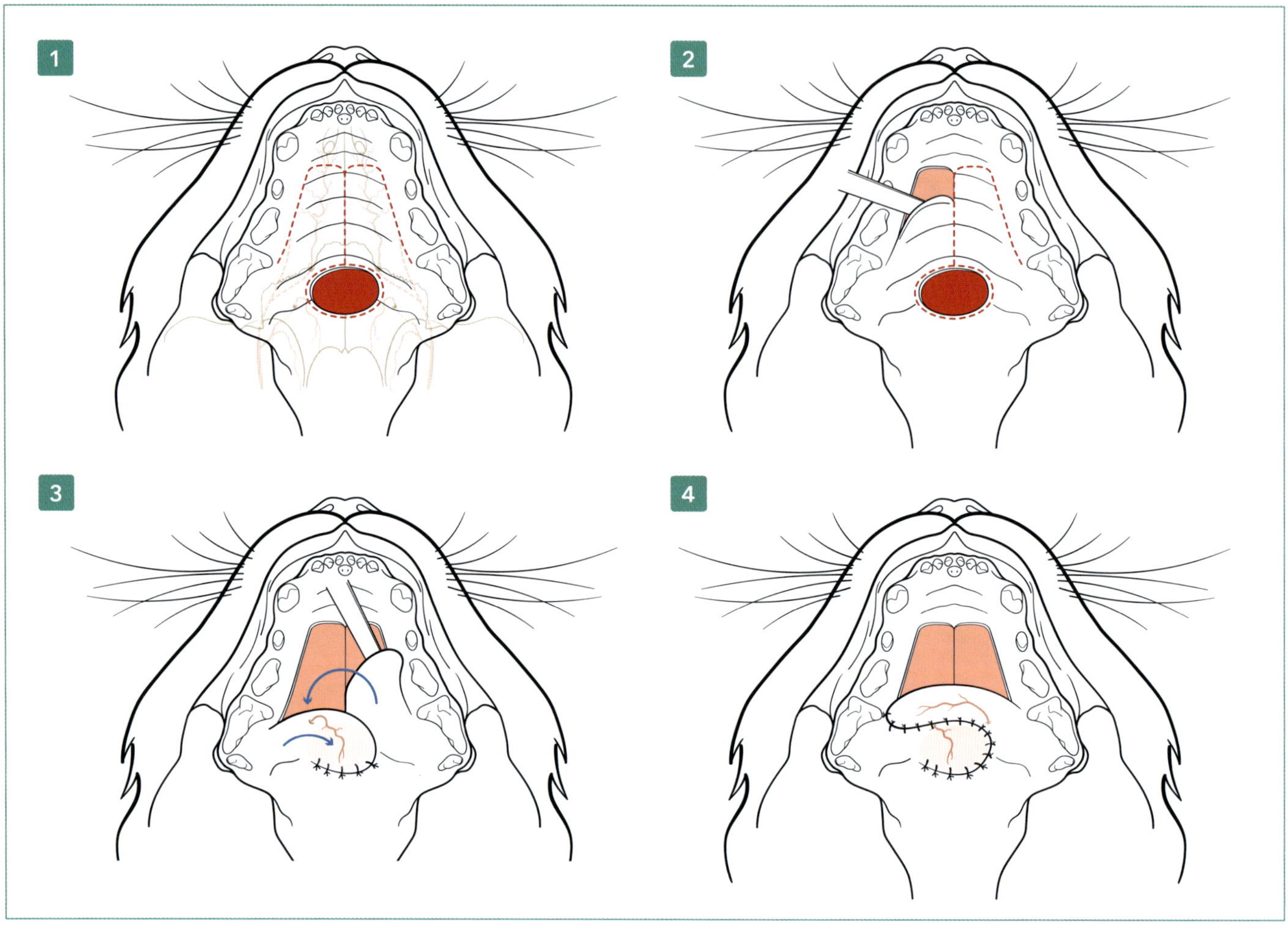

FIGURE 10. Steps of the split palatal U-flap technique.

1. The mucosa is incised to obtain the double split U-flap.
2. Dissection of the full thickness of both flaps, respecting the greater palatine arteries. The full thickness of the edge of the defect is also dissected or trimmed.
3. Transposition of one of the flaps towards the midline to cover the most caudal part of the defect. Monofilament suture in one or two layers (nasal and oral), if possible.
4. Rotation of the flap on the other side in the opposite direction as the first. It is sutured to the first rotated flap and to the opposite side of the dental arch. The exposed bony portion of the hard palate will heal by secondary intention.

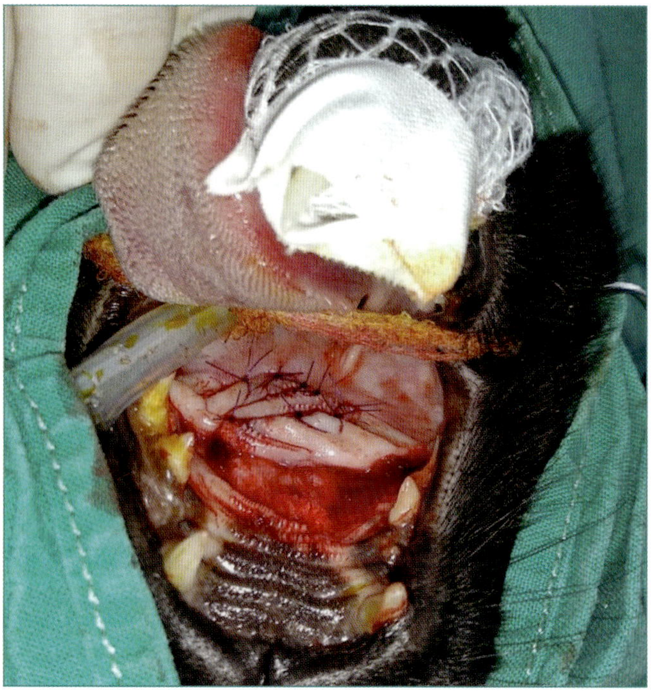

FIGURE 11. Intraoperative image of the patient in Figure 2 after performing a double split U-flap.

Double-layer flap (hinge flap + transposition flap)

This technique is used for the treatment of chronic dental oronasal fistulas, although it can be adapted for any focal defect of the hard palate. It consists of the combination of two flap types to first repair the nasal mucosa and then afterwards the oral mucosa.

The description corresponds to the procedure for the repair of an oronasal fistula located in the alveolus of the canine tooth.

Technique

1. The first step is to make a hinge flap that is rotated 180° to cover the entire fistula defect. To do so, we measure the defect width and dissect a flap of the mucosa of the hard palate the same shape as the defect, with the edge of the hinge coinciding with that of the fistula. The flap will cover one and a half times the width of the fistula so that it is not under tension once sutured. The other edge of the fistula is incised with a scalpel and the oral mucosa is dissected from the periosteum (Fig. 12.1).

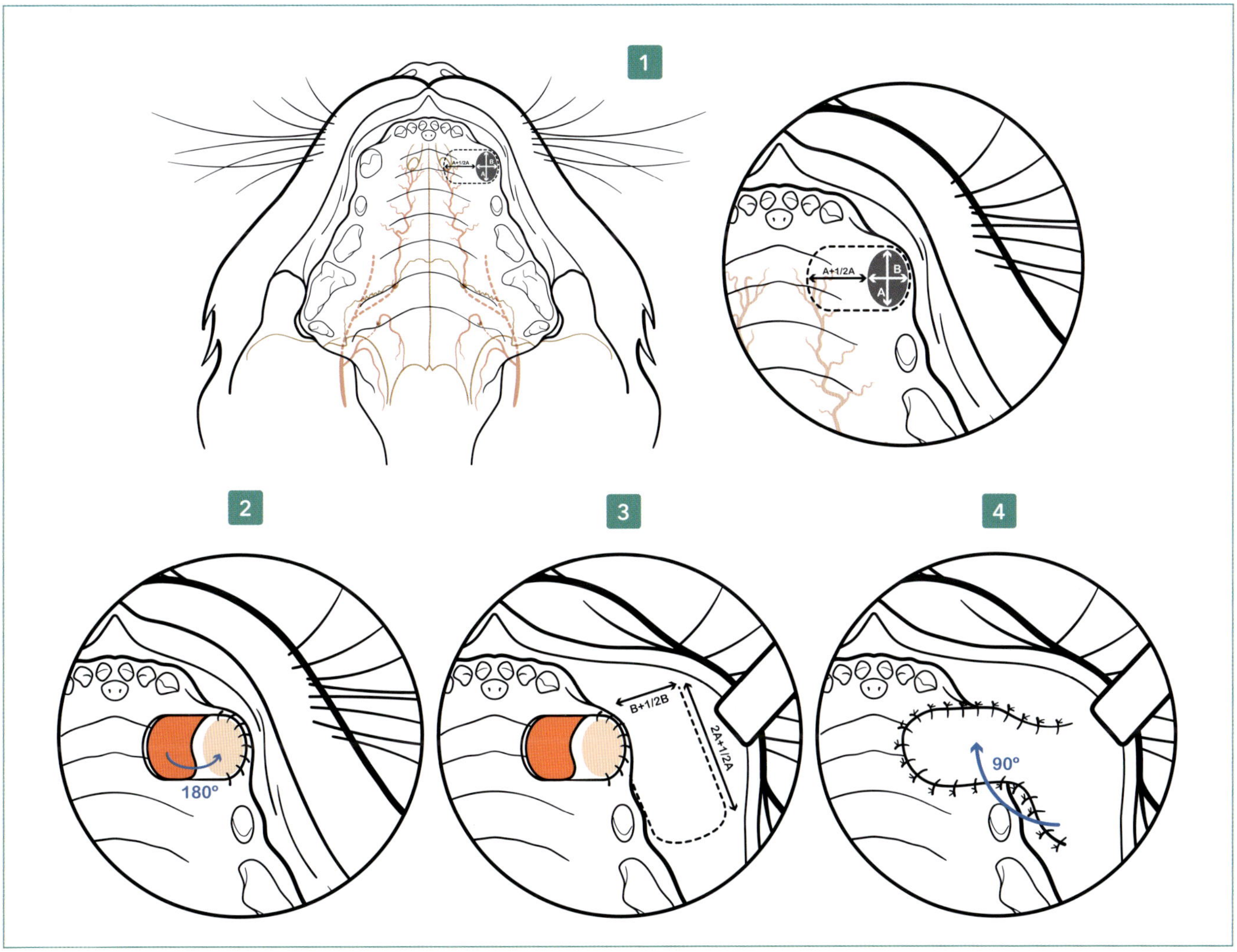

FIGURE 12. Steps of the double-layer flap technique (hinge flap + transposition flap).
1. Creation of a hinge flap that is rotated 180° to cover the entire fistula defect (1.5 times its width).
2. The flap is rotated over the edge of the defect to cover it. It is sutured in a simple interrupted pattern to the submucosal tissue at the opposite edge of the defect, avoiding any tension.
3. To make the transposition flap, use the mucosa of the internal aspect of the lip. The width of the flap should be 2.5 times the width of the defect, and the base, 1.5 times. The labial mucosa and submucosa are dissected.
4. The flap is rotated 90° and sutured to the edges of the defect and of the bed of the first flap. The lip bed defect is closed in a simple interrupted pattern, leaving only one suture line.

2. Once the entire edge of the flap is thoroughly dissected without tearing, the flap is rotated over the edge of the defect to cover it. The flap is sutured to the submucosal tissue at the opposite edge of the defect with simple interrupted sutures, avoiding any tension (Fig. 12.2).
3. To make the transposition flap the mucosa of the internal aspect of the lip is used. The shape should amply cover the hinge flap and the periosteum bed of hard palate that has been exposed. This will be about 2.5 times the width of the defect (measurement A, Fig. 12.1). The base of the flap should measure 1.5 times the width of the original defect (measurement B, Fig. 12.1). The labial mucosa and submucosa are dissected down to the base of the flap, so that it is free to be moved (Fig. 12.3).
4. The flap is rotated 90° and sutured to the edges of the defect and bed of the first flap until all the tissue is covered by the labial mucosa. The lip bed defect is closed with simple interrupted stitches, leaving only one suture line (Fig. 12.4).

Figures 13–16 show the application of this technique in a female cat with a severe maxillary injury due to an electrical burn.

Complications

One of the problems associated with chronic defects of the cat's palate is atrophy of the surrounding tissue. In the case of the alveolar arch, there is also the possibility of chronic osteomyelitis. This makes tissue dissection difficult and results in a very fibrous bed for the flaps. Suturing under these circumstances, with small-gauge needles, can be very difficult. It may be helpful in these cases to predrill with 21-gauge needles in the areas of the bed where the sutures will be placed.

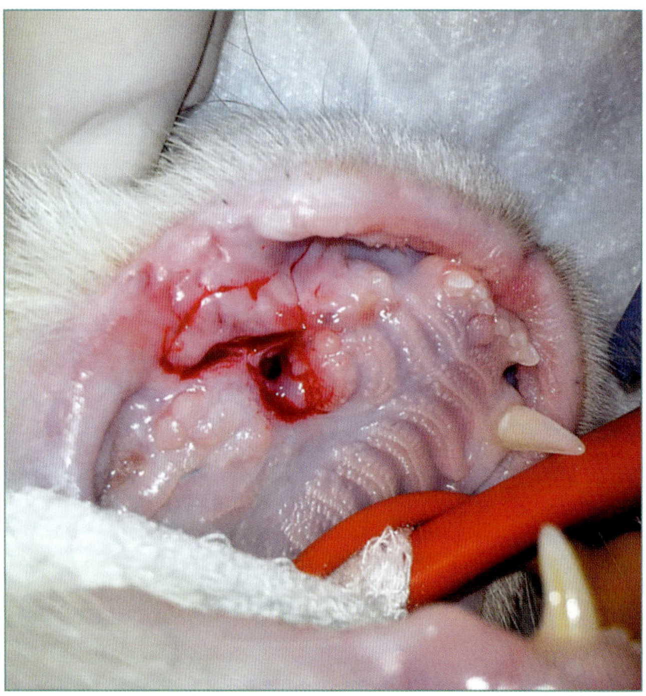

FIGURE 13. Planning of double hinge flap + transposition in a cat with a severe bone injury of the maxilla due to an electrical burn that caused an oronasal fistula at canine tooth 104.

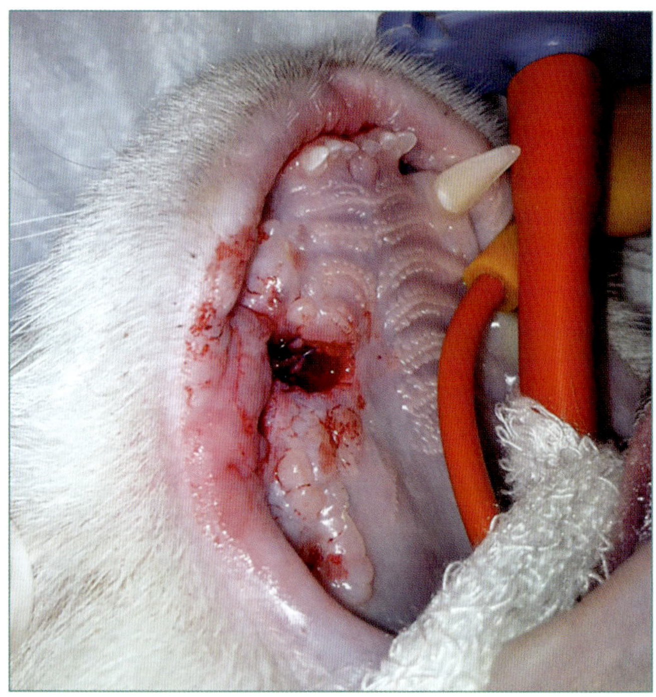

FIGURE 14. First the hinge flap is made to primarily close the defect.

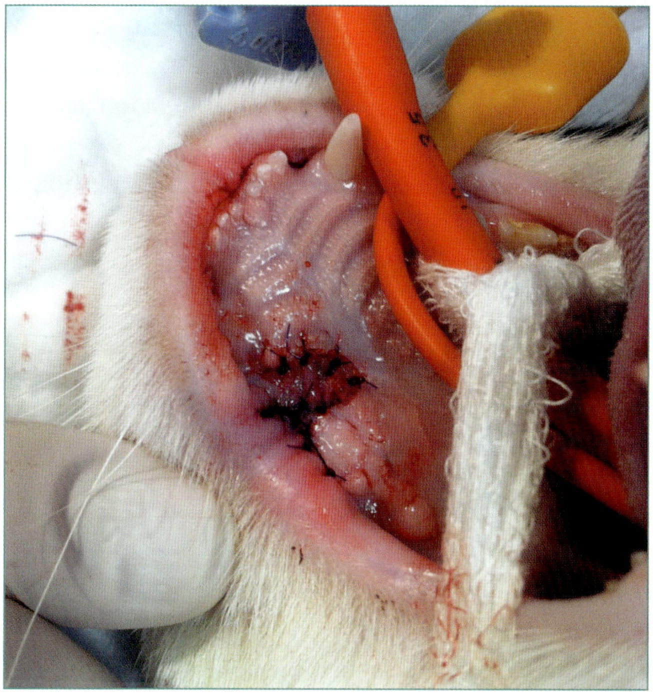

FIGURE 15. Second, the transposition flap from the labial mucosa is applied on top.

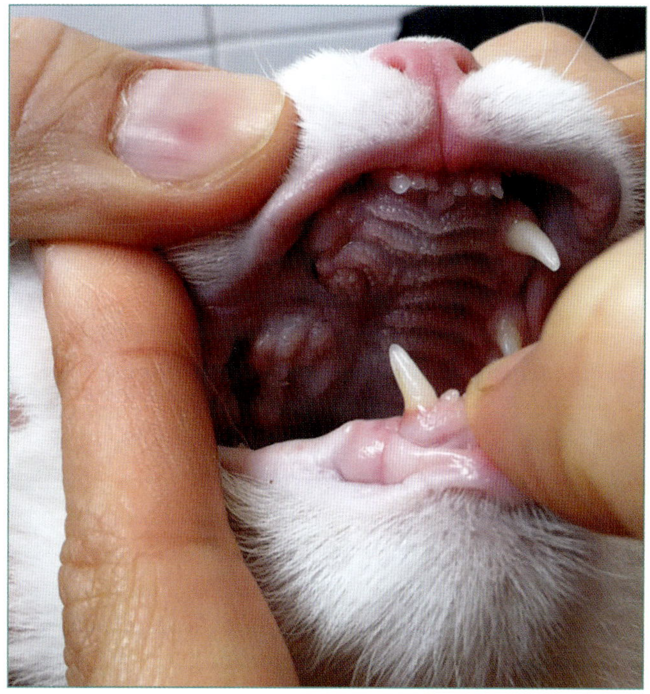

FIGURE 16. Healing of the defect after 2 months.

Bibliography

BECKMAN BW. Split palatal U-flap for repair of caudal palatal defects. *J Vet Dent*, 2006; 23(4):267–269.

COX CL, HUNT GB, CADIER MM. Repair of oronasal fistulae using auricular cartilage grafts in five cats. *Vet Surg*, 2007; 36(2):164–169.

ELLISON GW, MULLIGAN TW, FAGAN DA, TUGEND RK. A double reposition flap technique for repair of recurrent oronasal fistulas in dogs. *J Am Anim Hosp Assoc*, 1986; 22:803–808.

EUBANKS DL. Oral soft tissue anatomy in the dog and cat. *J Vet Dent*, 2007; 24(2):126–129.

HARVEY CE. Palate defects in dogs and cats. *Compend Contin Educ Pract Vet*, 1987; 9(4):404–418.

HEADRICK JF, MCANULTY JF. Reconstruction of a bilateral hypoplastic soft palate in a cat. *J Am Anim Hosp Assoc*, 2004; 40(1):86–90.

MARRETTA SM, GROVE TK, GRILLO JF. Split palatal U-flap: a new technique for repair of caudal hard palate defects. *J Vet Dent*, 1991; 8(1):5–8.

PETERSON NW, BUOTE NJ. Soft palate cyst in a cat. *J Feline Med Surg*, 2011; 13(8):594–596.

POPE ER, CONSTANTINESCU GM. Oral cavity. In: BOJRAB MJ (ed.). *Current Techniques in Small Animal Surgery*, 4th ed. Baltimore, MD: Williams & Wilkins, 1998; pp. 113–150.

REITER AM, SMITH MM. The oral cavity and oropharynx. In: BROCKMAN DJ, HOLT DE (eds.). *BSAVA Manual of Canine and Feline Head, Neck and Toracic Surgery*, 1st ed. Gloucester, UK: British Small Animal Veterinary Association, 2005; pp. 25–43.

SIVACOLUNDHU RK. Palate. In: LANGLEY-HOBBS SJ, DEMETRIOU JL, LADLOW JF (eds.). *Feline Soft Tissue and General Surgery*, 1st ed. Oxford, UK: Saunders Elsevier, 2014; pp. 683–690.

FELINE DENTAL EXTRACTIONS 14

Llibertat Real

Surgical anatomy

The **oral cavity** encompasses laterally the **cheeks**, ventrally the **tongue and intermandibular soft tissue**, dorsally the **palate** and extends from the **lips to the oropharynx** at the caudal border of the hard palate. The **vestibule** is the area between the lips, cheeks and dental arches. The surface is covered by the oral mucosa, consisting of nonkeratinized and keratinized squamous epithelium, under which we find the submucosa, consisting of connective tissue, lymphatic vessels, blood vessels, salivary ducts, salivary glands and muscle fibers. **Teeth** are hard anatomical organs located in the **alveoli** of the **mandibular and maxillary bone**, attached via the **periodontal ligament**, a dense connective tissue with the capacity to cushion the pressure received by the teeth.

Terms used for localization in the oral cavity

- **Mesial:** the side of the teeth toward the rostral area in the case of premolars, molars and canines, and the side toward the midline in the case of incisors.
- **Distal:** side facing the caudal portion of the dental arch and, in the case of the incisors, the lateral side.
- **Lingual or palatal (palatine):** side in contact with the tongue or palate, respectively.
- **Vestibular:** side in contact with the vestibule. The surface of canines and incisors located towards the lip can also be referred to as **labial** and the surface of molars and premolars on the cheek side can also be referred to as **buccal**.

The portion of keratinized oral mucosa that covers the alveolar bone and surrounds the dental neck is called the **gingiva**. Its function is to protect the underlying structures. Each tooth is divided into a **crown** (the part above the gums) and a **root** (the part that is in the socket). Teeth are composed of **dentin** (porous connective tissue, the second hardest substance in the body), covered by a layer of **enamel** (the hardest substance in the body) on the crown and a layer of **cementum** at the root. At the core of the crown and roots is the **dental pulp**, composed of blood vessels, connective tissue, collagen, nerves, lymphatic vessels and odontoblasts. The supporting apparatus of the tooth (**periodontium**) consists of the periodontal ligament, gingiva, cementum and alveolar bone.

Cats have **incisors**, **canines**, **premolars** and **molars**. The feline permanent dental formula is: I3/I3 C1/C1 P3/P2 M1/M1 on both sides of the mandible and maxilla. In the maxilla the first premolar we find is the second premolar, in the mandible it is the third premolar (there is no maxillary or mandibular first premolar, or mandibular second premolar). The canines and incisors have one root, the maxillary second premolars have one root, the maxillary third premolars have two roots and the maxillary fourth premolars have three roots. The maxillary third premolars may occasionally have a third root. Mandibular premolars have two roots and molars have two roots.

The teeth are identified using the modified Triadan system (Fig. 1). In this case, the right maxilla is quadrant 10, the left maxilla is quadrant 20, the left mandible is quadrant 30 and the right mandible is quadrant 40.

Sensory innervation comes from the maxillary and mandibular branches of the trigeminal nerve. These give rise to the **palatine nerves** (hard palate, soft palate and nasopharynx), **caudal maxillary alveolar nerve** (maxillary first molar, buccal gingiva, oral mucosa), **middle maxillary alveolar nerve** (maxillary premolars and associated oral mucosa), **rostral maxillary alveolar nerve** (canines, incisors and associated oral mucosa) and **mandibular nerve** (mandibular teeth to the symphysis). All these nerves are accessible and can be blocked by local anesthesia (see Ch. 2 "Feline sedation, anesthesia and analgesia").

The oral cavity is vascularized by the **maxillary artery** and the **mandibular inferior alveolar arteries**. The latter enter through the mandibular foramen on the medial aspect of the mandible,

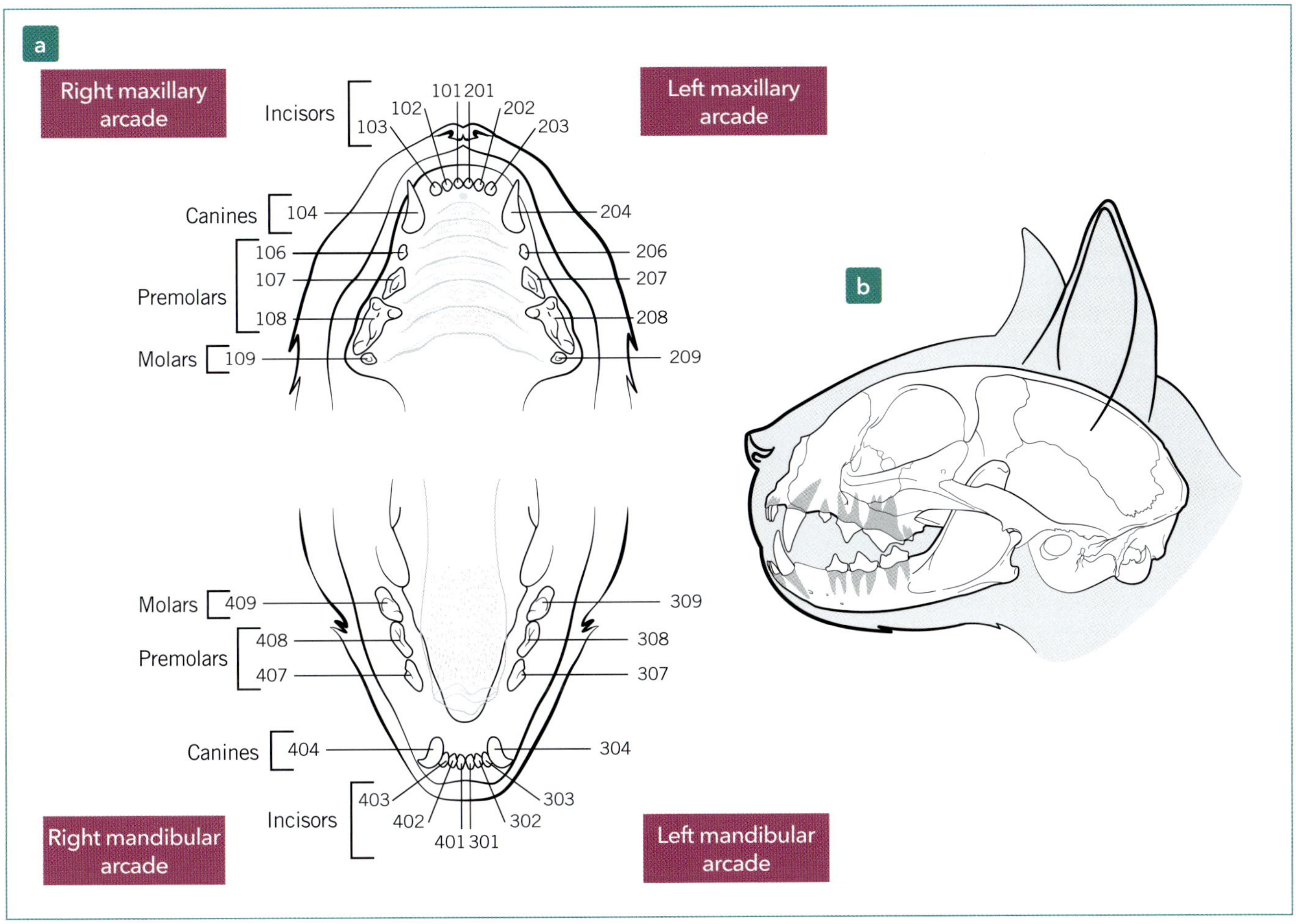

FIGURE 1. (a) Triadan numbering of the cat's permanent teeth. (b) Tooth roots.

travel along the mandibular canal and exit through the mental foramen. In addition to the mandibular, parotid, sublingual and zygomatic salivary glands, cats have four molar salivary glands (lingual and vestibular or buccal). Of these, the two lingual molar glands are located linguodistal to the mandibular first molar under the molar pad (structure covered by the oral mucosa where the molar salivary gland is located).

Surgical diseases of the oral cavity

Oral diseases in cats that may require surgical treatment include:

- Feline chronic gingivostomatitis
- Periodontal disease
- Dental resorption
- Dental fractures and luxations/subluxations
- Pyogenic granuloma
- Presence of persistent deciduous teeth, supernumerary teeth and impacted teeth

The diagnosis of the various diseases of the oral cavity that may require dental extractions is based on medical history, examination of the oral cavity under anesthesia, in some cases biopsy of the affected tissues and intraoral X-rays.

It is important to note that without intraoral X-rays (or another imaging test such as a CT scan) it is not possible to perform dental extractions safely or correctly.

Feline chronic gingivostomatitis

Feline chronic gingivostomatitis (Fig. 2) is a very painful multifactorial chronic oral disease characterized by severe inflammation of the oral mucosa, sometimes with hyperplasia of the tissues that can be confused with a neoplasm. Its causes are multifactorial, it is a combination of:

- A dysregulated immune system (with an inability to deactivate the inflammatory cascade and return to a resting state).
- A decreased oral tolerance to the presence of various antigens.
- The persistent presence of feline calicivirus (especially in cats with caudal oral mucosal involvement).
- The presence of bacterial plaque.
- Other individual factors that are more difficult to identify contribute to the perpetuation of inflammation.

Cats show clinical signs of dysphagia, self-trauma and drooling, poor coat and mild weight loss. In some cases, their feeding habits (they spend a lot of time near the feeder, but eat little) and their food preferences change (from wet only to dry only, or vice versa). The latter is due to the fact that it can be very painful to chew dry food (they prefer wet food) or it hurts them a lot to clean the remains of wet food inside the mouth with the tongue (they prefer to eat dry food without chewing, "sucking" it). We will typically observe this disease in cats living in a multicat environment or in solitary cats coming from a colony. **Biopsies from altered mucosa** usually show inflammation with a predominant presence of plasma cells, a variable number of lymphocytes, ulceration of the epithelium and in some cases necrosis. In many instances we will also find neutrophil infiltration due to the presence of a secondary infection by the oral flora.

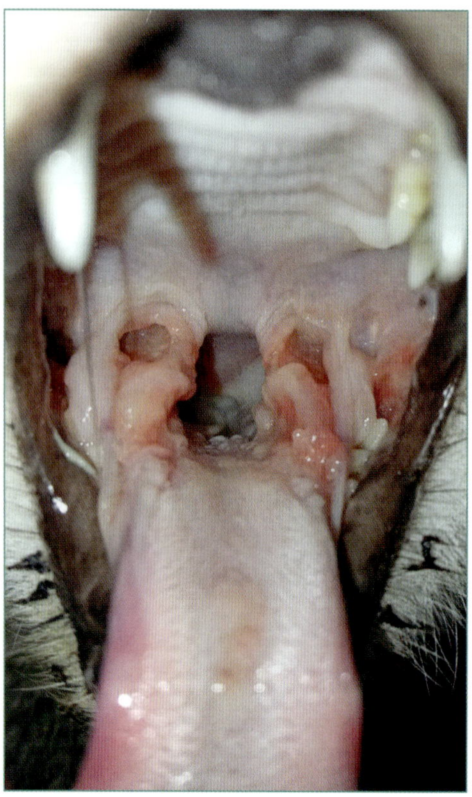

FIGURE 2. Feline chronic gingivostomatitis in a cat from a colony.

It is a complex disease to manage. The basis of the treatment is the extraction of all premolars and molars, which helps reduce the bacterial plaque and inflammation associated with the teeth. This results in recovery in approximately 50% of affected cats. The other 50% may require the extraction of canines and incisors if inflammation cannot be controlled without medication within a reasonable period of time, especially if they present alveolar mucositis around teeth that have not been extracted. This significantly improves the quality of life of patients and, in many cases, after a period of time, the disease remits. Approximately 5% of patients have a refractory disease that is extremely difficult to control and it is only through multiple treatments that they are able to maintain a reasonable quality of life.

Other adjuvant treatments (always combined with the dental extractions described above) such as oral, subcutaneous or intralesional feline interferon-ω, or oral cyclosporine have shown positive results, although their effect is slow and long term. Stem cell treatment has been described (always administered after tooth extractions), but it still needs to be perfected, as its effectiveness is very inconsistent. Another fundamental factor in disease management is stress control and preventing these cats from living in unstable environments with a constant influx of new cats. Although its clinical presentation is very characteristic, it should be differentiated from oral eosinophilic granuloma (more localized, pink lesions with fine whitish stippling; biopsy is diagnostic), oral squamous cell carcinoma (asymmetric lesions, lesions surrounding the teeth and affecting the bone, unilateral enlargement of the tonsils) and leishmaniasis, among other diseases.

Periodontal disease

Periodontal disease (Fig. 3) is the leading cause of oral disease in cats. It occurs in two phases, an initial phase, **gingivitis**, and, if not corrected, a second phase, **periodontitis** (inflammation and infection of the deeper supporting structures of the tooth: the periodontal ligament and the alveolar bone).

The gingival mucosa is closely attached to the neck of the tooth and, in conjunction with the periodontal ligament, prevents oral bacteria from penetrating into this space. The pathophysiology of this disease is related to individual predisposing factors and the presence of bacterial plaque and associated dental calculus. These conditions favor the appearance of inflammation, gingival recession and/or a periodontal pocket that allows the presence of this bacterial plaque below the free gingival margin and in the gingival sulcus. All this triggers a cycle of local inflammation that perpetuates itself and allows the bacterial population to penetrate in an apical direction, causing recurrent inflammation. The oral flora undergoes a change and the gram-negative bacteria increase, which causes more severe inflammation and destruction of the structures through the secretion of toxins and various metabolites. This leads to alveolar bone loss, gingival recession, increased tooth mobility and, in the most advanced stages, tooth loss.

There are four grades of periodontal disease:

- **Grade 1:** gingivitis without loss of dental attachment.
- **Grade 2:** periodontitis with a less than 25% loss of tooth attachment or stage 1 furcation involvement in multirooted teeth.
- **Grade 3:** periodontitis with 25%–50% loss of tooth attachment or stage 2 furcation involvement in multirooted teeth.

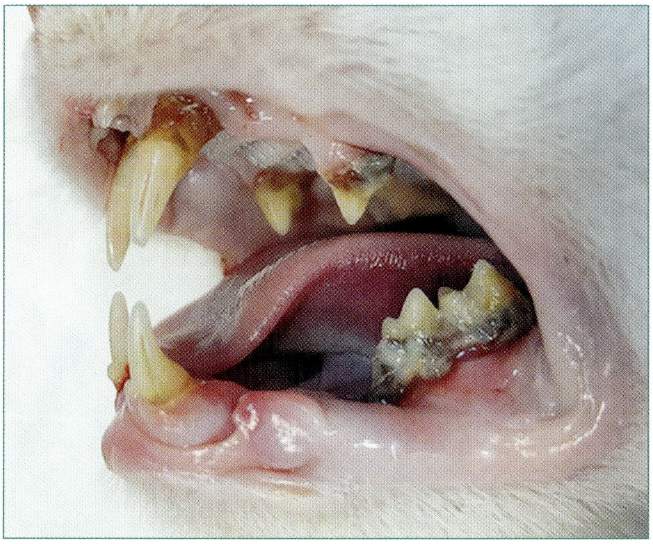

FIGURE 3. Grade 4 periodontal disease in a feline immunodeficiency virus (FIV)-positive cat.

- **Grade 4:** periodontitis with a loss of tooth attachment greater than 50% or stage 3 furcation involvement in multirooted teeth.

Diagnosis requires a complete examination of the oral cavity under anesthesia and **intraoral X-rays** to identify the degree of disease in each tooth and rule out the presence of teeth with resorptions or other damage associated with inflammation. These teeth require extraction:

- Those with a grade 3 mobility index (increased mobility in any direction except axial, a distance greater than 2 mm or any axial movement).
- When there has been a loss of dental attachment greater than 2/3.
- When periodontal disease has resulted in endodontic disease.

Whether or not other teeth with lesser degrees of disease need to be extracted will especially depend on the owner's ability to administer maintenance care at home.

Tooth resorption

Dental resorptions are defects that appear due to a loss of hard dental tissues due to the effect of odontoclasts. These defects may increase in size and depth, leading to the fracture of the tooth or its disappearance. They may be associated with the presence of severe inflammation (due to periodontal disease or another cause of local inflammation) or appear due to factors that are still unclear, although numerous hypotheses have been put forward over the years. In the latter case, defects usually appear on multiple teeth, often symmetrically, at the time of presentation or over time (Fig. 4). There are two types of tooth resorption in cats:

- **Type 1 tooth resorption:** alveolar bone loss occurs in a well-defined area of tooth resorption while the periodontal ligament space is maintained in the rest of the tooth. When these resorptions result in crown or root fractures, the apical fragments of the root or roots remain in the alveolus, causing intense inflammation.
- **Type 2 tooth resorption:** the roots undergo an ankylosis process leading to them becoming fused with the alveolar bone.

We can find both types in the same tooth (sometimes called **type 3 resorption**), which will require different approaches. Dental extraction is the only treatment.

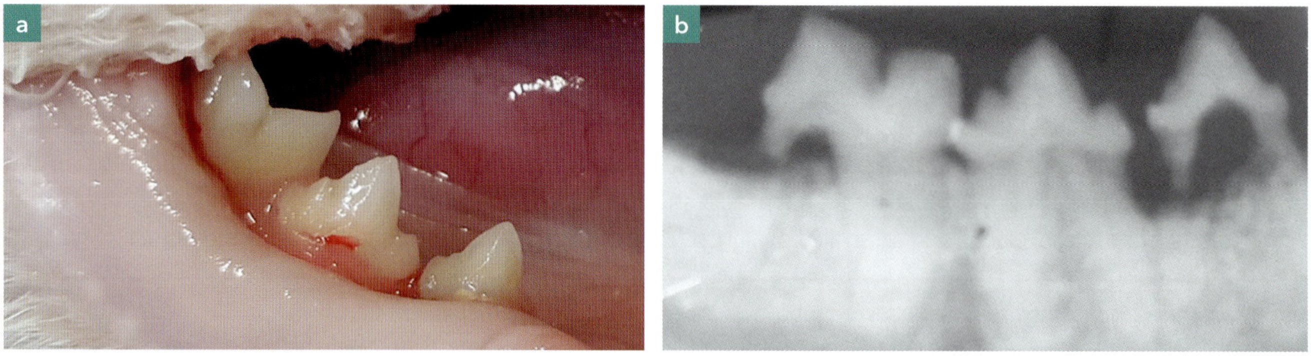

FIGURE 4. Type 1 and 2 dental resorptions in the premolars of a cat observed upon (a) oral examination and (b) intraoral X-ray. Comparing the two images, we can appreciate why intraoral X-rays are essential for the diagnosis and treatment of dental diseases.

All teeth with involvement above the gum, those associated with any degree of inflammation or periodontal disease and those visibly associated with signs of pain should be extracted.

The remaining teeth can only be kept if it is possible to closely monitor them by means of sedation and intraoral X-rays. If this is not the case, then they must also be extracted.

Dental fractures

Dental fractures affecting the crown can include:

- **Complicated:** with pulp exposure (Fig. 5).
- **Uncomplicated:** when the fracture does not expose the pulp, but extends to the dentin.

Dental fractures affecting the root may be coronal, medial or affect the apical third. The pulp is usually exposed. Fractures involving the crown and root may also occur. Whether a fracture requires tooth extraction will depend on the age of the patient, the type of fracture and whether or not endodontic treatment is possible. If this is not possible, we must extract the tooth, because whenever the dentin is exposed, bacteria can penetrate the pulp indirectly through its tubules and produce endodontic disease.

Dental luxations/subluxations are usually associated with trauma or severe periodontal disease and require tooth extraction in the vast majority of cases.

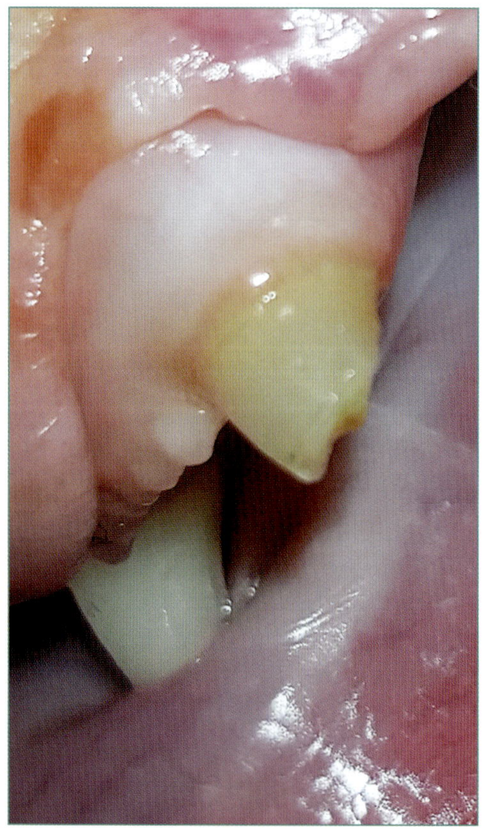

FIGURE 5. Complicated crown fracture of tooth 204.

Pyogenic granulomas

Pyogenic granulomas (Fig. 6) are inflammatory lesions produced in the oral mucosa by abnormal occlusal contact between molars, premolars and vestibular mucosa of opposing arches. The cause is not well known, but in many cases it is because this occlusion is not correct (due to multiple factors) or the occlusion changes due to pain, resulting in the perpetuation of trauma and inflammation. Treatment requires the extraction of the tooth or teeth responsible for the trauma, unless a crown reduction is sufficient, which is unusual if associated with a high degree of inflammation.

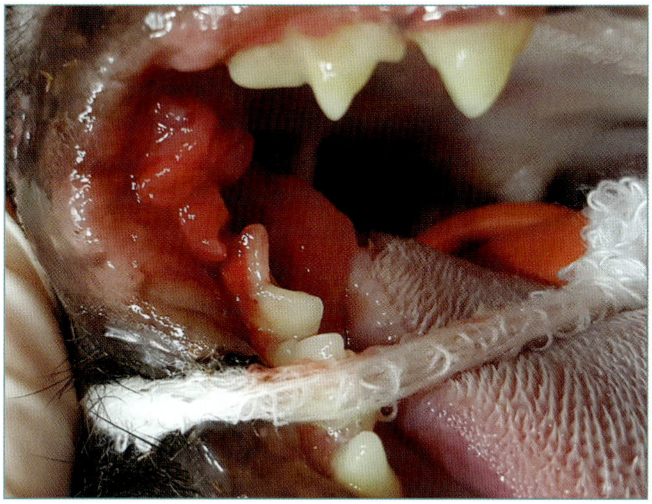

FIGURE 6. Pyogenic granuloma requiring the extraction of teeth 108 and 409 to prevent recurrence.

Dental anomalies

The presence of persistent deciduous teeth, supernumerary teeth or impacted permanent teeth is very rare in cats, but, if present, may require tooth extraction if they promote periodontal disease by accumulating food and tartar or cause problems associated with malocclusion or other causes.

We can detect a persistence of multiple deciduous teeth or the impaction of permanent teeth in cats presenting with acute lameness secondary to patellar fracture (uni- or bilateral). These cats may also present with fractures of other bones before or after the patellar fracture, paronychia and alterations in the maxillary and/or mandibular bone. This is known as **patellar fracture and dental anomaly syndrome** (PADS).

Preoperative and postoperative considerations

Before the procedure:

- We should examine the cat while awake to evaluate the occlusion, but we cannot determine exactly which tooth or teeth will require extraction until we have performed a complete examination of the oral cavity under anesthesia and intraoral X-rays. It is very important to convey this to cat guardian and to reflect it in the budget.
- To avoid unnecessary complications, we should pay special attention to the kidney function of cats with chronic oral inflammatory disorders. Also, many of these patients are cats over 8 years old and it is essential to do a complete geriatric blood test (including T_4 determination) within three months prior to surgery. If in doubt, a control analysis can be performed on the day of surgery. The thyroid hormone is important, as many early-stage hyperthyroid cats are asymptomatic, but may have cardiovascular adverse reactions under anesthesia.
- When dealing with a cat with oral and nasopharyngeal inflammatory disease, we must first resolve the dental disorder. This acts as an inflammatory focus for the nasopharyngeal condition, and we cannot adequately evaluate the success of any medical or surgical treatment for the resolution of nasopharyngeal disease without first eliminating the oral inflammation and infection.
- We must closely observe both the coloration and the appearance of the mucous membranes (surface, ulcers, hyperplasia) when performing an examination of the oral cavity of a sedated cat before deciding that this is not the cause of the cat's pain and clinical picture, especially if the cat has elevated globulin levels. Many sedation protocols produce vasoconstriction, causing the mucous membranes to present a deceptively normal color.

During the operation and in the postoperative period:

- Partial or complete tooth extraction surgery can take a long time, cats are continuously exposed to water/chlorhexidine from the dental unit, which can cause a significant decrease in body temperature, with all the negative effects that this entails. It is essential to apply all safe means at our disposal to maintain the patient's body temperature above 98.6°F (37°C) during surgery and in the postoperative period.
- It is advisable to use local blocks to better control intraoperative pain and reduce the concentration of anesthetic gases used. In addition, it is always a painful surgery and we must have a predetermined analgesic plan; however, we should be attentive to any sign of pain and modify this plan whenever necessary. We can use the grimace scale to evaluate the degree of pain, as it has been shown to be effective in this surgery.
- Some cats, especially Burmese and Burmilla breeds (but also European cats), may present postoperative orofacial pain syndrome. We must educate owners about the clinical signs and follow up appropriately in the days following surgery.
- On rare occasions, we may find excessive bleeding from the extraction site despite the use of an adequate technique; this may sometimes only be perceivable when the effects of the anesthesia on the cardiovascular system wear off, once

the cat has been extubated. We should monitor patients closely in the hour following surgery and it is useful to place white absorbent pads under the head for easy detection of bleeding. At this point it is still relatively simple to fix this complication.

Surgical tooth extraction techniques

The techniques described below must always be performed with the cat intubated and the pharynx protected. The basis for a correct dental extraction are technique, control of movement, patience, care and to never exert force. With the hand that is not in use, we must always hold the mandible or maxilla to keep the head stable. We should try to minimize surgical trauma whenever possible. Preferably, we should use a high-speed water-cooled handpiece enclosed in a high-pressure dental unit. Good lighting and, if necessary, magnifying glasses are also essential for a clear view of the structures and the area. The required material is described in Chapter 5 ("Surgical materials"). Once finished, intraoral X-rays should be taken to check that there are no root remnants.

Closed tooth extraction

Closed tooth extraction is used in those cases where, due to an advanced degree of periodontal disease and/or tooth mobility, the periodontal space is easily accessible for luxation and elevation of the tooth fragment. It is also used in teeth with a single root such as incisors (this is called simple closed extraction). This prevents the need for a mucoperiosteal flap or the removal of alveolar bone. Although on some occasions it is possible to extract a multirooted tooth without dividing it into single-root fragments, it is noteworthy that it is always advisable to divide teeth with multiple roots, since on many occasions one root is more attached than the rest and can easily be broken, unnecessarily increasing the extraction time and entailing an invasive procedure in order to recover it.

Technique

1. First, we make an incision around the perimeter of the gingival sulcus with a no. 11 scalpel blade until we reach the level of the alveolar bone (Fig. 7.1). This is done with the tip of the scalpel blade facing the tooth surface to avoid damaging the gingiva.
2. Using a fissure bur suitable for the feline oral cavity, the premolar or molar is sectioned in a furcation–crown direction until it is divided into two fragments. We should handle the bur with soft and short movements, like brushstrokes. In the case of teeth 108 and 208 we will first divide the two mesial roots (smaller) with respect to the distal root (larger) (Fig. 7.2).
3. We introduce a 1–2 mm luxator into the periodontal space to break the ligament. We should introduce it with a rocking motion, avoiding any rotating or wedging movements (the luxator could break, as it is not designed for this type of movements), little by little, holding close to the end with our hand (with the index finger and thumb) and with the tip at an angle of about 20° towards the surface of the tooth to avoid losing control of the instrument and causing any damage (Fig. 7.3). Never apply excessive force, only gentle pressure in a controlled manner. This movement is then repeated along the entire perimeter of the tooth. It is essential to ensure that the instrument is introduced into the periodontal space without unnecessarily traumatizing the alveolar bone.
4. Sometimes this previous step will be enough to free the fragment and we will be able to extract it directly. If this is not the case, once the periodontal space is luxated, we will introduce the elevator 1 to 4 mm depending on the size of the fragment to be elevated. The instrument should embrace the fragment without extending beyond it and comfortably enter the periodontal space. Apply sustained, controlled, slightly rotating pressure for 10–30 seconds (Fig. 7.4). This is repeated until the fragment is sufficiently mobile. It is better to apply moderate tension over a relatively long period than to apply very short and intense tension. The periodontal ligament is prepared to withstand continuous short pressures, but not sustained pressure over time, which will cause it to break more easily.
5. When the fragment is sufficiently mobile, we will extract it by holding it with the extraction forceps and making short, small rotary movements, rotating only the wrist (Fig. 7.5). This will be done carefully and without applying any force, only controlled tension. Special care must be taken to avoid breaking the fragment in teeth with resorptive lesions, with bulbous, convergent or excessively curved roots, very long roots or where there is a high degree of infection and inflammation. In the event that after a few brief moments we are not able to extract the fragment, it is better to luxate and elevate it again and, when the degree of mobility is deemed to be better, try again to extract it. This operation will be repeated with all fragments until all the necessary teeth are extracted. Then we will irrigate with 0.12% chlorhexidine solution followed by Ringer's lactate.

6. The gingiva should be sutured after extraction with a 4-0 or 5-0 absorbable monofilament suture, preferably with an atraumatic needle (Fig. 7.6). First, we scrape the alveolus, which allows us to eliminate granulation tissue and favors the formation of a fibrin clot that accelerates healing by first intention. If necessary, we perform an alveoloplasty with a round diamond-tipped bur to prevent irregularities in the alveolar bone and then proceed to suture the debrided edges of the gingiva where we initially made the incision using an envelope flap. This allows the cat to be more comfortable and return to normal more quickly. Also, healing will be faster, with fewer complications.

Open or surgical tooth extraction

This technique will be used on most occasions when the conditions for the previous technique are not met.

Technique

1. With a no. 11 scalpel blade we make a horizontal incision following the 360° of the gingival edge of the tooth or teeth to be extracted. Next, we make two vertical incisions in the alveolar mucosa on the distal side of the anterior tooth and the mesial side of the tooth posterior to the tooth or teeth to be extracted. Other flaps are possible, but this is the one we will use most often.
2. Using the periosteal elevator, we elevate the flap and expose the alveolar bone. We must be careful when making the flap so that it does not break and so we can suture it without tension, causing minimal trauma.
3. With a round bur, suitable for the feline oral cavity, we will remove the vertical alveolar bone covering the upper half of the roots, until the furcation is exposed, with gentle brush-like movements. We will then cut the tooth into fragments using the same method as in the previous technique.
4. We then proceed to luxate the periodontal ligament and elevate the fragment using the same procedure described above. In some fragments we can trim the crown to facilitate access to the periodontal space and minimize the possibility of root fracture.
5. If we find it difficult to introduce the luxator, we can increase the periodontal space with a 1/4 or 1/2 mm bur following the contour of the tooth to a depth of 1–2 mm. Once the fragment is sufficiently mobile (we must be able to extract it with few movements and without exerting force), we will remove it with extraction forceps. It is important not to make vigorous movements, especially in the distal root of 108 and 208 or the mesial root of 309 and 409 if they do not present sufficient mobility, since we could cause damage to the surrounding structures and it is easier to fracture the roots.
6. To extract the canines (104, 204, 304, 404) we will follow the same process. The flap will ideally start on the distal side of the third incisor and end on the mesial side of the second premolar to avoid suturing over the cavity. With a 1–2 mm round bur we will follow the mesial and distal contour of the tooth (along the periodontal ligament) and then remove the vestibular alveolar bone between these two cuts up to 1/3 or 1/2 of the root. We must dislocate them very carefully on the palatine or lingual side, because when the root is tilted we could damage the maxillary bone or the mandibular symphysis. We will always perform the greatest degree of luxation and elevation from the mesial and distal sides in 104 and 204 and from the vestibular (buccal) and dorsal sides in 304 and 404.
7. Once the extraction or extractions have been completed, we suture the flap with simple interrupted stitches (separation of approximately 2 mm) using 5-0 monofilament atraumatic suture. Before suturing the flap, we should make some incisions in the periosteum adhered to the maxillary mucosa, at the level of the mucogingival junction, to increase its flexibility and facilitate said suturing. Suturing should always be performed without tension. Avoid suturing over a cavity (try to suture over bone whenever possible) using nonepithelialized edges to minimize the possibility of dehiscence or necrosis.

Postoperative complications

Excessive bleeding at the extraction site

This complication is more frequent in 304 and 404 due to damage to the mandibular alveolar vessels that exit through the mental foramen when excessive alveolar bone is removed. It may also occur from the bottom of the alveolus due to excessive trauma, mildly reduced clotting ability or damage to soft tissues or vascular structures during extraction. The second most frequent area where we can see excessive bleeding is in 108 and 208.

The usual way to correct this is to redo the flap by closing the wound better. The hemostasis produced by the increased pressure of the stitches will be sufficient. If this is not successful, we can apply a few drops of adrenaline locally. In the case of persistent bleeding, a 2 mg/kg dose of intravenous prednisolone after resuturing, or even placing a biodegradable collagen implant in the area, may be an effective solution. Severe and persistent bleeding requires a transfusion of fresh plasma to correct the depletion of clotting factors.

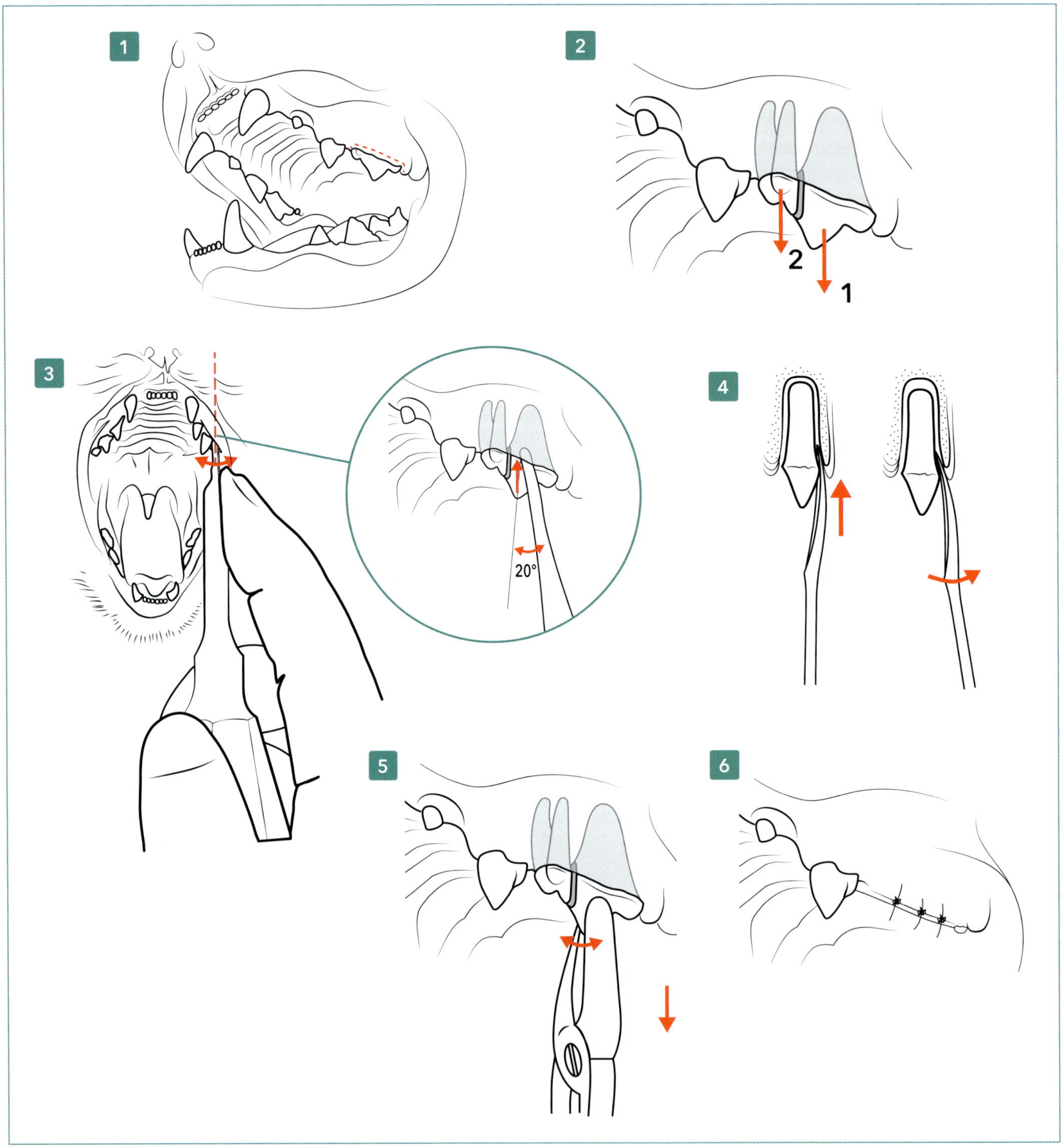

FIGURE 7. Steps of the closed dental extraction technique.

1. An incision is made around the perimeter of the gingival sulcus up to the level of the alveolar bone.
2. Using a suitable fissure bur, the premolar (or molar) is sectioned in a furcation–crown direction until it is divided into two fragments. The distal root is extracted first and then the two mesial roots.
3. The luxator is introduced into the periodontal space to break the ligament. The movement should be a rocking motion, with an instrument inclination of 20°.
4. Once the periodontal space has been luxated, if necessary, an elevator is introduced, applying sustained, controlled, slightly rotating pressure for 10–30 seconds.
5. When the fragment is sufficiently mobile, it is grasped with the extraction forceps and, with short, small rotating movements, with twists of the wrist, it is extracted.
6. Finally, the gingiva is sutured using 4-0 or 5-0 absorbable monofilament material and an atraumatic needle.

> Sometimes the bleeding is not detectable until the cat has been extubated, is waking up and blood flow in the area has improved. Therefore, we must closely monitor the patient until we are sure that they have woken up and there is no evidence of bleeding.

Acute pain or orofacial pain syndrome

It is essential to ensure proper analgesia and to carefully monitor for any signs of postoperative oral pain. Most cats already had oral pain, so in the postoperative period this will have diminished. But in some cases we can see acute pain that leads the cat to self-harm or to present with orofacial pain syndrome, where there is no correlation between the intervention performed and the degree of pain experienced by the cat. This pain is controlled with a multimodal analgesic approach and may even require the administration of phenobarbital.

Root remnants and root displacement

In order to avoid the presence of root remnants and the displacement of these remnants into the mandibular canal, nasal cavity or maxillary sinus we must use a careful technique, without excessive use of force, so that the roots do not break. If this happens, we must extract them in their entirety. The persistence of root remnants causes severe inflammation and is a frequent cause of inadequate responses to complete tooth extraction in cats with feline chronic gingivostomatitis. The only exception to this are roots with a type 2 resorptive lesion, in which case it is acceptable to perform a crown amputation. When root remnants need to be extracted, we must be careful when introducing the luxator/elevator into the periodontal space not to exert excessive apical pressure, as we can push the remnants into the mandibular canal, nasal cavity or maxillary sinus, from where they must be extracted in a much more complex and not risk-free procedure. We must be especially careful in cases with severe periodontal disease and osteomyelitis.

All these complications show that, as we said earlier, it is not possible to perform dental extractions safely and correctly if we do not have intraoral X-rays. Root remnants should never be atomized with a bur; it is very easy to remove too much (reaching the alveolar bone) or too little, which can lead to venous air embolization resulting in death, among other problems.

Lip entrapment

This is occasionally encountered when extracting the maxillary canines, such that the opposing mandibular canines traumatically contact the upper lip or rest on the lateral lip, potentially causing an ulcer. To prevent this from happening, we should try to remove as little vestibular alveolar bone as possible and be very careful with the mucoperiosteal flap with which we close the extraction area. If after a reasonable time it does not spontaneously resolve (some cats learn to position the lip properly) or the wound it produces is not acceptable in the short term, we should remove the mandibular canine causing the problem or perform a crown reduction and endodontic treatment.

Trauma to the eyeball

This occurs because the floor of the orbit is formed by soft tissues and can be easily penetrated due to incorrect technique when injecting local anesthesia in the maxillary nerve block or when handling the luxator and elevator when removing tooth 108 or 208. It may also be associated with an incorrect assessment of the degree of periodontal disease and associated osteomyelitis, or overlooking existing osteolytic lesions in the area. Therefore, we must be very familiar with the anatomy of the area, always control the pressure we exert and hold the extraction instrument with two fingers at the end to prevent it from moving in an uncontrolled manner.

Bone fractures and necrosis

Mandibular symphysis fracture is associated with an incorrect extraction technique, especially of teeth 304 and 404. It can also happen if we have not adequately evaluated the presence of osteolysis due to severe infection or neoplasia.

Maxillary or mandibular bone necrosis is seen more frequently in larger teeth (104, 204, 304, 404, 108, 208) when a fibrin clot has not formed properly. It is related to poor extraction technique and individual factors such as a state of immunosuppression. In order to avoid this very serious complication, in addition to a careful technique (with the minimum necessary trauma) and adequate patient management, it is recommended that the gum always be sutured in the extraction areas to protect the fibrin clot and ensure correct and rapid healing.

Bibliography

Bellows J. *Feline Dentistry.* Iowa: Wiley-Blackwell, 2011.

Blazejewski S 3rd, Lewis JR, Reiter AM. Mucoperiosteal flap for extraction of multiple teeth in the maxillary quadrant of the cat. *J Vet Dent*, 2006; 23(3):200–205.

Gracis M, Molinari E, Ferro S. Caudal mucogingival lesions secondary to traumatic dental occlusion in 27 cats: macroscopic and microscopic description, treatment and follow-up. *J Feline Med Surg*, 2015; 17(4):318–328.

Hennet P. Gingivo-stomatitis in cats: long-term follow-up of 30 cases treated by dental extractions. *J Vet Dent*, 1997; 14(1):15–21.

Jennings MW, Lewis JR, Soltero-Rivera MM et al. Effect of tooth extraction on stomatitis in cats: 95 cases (2000–2013). *J Am Vet Med Assoc*, 2015; 246(6):654–660.

Lee DB, Verstraete FJM, Arzi B. An update on feline chronic gingivostomatitis. *Vet Clin North Am Small Anim Pract*, 2020; 50(5):973–982.

Perry R, Tutt C. Periodontal disease in cats: back to basics—with an eye on the future. *J Feline Med Surg*, 2015; 17(1):45–65.

Reiter AM, Soltero-Rivera MM. Applied feline oral anatomy and tooth extraction techniques: an illustrated guide. *J Feline Med Surg*, 2014; 16(11):900–913.

Reyes NA, Longley M, Bailey S, Langley-Hobbs SJ. Incidence and types of preceding and subsequent fractures in cats with patellar fracture and dental anomaly syndrome. *J Feline Med Surg*, 2019; 21(8):750–764.

Smith MM. Extraction of teeth in the mandibular quadrant of the cat. *J Vet Dent*, 2008; 25(1):69–74.

Volk HA, Bayley KD, Fiani N, Billson FM. Ophthalmic complications following ocular penetration during routine dentistry in 13 cats. *N Z Vet J*, 2019; 67(1):46–51.

Volker MK, Luskin IR. Surgical extraction of the mandibular canine tooth in the cat. *J Vet Dent*, 2012; 29(2):134–137.

Watanabe R, Doodnaught GM, Evangelista MC et al. Inter-rater reliability of the feline grimace scale in cats undergoing dental extractions. *Front Vet Sci*, 2020; 7:302.

NASAL PLANUM AND NASAL CAVITY SURGERY 15

Alberto Barneto

Surgical anatomy

The function of the nasal cavity is to filter, warm, and moisten air that is inhaled and enters the lower respiratory tract. In cats there two distinct anatomical regions:

- **Nasal fossae:** include the nose itself (**nasal planum**) and the nasal orifices (**nostrils**). The nasal planum in cats has a triangular shape, is hairless and is covered with thick tough skin that may or may not be pigmented. Its epithelial surface has numerous small circular nodules that form a unique relief pattern which can be used to identify cats (**nose print**). A slight vertical indentation that divides the nasal planum into two equal parts, called the **nasolabial groove** (philtrum), goes from the upper lip over the lower half and the center of the nasal planum. The two nostrils, situated on either side of the nasal planum, are symmetrical. Each lateral portion is bordered by two wing-like **alar cartilages**, which enable the nasal fossae to remain passively open over a continuous period of time. Small muscles that insert into the alar cartilages enable voluntary movement of the opening when the cat sniffs up close or during forced breathing after exercise or resulting from disease. Each nasal orifice leads into a small chamber called the nasal vestibule.
- **Nasal cavity:** consists of two symmetrical halves divided by a partition known as the vertical midline **nasal septum**. The septum is composed of hyaline cartilage (cranial portion) and bone (caudal). Several bones of the face (nasal and frontal), and especially the superior maxillary bone, contribute to the lateral walls and roof of the nasal cavity. Meanwhile, the floor of the nasal cavity is composed of sections of the incisive, maxillary, palatine and vomer bones. The dorsocaudal part of the nasal cavity terminates in a bony partition that delineates the dome of the skull, while the ventrocaudal area is open and continues with the nasopharynx. The nasal cavity is itself divided into several parts:
  - **Nasal vestibule:** small space originating at the nostrils which houses the nasolacrimal ducts and the incisive canal. This canal belongs to the **vomeronasal organ**, which has the function of urinary pheromone recognition during the flehmen response, characteristic of this species.
- **Respiratory region:** the nasal cavity as such. It occupies the largest amount of space and is divided by the septum into right and left cavities. It houses several structures: the **nasal turbinates** (also known as nasal conchae) are structures formed by extremely thin sheets of convoluted bone anchored to the wall bones and which project towards the space of the cavity (Fig. 1). They are covered with a ciliated glandular epithelium with high vascularization, enabling them to warm and moisten air that passes through. They thus increase the surface area of the nasal cavity and optimize their function. The turbinates form the border of the nasal passages or **nasal meatuses**, which conduct air through the bony labyrinth towards the rest of the respiratory tree. Each half has several turbinates:
  - **Dorsal nasal concha:** the longest. Forms one part of the border of the **dorsal nasal meatus**, with the roof of the nasal cavity being the other part of the border, blind ended.
  - **Middle nasal concha:** the most extensive. The **middle nasal meatus**, also blind ended, extends between it and the dorsal concha.
  - **Ventral nasal concha:** small and cranial. The **ventral nasal meatus**, the largest and widest, passes below it. The nasopharynx is the continuation of this meatus.
  - **Ethmoidal conchae (ethmoidal labyrinth):** come from the ethmoid bone and are the most caudal within the nasal cavity. Covered with specialized nerve endings involved in olfaction. Continue caudally with the **cribiform plate**, through which the rootlets of the olfactory nerve pass toward the olfactory peduncles of the brain.
- **Choanae:** are two apertures bordered by bone at the far end of the hard palate, site of confluence of all the air from the nasal cavity. It serves as a passage for clean, warm and moist air towards the nasopharynx.

- **Paranasal sinuses:** are blind-ended pockets housed within certain bones of the head. They communicate with the nasal cavity through small openings. Cats have **frontal sinuses**, **sphenoid sinuses** and two small **maxillary recesses**.

The **maxillary artery**, which originates in the external carotid artery, irrigates the nasal cavity. It courses along both sides of the floor of the nasal cavity in a caudocranial direction, giving way to the **sphenopalatine**, **infraorbital** and **greater palatine arteries**, which are distributed through the different structures of the nasal cavity and fossae.

Innervation originates from the **cranial nerves I (olfactory) and V (trigeminal)**, specifically their maxillary and ophthalmic branches.

Surgical diseases

Diseases of the nasal planum and the nasal cavity usually share the same clinical signs (nonspecific): sneezing, nasal stertor, nasal discharge (from serous to mucopurulent, sometimes accompanied by epistaxis), facial deformities, anorexia and weakness. It is important to find out about the cat's lifestyle: if it goes outside, lives with other cats, sanitary conditions of the colony, etc. During the physical examination, we should not forget to examine the teeth, larynx and pharynx, the proper passage of air through the nasal fossae (a few cotton threads near the nostril can be used), drainage of the nasolacrimal duct, and depigmentation of the hair of the nasal planum (this occurs in colorpoint cats due to an increase in temperature in chronic rhinitis).

Main nasal conditions that may require surgery include:

- **Stenotic nostrils:** is the congenital narrowing of the nasal orifices, sometimes associated with misalignment of the maxillary lips, other times with alar cartilage deformities. It is characteristic of brachycephalic breeds: Persian, Exotic, Himalayan, and their crossbreeds. The passage of air generates noise, and sometimes there is serous discharge. Several surgical techniques have been described.
- **Nasal foreign bodies:** most often plant debris or toy packing material. It is more frequent in young cats. Produces sneezing and acute rhinitis, sometimes with blood. Ideally, once the foreign body is located, it is extracted with the help of rhinoscopy.
- **Tumors of the nasal planum:** the most common are squamous cell carcinomas, associated with white fur and high levels of exposure to ultraviolet radiation. The preferred location of these tumors is the pinnae and the nasal planum (Table 1). Other tumors that are diagnosed less frequently are hemangiosarcoma, basal cell carcinoma, and mast cell tumors. Superficial lesions with a thickness of less than 5 mm can very effectively be treated with electrochemotherapy or cryosurgery. Wider or deeper lesions require surgery (Fig. 2).

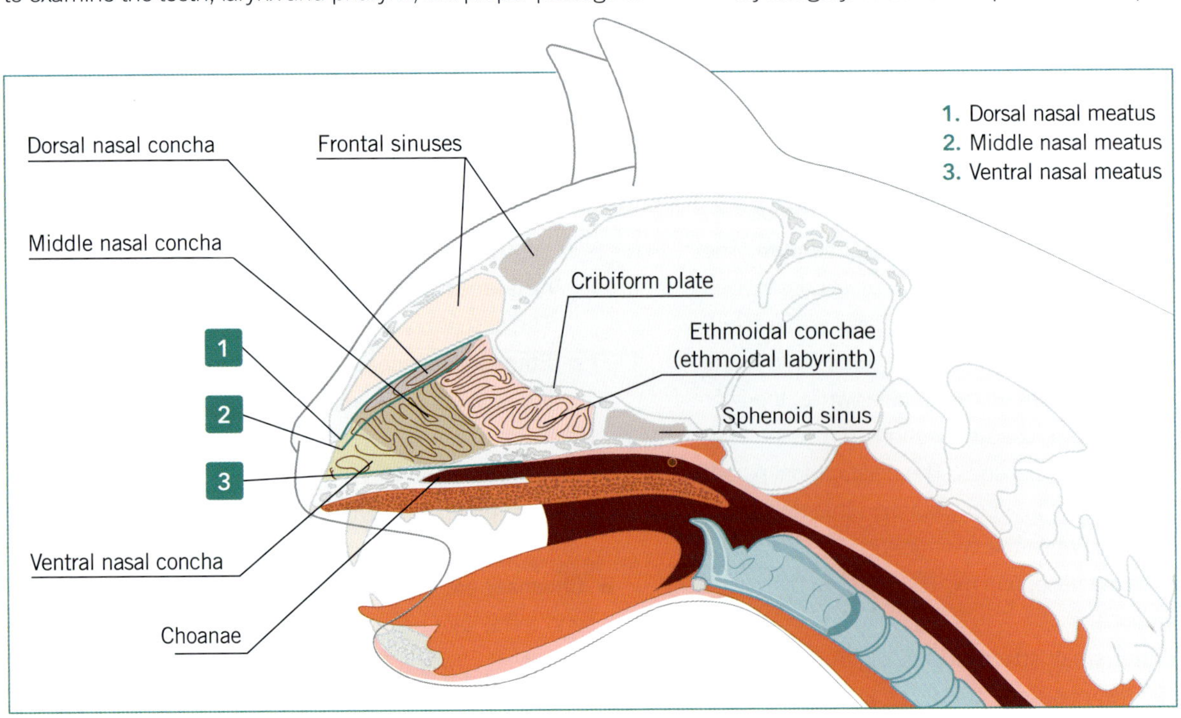

FIGURE 1. Structure of the feline nasal cavity.

TABLE 1. Staging of feline nasal squamous cell carcinoma according to the WHO (World Health Organization)

Stage	Description
Tis	Carcinoma in situ; superficial ulcerous/crusted lesion which does not extend beyond the basal lamina
T1a	Circumscribed, raised lesion, less than 1.5 cm
T1b	Superficial or minimally invasive lesion, 1.5 cm or larger
T2	Ulcerous or infiltrative lesion, 2 cm or larger
T3	Lesion larger than 5 cm or invaded the hypodermis
T4	Any size lesion that has invaded muscle, bone or fascia

- **Tumors of the nasal cavity:** the most common primary tumors of the nasal cavity are lymphoma (Fig. 3), adenocarcinoma, squamous cell carcinoma, and adenoma. With the exception of adenoma (not common), almost all of these tumors are malignant. Rare cases of benign mesenchymal tumors called hamartomas have also been described. These tumors consist of fibrous and osseous tissue. Nasal tumors produce nasal discharge, frequently with blood, as well as stertor, and deformity. Sometimes, a fragment of tumor is observed protruding from the nostrils.

- **Chronic rhinitis:** defined as having clinical signs that last longer than 4 weeks. It poses a diagnostic and therapeutic challenge. The cat presents with serous to purulent discharge (sometimes epistaxis) in one or both nostrils. The more chronic the condition, the more extensive the lesion in the turbinates and paranasal sinuses (Fig. 4). The primary causes are usually inflammatory (lymphoplasmacytic rhinitis), viral (FHV-1, FCV) or bacterial (*Chlamydia felis* or *Bordetella bronchiseptica*). But when the condition becomes chronic, bacteria from the nasal cavity (*Pseudomonas* spp., *Escherichia coli*, *Streptococcus* spp., *Staphylococcus* spp., *Klebsiella* spp., *Proteus* spp.) or, more rarely, fungi (*Cryptococcus* spp., *Aspergillus* spp.) multiply and the infection spreads to the turbinates and paranasal sinuses. Although medical treatment is frustrating in many cases, it is needed to manage chronic rhinitis. Most of the time, surgical techniques of last resort can only improve the clinical signs somewhat.

> Of nasal diseases, chronic rhinitis represents the biggest diagnostic and therapeutic challenge. Early diagnosis and treatment can prevent many of the effects that cannot be successfully addressed later.

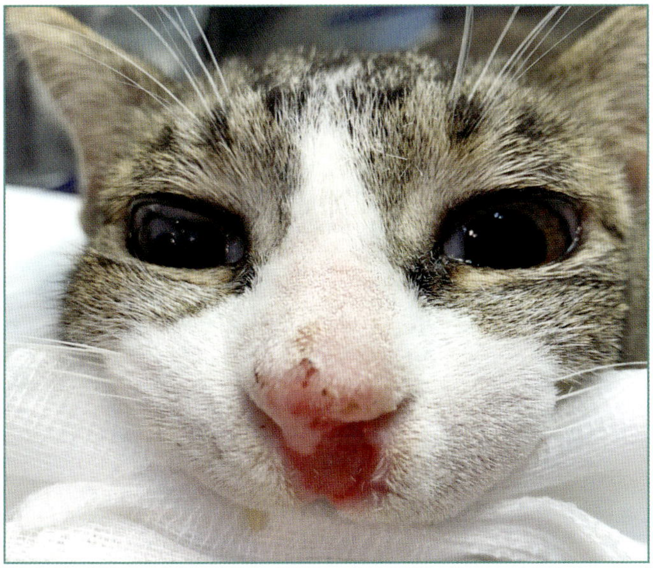

FIGURE 2. Squamous cell carcinoma in a cat's nasal planum. If not very extensive, this neoplasm can be treated with electrochemotherapy. A planectomy can be done in case of recurrence or as a first treatment option.

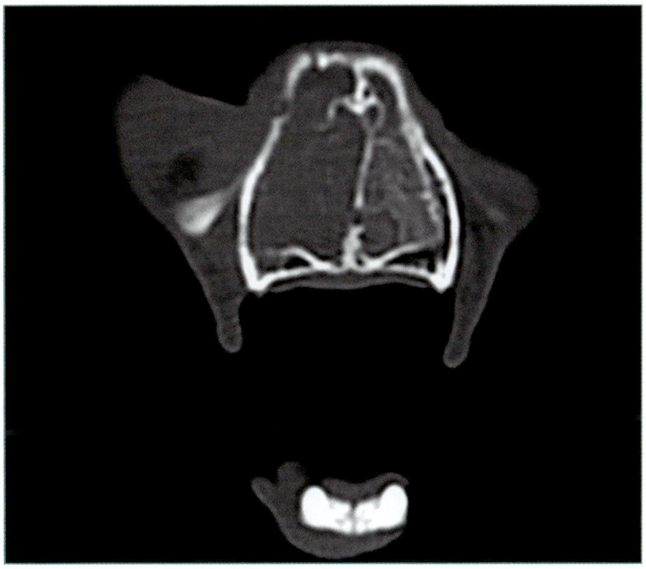

FIGURE 3. Computed tomography scan of a nasal tumor (lymphoma) that initially affected the right half of the nasal cavity, but has already started to invade the left half. In many cases, these tumors only cause moderate inspiratory dyspnea and epistaxis.

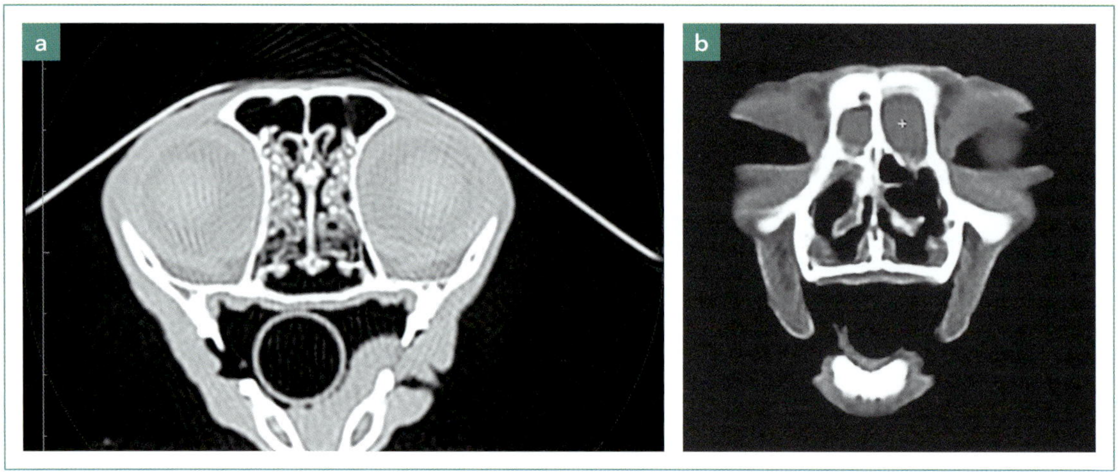

FIGURE 4.
(a) Computed tomography scan of the nasal cavity of a cat showing the normal appearance of the nasal turbinates, without fluid accumulation.
(b) Patient with chronic rhinitis, which has partially damaged and atrophied the rostral turbinates, with accumulation of fluid in the frontal sinuses.

Diagnosis

Advanced diagnostic imaging is an essential tool that allows us to locate and access lesions of the nasal cavity, while other diagnostic tests are needed to determine the cause (Table 2).

TABLE 2. Techniques and tests for the diagnosis of nasal cavity diseases

Diagnostic technique	Indications	Observations
Radiology	■ Chronic rhinitis ■ Radiopaque foreign bodies	Although X-rays are always obtained, they have low sensitivity and specificity to locate and diagnose the issue.
Computed tomography (CT)	All conditions	Gold standard for the diagnosis of diseases of the nasal cavity, specifically to locate the full area of the issue. Can also guide the taking of samples with other methods (rhinoscopy, fine needle aspiration —FNA—, swab sampling of exudates).
Rigid rhinoscopy	■ Examination ■ Biopsy ■ Extraction of foreign bodies	This is the other important diagnostic test for the nasal cavity. Although it enables the precise collection of samples, the configuration of the nasal cavity prevents the endoscope from having good access to all spaces (internal meatuses, nasal turbinates, paranasal sinuses, ethmoidal labyrinth). Accuracy is improved if accompanied by CT.
Flexible rhinoscopy	■ Examination ■ Biopsy ■ Extraction of foreign bodies	Has all the same uses as rigid rhinoscopy, but also enables better visualization of areas such as the choanae.
Biopsy	■ Chronic rhinitis ■ Tumors	■ A 2 mm punch biopsy of the nasal planum. ■ In the nasal cavity with the help of CT (FNA) or rhinoscopy (forceps).
Bacterial/ fungal culture	■ Bacterial rhinitis ■ Fungal rhinitis	Samples are obtained with the help of CT imaging, through rhinoscopy, guided with fluoroscopy, or through nasal flushing* (the patient should be anesthetized and intubated).
PCR	■ Viral rhinitis ■ *Chlamydia felis* ■ *Bordetella bronchiseptica*	Useful only in the early stages to learn the possible etiology. Difficult to interpret due to false positives (vaccinated animals) and false negatives (pathogen already eliminated or hidden). In cat colonies, it provides epidemiological data.
Serology	Fungal rhinitis	Supports the diagnosis in cases of cryptococcosis and aspergillosis.

* Lavage and irrigation with saline solution under moderate pressure.

How to perform a nasal flushing

Nasal flushing (lavage and irrigation technique using pressurized saline solution) is a very useful procedure for taking samples of any disease that entails nasal discharge. The material collected can be used to perform a culture, PCR, or cytology to help diagnose the primary cause.

To perform nasal flushing the following must be prepared:

- A piece of sterile rolled-up gauze held with an Allis forceps or tied to the edge of a dressing.
- 5 ml syringes with warm sterile isotonic saline solution.
- Culture media, microscope slides and sterile swabs for submission of samples for PCR.

Technique

1. The cat is anesthetized, intubated and placed in sternal recumbency.
2. The roll of gauze is moistened with sterile isotonic saline solution and inserted into the mouth up to the pharynx (it should not be lodged in the oral cavity if we wish to recover the sample).
3. The tip of a syringe with warm sterile isotonic saline solution is applied inside one of the cat's nostrils. The entire syringe tip should enter, running the length of the alar cartilage.
4. The other nostril is closed with a finger, the cat's head is lifted slightly, and the syringe plunger is depressed with force to discharge the liquid with pressure.
5. The roll of gauze is removed from the pharynx, being careful not to pull the tracheal tube in an outward direction. The sample is then processed for submission to the laboratory.
6. The procedure is repeated in the other nostril.

VIDEO

Nasal flushing performed on two feline patients

Preoperative and postoperative considerations

Things that should be kept in mind before and after the surgery:

- Nasal planum surgery can greatly affect the animal's appearance. We should inform owners of this and whenever possible show them images of cats that have had such operations, so that they can be aware beforehand.
- Both the nasal planum and the nasal cavity are highly irrigated and bleed profusely during the intervention. We should do clotting tests before the surgery and sometimes have bags of fresh plasma compatible with the patient's blood group to prevent postoperative anemia.
- Pain is controlled by infiltrating the maxillary nerve with bupivacaine or mepivacaine.
- To prevent blood from entering the digestive tract, we place a tied, rolled-up piece of gauze at one end of a gauze dressing to collect secretions during the surgery.
- Additional instruments used during this surgery are contra-angle dental burs and a Freer periosteal elevator (see Ch. 5). These instruments are used to access the nasal cavity and ensure that subsequent apposition of tissues is correct. It is useful to have microsurgery material available to work on such small tissues and in such small spaces.
- During the surgery, it is also important to have on hand cold sterile saline solution to irrigate and help stop bleeding. If the surgery is expected to result in too much loss of blood, the external carotid artery can be ligated on the side that will be operated on for a maximum of 40 minutes. However, it is rare to have to use this technique during feline nasal surgery.
- Loss of appetite for a period of time is common after nasal surgery. If necessary, an esophagostomy tube can be placed (see Ch. 3).

Surgical techniques

All surgical procedures involving the nasal cavity and planum are performed with the patient intubated in sternal recumbency and the head slightly elevated with a towel under the mandible.

Techniques for resolving stenotic nostrils

Wedge resection of the alar cartilage

This is the technique of choice when the issue of stenotic nostrils is a congenital medial dislocation of the alar cartilages. Surgical cleaning of the nasal planum is necessary, but the area does not need to be shaved.

Using an Adson forceps with teeth, the portion of the alar cartilage that will be sectioned is pinched **vertically** (Fig. 5). A vertical wedge is sectioned from the marked portion with a no. 11 scalpel blade, and a piece in the shape of an orange wedge is extracted. Bleeding is controlled by applying pressure for a few minutes, and the wound is closed with two 5-0 nylon stitches and a round needle, leaving the knots in the outer part of the alar cartilage (Fig. 6).

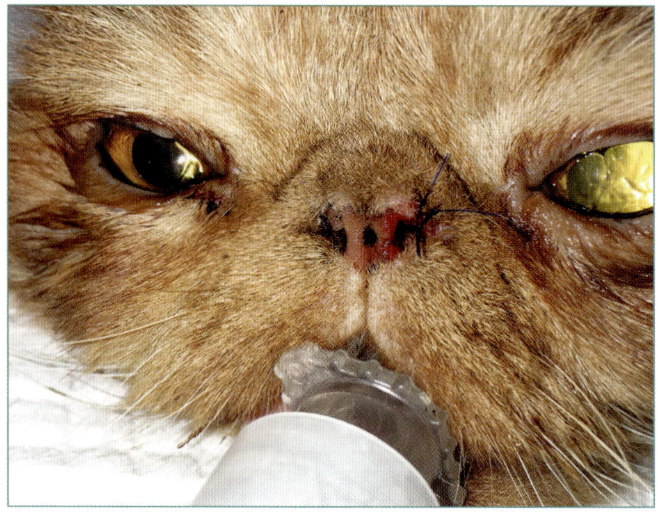

FIGURE 6. Wedge resection of the alar cartilage in a Persian cat. The technique has been completed on one side, while the other side has not yet been finished. The improvement in the opening on the operated side can be observed.

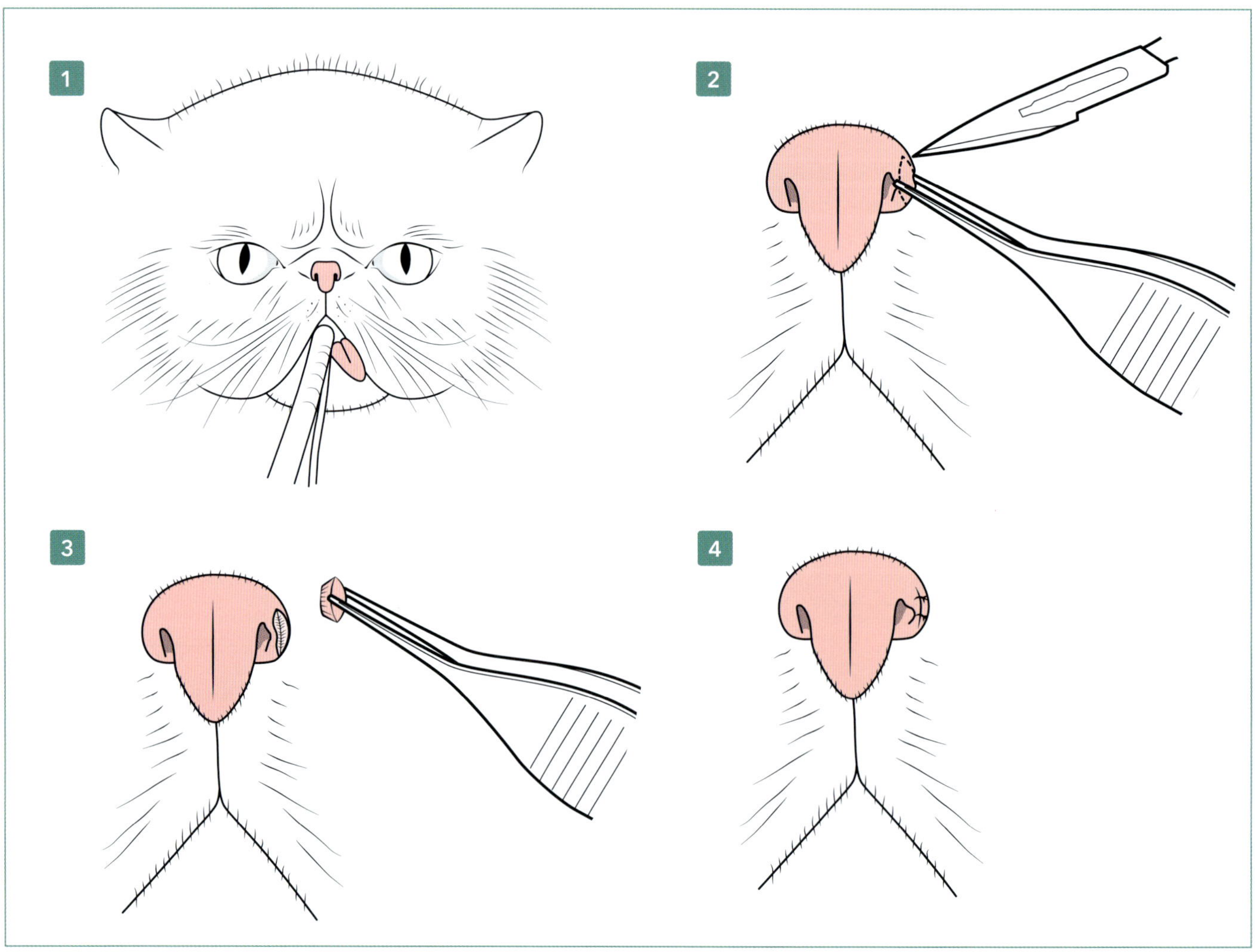

FIGURE 5. Technique for resolving stenotic nostrils through wedge resection of the alar cartilage.

Single pedicle advancement flap

Many brachycephalic cats have obstruction of the ventral part of the nostrils due to an excess of skin on the upper lip. This technique aims to open this stenosis with a flap that tightens the lip and opens the nostril (Fig. 7).

The maxillary lip area is shaved, leaving the whiskers intact. Povidone is used to disinfect. A rectangular flap is dissected, beginning around the maxillary lip at a distance of 3–5 mm ventrally to the nasal orifice. The dissection of the flap is carefully continued until reaching approximately 3–5 mm inside the nasal mucosa (Fig. 8). Traction is applied to the flap towards the cranioventral area. A stitch is placed going from the center of the flap to the vertex in the beginning of the square, and this process is repeated on the other side. We have thus tightened the skin of the flap over the maxillary lip, which tends to lower itself and open the nostrils. We are left with approximately half of the flap left over: it is cut and discarded. All that is left at this point is to finalize the

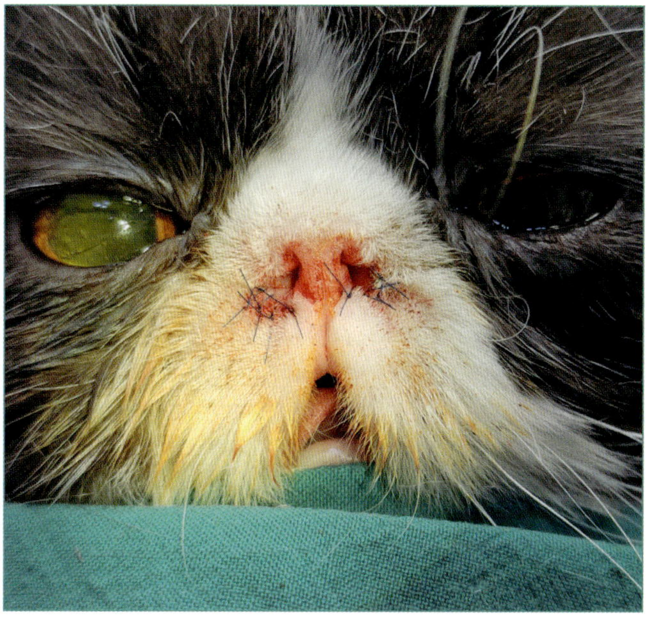

FIGURE 7. Resolution of stenotic nostrils due to an excess of skin on the upper lip in a Persian cat using a single pedicle advancement flap.

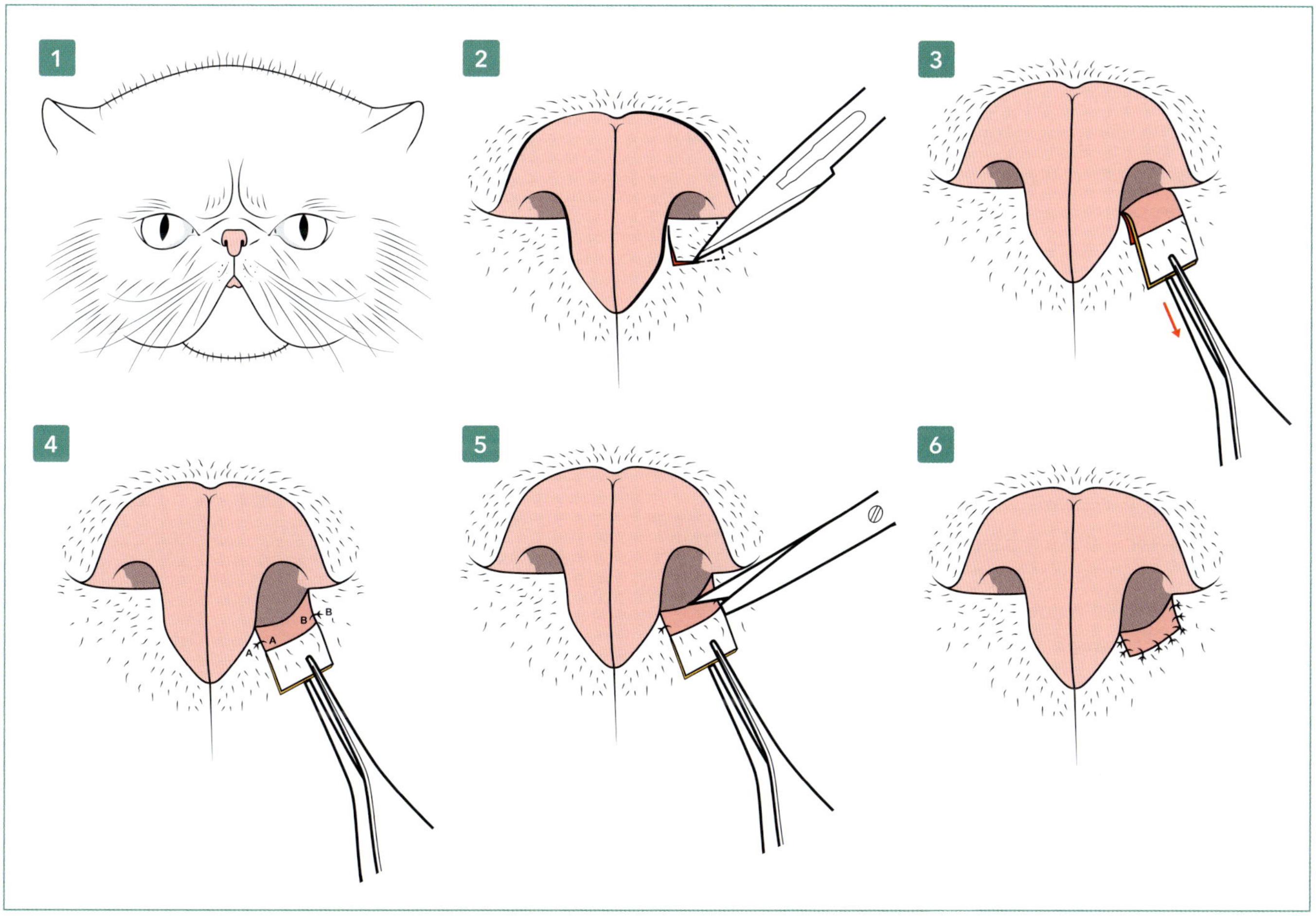

FIGURE 8. Technique for resolving stenotic nostrils through a single pedicle advancement flap.

suture with 5-0 nylon or absorbable monofilament, both in the mucosa inside the nasal orifice and in the maxillary lip. If necessary, this same technique is applied to the other side (it is usually always necessary).

Surgical treatment techniques for nasal planum tumors

Lip-to-nose flap

This is a simple flap technique used when the tumor only affects one part of the nasal planum (lateral or dorsal). When performing this surgery, the area around the corresponding maxillary lip is shaved. First the nasal tumor is removed with sufficient safety margins. Next, two parallel incisions are made at an oblique angle across the lip approximately 1 cm apart. The incisions begin near the lower eyelid and are directed ventally and rostrally toward the rostral edge of the upper lip, avoiding the whisker area (Fig. 9). The two incisions converge in the ventral area, and we dissect the flap, including the musculocutaneous tissue. If any skin is left between the base of the flap and the defect of the tumor, an incision is made across it, since there should be a continuous wound between the defect and the base of the flap. We transfer the flap to the area of the defect, covering it, and we suture, beginning as usual at the ends furthest from the base of the flap. We finish suturing the skin of the flap along the length of the open incision on the skin bridge. The defect of the maxillary lip which is the origin of the flap is also sutured with interrupted stitches. For this technique 4-0 nonabsorbable monofilament sutures are used. For treatment of tumors located at these sites, the use of angularis oris flaps has also been described (see Ch. 9).

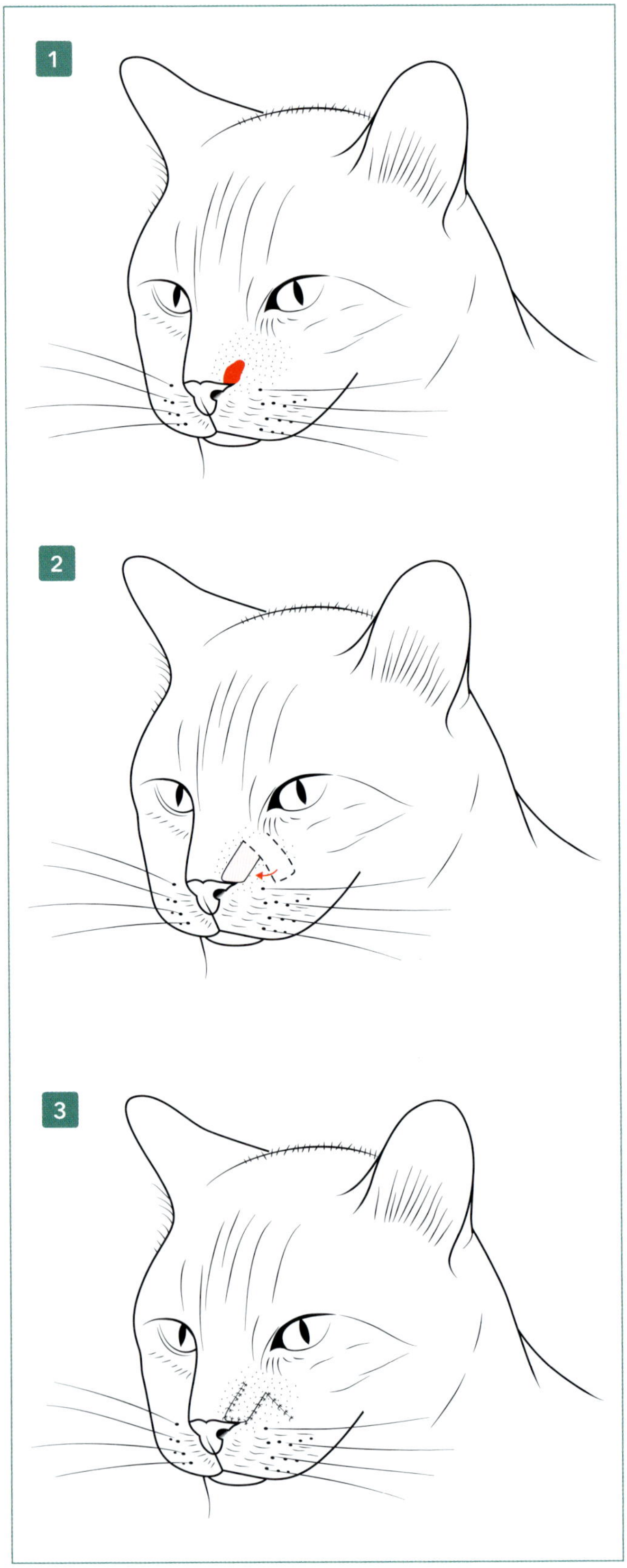

FIGURE 9. Lip-to-nose flap technique.

Total planectomy

This technique is used when the tumor affects nearly the entire nasal planum and the lesion is over 5 mm deep in the skin. It results in a major change in appearance of the cat's face, and this should be discussed with the owners beforehand. The area between the nose and the maxillary lips is shaved and disinfected. The mouth is kept slightly open with a 2 ml syringe barrel, and the mandible is fastened to the table with adhesive strip.

The surgical field includes the upper lips, upper jaw, canine teeth and the entire dorsal nasal area. Mini towel clamps are useful, or the surgical field can be sutured to avoid taking up too much space. A 360° incision is made including the entire

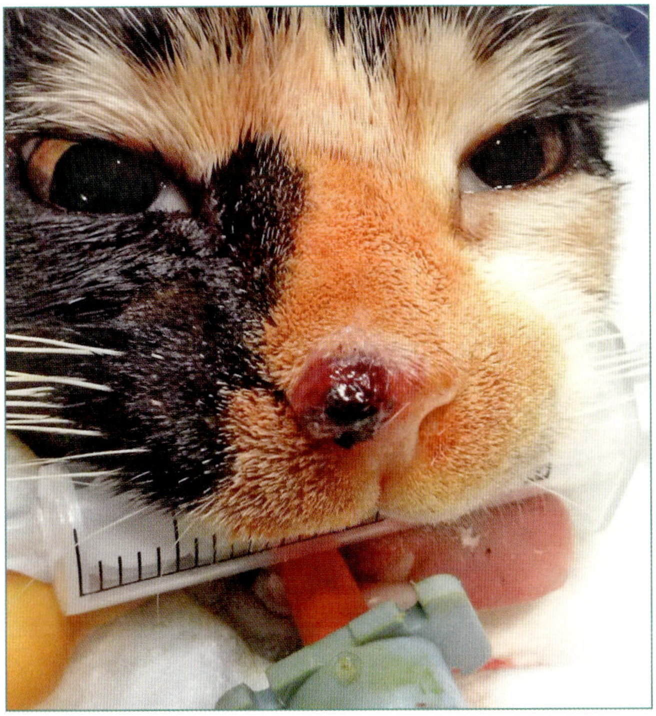

FIGURE 10. Preparation of the surgical field for a total planectomy in a cat suffering from hemangiosarcoma of the nasal planum. For solid support for the duration of the surgery and to avoid bite injuries on the tongue, the mouth is kept slightly open with the barrel of a 2 ml syringe.

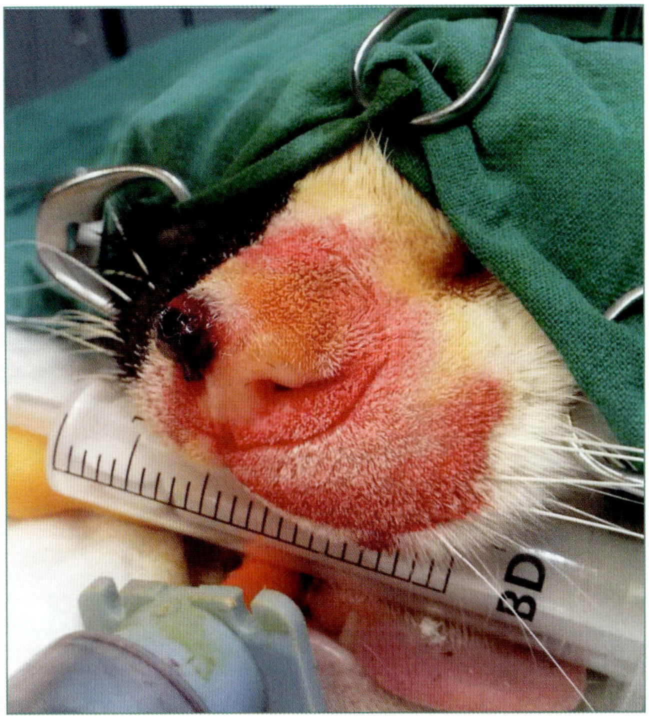

FIGURE 11. Beginning of the surgery with a 360° incision. The epidermis should protrude slightly more than the dermis so that after the subsequent suture, the latter can heal without forming keloid scars.

nasal planum with ample safety margins that include at least 1 cm of healthy tissue around the tumor. The incision can be drawn previously with a sterile skin marker. The scalpel blade is angled so that the epidermis is left protruding slightly more than the dermis (this facilitates suturing and wound healing later on). The incision should not extend to the edge of the upper lips so that later the philtrum, which will inevitably be removed, can be reconstructed. The tissue is dissected deeply in order to remove the entire tumor.

To prepare the suture, me make perforations in the visible nasal and maxillary bones, at a sufficient enough distance to ensure a good closure, using a Jacobs sleeve and 1 mm Kirschner wires. First, we suture the lips with 2–4 vertical stitches to reconstruct the philtrum. The sutures for the remainder of the 360° defect join nasal mucosa and skin. Bone may or may not be included in between, depending on the requirements of the area (Figs. 10–14). The suture material used is 4-0 nonabsorbable monofilament.

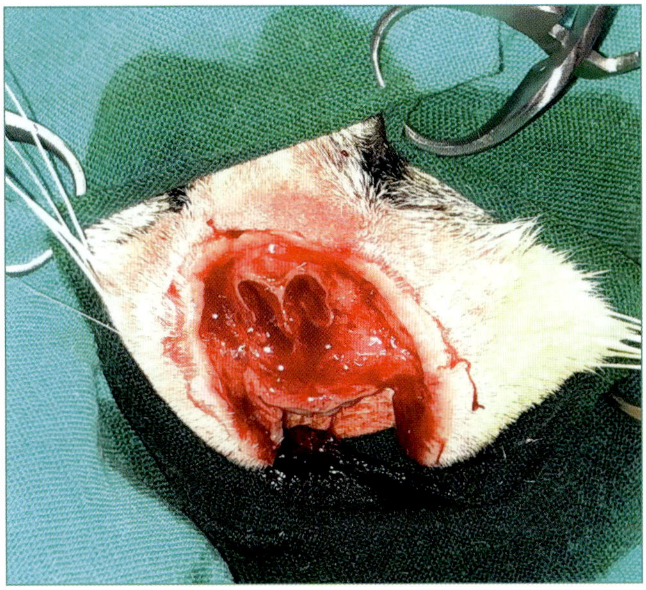

FIGURE 12. The entire nasal planum has been eliminated en bloc with a 1 cm margin of healthy tissue around the tumor. The philtrum and part of the maxillary lips were included. Later they will be remade with the suture.

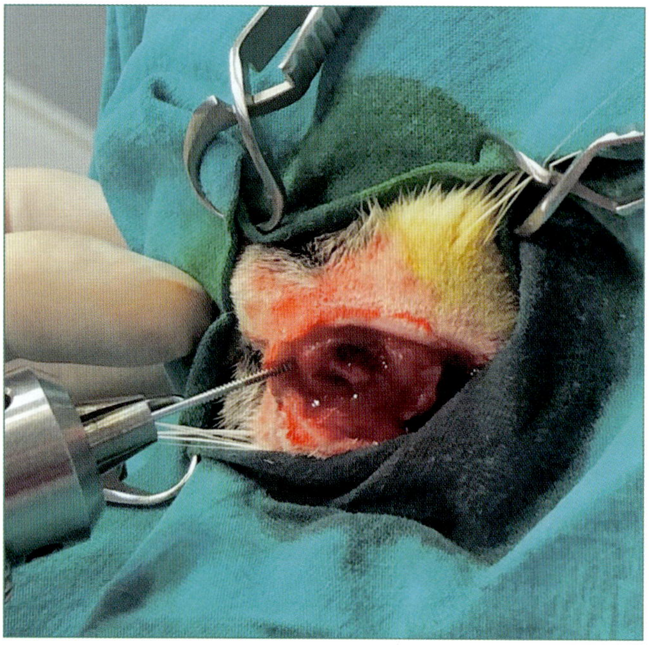

FIGURE 13. Using a threaded wire on the nasal bone, holes are made in the place where the sutures will later be anchored.

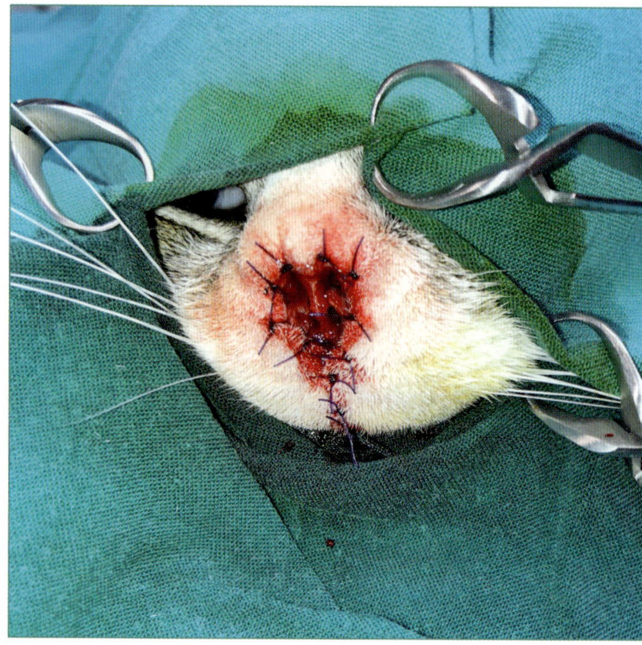

FIGURE 14. Appearance of the patient after completion of the suture and reconstruction of the lips and philtrum.

Nasal biopsies

When performing biopsies of the interior of the nasal cavity, we should always have CT image tests done beforehand. Rhinoscopes used for biopsies should preferably be flexible and be of a minimum caliber (up to 2.2 mm in diameter). If such a fine caliber prevents us from being able to insert instruments through the fiber endoscope, an effective technique is to use a urinary catheter for cats with the tip cut at an angle. The catheter is inserted parallel to the rhinoscope and the mass is incised for the biopsy (or the catheter is inserted into the sample of exudate or into the nasal mucosa). Suction is applied with the syringe and the material is prepared for the diagnostic laboratory. Bleeding tends to be minimal, and clotting is checked for with the rhinoscope itself.

Dorsal rhinotomy

Rhinotomies are not a very common surgery. It is considered a last-resort option for chronic conditions that cannot otherwise be treated from a medical perspective. There are two approaches to the nasal cavity: ventral (through an incision in the hard palate) and dorsal (through the frontal and nasal bones). We will describe the latter technique, since the former offers very limited access where it is difficult to work.

The surgical field is prepared for the dorsal rhinotomy by shaving the entire nasal region down the face to the upper lips. A midline incision is made at the medial canthus of the eye and continued until the end of the nasal bone. The periosteum is removed from the nasal bone with the help of a Freer periosteotome. With stay sutures or with Gelpi retractors, the skin and periosteum are displaced laterally.

Access to the nasal cavity can be gained using various techniques:

- A bur is used to drill through the nasal bone lengthwise, creating a 3–5 mm wide approach. Care must be taken to avoid causing injury at a depth with the bur.
- Two orifices are made with a hammer and Steinmann pin at the beginning and end of the planned incision. The two orifices are connected, eliminating any bone fragments with a rongeur forceps to open the access point.
- If the cat's nasal cavity were somewhat larger, a rectangular lid of nasal bone can be lifted off with an oscillating saw. This approach to the rhinotomy is no longer used for cats due to the small size of the nasal bone.

Once access to the nasal cavity is obtained, the foreign material, tumor or necrotic tissue is eliminated, depending on the reason for the rhinotomy. Cold saline solution is used liberally to wash the area, remove debris and stop bleeding of the turbinates.

Closure is performed in two layers: first the periosteum is sutured with a long-lasting absorbable monofilament (e.g., polydioxanone). The skin is sutured separately with continuous or interrupted stitches. If we want to place a drain to decrease the risk of postoperative subcutaneous emphysema, a stoma outside of the wound is opened in the skin before closure. A section of sterile silicone tube is passed through the stoma (such as is done with venipuncture with butterfly needles) and it is housed in the nasal cavity. The tube is attached to the skin with a Roman sandal suture, and it is removed in 5–7 days (Figs. 15–17).

Complications

Nasal surgery always involves several hours or days of light bleeding, more pronounced if there is sneezing. This occurs more often in surgeries that affect the rostral nasal cavity (respiratory area).

Dorsal rhinotomies can result in subcutaneous emphysema, but the risk of this can be reduced with the use of postoperative drains (Fig. 17).

In planectomies, especially those that affect the maxilla, dehiscence of sutures of the oral mucosa can occur. This must be detected and resolved to avoid chronic oronasal fistulas.

Both nasal tumors and chronic bacterial rhinitis can recur despite using the proper surgical technique.

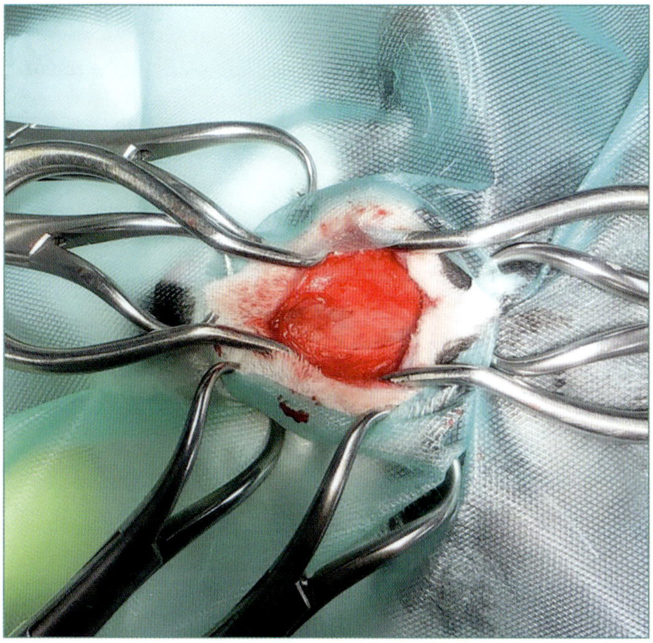

FIGURE 15. Access to the nasal bone for trephination and dorsal rhinotomy. Gelpi self-retaining retractors widen the surgical area and facilitate removal of the periosteum.

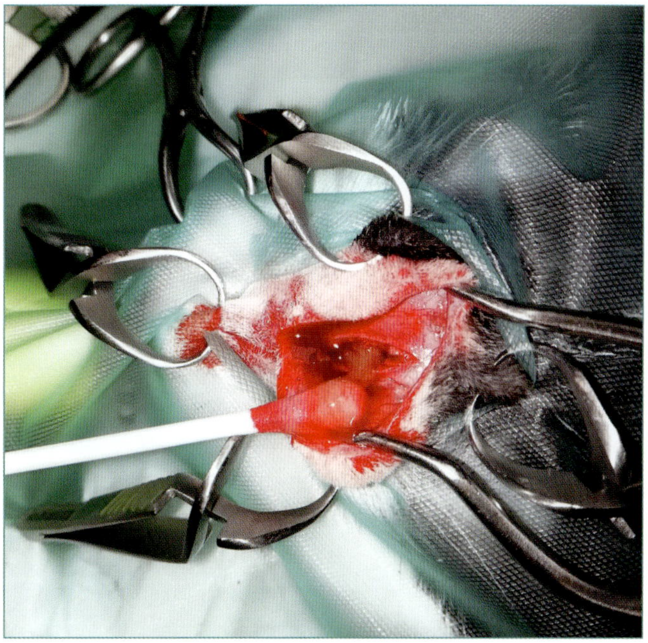

FIGURE 16. Once the rhinotomy is complete, a sample of mucus is taken for a culture and antibiogram (even if this has been done previously). The characteristically dense mucus points to how difficult it is to medically treat some of these cases.

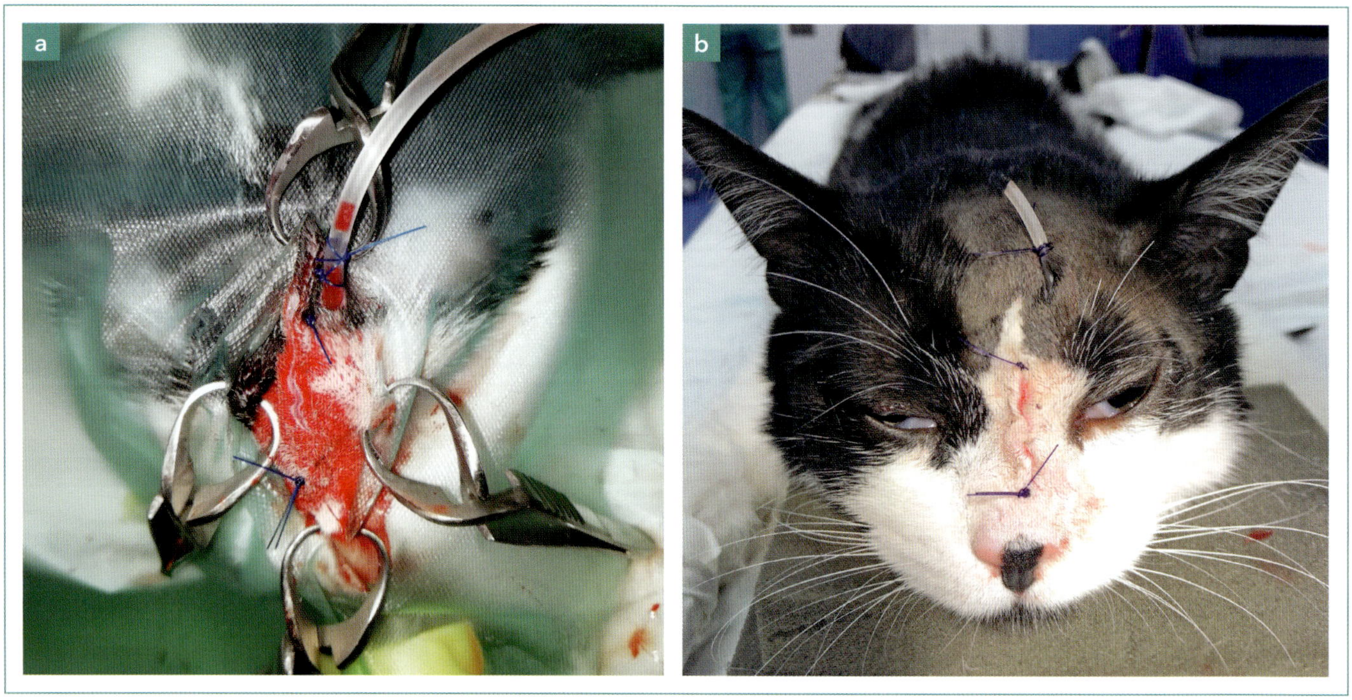

FIGURE 17. (a) After finishing the surgery, a drainage tube is placed inside the nasal cavity. This prevents subcutaneous emphysema in the postoperative period. (b) Final appearance of the patient.

Bibliography

Ashbaugh EA, McKiernan BC, Miller CJ, Powers B. Nasal hydropulsion: a novel tumour biopsy technique. *J Am Anim Hosp Assoc*, 2011; 47(5):312–316.

Berns CN, Schmiedt CW, Dickerson VM, Murphy SM. Single pedicle advancement flap for treatment of feline stenotic nares: technique and results in five cases. *J Feline Med Surg*, 2020; 22(12):1238–1242.

De Lorenzi D, BertoncelloD, Bottero E. Squash-preparation cytology from nasopharyngeal masses in the cat: cytological results and histological correlations in 30 cases. *J Feline Med Surg*, 2008; 10(1):55–60.

Demko JL, Cohn LA. Chronic nasal discharge in cats: 75 cases (1993–2004). *J Am Vet Med Assoc*, 2007; 230(7):1032–1037.

Harvey CE. Surgical correction of stenotic nares in a cat. *J Am Anim Hosp Assoc*, 1986; 22:31–32.

Lamb CR, Richbell S, Mantis P. Radiographic signs in cats with nasal disease. *J Feline Med Surg*, 2003; 5(4):227–235.

Massari F, Chiti LE, Lisi MLP et al. Lip-to-nose flap for reconstruction of the nasal planum after curative intent excision of squamous cell carcinoma in cats: description of technique and outcome in seven cases. *Vet Surg*, 2020; 49:339–346.

Mukaratirwa S, van der Linde-Sipman JS, Gruys E. Feline nasal and paranasal sinus tumours: clinicopathological study, histomorphological description and diagnostic immunohistochemistry of 123 cases. *J Feline Med Surg*, 2001; 3(4):235–245.

Reed N, Gunn-Moore D. Nasopharyngeal disease in cats: 1. Diagnostic investigation. *J Feline Med Surg*, 2012; 14(5):306–315.

Reed N, Gunn-Moore D. Nasopharyngeal disease in cats: 2. Specific conditions and their management. *J Feline Med Surg*, 2012; 14(5):317–326.

Schoenborn WC, Wisner ER, Kass PP, Dale M. Retrospective assessment of computed tomographic imaging of feline sinonasal disease in 62 cats. *Vet Radiol Ultrasound*, 2003; 44(2):185–195.

Spugnini EP, Vincenzi B et al. Electrochemotherapy for the treatment of squamous cell carcinoma in cats: a preliminary report. *Vet J*, 2009; 179(1):117–120.

Winstanley EW. Trephining frontal sinuses in the treatment of rhinitis and sinusitis in the cat. *Vet Rec*, 1974; 95(13):289–292.

NASOPHARYNGEAL POLYPS AND STENOSIS

16

Alberto Barneto

Surgical anatomy

The nasopharynx in the cat is a narrow, partially bony but predominantly soft-tissue passageway where air from the nasal cavity converges and is then directed towards the larynx and lower respiratory tract.

The width of the **nasopharyngeal airway** ranges between 5 and 10 mm in cats. Its rostral portion begins in the **choanae**, which are still divided in two by the nasal septum. This portion maintains its bony structure and measures approximately 1 cm. The hard palate continues caudally to the choanae. Its base (the **vomer bone**) is the floor of the nasopharyngeal airway in this section. Now a single passageway, the hard palate turns into the **soft palate**. This is the longest part of the nasopharynx, between 2 and 3 cm, depending on the breed and the length of the soft palate. Finally, the soft palate makes contact with a flap of cartilage known as the **epiglottis**, then continues essentially as the laryngeal lumen. This enables the passage of air and separates the nasopharynx from the pharynx and the opening of the esophagus (Fig. 1).

The mucosa is highly vascularized and innervated, and incorporates lymphoid tissue structures known as the **pharyngeal tonsils**. Midway through the nasopharynx on both sides, the **nasopharyngeal openings** of the **Eustachian tubes** (or auditory tubes) connect the nasopharynx to the middle ear. The innervation is significant and arises from branches of the cranial nerve V (the trigeminal nerve and its branches, the **maxillary and ophthalmic nerves**). The vascularization comes from arterioles originating in the maxillary artery (Fig. 2).

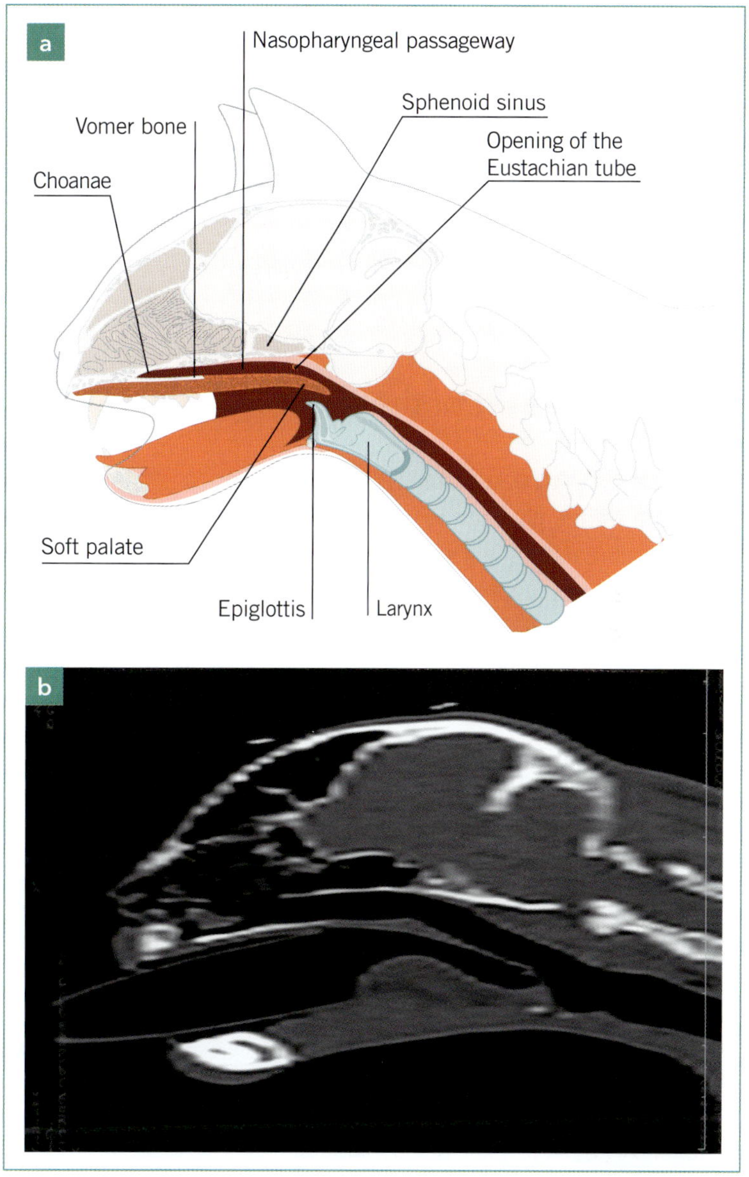

FIGURE 1. (a) Structures of the nasopharynx. (b) Computed tomography scan of the area.

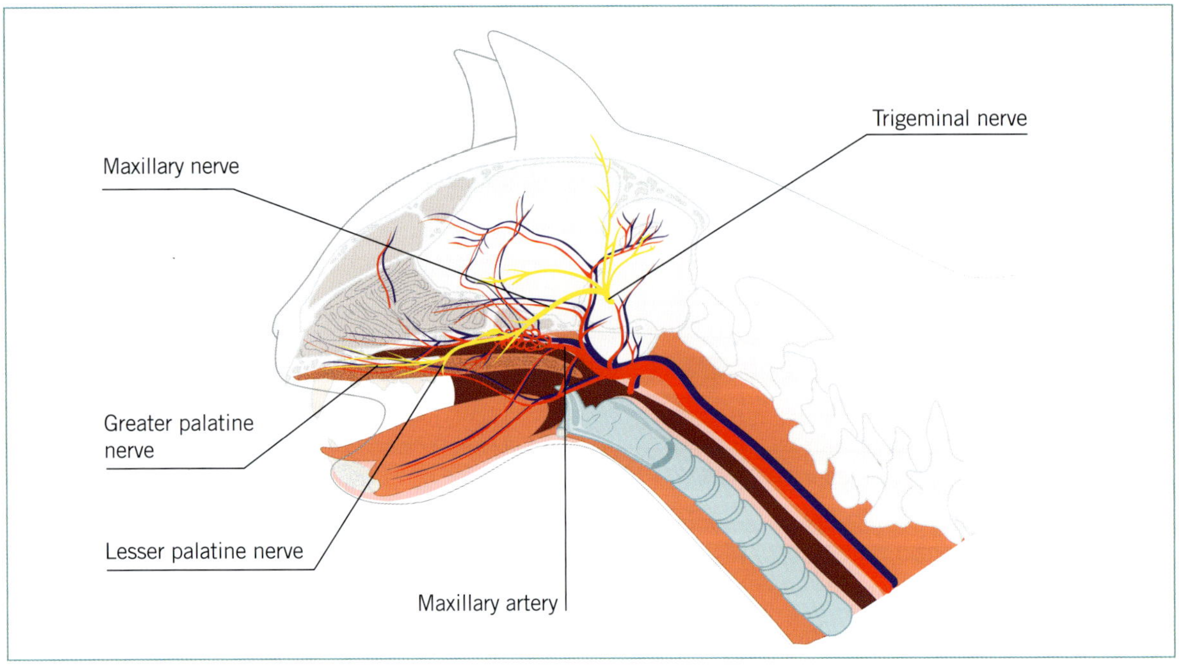

FIGURE 2. Vascularization and innervation of the nasopharynx.

Surgical diseases of the nasopharynx

Nasopharyngeal foreign bodies

These are frequently seen in outdoor cats. These patients present a clinical picture of acute stertor (easily audible forced breathing sound during inhalation) and forced swallowing movements depending on the size and location of the object. They usually consist of awns or blades of grass of various length (Fig. 3). If protruding from the soft palate towards the pharynx, they can often be extracted under anesthesia without the need for rhinoscopy.

Nasopharyngeal tumors

Although lymphoma is the most frequent tumor found in nasal passages, very few cases of lymphoma affect the nasopharynx (less than 20%). Likewise, squamous cell carcinoma is more typical of the oral mucosa and only occasionally affects the pharynx and soft palate. **Nasopharyngeal polyps** are the most common nasopharyngeal tumor. These are benign inflammatory masses that originate in the Eustachian tube mucosa and, as they grow, they invade the nasopharynx, especially caudally, eventually obstructing it. Their origin is unknown, although it is suspected that the cause could be chronic infection or

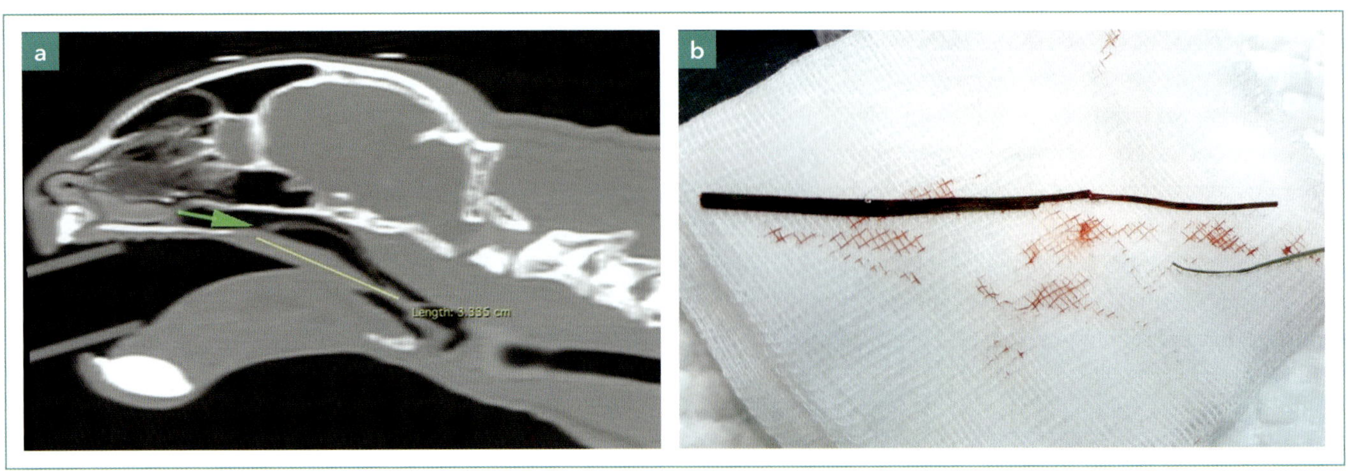

FIGURE 3. (a) Computed tomography scan in which a foreign body is observed (grass stem, green arrow) in the nasopharynx of a cat. (b) Foreign body after extraction.

inflammation. The incidence is higher in young kittens that live in colonies (Fig. 4), but cats up to 15 years of age have been diagnosed. When polyps grow towards the middle ear, they are called **aural polyps**, and they affect the sympathetic nerves there, producing Horner syndrome (see Ch. 18 "Ear canal and middle ear surgery"). Cases of cats with a nasopharyngeal polyp and an aural polyp at the same time have been described.

Nasopharyngitis

Inflammation of the nasopharynx in cats is frequently triggered by rhinitis, gingivostomatitis, or chronic regurgitation. Nasopharyngitis can also occur as an independent condition. Several infectious causes have been described as the origin of the condition, with herpesvirus (FHV-1) and calicivirus (FCV) occurring most often. In these cases, bacterial contamination is common. Reverse sneezing, stertor, and chronic sneezing are the most frequent clinical signs.

> Many infections of the nasopharynx coexist with foreign bodies, polyps or nasopharyngeal stenosis; therefore, it is essential to diagnose and treat these infections beforehand or at the same time as the other pathologies.

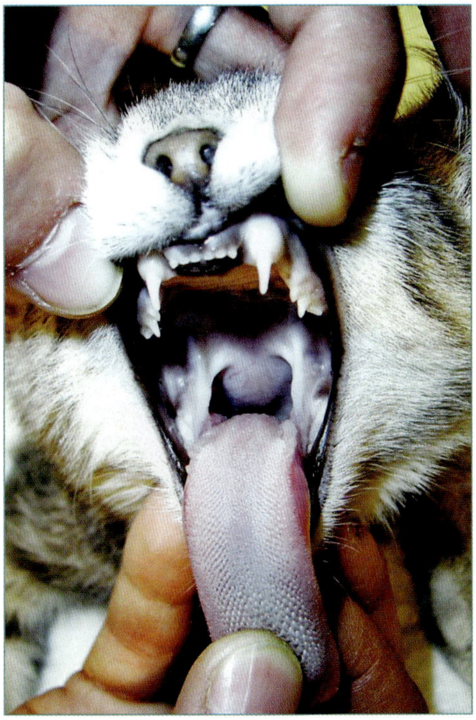

FIGURE 4. Nasopharyngeal polyp in a 4-month-old kitten. The abnormally convex shape of the soft palate is seen.

Nasopharyngeal stenosis

After bouts of chronic infection and inflammation (although stenosis may also be congenital), some cats undergo a narrowing of the mucosa and even have membranes, which obstructs the passage of air through the nasopharynx. Chronic regurgitation, foreign bodies, oronasal fistulas, severe gingivostomatitis, polyps and any chronic infectious condition that affects the nasal cavity, pharynx, middle ear or mouth can cause **nasopharyngeal stenosis** (Fig. 5). When the origin is a bacterial infection, the stenosis perpetuates rhinitis and makes it chronic. In such circumstances, the cat sneezes, breathes through its mouth, discharges mucus chronically through the nostrils, and produces easily audible stertor during expiration.

Diagnosis

Presentation of nasopharyngeal disease tends to occur at an early age. Patients are young cats that have spent their first few months of life in colonies without adequate health checks. The most frequent clinical signs are stertor upon inspiration (a very evident noise made as air passes through a narrow passageway, more audible while eating and swallowing), regular and reverse sneezing (especially if there is associated rhinitis), dysphagia, open-mouth breathing and nasal discharge.

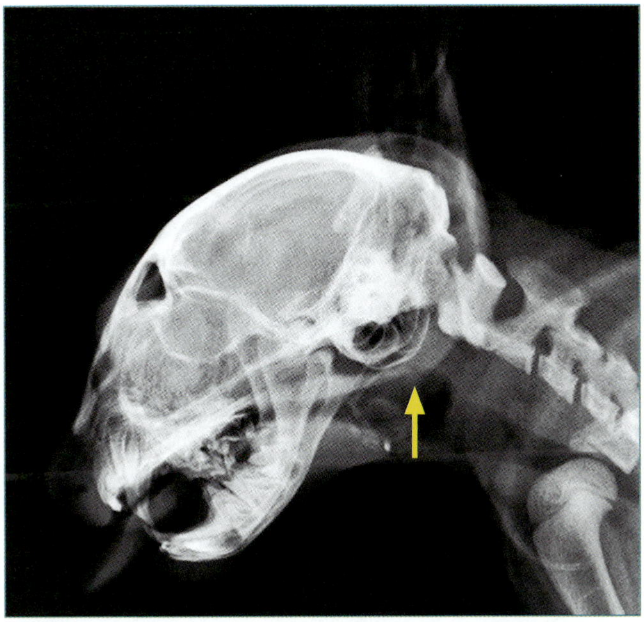

FIGURE 5. Laterolateral X-ray of the head of a cat with nasopharyngeal stenosis. The end of the soft palate has adhered to the roof of the nasopharynx, obstructing the flow of air (arrow).

VIDEO

Kitten with nasopharyngeal stertor. This clinical sign helps pinpoint the location of the issue, but it does not help narrow down whether it is due to a nasopharyngeal polyp or nasopharyngeal stenosis. Imaging tests are needed to diagnose the cause.

Given this clinical picture, advanced imaging tests under sedation/anesthesia are always required to diagnose the condition (Figs. 6–8). Table 1 details the diagnostic protocol for nasopharyngeal disease.

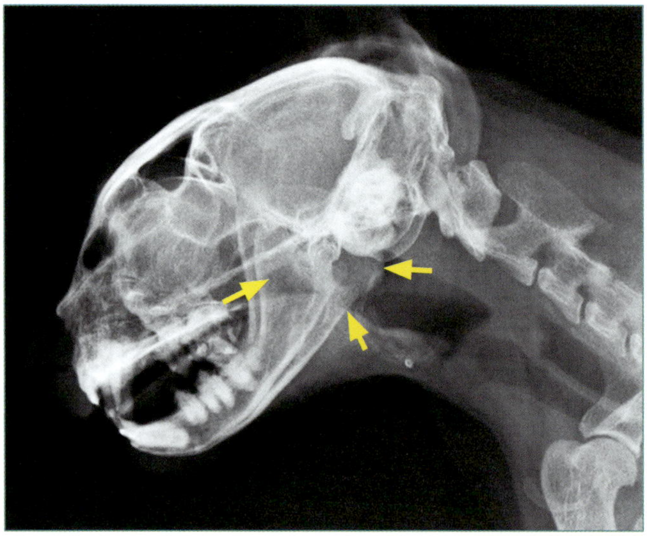

FIGURE 6. Laterolateral X-ray of the cranium of a cat with a nasopharyngeal polyp that dilates the nasopharynx and occupies the central portion of the passageway (yellow arrows). Dilation of the pharynx is seen, along with the presence of air in the esophagus, both of which are the consequence of forced breathing and aerophagia.

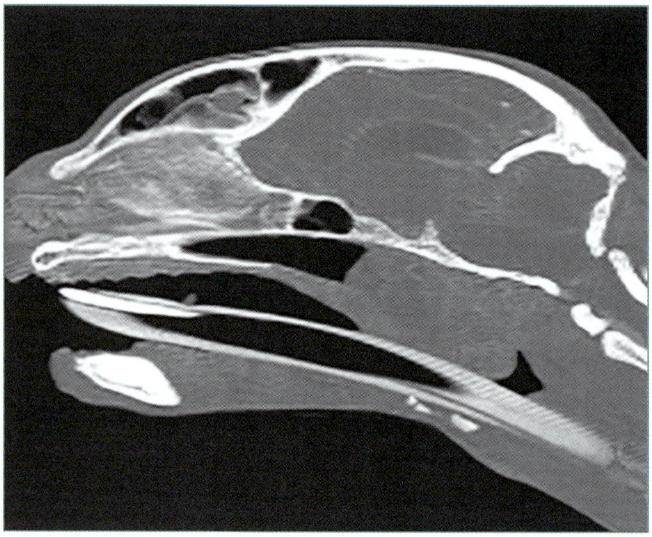

FIGURE 7. Computed tomography scan of a cat with a nasopharyngeal polyp in the distal portion of the nasopharynx. This location severely compromises breathing. Therefore, the patient should be intubated for the imaging tests, as seen in this case.

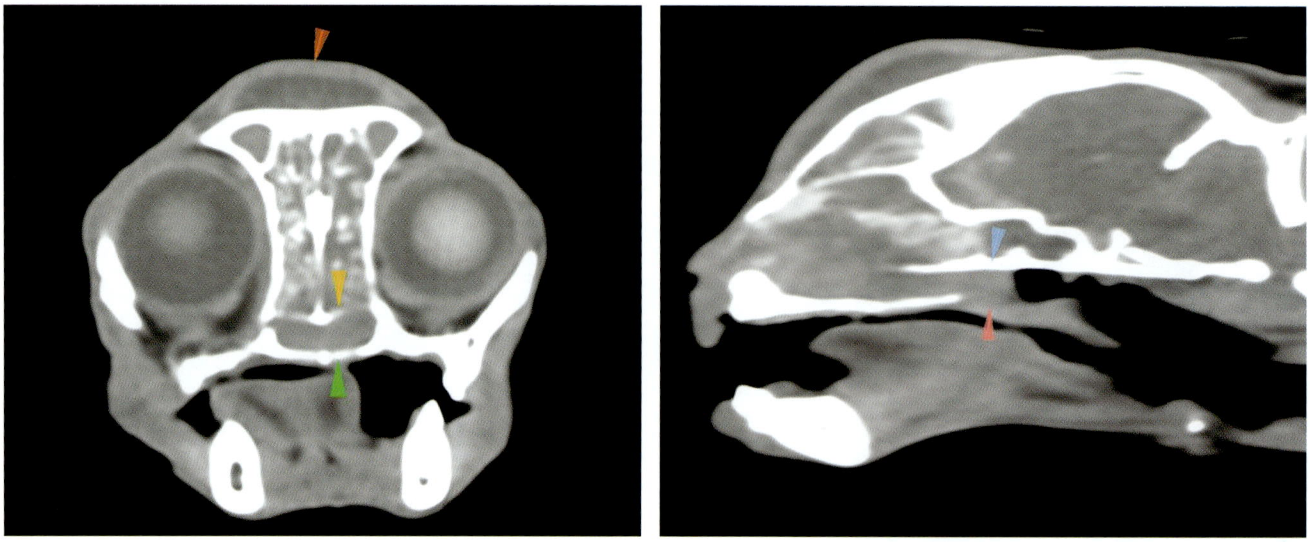

FIGURE 8. Computed tomography scan of a nasal lymphoma, the growth of which has partially invaded the nasopharynx, producing stenosis (arrows). Nasal flushing releases sufficient tissue material of such tumors to enable a good cytological diagnosis.

TABLE 1. Diagnostic protocol for nasopharyngeal disease

Diagnostic test	Indications	Observations
Physical examination	■ Nasopharyngeal polyps ■ Caudal stenosis ■ Some foreign bodies	■ With the cat sedated, the mouth is opened widely, and the soft palate is retracted cranially with a surgical hook, traction suture or an Adson forceps with teeth. ■ The caudal nasopharynx can be examined with a lighted laryngoscope.
Radiography under sedation	■ Nasopharyngeal polyps ■ Nasopharyngeal stenosis ■ Radiopaque foreign bodies ■ Some nasopharyngitis	■ Laterolateral projection of the cranium with the two auditory bullae overlaid. ■ We should look to see that the line of the soft palate has a smooth curve and is parallel to the roof of the nasopharynx.
Bacterial culture (flushing under anesthesia)	■ Nasopharyngitis ■ Bacterial rhinitis	■ Nasal flushing is done under anesthesia, and the material at the back of the pharynx is collected with a gauze swab. ■ If the nasopharynx is obstructed, the sample is collected through the nostrils .
Rigid or flexible (retrograde) rhinoscopy	■ Nasopharyngeal stenosis ■ Neoplasm ■ Nasopharyngitis ■ Foreign bodies	■ Very useful in diagnosis and sometimes in treatment. ■ Difficult space to work in, especially in the retrograde direction.
Computed tomography	■ Nasopharyngeal polyps ■ Nasopharyngeal stenosis ■ Foreign bodies ■ Nasopharyngitis ■ Neoplasm	■ Technique of choice for diagnosing conditions of the nasopharynx. ■ Helps pinpoint the area to be surgically biopsied or treated.
Fluoroscopy	Nasopharyngeal stenosis	Very useful technique to support the treatment of nasopharyngeal stenosis.

Preoperative and postoperative considerations

Things that should be kept in mind before and after the surgery:

- Use of local anesthesia, whether instilled in the nostrils for rhinoscopy or injectable for maxillary nerve block.
- For many techniques such as nasal flushing or rigid rhinoscopy, it is useful to prepare a gauze swab moistened with sterile isotonic saline solution tied to a sufficiently long piece of gauze (Fig. 9). With the patient always intubated, the swab is inserted into the pharynx to absorb any bleeding or material obtained with the nasal flushing. The swab is recovered later by pulling the previously tied gauze.
- To facilitate work in the nasopharynx, an assistant should firmly hold the patient's head in place and keep the mouth open by applying traction to the tongue (see Fig. 3). We will also need good lighting from a laryngoscope or similar tool, and an Adson forceps or 3-0 nylon stay suture to apply traction to the palatal veil in a rostral direction (Fig. 10).
- Due to the position in which the patient is held, intubation with either thermosensitive PVC tubes or, preferably, caliber 14 Fr or 18 Fr silicone tubes is advised, since they provide good support at this angle without collapsing.

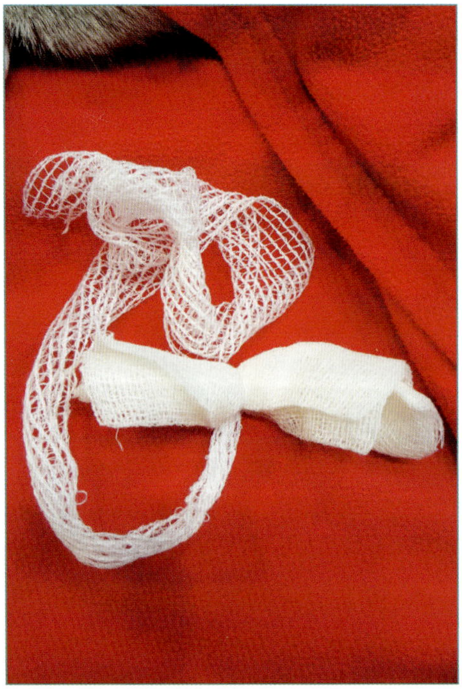

FIGURE 9. To collect the material of the nasal flushing, a sterile gauze pad is moistened and tied with a piece of gauze. After it is inserted into the back of the pharynx, saline solution is infused under pressure in the nostrils. The material collected from the nasopharynx and nasal cavity is sent to a laboratory for bacterial culture and cytology.

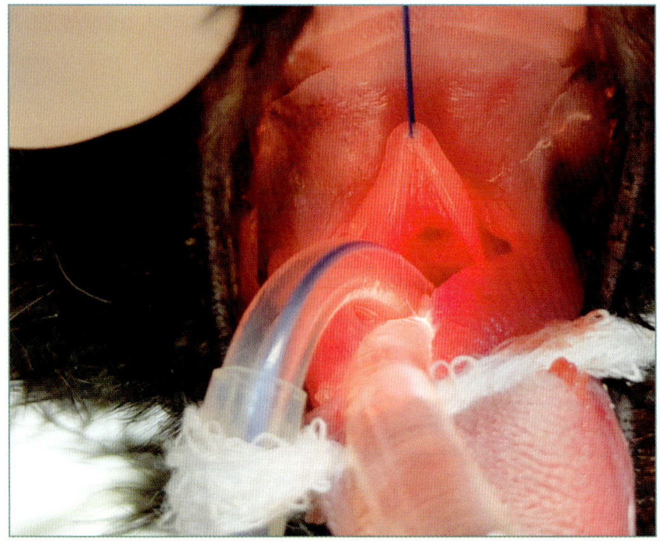

FIGURE 10. Proper position for examination of the nasopharynx. An assistant holds the intubated patient, gripping by the gums at the maxillary canines and applying traction to the tongue. The nylon stay suture helps with the rostral and upward traction of the palatal veil, which enables examination of the most caudal part of the nasopharynx.

Surgical techniques

Removal of a nasopharyngeal polyp via traction-avulsion

- **Patient positioning:** sternal recumbency, with the mouth held open by an assistant, with bilateral local anesthesia of both maxillary nerves.
- **Surgical field:** asepsis is not required. Visualization of the nasopharynx is aided by one or two stay sutures with traction applied at the edge of the soft palate in a cranial direction. The assistant can maintain this traction while holding the maxilla in place. An Adson forceps with teeth can also be used to hold the soft palate.
- **Technique**
  1. Cranial traction of the soft palate should be sufficient to be able to see 50%–75% of the mass of the reddish gray polyp. If we apply traction firmly, this is usually the amount that is visible (Fig. 11).
  2. Using an Allis forceps, the polyp is grasped, attempting to reach as far to the base as possible (craniodorsally in the position we are working). Once firmly grasped, we effectuate a **combined rotation and traction movement on the polyp**. The tearing of the tissue that holds the polyp to the tubal mucosa is clearly noted; therefore, the entire mass of the tumor can be extracted towards the oral cavity (Fig. 12).

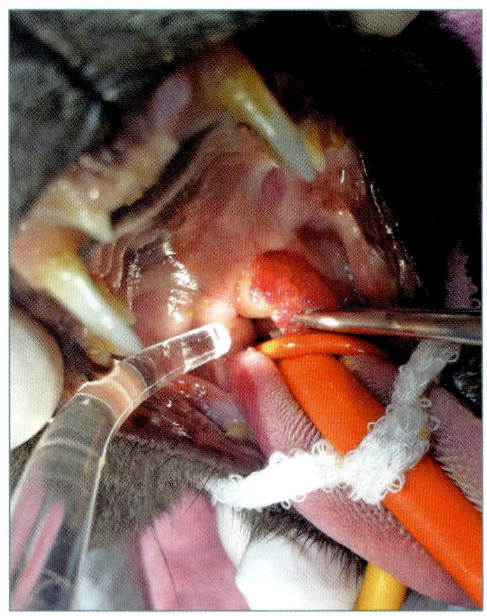

FIGURE 11. Nasopharyngeal polyp exposed after retraction of the soft palate and ready for extraction with Allis forceps using the traction–avulsion technique (see video).

VIDEO

Traction-avulsion technique to remove a nasopharyngeal polyp in a cat. The assistant's role in holding the patient in place is essential. They should keep the patient's mouth open and the tongue pulled out.

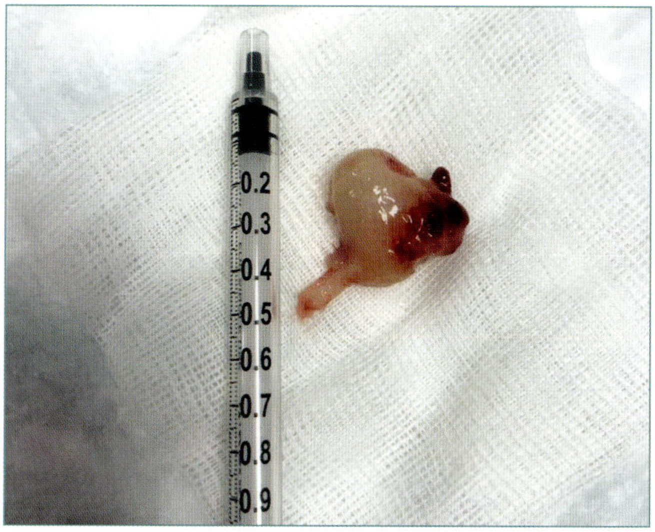

FIGURE 12. Extracted polyp with visible pedicle that originated in the Eustachian tube. To avoid recurrence, it is important to confirm the complete removal of the polyp, including the pedicle.

3. It is recommended to examine the nasopharynx after 5–10 minutes and clear away any remaining blood. An anti-inflammatory dose of prednisolone (2 mg/kg) is administered and continued for 15 days.
4. If there is an aural polyp (in the middle ear), in addition to the nasopharyngeal polyp, a bulla osteotomy can be planned for the same surgery (see Ch. 18 "Ear canal and middle ear surgery").
5. If the polyp is very cranial or very small, the patient can be placed in dorsal recumbency, and their nasopharynx can be accessed via an incision in the midline of the soft palate, **without the incision reaching the caudal edge**. Once the mass of the polyp has been exposed, traction–avulsion is firmly effectuated using an Allis forceps. Any bleeding is controlled and the soft palate wound is closed with a double continuous suture using 4-0 absorbable monofilament material (first the nasal mucosa, followed by the oral mucosa).

Resolution of nasopharyngeal stenosis

Nasopharyngeal stenosis is a typical condition of cats that are very frequently affected by a chronic infectious or inflammatory condition (nasal or oral). For this reason, the likelihood of correcting the stenosis is increased **if the underlying condition that caused the stenosis is treated before and after**. A culture of the nasal exudate and a biopsy of the nasopharyngeal mucosa guide preoperative and postoperative medical treatment.

A completely successful surgical technique that can resolve this disease in every case does not yet exist. The three most described techniques are set out below.

Removal of the stenotic tissue

One of the techniques initially used in the surgical treatment of nasopharyngeal stenosis was the elimination en bloc of the stenotic tissue, along with an advancement flap of mucosa. In recent years, a second technique has been described:

- **Advancement flap of nasal mucosa:** with the patient anesthetized and in dorsal recumbency, the mouth is kept open for good visualization of the entire soft palate. A solution of povidone-iodine is used to disinfect, and the midline of the soft palate is incised up to the area of the stenosis. A circular cut is made around the stenotic tissue with Iris scissors. The defect in the dorsal wall of the nasopharynx is repaired with an advancement flap of mucosa and submucosa sutured in two layers with a 5-0 absorbable monofilament suture. The defect in the soft palate is closed firstly by suturing the mucosa of the nasal planum, followed by the full thickness of the palate, and finally, the oral mucosa. A 4-0 absorbable monofilament suture is used for this (Fig. 13).
- **Palatoplasty:** in this case, the stenotic tissue is removed via an incision in the distal portion of the soft palate, just anterior to the palatine tonsils. This incision should be performed in the shape of an arc using a monopolar electric scalpel, such that the stenotic membrane tissue is included in the removal (Fig. 14). Given the cut technique used, suturing will not be necessary.

Dilation of the stenosis

Stenotic tissue usually has a central region, and although this region is sometimes very narrow, an instrument can be passed through it to dilate it so that it once again has the proper diameter for the passage of air. Several techniques have been described for the dilation of nasopharyngeal stenosis:

- **Dilation with forceps:** possibly the first technique described for treatment of stenosis. With the patient intubated, in sternal recumbency, and with the mouth held open by an assistant, traction is applied to the soft palate in a rostral direction, using one or two stay sutures or an Adson forceps with teeth. Once the opening of the stenosis becomes visible, the tip of a forceps or a mosquito forceps can be inserted into it. The stenosis is dilated in several directions, trying not to cause too much bleeding, so that subsequent restenosis is minimized (Fig. 15).

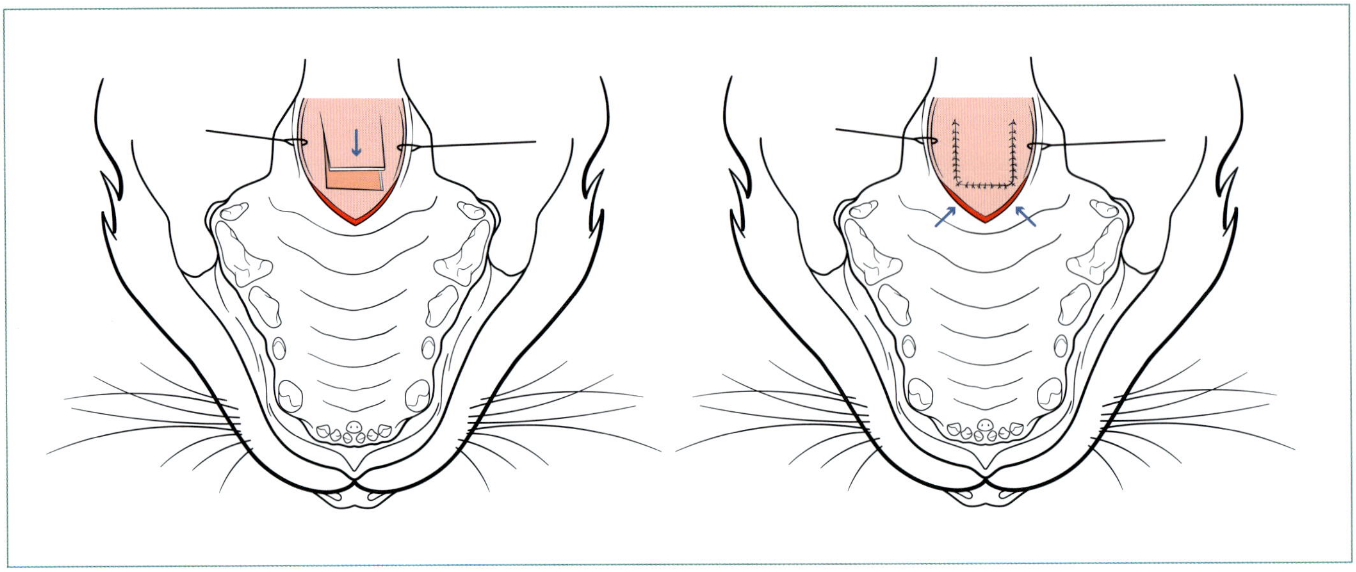

FIGURE 13. Advancement flap of nasal mucosa. The approach is through an incision in the midline of the soft palate, which is subsequently closed with a double continuous suture using absorbable material (direction of the closure marked with blue arrows).

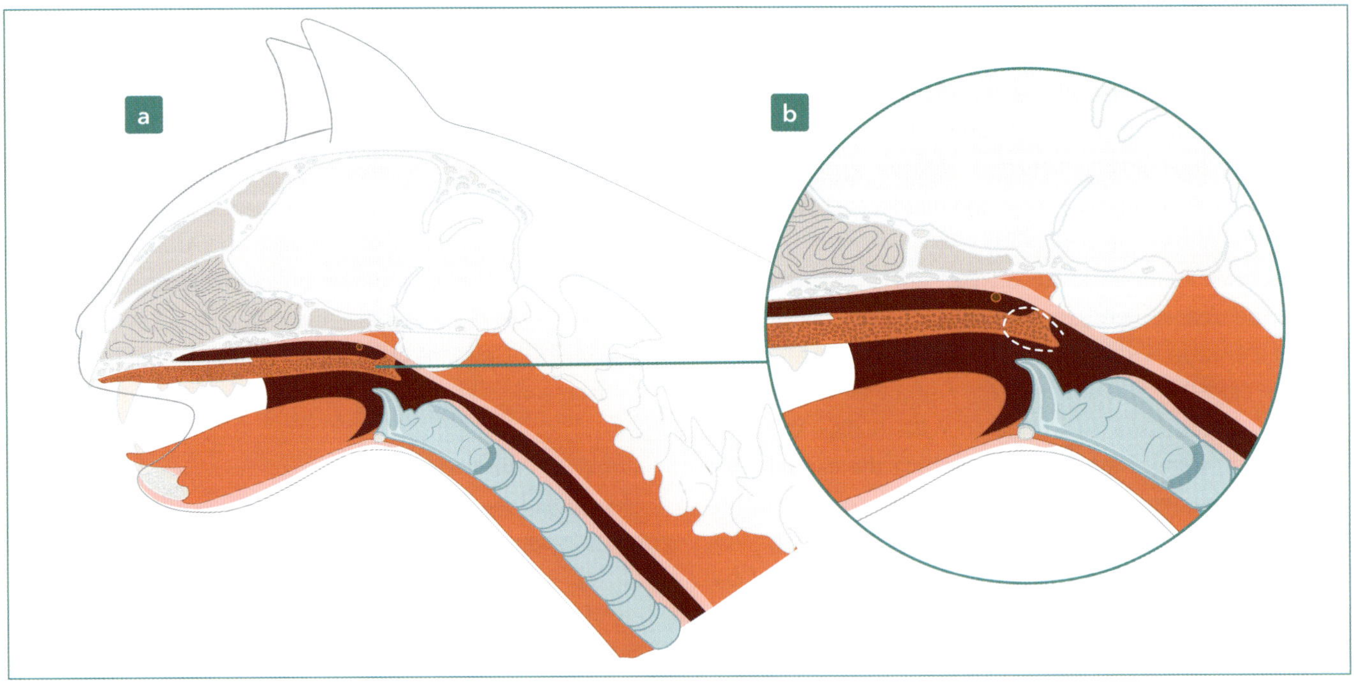

FIGURE 14. Palatoplasty. (a) Presence of stenotic tissue narrowing the soft palate. (b) The dashed line indicates the stenotic tissue that must be removed.

- **Balloon dilation:** the use of C-arm **fluoroscopy** is required for this technique, along with personal protective equipment (the use of **flexible retrograde rhinoscopy** has also been described, but visibility is reduced). With the cat intubated and positioned in lateral recumbency, a 0.035 inch **guidewire** is moistened, and, guided by the fluoroscopy image, it is inserted through the ventral nasal meatus toward the site of nasopharyngeal stenosis. Once the guidewire is in the pharynx, it is retracted with the help of mosquito forceps and the soft palate is pulled back rostrally. Enough of the guidewire is pulled out to be able to place a 6–12 mm **balloon catheter** along its full length (depending on the size of the cat).

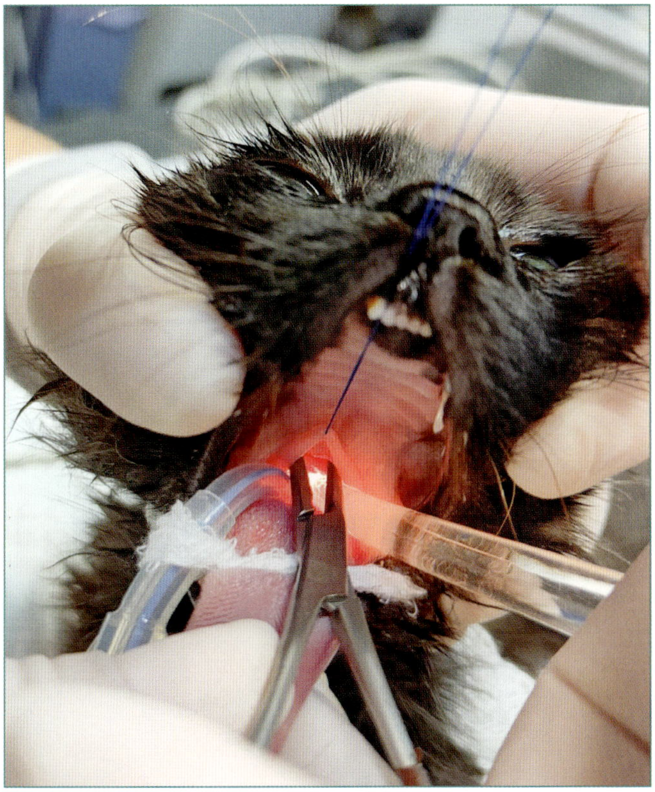

FIGURE 15. Dilation of a nasopharyngeal stenosis using forceps technique (with mosquito forceps). The less inflammation we cause, the lower the risk of recurrence, although recurrence is frequent with this technique.

This guidewire should be previously moistened for lubrication. With the help of fluoroscopy, the catheter plus guidewire is moved along the nasal cavity and nasopharynx such that the marks on the balloon area are aligned with the area to be dilated. At this time, an assistant holds both ends of the guidewire so that the surgeon is freed to focus only on the dilation. This maneuver is very important and should be done in coordination, and under fluoroscopy. If the balloon catheter is not positioned and set in place properly, it will slip outside the stenosis when it is inflated. Once everything has been prepared, the balloon is filled with 5–10 ml of **iodinated contrast media** to dilate the stenosis to the desired caliber (8–12 mm depending on the size of the cat). This operation should be repeated once or twice until the fluoroscopic image shows a resolved stenosis (no indentations of any kind should be visible in the inflated balloon) (see video).

Endoprosthesis (stent) placement

Because it is not very invasive and can be repeated, stenosis dilation is the technique most often used. Unfortunately, some

VIDEO

Fluoroscopy of a balloon dilation to resolve a nasopharyngeal stenosis. The nitinol guidewire that enters through the nostril and exits through the mouth should be firmly grasped during the entire process in order to center the point of maximal dilation in the stenosis (an indentation is seen in the balloon, which quickly cedes to pressure).

cats are prone to recurrence of stenoses. Therefore, several techniques have been described over the past few years on the use of dilation devices (stents) to keep the tissue dilated for a period of time and avoid restenosis:

- **Permanent metallic (coated or uncoated) stent:** in cases that continue to recur after several balloon dilations, this technique has been described as the only remaining treatment or as a salvage treatment. Metallic stents (coated or uncoated) are applied using the same technique as for balloon dilation, although it may require the additional support of flexible retrograde rhinoscopy to better pinpoint the ideal location for the stent. Once the applicator is set in place through the nasopharyngeal stenosis with the help of fluoroscopic imaging or rhinoscopy, the next step is to dilate the stent to its maximum, thus distending the stenotic tissue. If placement is correct, the applicator is turned to release the stent in place (Fig. 16).
- **Temporary silicone stent:** this technique consists of dilating the stenosis with forceps or a balloon catheter using images obtained through computed tomography. After measuring the area of the stenosis and pinpointing its location, a piece of 24–28 Fr silicone tube is cut, depending on the size of the cat. Two stay sutures are placed at the caudal end of the soft palate to facilitate its retraction. Another suture is placed at the end of the silicone stent so that the device can be recovered or repositioned once it is set in place. For a good grip on the end of the stent, it is useful to use **right-angle hemostatic forceps** to advance it rostrally through the nasopharynx to the level of the choanae. Once placed in the area of the stenosis, it is fixed in place with a transfixion suture through the soft palate (Fig. 17). A 3-0 nonabsorbable suture is used, and before knotting, a silicone pin is placed (made from butterfly needle tubing) to avoid tearing the mucosa of the palate. The suture is removed in 3–4 weeks, along with the silicone stent.

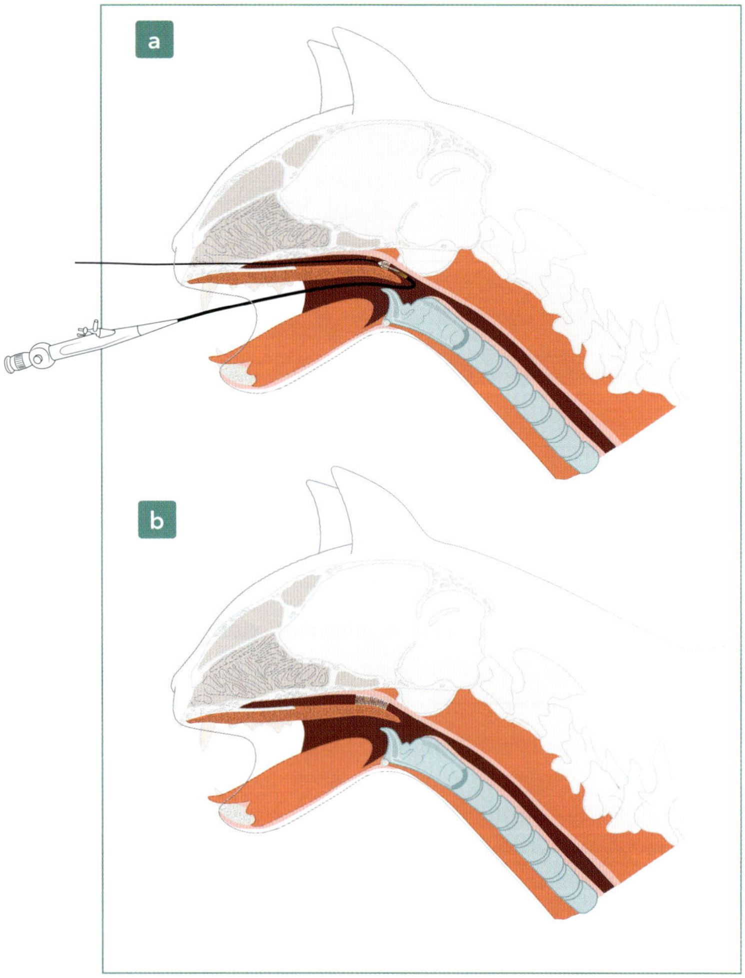

FIGURE 16. (a) Application of a metallic stent through flexible retrograde rhinoscopy. (b) Dilated stent placed in the correct position to correct the stenosis.

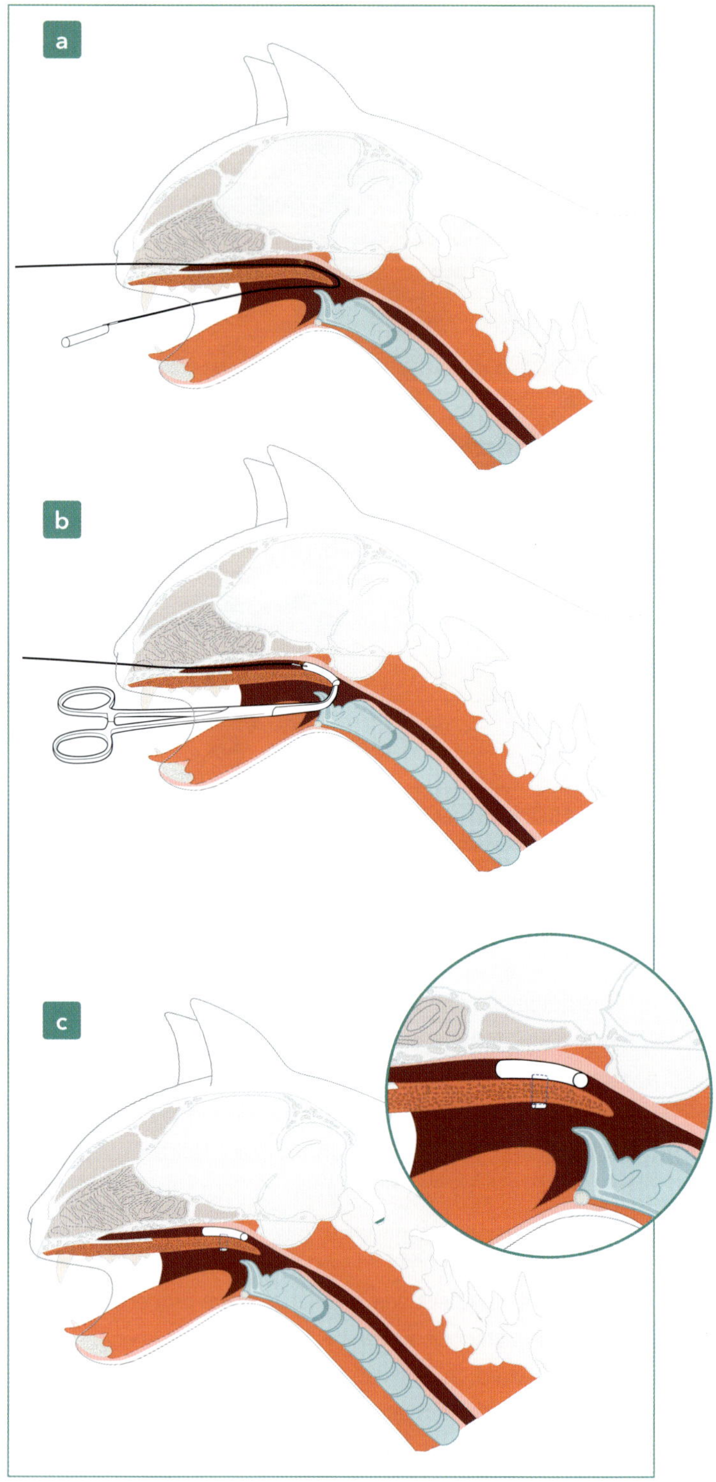

FIGURE 17. (a) Application of a nonpermanent silicone stent with endoscopic biopsy forceps inserted through the nasal passageway. (b) Proper placement of the tube with the help of right-angle hemostatic forceps. (c) Securing the silicone stent in place by placing a transfixion suture through the soft palate.

Postoperative care and complications

For 2 weeks following surgery, a 2 mg/kg dose of prednisolone is administered every 24 hours, along with antibiotic therapy based on the results of the preoperative culture.

Stenotic tissue removal techniques have been successful, but very few case studies have been published. As in any invasive surgical intervention on the nasopharyngeal mucosa, we should exercise extreme caution regarding associated infections and inflammation in the area.

The clinical signs should be under control before proceeding to the intervention.

Dilation with forceps and balloon dilation have both been associated with recurrence. The more traumatic the technique and the less controlled the infection and inflammation, the more this holds true. The best results have been obtained with balloon dilation (50% success rate after two dilations several weeks apart). If the stenosis has recurred after two dilations, placement of a stent is advised to maintain the nasopharyngeal passageway open in the long term.

Dilation with permanent metallic stents is controversial in cats. In one retrospective article, up to 68% of cats with such stents had complications, notable among these being overgrowth of inflammatory tissue through the mesh of the device, infections, stent fracture and oronasal fistulas. Eventually, all cats with these complications had to have the device removed. In the published series of case studies in which the cats were treated with temporary silicone stents, treatment success was achieved in all cases. Nevertheless, subsequent data from other authors do not reproduce these results. Currently dilation with temporary silicone stents is the most commonly used technique.

Bibliography

Berent AC, Weisse C, Todd K et al. Use of a balloon-expandable metallic stent for treatment of nasopharyngeal stenosis in dogs and cats: six cases (2005–2007). *J Am Vet Med Assoc*, 2008; 233(9):1432–1440.

Berent AC. Diagnosis and management of nasopharyngeal stenosis. *Vet Clin North Am Small Anim Pract*, 2016; 46(4):677–689.

Boswood A, Lamb CR, Brockman DJ et al. Baloon dilatation of nasopharyngeal stenosis in a cat. *Vet Radiol Ultrasound*, 2003; 44(1):53–55.

Brown JD, Woerde DJ, Hoffmann KL et al. Partial resolution of chronic unilateral sinonasal obstructive disease in a cat using a temporary polyvinylchloride stent. *JFMS Open Rep*, 2020; 6(2):1–8.

Burdick S, Berent AC, Weisse C et al. Interventional treatment of benign nasopharyngeal stenosis and imperforate nasopharynx in dogs and cats: 46 cases (2005–2013). *J Am Vet Med Assoc*, 2018; 253(10):1300–1308.

De Lorenzi D, Bertoncello D, Comastri S, Bottero E. Treatment of acquired nasopharyngeal stenosis using a removable silicone stent. *J Feline Med Surg*, 2015; 17(2):117–124.

Dorn ES, Tress B, Suchodolski JS et al. Bacterial microbiome in the nose of healthy cats and in cats with nasal disease. *PLoS ONE*, 2017; 12(6):e0180299.

Glaus TM, Gerber B, Tomsa K et al. Reproducible and long-lasting success of balloon dilation of nasopharyngeal stenosis in cats. *Vet Rec*, 2005; 157(9):257–259.

Greci V, Mortellaro CM. Management of otic and nasopharyngeal, and nasal polyps in cats and dogs. *Vet Clin North Am Small Anim Pract*, 2016; 46(4):643–661.

Griffon DJ, Tasker S. Use of a mucosal advancement flap for the treatment of nasopharyngeal stenosis in a cat. *J Small Anim Pract*, 2000; 41(2):71–73.

Johnson KL, James MD, Carrera-Justiz S. What is your neurologic diagnosis? *J Am Vet Med Assoc*, 2017; 251(6):653–656.

Kmieciak L, Hague DW, Neumann ZL, Joslyn S. What is your neurologic diagnosis? *J Am Vet Med Assoc*, 2016; 248(6):613–616.

Michiels L, Day MJ, Snaps F et al. A retrospective study of non-specific rhinitis in 22 cats and the value of nasal cytology and histopathology. *J Feline Med Surg*, 2003; 5(5):279–285.

Osinchuk SC, Zwueste DM, Grahn BH. Peripheral cranial neuropathies consistent with cavernous sinus syndrome caused by extracranial nasopharyngeal lymphoma in a cat. *Can Vet J*, 2019; 60(11):1156–1160.

Reed N, Gunn-Moore D. Nasopharyngeal disease in cats 1. Diagnostic investigation. *J Feline Med Surg*, 2012; 14(5):306–315.

Reed N, Gunn-Moore D. Nasopharyngeal disease in cats 2. Specific conditions and their management. *J Feline Med Surg*, 2012; 14(5):317–326.

Sériot P, Gibert S, Poujol L et al. Extended palatoplasty as surgical treatment for nasopharyngeal stenosis in six cats. *J Small Anim Pract*, 2019; 60(9):559–564.

Takahashi K, Baba T, Hirokawa M et al. Long-term management of a cat with nasopharyngeal lymphoma by chlorambucil. *Open Vet J*, 2021; 11(2):217–221.

Tollefson CR, Hiebert EC, Lee AM, Gambino JM. What is your diagnosis? *J Am Vet Med Assoc*, 2018; 253(11):1405–1407.

Weeden AM, Degner DA. Surgical approaches to the nasal cavity and sinuses. *Vet Clin North Am Small Anim Pract*, 2016; 46(4):719–733.

Wong VM, Jaffe MH. Pathology in practice. *J Am Vet Med Assoc*, 2018; 252(3):297–299.

EYELID AND ORBITAL SURGERY 17

Alberto Barneto

Surgical anatomy

The two **main eyelids (upper and lower)** make contact with the surface of the eye by means of two elongated membranes composed of dense connective tissue (palpebral tarsus). Dozens of **meibomian glands** open at its margin, which are responsible for secreting the lipid portion of the tears. Feline eyelids do not usually have eyelashes (cilia), although sporadically there is a case of distichiasis (cilia that incorrectly protrude out of the meibomian orifices and cause rubbing and irritation of the cornea). The inner tissue layer in contact with the eye is the **conjunctiva** (Fig. 1), a highly vascularized epithelium that possesses abundant goblet cells that produce mucin, the protein component of the tears. The eyelid is covered with thin, hairy, highly mobile skin over a subcutaneous layer that is deeply attached to the orbicularis oculi muscles. They are responsible for the actual movement of the eyelids. Each eyelid has an orifice (lacrimal punctum) that drains tears into the upper and lower canaliculi, which join to form the **nasolacrimal duct**. This carries the tears to the nasal vestibule.

Each eye has a **third eyelid** or **nictitating membrane** inserted into the ventromedial area of the orbit, with T-shaped supporting cartilage at its base where it joins a lacrimal gland.

The eyelids physically protect the eyeball thanks to the menace response, remove contaminated debris from the ocular surface and distribute tears as they move, in addition to contributing to the formation of tears.

The branches of the **superficial temporal, external ethmoidal and infraorbital arteries** enter through the lateral and medial canthi and supply blood to the eyelids. Their innervation comes from branches of the **facial nerve** (motor functions) and the **trigeminal nerve** (sensory).

The eyeball occupies the entire orbit and the part that is not encompassed by the orbit (approximately 40% of the sphere) is covered by the eyelids and their adjacent tissues (lacrimal glands, zygomatic salivary gland). We will not make an exhaustive anatomical description of the feline eye because we will not be dealing with specialized ophthalmologic surgery in this work.

The **feline orbit** is relatively deep and is not completely comprised of bone, although it provides considerable protection to the eye. It is made up of portions of seven craniofacial bones:

- Sphenoid bone
- Maxillary bone
- Lacrimal bone
- Zygomatic bone
- Frontal bone
- Ethmoid bone
- Palatine bone

These seven bones form a concavity that is incomplete in the caudoventral and lateral aspects. On the lateral aspect, support is provided by the orbital ligament, while the masseter, temporalis and pterygoid muscles contribute to this same lateral wall and to the caudoventral wall.

The orbit contains the eyeball and its muscular attachments, which arise from the orbital apex and pass through the orbital space to attach before the equator of the sphere of the eye (Fig. 2). At the back of the orbit, the **optic canal (foramen)** opens in the sphenoid bone, through which the **optic nerve** (cranial nerve II) exits. There are three types of orbital muscles:

- **Eye retractor (retractor oculi/bulbi) muscle:** has four bellies that envelop the optic nerve after emerging through the optic canal.
- **Orbital rectus muscles:** there are four, the dorsal, lateral, ventral and medial.
- **Orbital oblique muscles:** there are two, the dorsal and ventral.

Vascularization arises from branches of the maxillary artery, which emerges from the rostral alar foramen, and the internal ophthalmic artery (enters the orbit together with the optic nerve through the optic foramen). The innervation of the eye is complex and arises from several branches of cranial nerves III (oculomotor), IV (trochlear), V (trigeminal) and VI (abducens). They all exit through the **orbital fissure** and distribute giving motor function (to the muscles) and sensory function (to the eye and appendages) (Fig. 3).

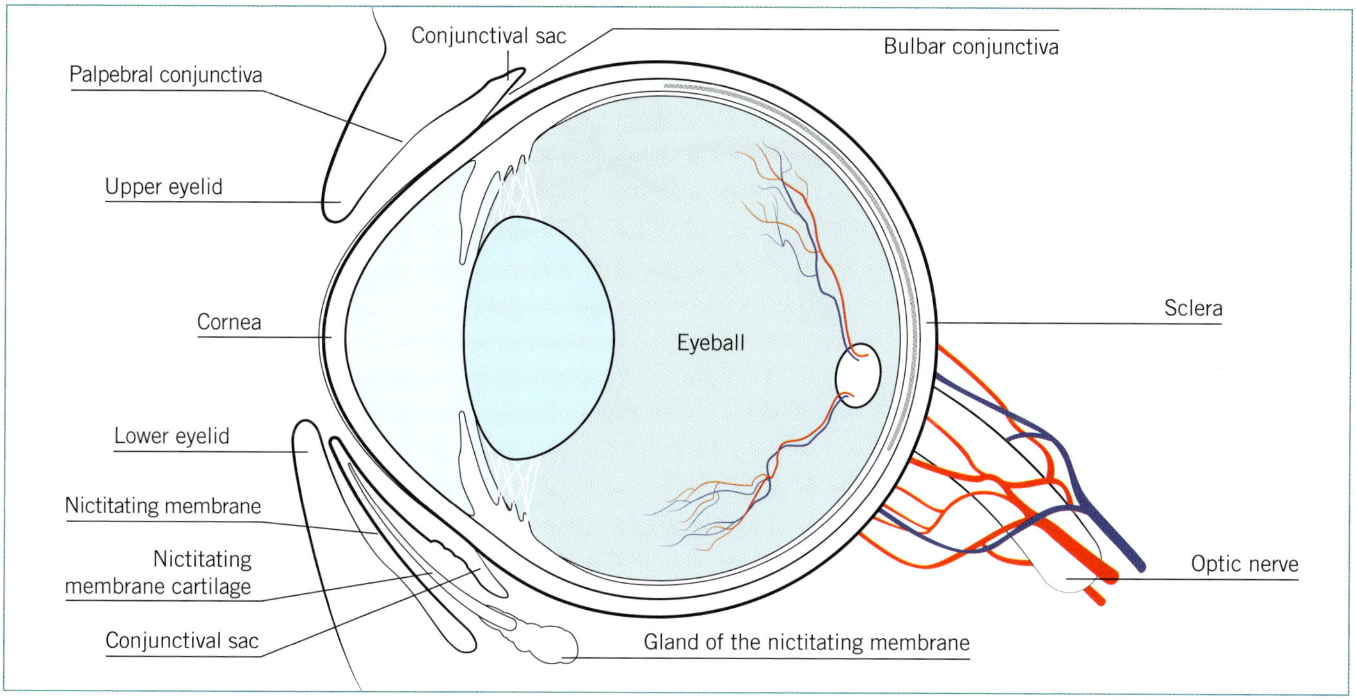

FIGURE 1. Structure of the eyeball and its appendages.

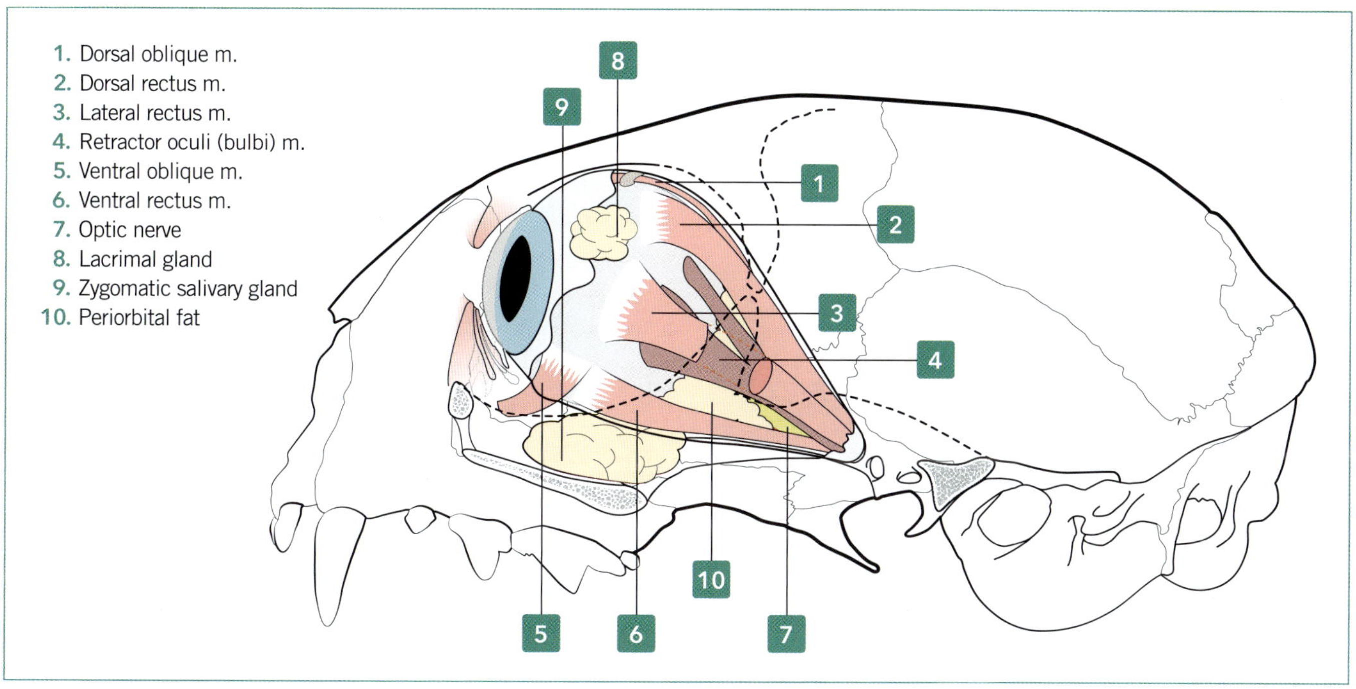

FIGURE 2. Structures of the orbit of the feline eye.

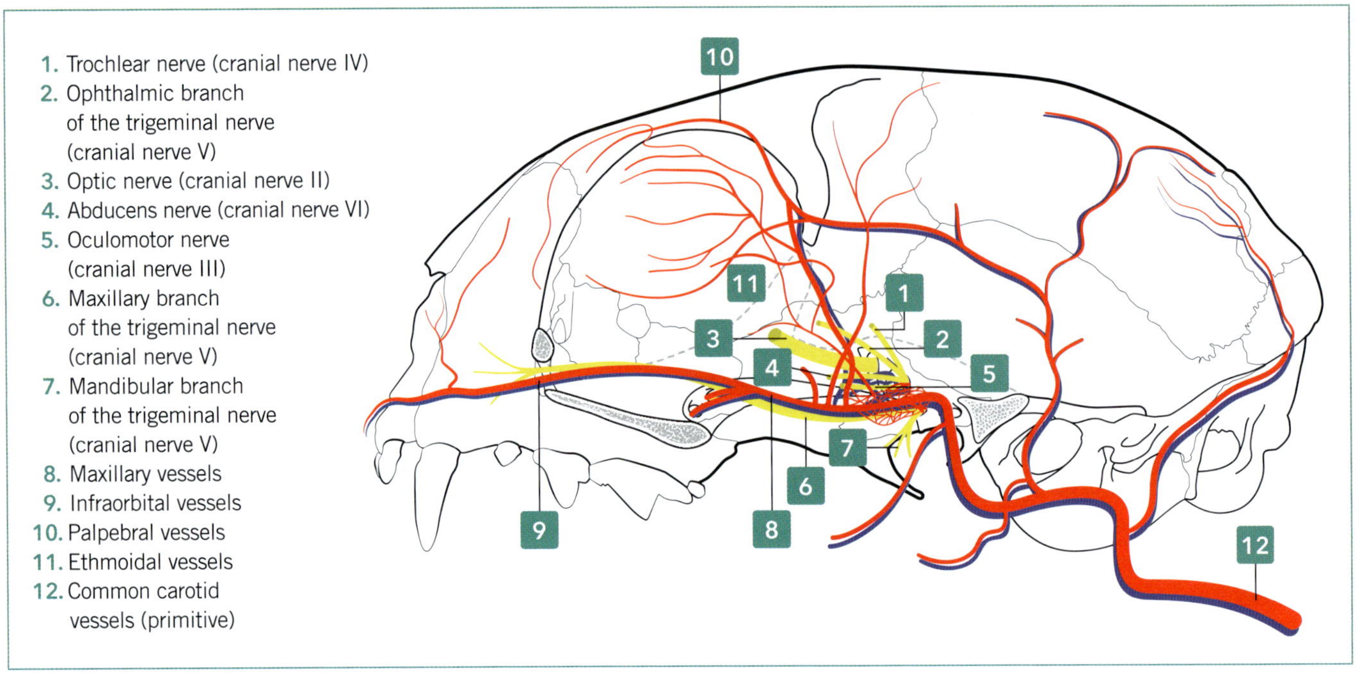

FIGURE 3. Feline orbital vascularization and innervation.

Surgical diseases

Ankyloblepharon

The palpebral rims open physiologically two weeks after birth. Sometimes there is incomplete development or conjunctivitis (during or after delivery) resulting in abnormal fusion of the palpebral tarsi. The eye will remain closed for too long and will sometimes even have a purulent infection that can affect and destroy the ocular structures (**neonatal ophthalmia**—ophthalmia neonatorum—which can degenerate into **panophthalmia** and loss of the eyeball) (Figs. 4 and 5). In these circumstances, the problem should be detected and prompt action should be taken by opening the palpebral fissure. Avoid the use of sharp instruments that may destroy the palpebral tarsus. Ideally, moisten the eyelids and use mosquito forceps to open the fissure. Abundant irrigation with saline will remove all traces of infection and will allow treatment of the eyeball and conjunctiva in the case of corneal ulcers and **symblepharon** (adhesions of the conjunctiva to the eyeball due to loss of corneal epithelium).

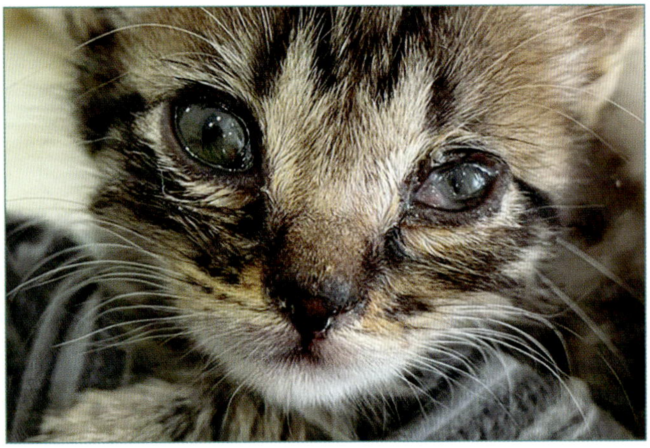

FIGURE 4. Neonatal ophthalmia (ophthalmia neonatorum) in a kitten after opening of the ankyloblepharon. Because it was performed in time, the adhesions were removed and the eye was saved.

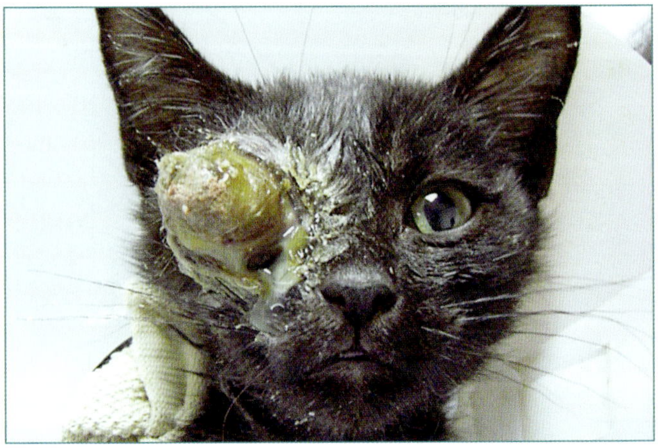

FIGURE 5. Panophthalmia in a kitten that suffered from untreated ankyloblepharon.

Coloboma

Coloboma is the agenesis of the eyelid edge. In cats it usually affects the outer canthus of the upper eyelid, where it causes the skin hair to invade the corneal surface in that area. Surgical reconstruction using flap techniques is the indicated treatment.

Entropion

Entropion consists of a malformation of the orbicularis oculi muscle that causes a rolling or inversion of the eyelid margin towards the eyeball. As a consequence, the hair of the eyelid skin rubs against the cornea as the eyelid moves. The cat presents with conjunctivitis, blepharospasm (reduced opening of the palpebral fissure) and chronic corneal ulcers. A slight entropion of the medial angle is considered physiological in brachycephalic breeds (Persian, Himalayan, Exotic). The most frequent location of pathologic entropion is the edge of the lower eyelid, sometimes extending to the outer canthus, the solution for which is always surgical (Fig. 6).

Palpebral neoplasia

The most common eyelid tumor in cats is squamous cell carcinoma. Cats are predisposed to this if they have white coats or white hair around their eyes and are overexposed to the damaging effect of ultraviolet light (Fig. 7). It is locally aggressive and should always be treated, once diagnosed by biopsy, either using electrochemotherapy or surgical techniques. Other less common palpebral tumors in cats are mast cell tumors, hemangiosarcomas and lymphomas. Some benign tumors such as apocrine cysts or epitheliomas can also affect the palpebral rim and generate chronic corneal lesions due to rubbing; therefore, surgery will always be the treatment of choice.

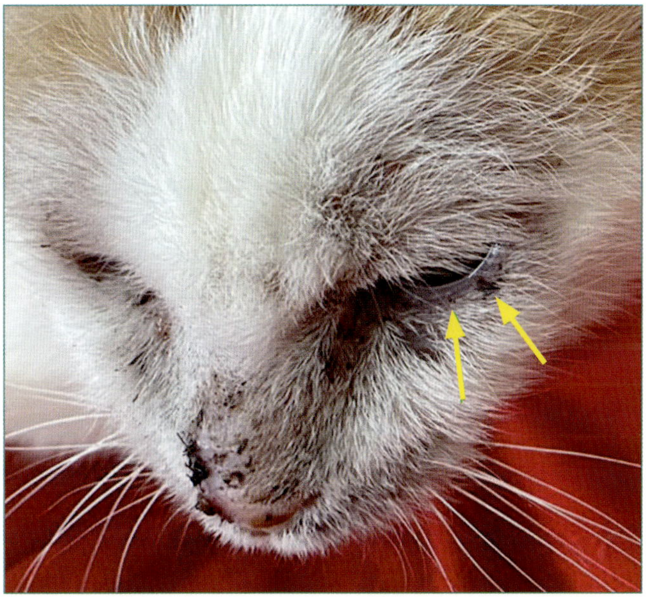

FIGURE 7. Palpebral squamous cell carcinoma (arrows). It appears as desquamative or ulcerated lesions of the palpebral margin in white-coated cats with high UV exposure. In this case, the patient had already undergone amputation of both pinnae due to the same disease.

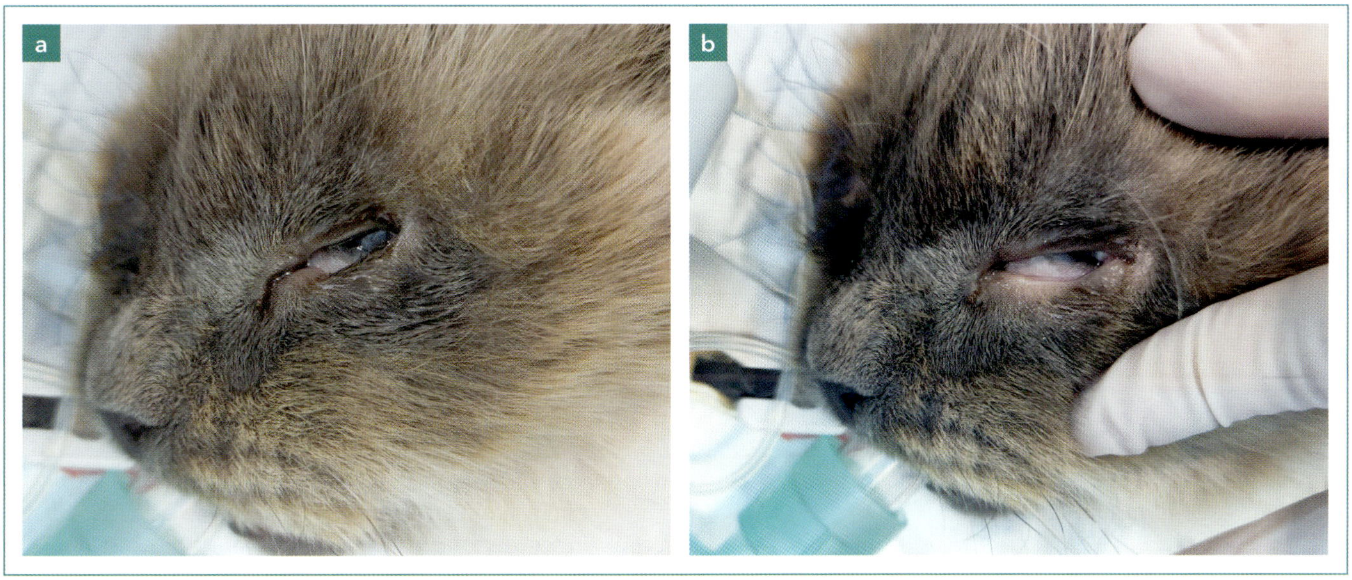

FIGURE 6. (a) Entropion at the lateral margin of the lower eyelid. (b) In order to evaluate the amount of tissue to be removed, the defect must be unrolled until the palpebral canthus is visible.

Corneal ulcer

Of a viral (herpetic) or mechanical origin, a corneal ulcer that does not respond well to medical treatment usually requires mechanical protection and vascular support of the conjunctiva to aid healing. In feline medicine, treatment has been described with the application of different conjunctival flaps and even corneal transplants, although sometimes a simple tarsorrhaphy technique can solve many cases of chronic corneal ulcers.

Orbital neoplasia

Feline orbital neoplasms are usually malignant and have a grave prognosis. The most common cases are lymphomas (Fig. 8), carcinomas, osteosarcomas and fibrosarcomas, all of which are metastatic with invasion of the surrounding bone tissue (nasal cavity, maxilla and retrobulbar space). The diagnostic modality of choice is a computed tomography (CT) scan or magnetic resonance imaging (MRI).

Inflammatory diseases of the orbit

Retrobulbar abscesses and cellulitis are rare but very characteristic of some brachycephalic feline breeds. Bacterial (*Bacteroides* spp., *Pasteurella* spp.) and fungal (*Aspergillus* spp.) causes have been described, which gain access either via hematogenous or external traumatic routes. The globe is eccentric, the nictitating membrane is protruded and the cat presents with weakness and anorexia. The diagnosis should always be confirmed by ultrasound or, ideally, a CT scan or MRI. To drain the abscess and take samples, needle aspiration of the pterygopalatine (retromaxillary) fossa is a very useful technique.

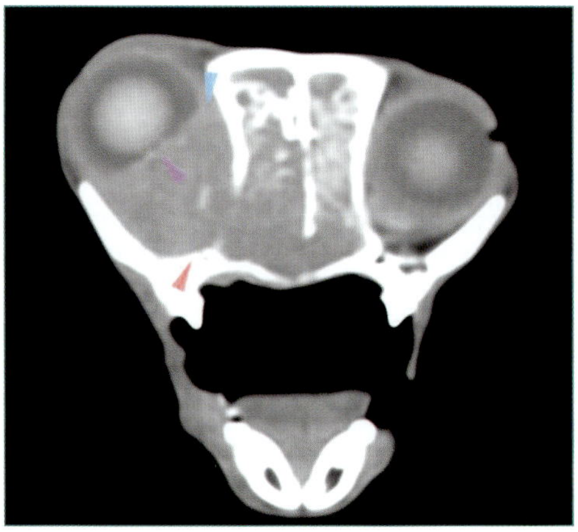

FIGURE 8. CT scan of a nasal lymphoma infiltrating the right orbit in a cat. The eyeball is eccentric with respect to the orbital cavity.

Proptosis/exophthalmos

Is the anterior dislocation of the eyeball, produced acutely by trauma (proptosis) or chronically when the globe is pushed out of the orbit by tumor or inflammatory masses that occupy that space (exophthalmos). Regardless of the cause, this is an ophthalmologic emergency that, if it is not treated in the short term, will result in a loss of function of the eye due to secondary glaucoma and will require enucleation.

Diagnosis

Apart from ophthalmologic diagnostic techniques for specific diseases, which are not described in this book, diseases of the eyelids and orbit require that different diagnostic tests be performed before surgical decisions are made (Table 1).

TABLE 1. Main diagnostic tests for ocular and periorbital diseases

Diagnostic test	Indications	Observations
Cytology/biopsy	Palpebral tumors	Most cases will involve excisional biopsies to remove the lesion.
	Orbital masses	Ultrasound-guided or CT-guided cytology.
Ultrasound	Internal diseases of the eyeball and orbit	It also allows for ultrasound-guided needle aspiration for diagnosis or treatment.
CT scan/MRI	Diseases of the orbit	Method of choice for the diagnosis of orbital diseases and their relationship to adjacent structures.
Retrobulbar needle aspiration	Retrobulbar lesions (inflammation, tumors)	Can be approached either from the skin (following the orbital ligament) or from the retromaxillary space behind the last molar (especially in abscesses, to take samples and relieve pressure).

Preoperative and postoperative considerations

Aspects to be taken into account before and after the intervention:

- Any eye surgery involves delicate, very fine-gauge sutures. The necessary analgesia does not prevent the use of an Elizabethan collar during the postoperative period.
- Good eye hygiene and asepsis are essential. Therefore, we will apply a good layer of artificial tear gel before shaving the area to minimize corneal irritation. Once shaved, the eye should be thoroughly washed with physiological saline or Ringer's lactate. As an antiseptic, the use of povidone-iodine solutions (10%, diluted in saline at a 1:50 ratio for the eyeball and a 1:20 ratio for the eyelids) is safer, as it does not interfere with the tear film.
- Topical analgesia containing 0.5% proparacaine, applied 5 times at 20-second intervals between each drop, confers superficial analgesia lasting up to 25 minutes, which is sufficient for many surgical procedures. The use of opioids during and after surgery as systemic analgesics should also be evaluated (see Ch. 2).
- Adhesive surgical drapes are a good option in ocular surgery, as they prevent folds and lacerations due to the use of towel clamps.
- A large number of ophthalmologic procedures require magnifying instruments to improve visibility of the structures, as well as specific surgical material and sutures. In most of the interventions described in this chapter, a ×2.5–×3.5 magnification is sufficient.
- Any eyelid surgery involving the use of a scalpel will require that the eyeball be protected during the incision. The use of a no. 3 scalpel handle in the conjunctival sac or, preferably, a Jaeger eyelid plate, will give solid support to the incision and improve our accuracy, as well as prevent corneal lacerations.

> Alcohol or soap solutions should never be used on the surface of the eye for surgical disinfection.

Surgical techniques

Tarsorrhaphy

Tarsorrhaphy is the temporary fixation by suture of one or more eyelids to each other so that the palpebral conjunctiva protects and helps repair injuries to the eyeball, usually the cornea (ulcers, bullous keratopathy). There are two techniques for tarsorrhaphy in cats, which are described below.

Tarsorrhaphy of the nictitating membrane

It is the most commonly used technique, and if well performed can be maintained for weeks with little or no discomfort to the cat. We will choose this technique when chronic corneal wounds are present that require protection in addition to medical treatment. By exposing the conjunctiva of the nictitating membrane, the treatment indicated for the wound can be continued.

For the technique, the upper eyelid is aseptically cleaned and two 5–8 mm silicone tube fragments are prepared (venipuncture tubes are ideal). We place a U-shaped stitch with 3-0 nylon in the following order (Fig. 9):

- First, we pierce the silicone tube near one end.
- The thickness of the upper eyelid is then spanned approximately 1 cm from the palpebral margin.
- Next, a wide, nontransfixing stitch is made on the external aspect of the conjunctiva of the third eyelid.
- We stitch again along the entire thickness of the upper eyelid, this time from the conjunctiva to the skin, approximately 5–8 mm from the previous one.
- Finally, we pass through the silicone tube again about 5 mm from the previous point and near the other end. Knot the stitch with 3–5 loops (Fig. 10).

Tarsorrhaphy of the main eyelids

This is a more uncomfortable technique for the patient, since both eyelids are subjected to the pressure of the stitches. It is more indicated in kittens, in which the mucosa of the third eyelid is very weak and conventional tarsorrhaphy would cause it to loosen prematurely. It is also employed in situations where the volume of the eyeball has increased (e.g., recovery from neonatal ophthalmia), as the excess pressure of the globe on the suture would tear the conjunctival mucosa.

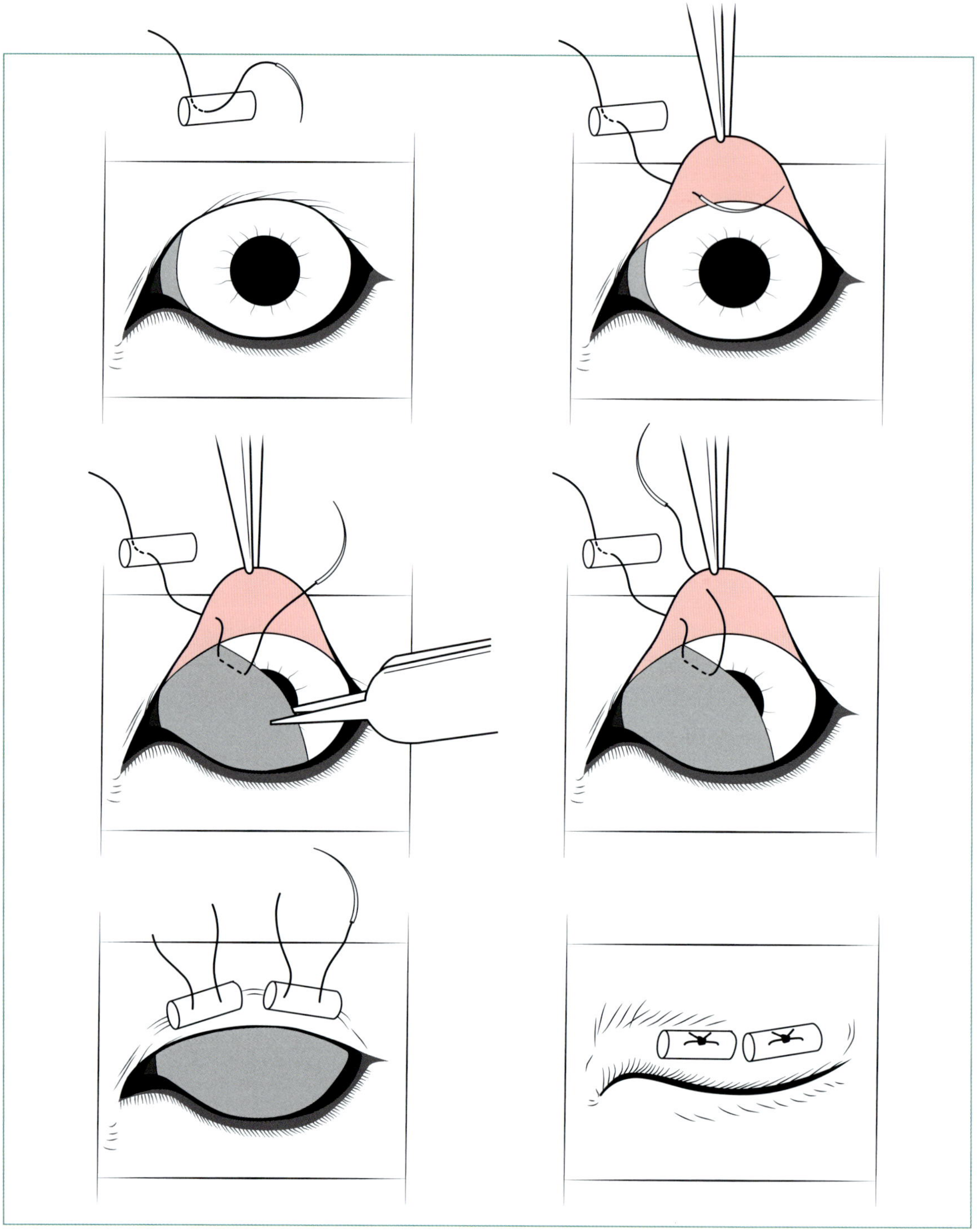

FIGURE 9. Technique for tarsorrhaphy of the nictitating membrane

Both the suture technique and the concept are very similar to nictitating membrane tarsorrhaphy. In this case, two silicone tubes will be used at each U-point. The suture order is as follows (Fig. 11):

- End of the upper silicone tube.
- Upper eyelid skin, exiting through the palpebral conjunctiva.

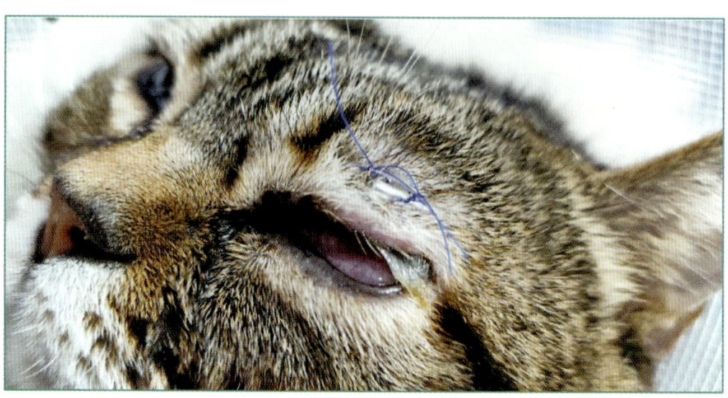

FIGURE 10. Tarsorrhaphy of the nictitating membrane. The suture is anchored in the upper eyelid and includes the external mucosa of the third eyelid.

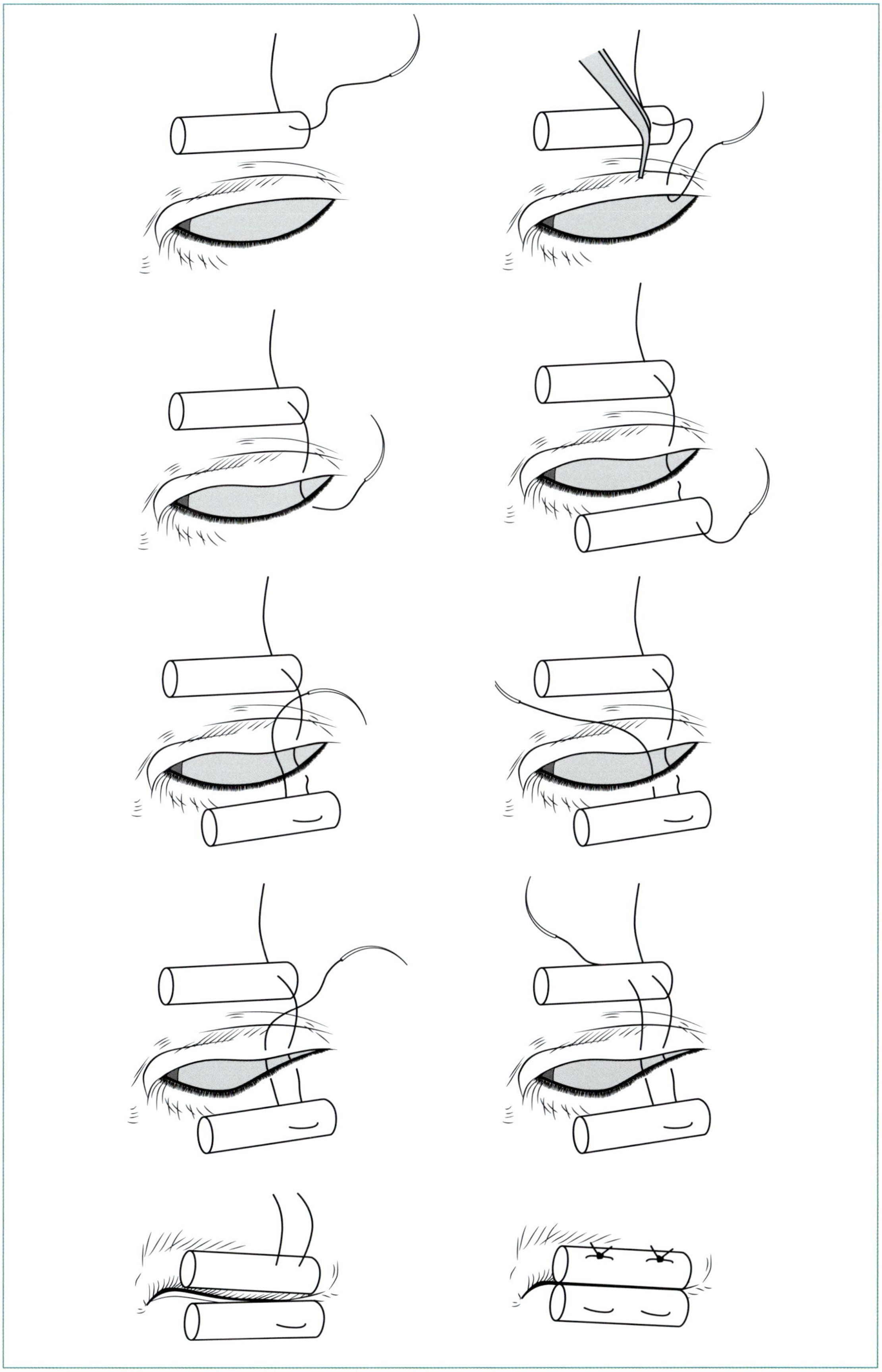

FIGURE 11. Technique for tarsorrhaphy of the main eyelids.

- Palpebral conjunctiva of the lower eyelid, with the needle exiting through the skin.
- End of the lower silicone tube.
- Opposite end of the lower silicone tube.
- Lower eyelid skin, exiting through the palpebral conjunctiva.
- Palpebral conjunctiva of the upper eyelid, exiting through the skin.
- Opposite end of the upper silicone tube (Fig. 12).

As there is a lot of suture handling, the authors recommend holding the free end of the suture with mosquito forceps from the outset to prevent the thread from being pulled out of the silicone tube due to traction, which would force us to repeat the whole process.

Depending on the size of the eye, a second stitch can be placed or it can be left as a single stitch. In this case, topical treatment may be applied through the remaining palpebral fissure.

Resection of palpebral tumors

Palpebral tumors in cats are relatively common. From most to least likely, squamous cell carcinoma, mast cell tumor, basal cell carcinoma, hemangiosarcoma, fibrosarcoma and lymphoma have been described. Because they are easily detectable, surgical resection is often the therapeutic technique of choice. Several resection techniques have been described.

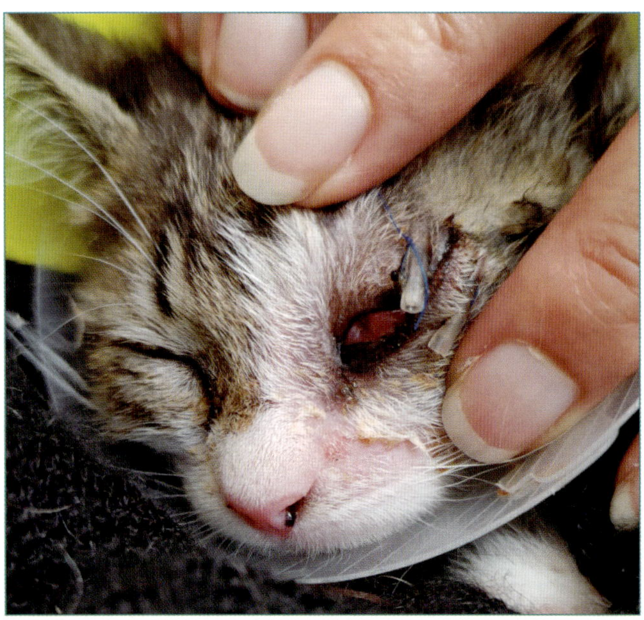

FIGURE 12. Tarsorrhaphy of the main eyelids in a kitten with panophthalmitis as a technique to help recover the eyeball.

Simple wedge resection technique

It is used to remove small tumors affecting the palpebral rim. The affected eyelid margin is sectioned with Spencer tenotomy scissors with two cuts forming a wedge (Fig. 13). The stitch closest to the palpebral edge is the first stitch we will place (4-0 nylon), with a **figure of eight pattern** whose knot is on the side farthest from the tarsal plates. This will prevent the knot from moving towards and irritating the cornea. Another way to avoid corneal trauma due to suture rubbing is to leave 4–5 cm of thread length at each stitch.

H-plasty technique

Tumors covering a considerable length of the eyelid cannot be resected with the wedge technique, as the size of the palpebral fissure would be excessively reduced. For this, the sliding flap technique or H-plasty is used. The tumor resection is in the shape of a rectangle. Once removed, the eyelid skin is then incised, creating a piece identical to the excised fragment (Fig. 14). On both sides of this rectangle we resect triangular wedges with bases equal to the length of the excised piece (Burow's triangles), which will allow us to advance the piece of skin by sliding it to the palpebral margin. The stitches closest to the cornea will both be placed in a figure of eight pattern using a 4-0 monofilament suture. The rest will be simple stitches, with the ends left very long.

Entropion correction technique

Entropion in cats most commonly occurs in the lower eyelid. Calculation of the skin width necessary to correct the entropion will be done before anesthetizing the patient. Thus, it will be possible to check the tension exerted by the orbicularis oculi muscle to roll the palpebral margin. Once the patient is anesthetized, we can draw on the eyelid skin to indicate the length and width of the skin fragment to be excised.

The most frequent resolution is by means of the **Hotz–Celsus technique**. Once the eyelid is prepared for surgery, we will use a Jaeger eyelid plate to make a 3 mm long incision along the palpebral margin. A second spindle-shaped incision almost parallel to the previous one, with the initially calculated width, will allow us to remove the portion of skin necessary to correct the entropion. Next, we will proceed to perform the key part of the technique: we will dissect and remove a band of equal width and

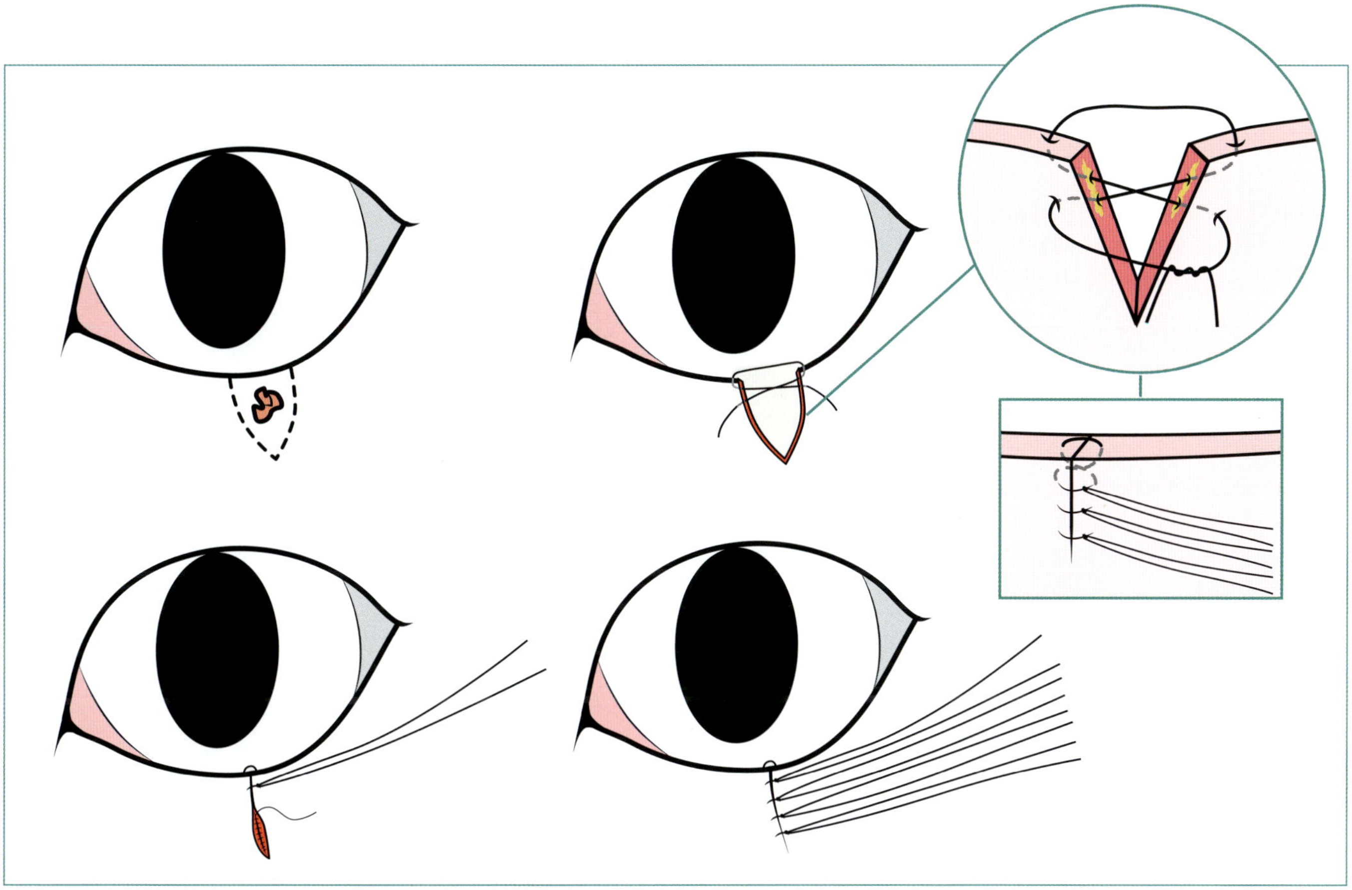

FIGURE 13. Simple wedge resection technique. Detail of the figure of eight suture.

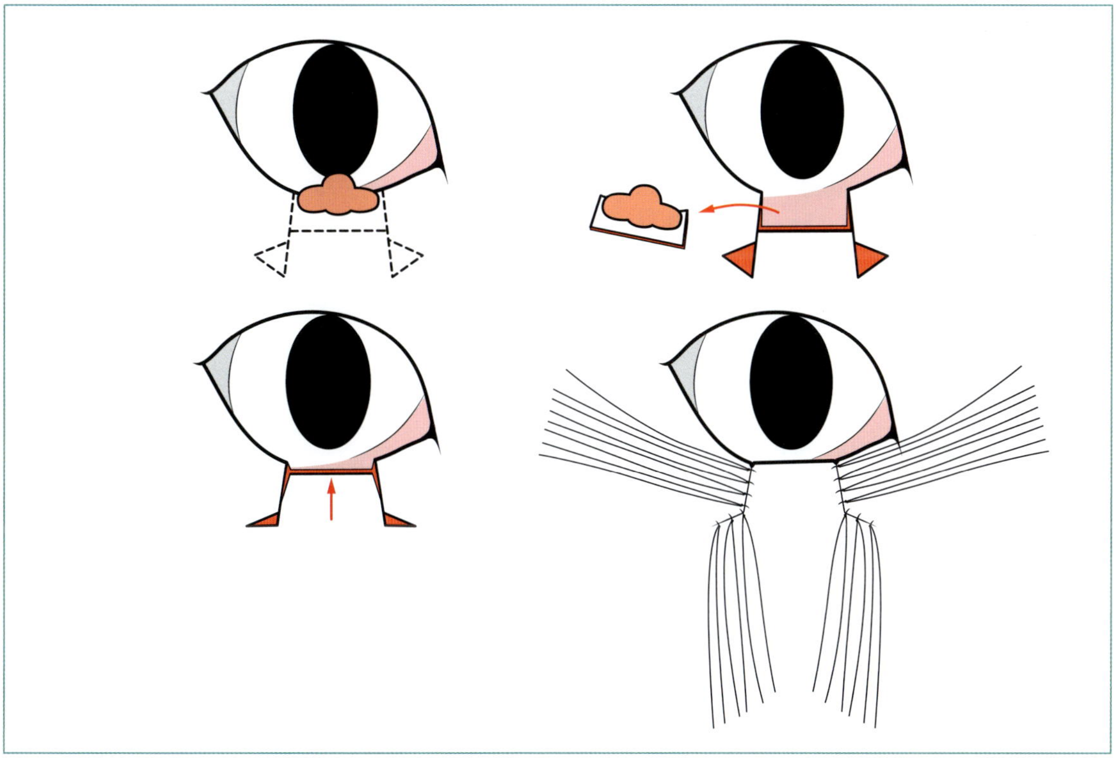

FIGURE 14. H-plasty resection technique.

length of the orbicularis oculi muscle with tenotomy scissors. The wound bed should not have any muscle remnants, it will be composed only of the inner layer of the palpebral conjunctiva. Thus, the suture will not have any tension and the traction of the stitches will undo the pathologic rolling of the palpebral margin. The suture pattern is simple interrupted stitches using 5-0 monofilament, leaving the ends very long to minimize corneal irritation (Fig. 15).

Successful corrective surgery for entropion involves the removal of a sufficiently wide band of orbicularis oculi muscle to release tension from the palpebral margin.

Reconstructive flaps

Severe eyelid lacerations, large tumors or congenital defects (colobomas) require plastic surgery, and various flap techniques have been described. Some of these have already been explained in Chapter 9. The specialized nature of these methods means that we will not expand on them in this book. Suffice it to say that the most commonly used technique is lip-to-lid plasty, in which a flap that starts at the lip margin is rotated towards the defect of the palpebral margin where it is sutured to repair it without losing the length of the fissure.

Enucleation

Enucleation involves the removal of the entire eyeball as a consequence of any traumatic disease, neoplastic disease or glaucoma that cannot be controlled with medical therapy and that results in a loss of vision and the viability of the organ. Two enucleation techniques have been described: transpalpebral and transconjunctival.

Transpalpebral enucleation

This is the technique most used by the author. It is started by closing the palpebral fissure with a continuous suture or, more simply, by clamping both eyelids closed with two Allis forceps. We draw a tapered incision around both eyelids, about 5 mm from them. We start a deep dissection of the conjunctival tissue following the curvature of the eyeball and avoiding penetration of the conjunctival sac. There is a branch of the maxillary artery in the dorsomedial canthus that must be ligated to minimize bleeding on the surgical field. Towards approximately the equator of the globe, the insertions of the different muscle bellies begin to emerge, which will be sectioned with tenotomy scissors

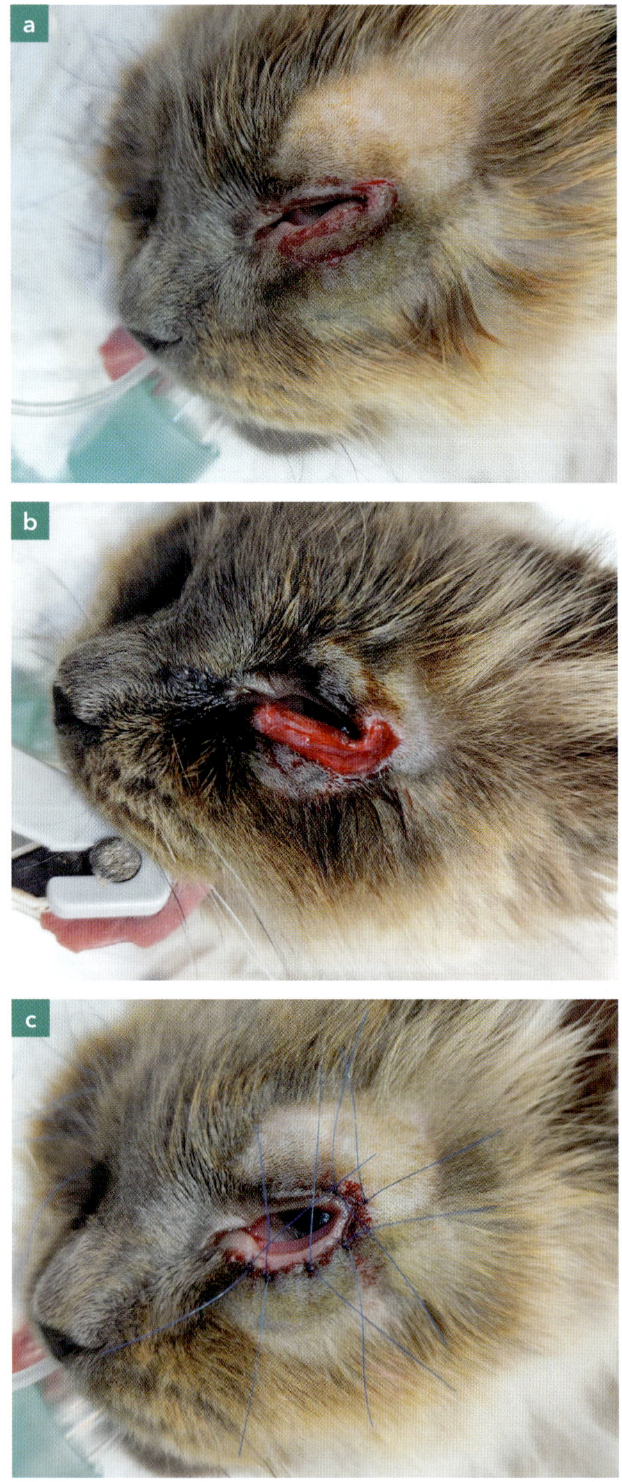

FIGURE 15. Resolution of entropion in a cat using the Hotz–Celsus technique. (a) Once the amount of tissue that needs to be removed has been calculated, the skin incision is marked on the skin. In this case, the lateral canthus has also been included. (b) Image after dissection of the entire skin and deep removal of the corresponding band of orbicularis oculi muscle. (c) Simple interrupted suture with very long ends to avoid corneal trauma in the postoperative period.

while blunt dissection is continued up to the ophthalmic pedicle (optic nerve, origin of orbital muscles and ocular vessels) (Fig. 16). The external insertion of the nictitating membrane at the medioventral canthus is also removed. All this should be performed as close as possible to the sclera until isolating the optic nerve, which will be gently tractioned to avoid injuring the optic chiasm, causing blindness in the contralateral eye. Once the optic nerve has been sectioned, we will proceed to close the orbit. For this purpose, a double suture can be performed, first an approximating suture and finally the skin closure. The author prefers to integrate the two by first making a continuous suture net by passing threads from one edge of the orbital ligament to the other. This net is made in a back-and-forth fashion, thus providing a flat support for the remaining eyelid skin (Fig. 17). Upon completion of the second subcutaneous net, a continuous intradermal suture is made, which will be used for the definitive closure of the incision.

Transconjunctival enucleation

In this case, the technique is started with a lateral canthotomy of about 10 mm. The conjunctiva is incised a few millimeters from the corneal limbus in a 360° cut. By means of blunt dissection, the orbital muscles are reached and cut to reach the optic nerve, which is also cut with curved iris scissors. All this dissection–incision should be performed without traction of the eyeball, working close to the sclera. The remaining fascial tissues and eyelid margins are trimmed and wound closure is initiated with the same technique used for transpalpebral enucleation.

Complications

The most frequent complications of reconstructive surgeries around the eyeball are related to corneal injuries. These may be due to:

- Inadequate protection technique: the use of tear gels on the cornea is mandatory in anesthesia procedures. In anesthetized cats, the eyeball does not roll down and the nictitating membrane does not protrude. The cornea is exposed and may dry out if we do not protect it.
- Lacerations with instruments during surgery: this can be avoided by inserting a scalpel handle or a Jaeger eyelid plate between the eyelid and the eyeball when using a scalpel or sharp instruments. The use of magnifying loupes also minimizes the risk of accidents.
- Suture friction on the cornea in the postoperative period: the stitches closest to the palpebral margin should be made in a figure of eight pattern. All sutures should be left with very long ends (approximately 4 cm), so that even if they enter the eye they do not have a puncturing effect on the cornea.

Another type of complication is caused by suture dehiscence due to insufficient suture protection (good analgesia, use of Elizabethan collars) or failure of the technique due to lack of experience (entropion can recur if not enough muscle tissue has been removed. In any case, it is better to have to repeat the entropion technique than to cause an ectropion by removing too much tissue).

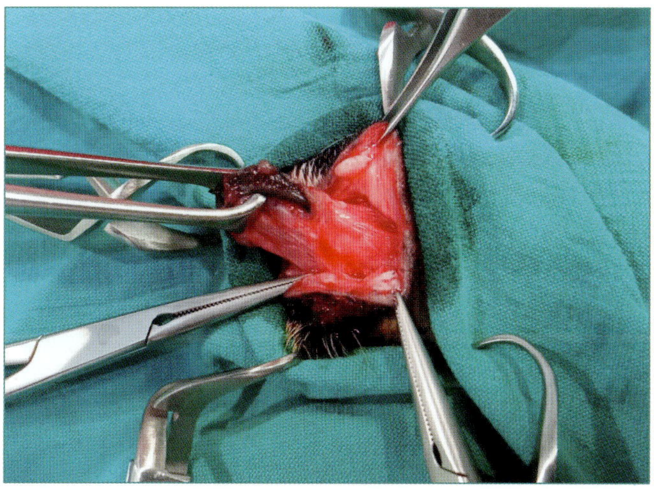

FIGURE 16. Transpalpebral enucleation: the connective tissue around the eyeball has been dissected and the eyelids are clamped closed with an Allis clamp (left). Next to it, mosquito forceps close the palpebral branch of the maxillary artery to prevent bleeding.

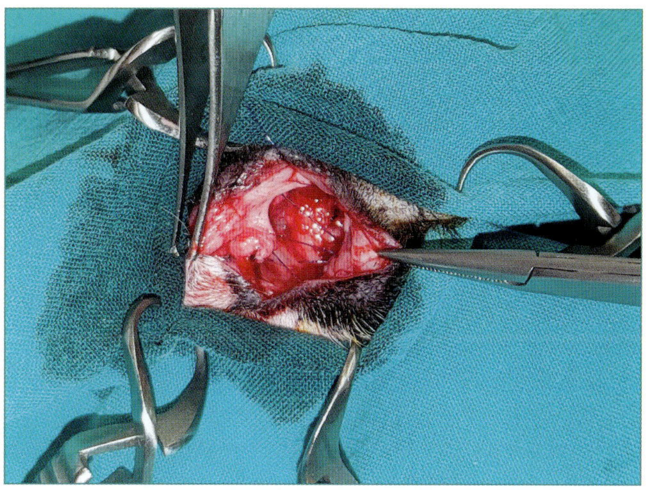

FIGURE 17. Once the eyeball has been removed, the orbit is closed. The image shows the first layer (net pattern, between the edges of the orbital ligament) of the three that will form the complete suture.

Finally, in enucleations, the accumulation of serohemorrhagic fluid inside the orbit is frequent and some of this exudate may even come out through the nostril via the nasolacrimal duct remnant. Normally, the vessels associated with the optic nerve are not sutured to avoid irritating the nerve tissue. The hemorrhage quickly forms a clot that does not cause complications if the skin suture is sufficiently tight.

Bibliography

Apt L, Isenberg S, Yoshimori R, Paez JH. Chemical preparation of the eye in ophthalmic surgery. III. Effect of povidone-iodine on the conjuntiva. *Arch Ophthalmol*, 1984; 102(5):728–729.

Attali-Soussay K, Jegou JP, Clerc B. Retrobulbar tumors in dogs and cats: 25 cases. *Vet Ophtalm*, 2001; 4(1):19–27.

Barrs VR, Beatty JA, Dhand NK et al. Computed tomographic features of feline sino-nasal and sino-orbital aspergillosis. *Vet J,* 2014; 201(2):215–222.

Binder BR, Herring IP. Duration of corneal anesthesia following topical administration of 0.5 % proparacaine hydrochloride solution in clinically normal cats. *Am J Vet Res*, 2006; 67(10):1780–1782.

Gelatt KN, Gelatt JP. *Small Animal Ophthalmic Surgery.* Oxford: Butterworth-Heinemann, 2001; pp. 46–124.

Gilger BC, Hamilton HL, Wilkie DA et al. Traumatic ocular proptoses in dogs and cats: 84 cases (1980–1993). *J Am Vet Med Assoc*, 1995; 206(8):1186–1190.

Gilger BC, McLaughlin SA, Whitely RD, Wright JC. Orbital neoplasms in cats: 21 cases (1974–1990). *J Am Vet Med Assoc*, 1992; 201(7):1083–1086.

Hudson LC, Hamilton WP. Musculoskeletal system. In: Hudson LC, Hamilton WP (eds.). *Atlas of Feline Anatomy for Veterinarians*, 2nd ed. Jackson (WY): Teton Newmedia, 2010; pp. 23–78.

Hudson LC. Chapter 11. Part 2: Eye. In: Hudson LC, Hamilton WP (eds.). *Atlas of Feline Anatomy for Veterinarians*, 2nd ed. Jackson (WY): Teton Newmedia, 2010; pp. 240–254.

Hunt GB. Use of the lip-to-lid flap for replacement of the lower eyelid in five cats. *Vet Surg*, 2006; 35(3):284–286.

Kafarnik C, Allgoewer I, Reese S. Innervation of the feline and canine cornea in correlation to corneal sensitivity (abstract). International Veterinary Ophthalmology Meeting (DOK/ECVO/ESVO), Munich, 2004.

McLaughlin SA, Whitely RD, Gilger BC et al. Eyelid neoplasia in cats: a review of demographic data (1979–1989). *J Am Anim Hosp Assoc*, 1993; 29:63–67.

Mitchell N, Oliver J. The eyelids, nictitans and lacrimal system. In: Mitchell N, Oliver J (eds.). *Feline Ophthalmology. The Manual.* Zaragoza: Servet–Grupo Asís, 2015; pp. 61–88.

Mitchell N, Oliver J. The orbit and globe. In: Mitchell N, Oliver J (eds.). *Feline Ophthalmology. The Manual.* Zaragoza: Servet–Grupo Asís, 2015; pp. 41–60.

Murphy S. Cutaneous squamous cell carcinoma in the cat: current understanding and treatment approaches. *J Feline Med Surg*, 2013; 15(5):401–407.

Newkirk KM, Rohrbach BW. A retrospective study of eyelid tumors from 43 cats. *Vet Pathol*, 2009; 46(5):916–927.

Plummer CE. Eyelids and orbit. In: Langley-Hobbs SJ, Demetriou JL, Ladlow JF (eds.). *Feline Soft Tissue and General Surgery.* Philadelphia, PA: Saunders Elsevier, 2014; pp. 691–705.

Schlueter C, Budras KD, Ludewig E et al. Brachycephalic feline noses: CT and anatomical study of the relationship between head conformation and the nasolacrimal drainage system. *J Feline Med Surg*, 2009; 11(11):891–900.

Spugnini EP, Vincenzi B, Citro G et al. Electrochemotherapy for the treatment of squamous cell carcinoma in cats: a preliminary report. *Vet J*, 2009, 179(1):117–120.

Stiles J, Townsend WM. Feline ophthalmology. In: Gelatt KN (ed.). *Veterinary Ophthalmology.* Ames, IA: Blackwell, 2007; pp. 1095–1164.

van der Woerdt A. Orbital inflammatory disease and pseudotumor in 7 cats. *Vet Clin North Am Small Anim Pract*, 2008; 38(2):389–401.

White JS, Grundon RA, Hardman C et al. Surgical management and outcome of lower eyelid entropion in 124 cats. *Vet Ophtalm*, 2012; 15(4):231–235.

Williams D, Kim J-Y. Feline entropion: a case series of 50 affected animals (2003–2008). *Vet Ophtalm*, 2009; 12(4):221–226.

Wolf E. Enucleation of the globe. In: Bojrab M (ed.). *Current Techniques in Small Animal Surgery.* Philadelphia: Lea & Febiger, 1990; pp. 119–123.

EAR CANAL AND MIDDLE EAR SURGERY 18

Alberto Barneto

Surgical anatomy

The ear, and particularly the inner ear, is where the receptors for the senses of hearing and balance (extremely developed in the cat) reside. The ear is anatomically divided into three zones: outer ear, middle ear and inner ear (Fig. 1).

Outer ear

The outer ear is formed by the **pinnae**, one on each side of the head, flat and convex, and the **external auditory canals**, short and cartilaginous, which conduct sounds to the auditory organ. The pinna has a wide, triangular surface (**scapha** or scaphal fossa), with two borders (the **helix** and the **antihelix**). The lateral and medial **auricular arteries** run superficially along the entire margin, while the intermediate auricular artery runs through the center.

The most dorsal portion of the pinna is formed by the **auricular cartilage** and is covered externally by more or less hair (in some breeds, the tip has a characteristic **tuft**).

> Movement and postures are important for sound reception (in the cat both pinnae can move independently), but also for behavioral and communication functions between cats and with other species.

With varying positions of the pinnae, the cat can show fear, anger, happiness or curiosity. To do so, they move them by means of several groups of extrinsic muscles (those that connect the outer ear cartilages with other parts of the head) and intrinsic muscles (interconnecting the outer ear cartilages themselves).

The base of the scapha joins the auricular cartilage on the lateral aspect. On the medial aspect, the auricular cartilage forms several folds (the **tragus**, the **antitragus** and the **antihelix**), which descend and join at depth to the **annular cartilage**. The auricular cartilage and the annular cartilage form the vertical portion and the horizontal portion of the external auditory canal, respectively. The skin inside the ear canal is lined with ceruminous glands, which function to lubricate and protect against physical and bacterial insults. The innermost part of the annular cartilage attaches to a small medial bony tunnel that penetrates the petrous portion of the temporal bone, the **external auditory meatus**. The skin of the ear canal continues through the meatus until it ends at the **tympanic membrane**, the end of the outer ear.

Middle ear

It begins at the **tympanic membrane**, connected at the external end to the auditory ossicles (**malleus**, **incus** and **stapes**), which in turn are connected to each other and to the **vestibular (oval) window** at the internal end. This opening together with the **cochlear (round) window** define the limit between the middle ear and the inner ear. All these structures are housed in a bony compartment of the temporal bone, the **tympanic bulla**.

The middle ear has three spaces or subdivisions:

- The smallest and most dorsal portion, the epitympanic recess, houses the malleus and incus ossicles, as well as the **facial nerve**.
- The **mesotympanum** or tympanic cavity proper, ventral to the previous one, includes the four orifices of the middle ear:
  - The tympanic membrane, adjacent to the manubrium of the malleus.
  - The vestibular (oval) window, with the stapes, the first communication with the inner ear.
  - The cochlear (round) window, the second connection to the inner ear.
  - The auditory (or Eustachian) tube, which is the communication between the middle ear and the pharynx.

  At the bottom of the mesotympanum, in a dorsomedial position, we find the **promontory**. This is a bony eminence of

1. Pinna
2. External auditory canal
3. Helix
4. Antihelix
5. Tragus
6. Antitragus
7. Scapha
8. Auricular cartilage
9. Annular cartilage
10. External auditory meatus
11. Tympanic membrane
12. Malleus (hammer)
13. Incus (anvil)
14. Stapes (stirrup)
15. Tympanic bulla
16. Cochlea
17. Vestibulocochlear nerve
18. Sympathetic branches of the cervical trunk
19. Eustachian tube
20. Inner septum of the tympanic bulla

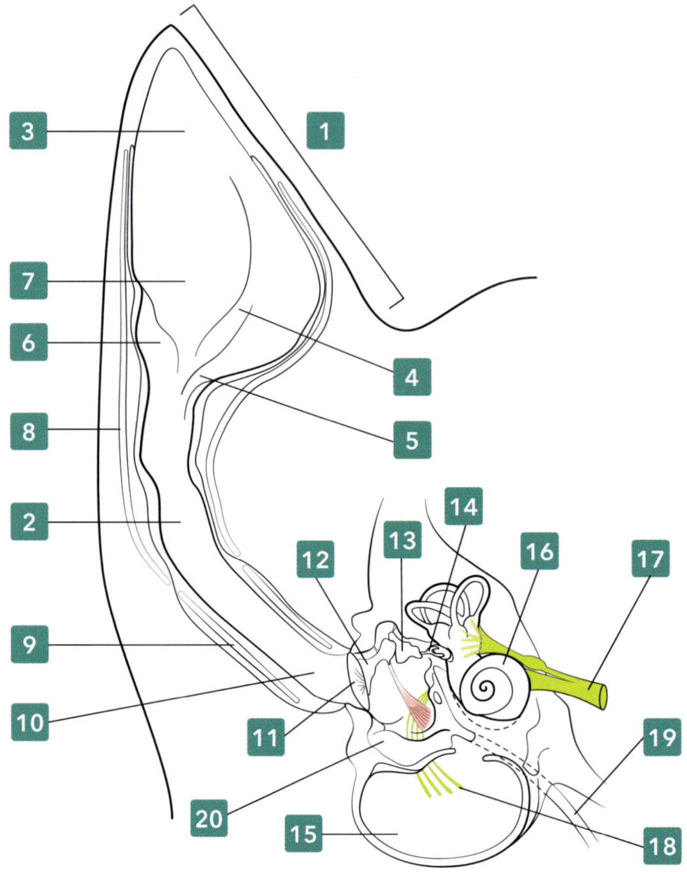

FIGURE 1. Anatomy of the cat ear.

the temporal bone, at the sides of which open the windows that communicate with the inner ear (vestibular and cochlear windows). Several **sympathetic branches of the cervical trunk** pass over the promontory. It is therefore a sensitive and delicate area that should never be injured in the various surgical procedures involving the middle ear (lavage, scraping, sampling).

- The **hypotympanum or tympanic bulla** is the largest cavity and is located ventrolaterally to the other two. It is separated from the mesotympanum by an incomplete **internal septum**, which is also crossed by cervical sympathetic branches. The tympanic bulla has an oval shape, a convex surface, is thin-walled and filled with air.

Inner ear

It consists of a network of canals, some snail-shaped (**cochlea**) and others semicircular within the temporal bone. This group of bony canaliculi houses the sensory organs for hearing and balance, as well as the vestibular and cochlear branches of cranial nerve VIII (**vestibulocochlear nerve**). It communicates with the middle ear through the oval and round windows.

Surgical diseases

In the **pinna**:

- **Otohematoma:** is an accumulation of blood or serohemorrhagic fluid between the skin and the cartilage of the pinna. The causes are varied: trauma (usually self-inflicted), infected bites, immune-mediated diseases, etc. The first objective is to empty the contents, usually by needle aspiration, appropriately treat the cause, control pain and inflammation with corticosteroids and protect the pinna with an Elizabethan collar to prevent self-injury until the underlying disease is controlled. This way we will avoid the chronification of the disease ("cauliflower ear").
- **Neoplasms of the pinna:** the most frequent is squamous cell carcinoma (SCC), a malignant tumor closely related to ultraviolet exposure and white pigmented areas with little hair (eyelids, nose and pinnae). It is 13 times more frequent in countries with longer hours of sun exposure. Although the surgical solution is always at our disposal, electrochemotherapy treatments are increasingly used to help cure this disease (Fig. 2).

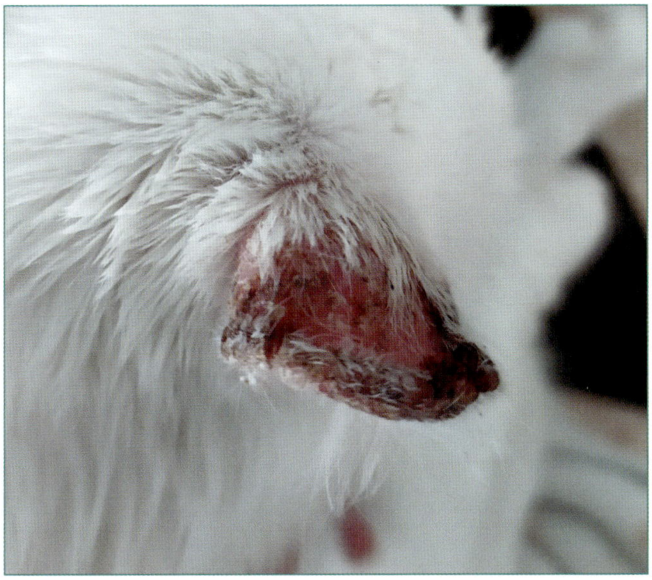

FIGURE 2. Squamous cell carcinoma (SCC) in the pinna of an outdoor white cat.

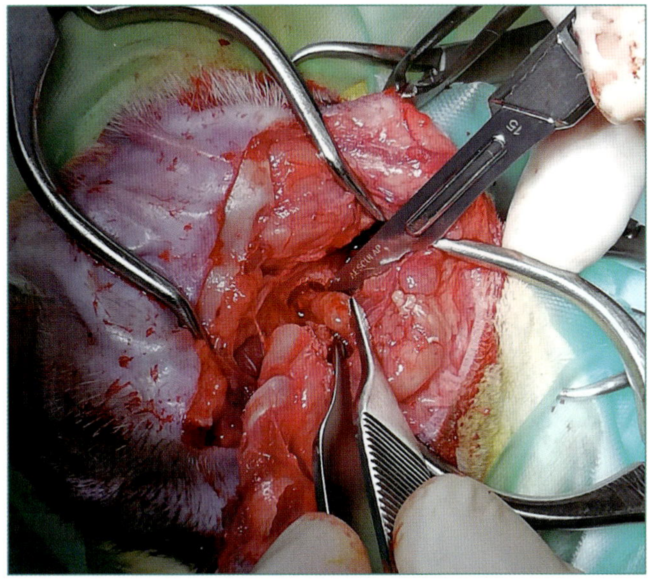

FIGURE 3. Surgical removal of a polyp within the horizontal ear canal after ablation of the vertical canal.

In the **auditory canal**:

- **Chronic otitis:** there are determining factors such as parasites (*Otodectes cynotis*, *Demodex cati* or *Notoedres cati*, which cause up to 50% of otitis in young cats), hypersensitivity and autoimmune diseases. But what makes the disease chronic and medically difficult to treat are perpetuating factors such as yeasts (*Malassezia pachydermatis*, *Candida* spp.) and bacteria (*Pseudomona* spp., *Enterococcus* spp., *Escherichia coli*).
- **Obstructive otitis:** there can be several causes of obstructive growth within the feline ear, the most frequent being ceruminous cystomatosis (multiple degenerated ceruminous glands with bluish-gray contents that can obstruct when they occur in large numbers) and tumors (ceruminous gland adenocarcinoma, SCC and benign inflammatory polyps). The solution is the removal of the cause or, if this is not possible, ear canal ablation (see under surgical techniques) (Fig. 3).

In the **middle and inner ear**:

- **Otitis media:** is an underdiagnosed disease (only 10% of cases present clinical signs) that is increasingly being discovered with the use of advanced imaging techniques (computed tomography, magnetic resonance). Neurological clinical signs are the most common (peripheral vestibular syndrome, Horner syndrome). The correct treatment is described below.
- **Tumors:** the most frequent are benign aural polyps, which usually cause otitis media due to the accumulation of secretions. They are always treated surgically by ventral bulla osteotomy or, sometimes, total ablation of the external auditory canal (see surgical techniques).

Therapeutic protocol for otitis media

- With the cat anesthetized and in lateral recumbency, a soft elevating roll is placed under the neck.
- The tympanic membrane is examined with an otoscope; if it is intact we perform a **myringotomy** (perforate the eardrum with a 20–22-gauge spinal needle, at least 4 cm deep) in a caudoventral direction.
- Samples of the contents are taken for cytology and culture with antibiogram.
- This is followed by flushing with an EDTA solution, with the possible use of nonototoxic antibiotics (e.g., enrofloxacin) and/or dexamethasone, depending on the causes. We can perform it with a sterile urethral catheter of 3.5 Fr (approx. 1 mm).
- Based on the results of diagnostic tests, appropriate systemic therapy will be added to the topical treatment.
- Analgesia should always be administered, pre- and postoperatively.
- Otitis should be treated for at least 1–2 months and followed-up weekly.

Diagnosis

The methods for diagnosing ear disease are varied and the protocol must be followed correctly in order to provide the most appropriate treatment. Table 1 lists the techniques and their indications.

TABLE 1. Techniques and tests for the diagnosis of ear disease

Diagnostic technique	Indications	Observations
Clinical examination with otoscope	■ Any disease of the external auditory canal. ■ Evaluation of the tympanic membrane and sometimes the inner ear.	The authors recommend a high-end otoscope, with a magnifying lens and the ability to work through the cone with the help of the lens.
Cytology/biopsy	■ Evaluation of any type of discharge from the outer and middle ear. ■ Scrapings or biopsies of lesions of the pinna.	■ This technique is essential to know the etiology and complications of any ear disease. ■ Very sebaceous secretions should be fixed with heat, avoiding alcohol solutions.
Culture and antibiogram	Bacterial complication of any ear disease.	■ Cats do not often have primary bacterial ear diseases, but, if left untreated, surgical treatment will be complicated. ■ We must have this information before the operation or, at the latest, during the surgical procedure.
X-ray	Useful, but with new diagnostic imaging techniques it is no longer as relevant.	■ The most useful projection is the rostrocaudal with the mouth open and ventral flexion of the neck (Fig. 4) to see the symmetry and the contents of the tympanic bullae. ■ The laterolateral projection also helps in viewing the bullae. ■ The ventrodorsal projection allows for evaluation of the external auditory canal.
CT scan	The test of choice for any solid or liquid content in the external auditory canal and middle ear.	■ There may be limitations in assessing tissue density. ■ As the cat is sedated, the tissues of the external auditory canal undergo anatomical variations that the surgeon will have to interpret (Fig. 5).

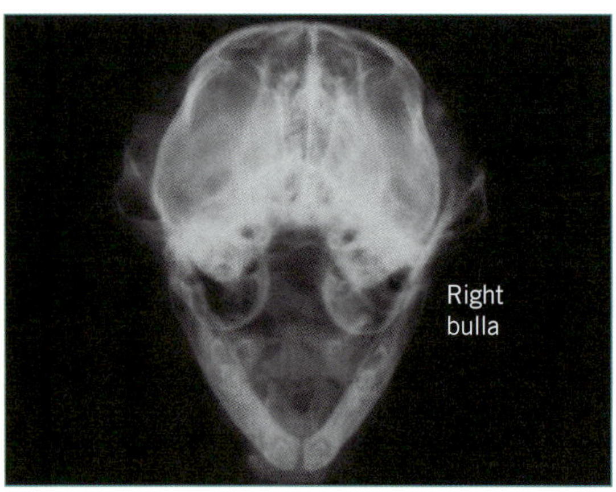

FIGURE 4. Open-mouth rostrocaudal X-ray of a kitten with a denser right tympanic bulla, indicative of otitis media (in this case due to a polyp). Radiographic positioning is very important to be able to interpret the images well.

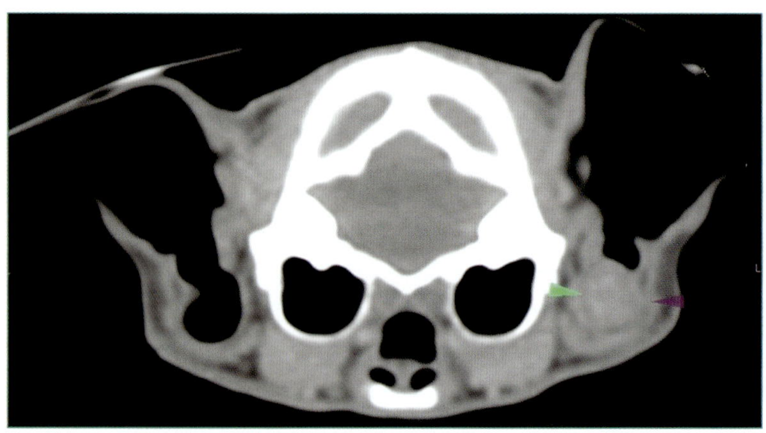

FIGURE 5. CT scan of a tumor in the left vertical ear canal (arrowheads). Although it initially seemed to occupy the horizontal canal as well, the tissue image after sedation was misleading and during surgery only the vertical portion of the affected ear canal had to be removed. Image courtesy of Diagnosfera.

Preoperative and postoperative considerations

Aspects to be taken into account before and after the intervention:

- Shaving and asepsis of the pinna and surrounding area can be successfully completed. We must protect the eyeball from the toxic effect of antiseptics with abundant artificial tear gel.
- Asepsis of the ear canal is not effective, especially in chronic infectious processes. Ear canal surgery is considered contaminated or clean–contaminated.
- If possible, infection should be controlled prior to surgery. If not, samples of the exudate should be taken during the intervention for culture and antibiogram.
- If the eardrum is ruptured or the middle ear has to be entered, a sterile gauze pad moistened and tied with a piece of bandage will be prepared and introduced into the pharynx to collect possible fluids through the Eustachian tube during surgery.
- After surgery, especially in total ear canal ablation and in bulla osteotomy, a Penrose drain should be applied to prevent the accumulation of fluids and secretions, which may hinder healing.
- A good analgesia protocol with buprenorphine or methadone should be established before, during and after surgery.

Surgical techniques

Pinnectomy

- **Patient positioning and preparation:** in sternal recumbency if the operation is bilateral, or in lateral recumbency if only one side is to undergo the intervention. All the hair on the pinna is clipped and the skin is disinfected on both sides and in the surrounding area. The inside of the ear canal is protected with a cotton swab.
- **Technique**
  1. The lesion is located and the pinna is cut at least 1 cm from the margin of the lesion. If it is a SCC and the cat will continue to be in contact with UV light, the authors recommend cutting both pinnae to the base (Fig. 6). As much as possible, we will avoid going as far as the antitragus, helix and antihelix cartilages in order to facilitate the symmetry of the subsequent suture.
  2. Before suturing the skin, we will ligate the main vessels of the pinna to reduce postsurgical bleeding in the subcutaneous tissue (branches of the caudal auricular and superficial temporal arteries).
  3. Suturing of the skin edges is performed with a continuous technique using closely spaced stitches to avoid suffusive hemorrhage and dehiscence. The preferred material is 4-0 or 5-0 nylon or absorbable monofilament.

> The secret to the good healing of this suture is to ensure the symmetrical apposition of the corresponding stitches between the external and internal edges of the base of the ear.

Vertical or total ear canal ablation

- **Patient positioning and preparation:** in lateral recumbency with a small towel roll under the neck at the level of the atlas joint. We should protect the cornea of the corresponding eye with abundant gel before surgical cleaning. The entire area of the face, skull and throat up to the pharyngeal midline, as well as the pinna, is depilated and disinfected. Since this cannot be done properly inside the ear canal, it is considered a clean–contaminated intervention.

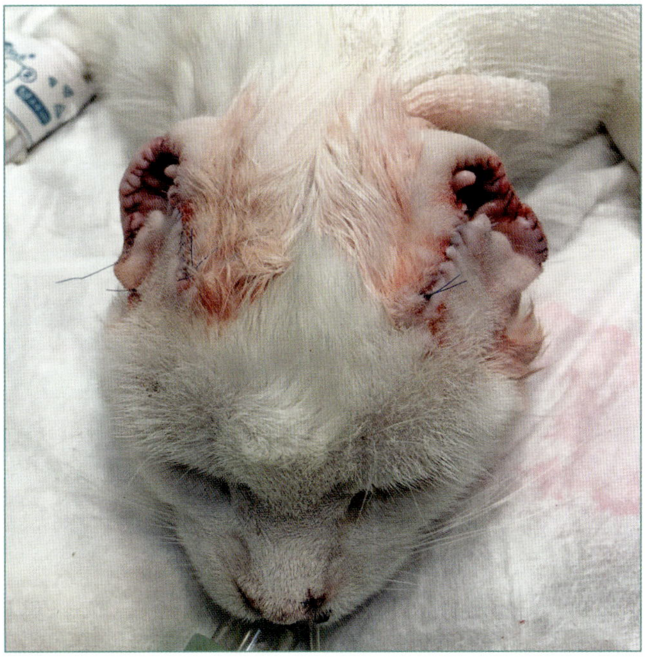

FIGURE 6. Cat after double pinnectomy due to bilateral squamous cell carcinoma.

- **Technique**

1. An incision is made around the entire external auditory meatus, including the tragus, antitragus, helix and antihelix folds, in order to remove them. We dissect the connective tissue around the entire circumference, taking special care not to damage the auricular cartilage. Once this is done, we make a second incision, this time vertical from the edge of the tragus along the entire length of the vertical ear canal (Fig. 7).
2. All the connective tissue around the vertical auditory canal is bluntly dissected, sticking as close as possible to it (it is very easy to see because of its characteristic yellowish color) (Fig. 8). On the external side we will find the glandular tissue of the parotid gland, which we will carefully separate from the ear canal. At this point we can already see the entire circumference of the vertical canal.
3. **If the ablation will only involve the vertical ear canal**, the vertical canal is cut transversely and a sample is taken of any exudate that may be inside the horizontal ear canal. The remaining canal is double incised so that it becomes two semicircular flaps, one dorsal and one ventral. Both flaps are sutured to the edges of the skin incision with 5-0 nylon suture. We continue closing the entire wound with this suture, leaving a T-shape (Fig. 9).
4. **If the ablation is of the entire auditory canal**, we must locate in this area the **facial nerve** pathway (around and ventrally bordering the auditory canal) and the **maxillary and superficial temporal arteries**, which are slightly deeper than the facial nerve, but have the same pathway (Figs. 10 and 11). We continue the blunt dissection of the horizontal canal, very close to it, until we reach the insertion at the **external auditory meatus**.
5. We section the insertion of the canal into the meatus with a no. 11 scalpel blade, carefully protecting the facial nerve and the vessels. We remove the remains of the canal with rongeurs and ventrally enlarge the auditory meatus. The bony internal septum that separates the dorsolateral and ventromedial compartments of the tympanic bulla is removed. A sample of the contents of the middle ear is taken, the epithelium is removed with a scraper and the contents are lavaged with warm saline several times. We must avoid the dorsomedial area of the small compartment of the bulla in order not to damage the auditory ossicles or the sympathetic neurological pathways (if we do so, we would cause a permanent Horner syndrome).
6. The deep tissues are sutured by apposition, avoiding the facial nerve and the vessels, a Penrose drain is kept in place for 5 days, if required (e.g., infection), and the skin wound is closed as in the case of partial ear canal ablation.

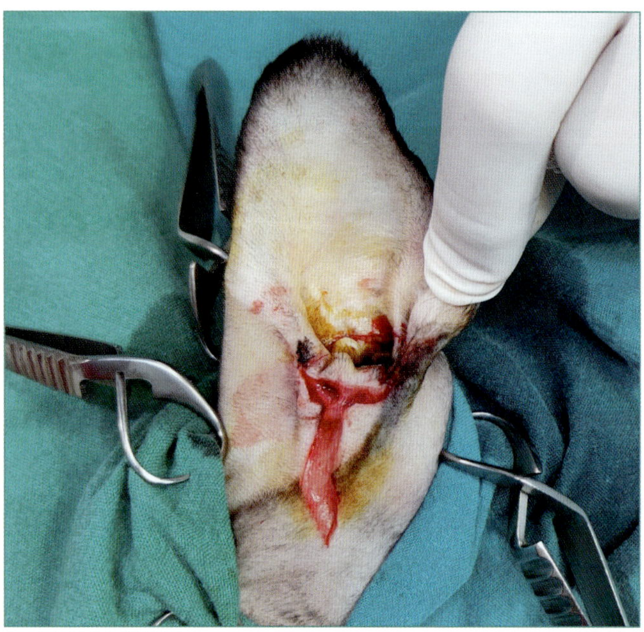

FIGURE 7. Double incision (circumferential and vertical from the tragus over the ear canal) in ear canal ablation surgery.

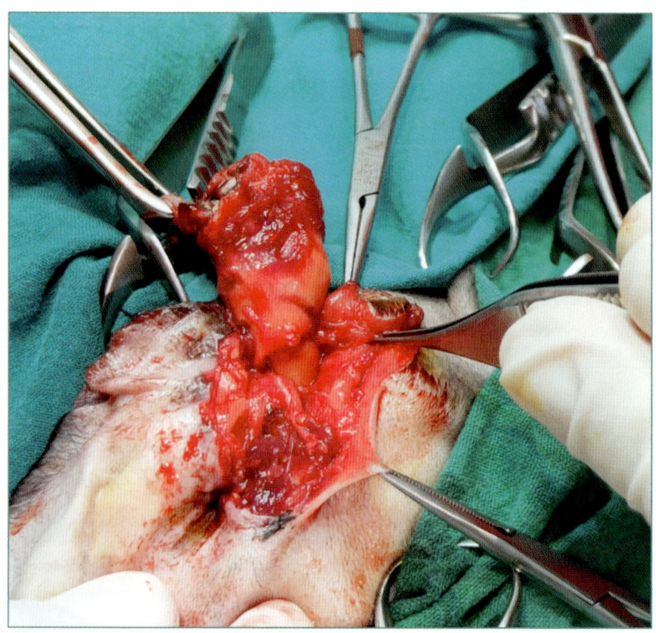

FIGURE 8. Dissection of the vertical ear canal in ablation surgery. The yellowish color of the cartilage is very clearly visible once all the surrounding connective tissue has been dissected.

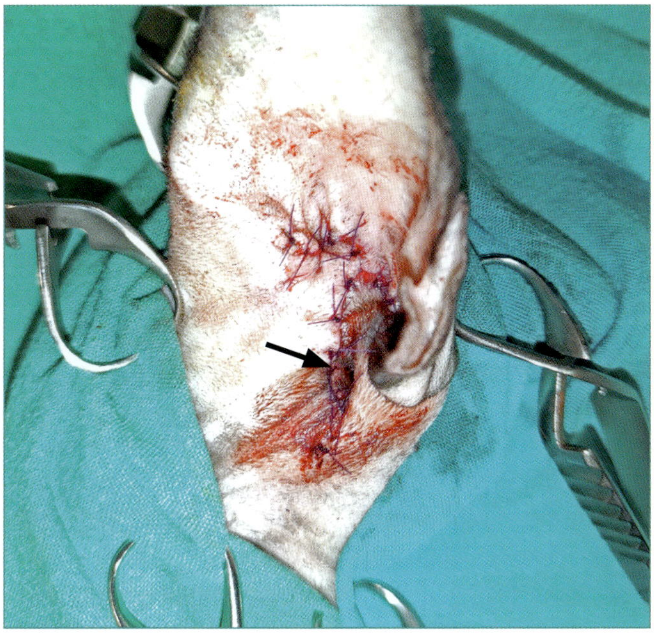

FIGURE 9. T-shaped suture after ear canal ablation surgery. The arrow indicates the location of the horizontal canal opening once sutured to the skin.

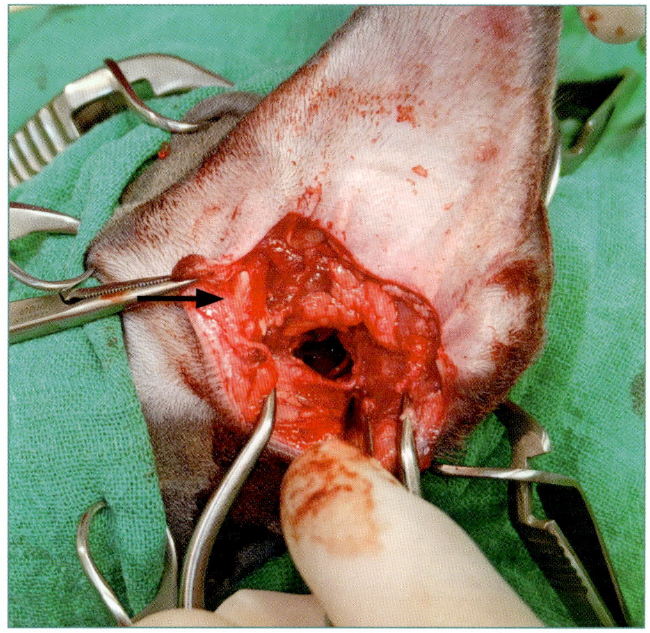

FIGURE 10. Total ablation of the external ear canal in a cat with an aural polyp. The canal has already been completely excised and the external auditory meatus can be seen inside. Slightly more superficial, bordering the ventral area in a rostral direction, the facial nerve can be seen in its pathway around the auditory canal (arrow).

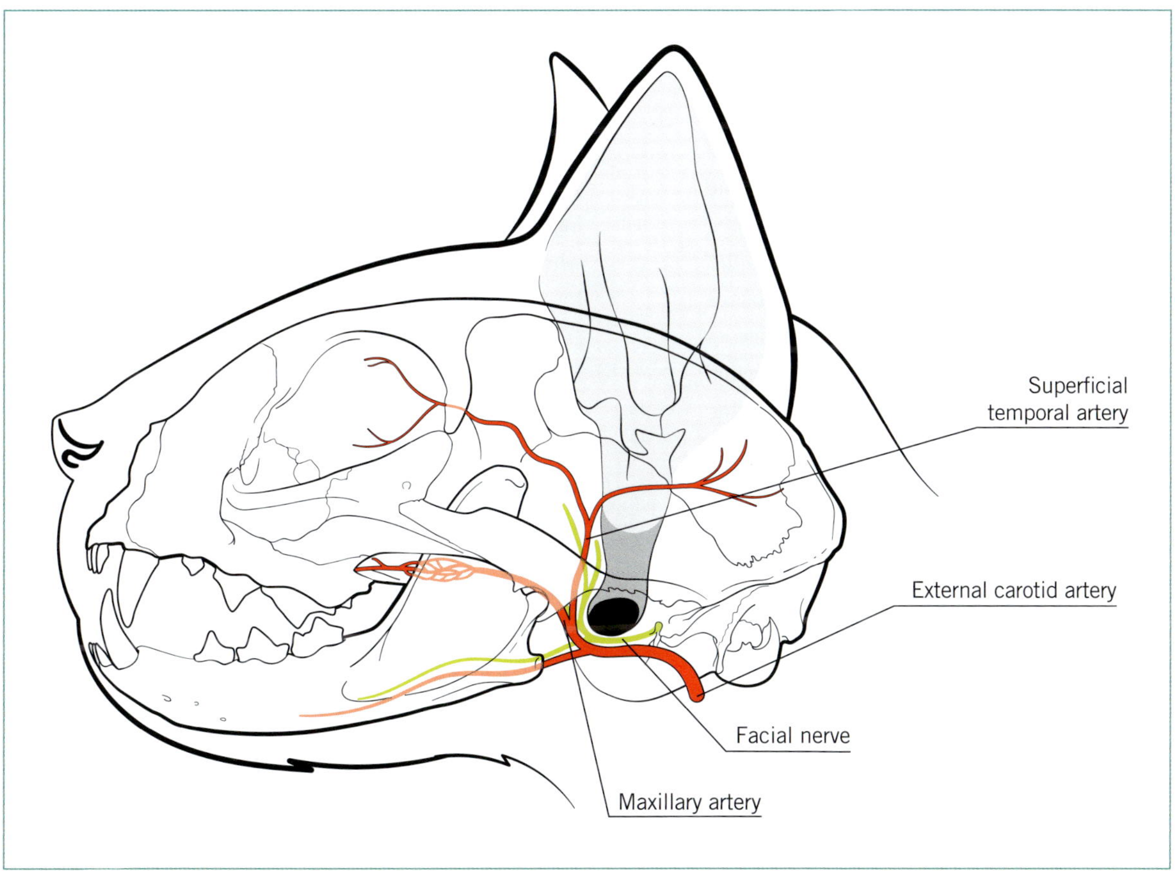

FIGURE 11. Vascularization and innervation of the ear canal.

Ventral bulla osteotomy

- **Patient positioning and preparation:** in dorsal recumbency, with the thoracic limbs held caudally and the head extended. A small towel roll under the nape of the neck and fixation of the maxillary canines to the table with adhesive bands will keep the area undergoing the intervention stable. A surgical clip is made from the mandibular symphysis to the sternal manubrium and laterally to the ear canal openings.
- **Technique**
  1. Anatomical landmarks are located: the **wing of the atlas**, the **mandibular angular process** and the **mandibular ramus**, the **midline** and the **digastric muscle** (a tubular belly between the wing of the atlas and the caudoventral aspect of the mandibular ramus). In this position, the **tympanic bulla** can be thoroughly palpated as a rounded convex protrusion between the midline and the mandibular ramus, caudal to the latter. Although the incision will be parallel to the midline, it is very important to know and mentally retain the actual orientation of the tympanic bulla in the cat, which is slightly divergent from the midline in a craniomedial to caudolateral direction. The incision is made paramedially, midway between the midline and the mandibular angular process, just medial to the belly of the digastric muscle. The incision should begin at a distance of 1 cm cranial to the mandibular angular process and extend to the wing of the atlas (Fig. 12.1).
  2. After incising the skin, we will proceed with the blunt dissection of the flat, subcutaneous muscles (**platysma and sphincter muscle of the neck**), continuing with the same technique between the digastric muscle (which we will leave laterally in the surgical field) and the **styloglossus and hyoglossus muscles**. Here we will find four structures: the **linguofacial vein**, from which arises the **hyoid venous arch** that joins the medial border of the digastric muscle and runs perpendicular to the incision (we will retract it caudally), the **lingual artery** and the **hypoglossal nerve**, which run lateral to the hyoglossus muscle and should be retracted and protected medially next to it. For this and to maintain a good surgical field opening, two Gelpi self-retaining retractors are placed. We will continue the deep blunt dissection to widen the field, always palpating the convex surface of the bulla in order not to lose the landmark. With the help of a periosteotome we will clean the remains of muscle fibers and connective tissue from the convex wall of the tympanic bulla (ventral and lateral areas) (Fig. 12.2).
  3. To penetrate inside the bulla we will make two equidistant holes 1–2 mm apart. We can use several techniques: a Steinmann pin mounted in a Jacobs hand chuck, a bur in a turbine or a Steinmann pin and a mallet. The authors prefer the latter technique because, when carefully performed, it allows controlled entry into the cavity through the thin wall of the bulla (Fig. 12.3). If we use a bur we must be careful because the vibration can damage the cochlear system and affect hearing. This allows access to the larger compartment. We will take the opportunity to take a sample of the accumulated mucus for bacterial culture.
  4. From the two holes we will expand the osteotomy by removing fragments with rongeurs, first expanding the surface and then moving towards the lateral area of the bulla. The next wall we will encounter is the internal septum, which separates the major and minor compartments. We will advance with the rongeurs in a lateral and dorsal direction, breaking the septum to access the dorsolateral compartment of the bulla (Fig. 12.4). This is where most aural polyps originate, so we can remove them with the help of mosquito forceps and spoon curettes if this is the objective of the intervention. After that we will lavage the bulla carefully using warm sterile saline. When working inside the tympanic bulla, we must avoid damaging the dorsomedial surface, in the minor compartment, where the most delicate structures are located: the auditory ossicles, the round and oval windows and the sympathetic nerve branches of the cervical trunk (Fig. 12.5).
  5. Prior to closure, we will place an active drain (with a butterfly catheter connected to a vacuum tube) or passive drain inside the cavity to help eliminate exudates in the postoperative period, if we expect them to accumulate. To allow the drain to exit, we will make a hole outside the wound and suture the drain to the skin of the neck. The apposition of the muscular structures is done with 4-0 absorbable suture by planes and we will close the skin wound with an intradermal suture.

Figures 13, 14 and 15 show intraoperative images of this technique in different patients.

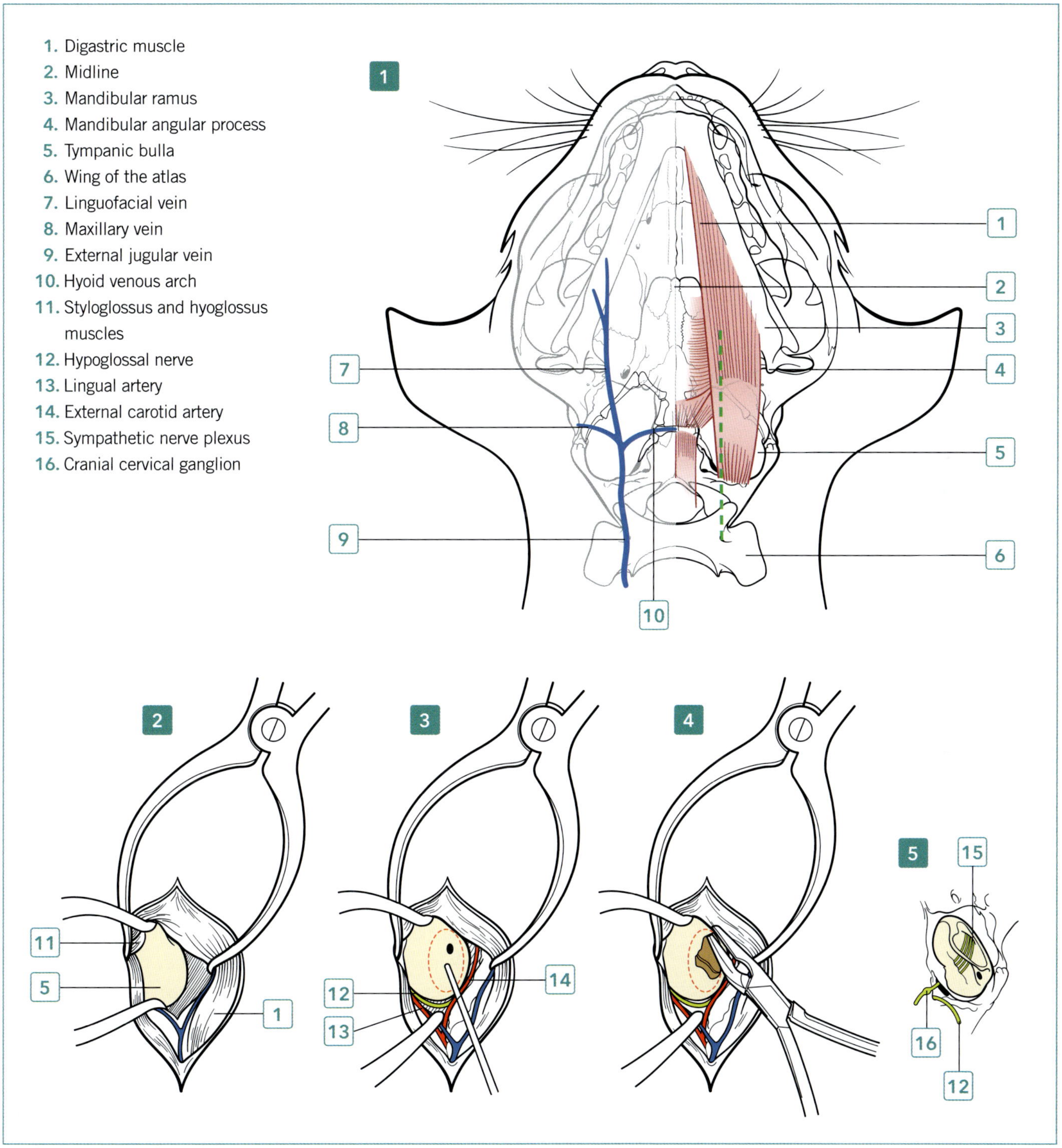

FIGURE 12. Steps of the surgical technique to perform a ventral bulla osteotomy (left bulla in this case).

1. Anatomical landmarks and incision line (green dashed line).
2. Blunt dissection of the flat, subcutaneous muscles, dissection and lateral retraction of the digastric muscle, medial retraction of the styloglossus and hyoglossus muscles and retraction of the linguofacial vein and the hyoid venous arch. For this purpose, two Gelpi self-retaining retractors are used.
3. Perforation of the bulla using a Steinmann pin, with two equidistant holes 1–2 mm apart, to access the larger compartment.
4. From the two holes, the osteotomy is expanded by removing fragments with rongeurs, first expanding the surface and then moving towards the lateral aspect of the bulla.
5. Special caution should be taken with the structures on the dorsomedial surface of the lesser bulla compartment: the auditory ossicles, the round and oval windows and the sympathetic nerve branches of the cervical trunk.

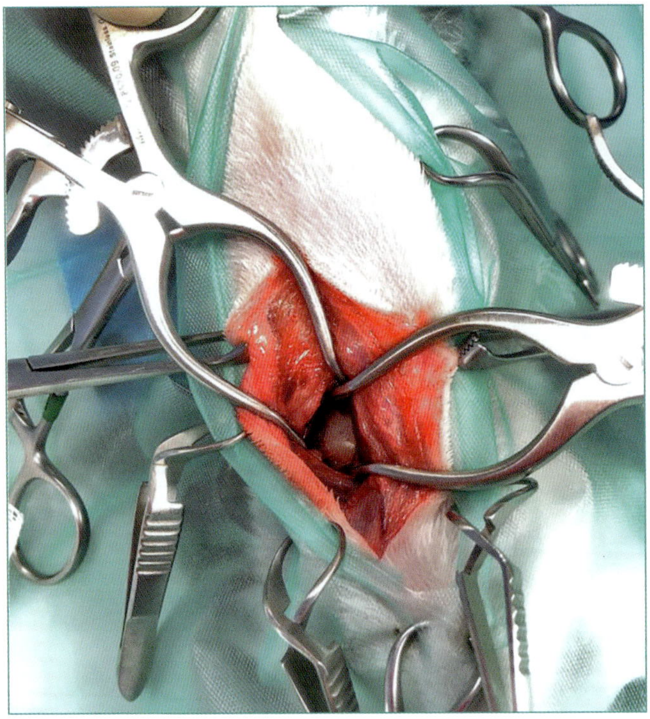

FIGURE 13. After dissection of the styloglossus and hyoglossus muscles, the smooth, convex surface of the tympanic bulla of a cat is visible. It is essential to use two Gelpi self-retaining retractors to work comfortably at depth.

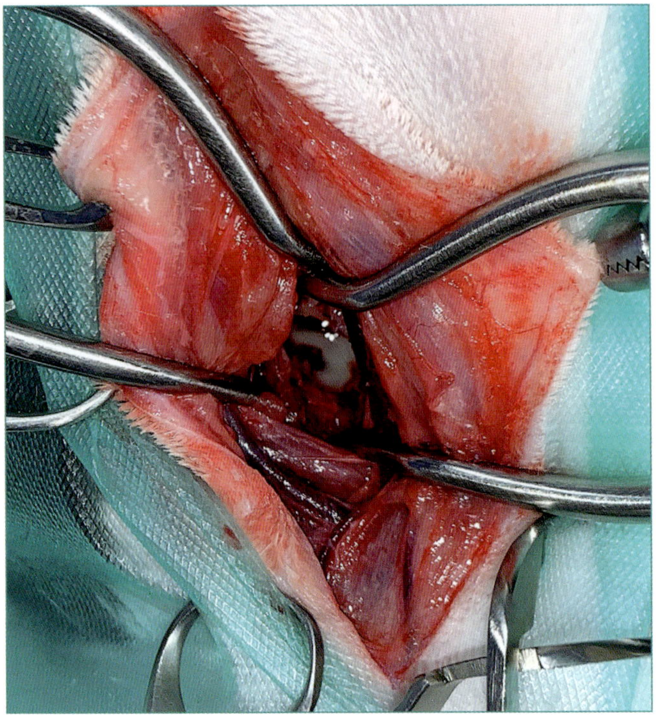

FIGURE 15. In this case, bulla osteotomy revealed a purulent otitis media without the presence of tumor material. In these cases, we should take samples for culture and antibiogram and leave a drain after repeated lavages with warm sterile saline.

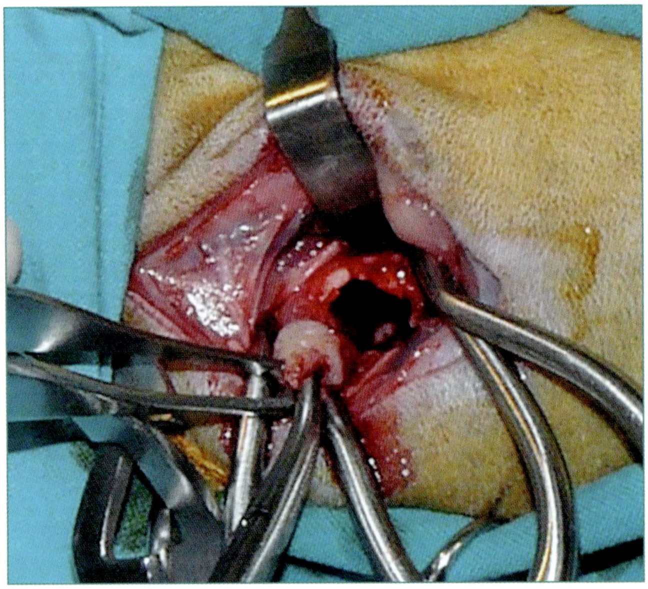

FIGURE 14. Removal of an aural polyp in the dorsolateral compartment after bulla osteotomy and removal of the internal septum dividing the tympanic bulla in cats.

Complications

Hemorrhages and exudates may occur, which will be well controlled with postsurgical drains. Infections should not be a complication if the correct systemic treatment has been administered prior to surgery, based on culture and antibiogram.

Facial nerve damage (Horner syndrome) is common in the postoperative period in cats, although they usually recover in 3–4 weeks. The way to avoid this is a combination of anatomical knowledge and good surgical technique.

Deafness may occur after surgery, more frequently in cats that have undergone middle ear surgery.

Another complication is due to poor control of the initial disease after surgery: this is usually more frequent in surgeries involving lateral wall resection or partial ear canal ablation.

Bibliography

Bacon NJ, Gilbert RL, Bostock DE, White RA. Total ear canal ablation in the cat: indications, morbidity and log-term survival. *J Small Anim Pract*, 2003; 44(10):430–434.

Baines SJ. Ear. In: Langley-Hobbs SJ, Demetriou JL, Ladlow JF (eds.). *Feline Soft Tissue and General Surgery*, 1st ed. Oxford: Saunders Elsevier, 2014; pp. 587–615.

Barnes JA. Cardiovascular system. In: Hudson LC, Hamilton WP (eds.). *Atlas of Feline Anatomy for Veterinarians*, 2nd ed. Jackson (WY): Teton Newmedia, 2010; pp. 79–114.

Barthez PY, Koblik PD, Hornof WJ et al. Apparent wall thickening in fluid filled versus air filled tympanic bulla in computed tomography. *Vet Radiol Ultrasound*, 1996; 37(2):95–98.

Bischoff MG, Kneller SK. Diagnostic imaging of the canine and feline ear. *Vet Clin North Am Small Anim Pract*, 2004; 34(2):437–458.

Callaghan D, Culley CD. Ototoxicity in the dog and cat. *Vet Rec*, 1985; 117(11):291.

Cook LB, Bergman RL, Bahr A, Boothe HW. Inflammatory polyp in the middle ear with secondary suppurative meningoencephalitis in a cat. *Vet Radiol Ultrasound*, 2003; 44(6):648–651.

de Lorimier LP, Alexander SD, Fan TM. T-cell lymphoma of the tympanic bulla in a feline leukemia virus-negative cat. *Can Vet J*, 2003; 44(12):987–989.

Detweiler DA, Johnson LR, Kass PH, Wisner ER. Computed tomographic evidence of bulla effusion in cats with sinonasal disease: 2001–2004. *J Vet Intern Med*, 2006; 20(5):1080–1084.

Fan TM, de Lorimier LP. Inflammatory polyps and aural neoplasia. *Vet Clin North Am Small Anim Pract*, 2004; 34(2):489–509.

Gotthelf LN. Diagnosis and treatment of otitis media in dogs and cats. *Vet Clin North Am Small Anim Pract*, 2004; 34(2):469–487.

Hofer P, Meisen N, Bartholdi S, Kaser-Hotz B. A new radiographic view of the feline tympanic bullae. *Vet Radiol Ultrasound*, 1995; 36(1):14–15.

Hudson LC, Hamilton WP. Musculoskeletal system. In: Hudson LC, Hamilton WP (eds.). *Atlas of Feline Anatomy for Veterinarians*, 2nd ed. Jackson (WY): Teton Newmedia, 2010; pp. 23–78.

Hudson LC. Special sensory organs. In: Hudson LC, Hamilton WP (eds.). *Atlas of Feline Anatomy for Veterinarians*, 2nd ed. Jackson (WY): Teton Newmedia, 2010; pp. 231–242.

Indrieri RJ, Taylor RF. Vestibular dysfunction caused squamous cell carcinoma involving the middle ear and inner ear in two cats. *J Am Vet Med Assoc*, 1984; 184(4):471–473.

King AM, Weinrauch SA, Doust R et al. Comparison of ultrasonography, radiography and a single computed tomography slice for fluid identification within the feline tympanic bulla. *Vet J*, 2007; 173(3):638–644.

Lane IF, Hall DG. Adenocarcinoma of the middle ear with osteolysis of the tympanic bulla in a cat. *J Am Vet Med Assoc*, 1992; 201(3):463–465.

LeCoteur RA, Vernau KM. Feline vestibular disorders. Part I: anatomy and clinical signs. *J Feline Med Surg*, 1999; 1(2):71–80.

LeCoteur RA. Feline vestibular diseases-new developments. *J Feline Med Surg*, 2003; 5(2):101–108.

Little CJL, Lane JG. The surgical anatomy of the feline bulla tympanica. *J Small Anim Pract*, 1986; 27(6):371–378.

Negrin A, Cherubini GB, Lamb C et al. Clinical signs, magnetic resonance imaging findings and outcome in 77 cats with vestibular disease: a retrospective study. *J Feline Med Surg*, 2010; 12(4):291–299.

Ruberte J, Sautet J. *Atlas de anatomía del perro y del gato. Cabeza y cuello.* Sant Cugat del Vallès (Barcelona): Ed. Multimédica, 1995.

Schlicksup MD, Van Winkle TJ, Holt DE. Prevalence of clinical abnormalities in cats found to have nonneoplastic middle ear disease at necropsy: 59 cases (1991–2007). *J Am Vet Med Assoc*, 2009; 235(7):841–843.

Tobias KM, Morris D. The Ear. In: Brockman DJ, Holt DE (eds.). *BSAVA Manual of Canine and Feline Head, Neck and Toracic Surgery*, 1st ed. Gloucester: British Small Animal Veterinary Association, 2005; pp. 56–72.

Trevor PB, Martin RA. Tympanic bulla osteotomy for treatment of middle-ear disease in cats: 19 cases (1984–1991). *J Am Vet Med Assoc*, 1993; 202(1):123–128.

Vernau KM, LeCoteur RA. Feline vestibular disorders. Part II: diagnostic approach and differential diagnosis. *J Feline Med Surg*, 1999; 1(2):81–88.

Williams JM, White RAS. Total ear canal ablation combined with lateral bulla osteotomy in the cat. *J Small Anim Pract*, 1992; 33(5):225–227.

Woodbridge NT, Baines EA, Baines SJ. Otitis media in five cats associated with soft palate abnormalities. *Vet Rec*, 2012; 171(5):124.

THYROID AND PARATHYROID SURGERY 19

Alberto Barneto

Surgical anatomy

The feline **thyroid gland** is composed of two independent lobes, one on either side of the ventral aspect of the **tracheal cervical fascia**, immediately caudal to the larynx. In normal conditions each lobe is 1–2 cm long, 4–8 mm wide and 2 mm thick, and is located between the sternohyoid and sternothyroid muscles. The gland is not palpable externally. It has an oval shape and a cinnamon-like coloration. Each lobe is associated with two small **parathyroid glands**: the **external parathyroid gland** at the cranial pole, on the external thyroid capsule; and the **internal parathyroid gland**, which is usually embedded within the thyroid parenchyma and therefore not visible. They have a paler, whitish color. The location of the external parathyroid glands can vary: they are most commonly located at the cranial end, but can be situated along the thyroid lobe or even independent of it.

The blood supply to each thyroid lobe is provided by the **common carotid artery**, from which arises the **cranial thyroid artery**. The cranial thyroid artery supplies the thyroid lobe, from the cranial end, and emits a small branch towards the external parathyroid gland. Some cats also have a **caudal thyroid artery**, which helps supply the thyroid lobe from the posterior pole. The **cranial and caudal thyroid veins** flow into the **internal jugular vein**. Parallel to the carotid arteries and internal jugular veins are the **vagosympathetic trunks**; and on each side, adjacent to the tracheal fascia, the **recurrent laryngeal nerves**. All these structures must be well identified to avoid damaging them during surgery (Fig. 1).

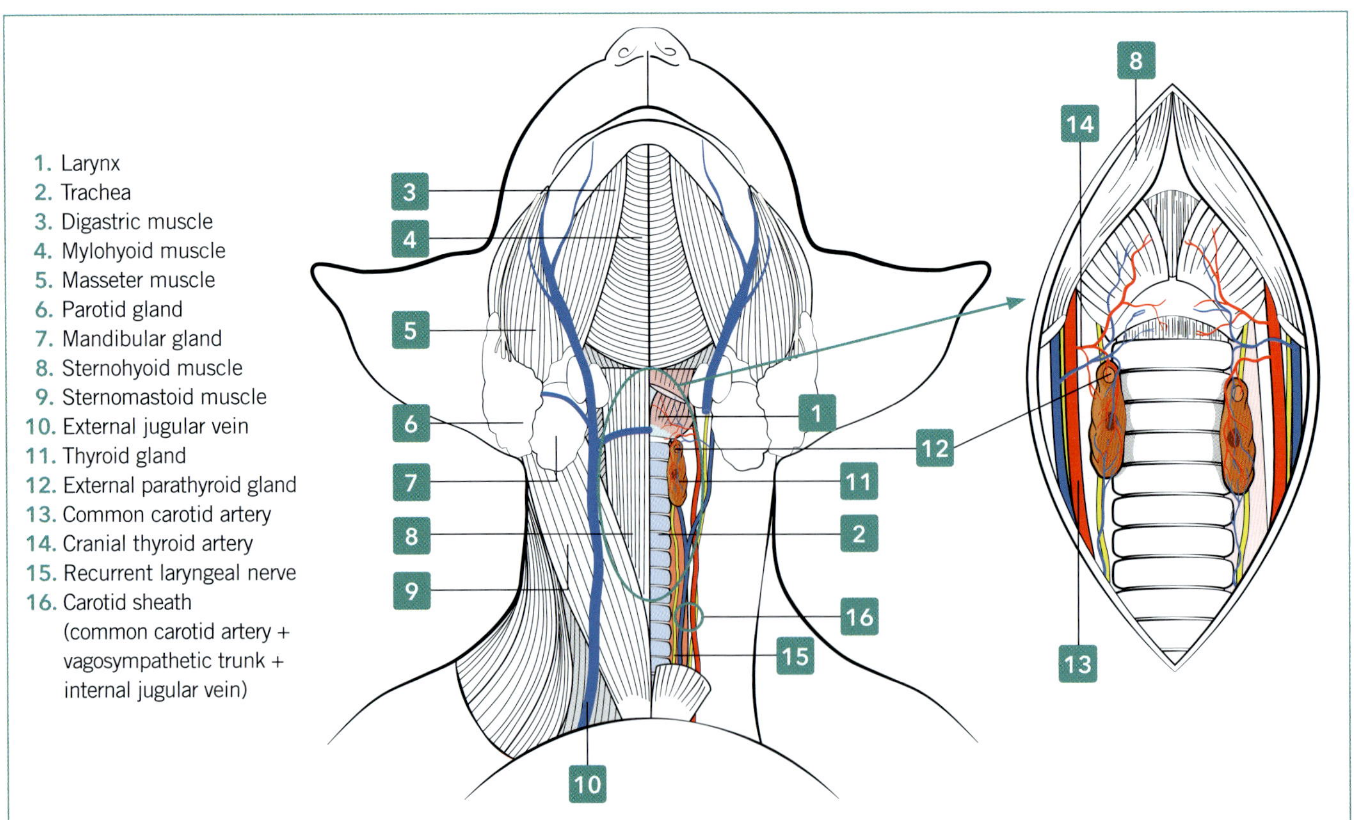

FIGURE 1. Anatomical relationships in the thyroid gland area.

Embryologically, the thyroid gland is derived from the endoderm of the first pharyngeal pouch. In some cats, migration of some of the thyroid tissue occurs during embryonic development, resulting in the presence of **ectopic thyroid tissue** in different locations along the trachea and thorax (approximately in 4% of hyperthyroid cats).

Surgical diseases of the thyroid gland

Feline hyperthyroidism is the thyroid disease that most commonly requires surgical treatment. It is a frequent condition in older cats (mean age at initial diagnosis, 12.5 years). It is usually caused by benign thyroid hormone–producing tumors in one or both gland lobes (**thyroid adenoma**). Unilateral disease occurs in less than a third of cases, while bilateral disease is much more common (>50% of feline hyperthyroidism cases). Only in a very small proportion of cases (1%–2%) are thyroid carcinomas diagnosed.

Diagnosis and the selection of the most appropriate treatment are based on clinical signs together with diagnostic test results (Table 1).

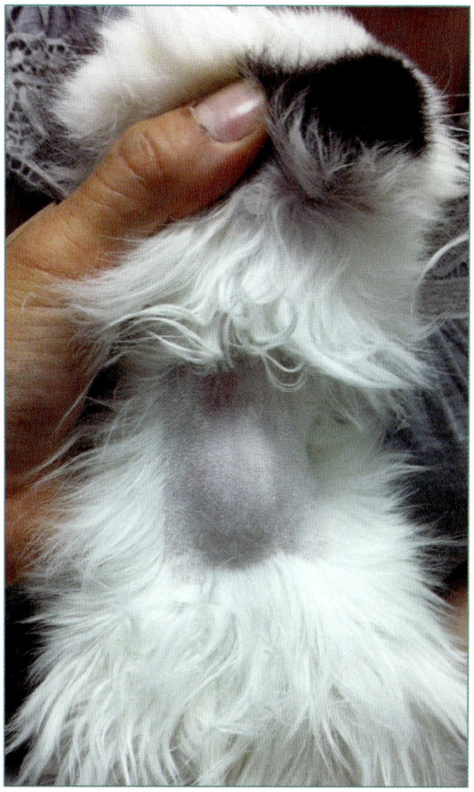

FIGURE 2. Correct positioning to detect a thyroid nodule in the cat. In this case, after shaving the hair, the bulk of the nodule is visible with the naked eye.

TABLE 1. Tests for the diagnosis and clinical evaluation of cats with hyperthyroidism

Diagnostic test	Results	Observations
Clinical signs	■ Weight loss, polyphagia, vomiting, polydipsia–polyuria syndrome, hyperactivity ■ Palpable nodule, thinness, heart murmur, tachycardia, poor haircoat condition ■ Systemic hypertension >160 mmHg	■ The relevant diagnostic tests are carried out based on the patient's clinical signs and age. ■ To detect a thyroid nodule, extend the patient's neck and palpate with the pads of the thumb and index finger along the trachea, both above and below (Fig. 2; see video). ■ It is important to **avoid stress** when handling these patients, as this can result in sudden worsening of their condition (**thyroid storm**).
Laboratory tests	■ Total thyroxine (TT_4) >4.5 μg/dl ■ TSH <0.03 ng/ml ■ High renal function parameters ■ Elevated ALT (alanine aminotransferase) levels	■ Most hyperthyroid cats have TT_4 levels above the reference interval (1–4.5 μg/dl). ■ In cases of subclinical hyperthyroidism TT_4 levels are normal and TSH levels decreased. ■ 25% of cats are azotemic, but nearly all have some degree of kidney disease. ■ More than 80% of hyperthyroid cats show elevated ALT.
Echocardiography	■ Hypertrophic cardiomyopathy ■ Anterior systolic movement (ASM) of the mitral valve	■ Hypertrophic cardiomyopathy is secondary to hypertension and the action of TT_4 on myocytes. ■ ASM produces a murmur and gallop on auscultation.
Ultrasound/CT scan	Increase in the size of one or both thyroid lobes (Figs. 3 and 4)	In unilateral cases, the other lobe will be atrophied. If it is normal in size, hyperthyroidism is considered bilateral.
Scintigraphy	Excessive radioactive iodine uptake by tumor thyroid tissue (Fig. 5)	If possible to perform, this is the most sensitive test to discriminate between unilateral and bilateral hyperthyroidism and to detect tumoral ectopic thyroid tissue (caudal cervical, thoracic).

VIDEO

Physical examination of the neck of a cat to detect a thyroid nodule. The atlantoaxial joint is extended, immobilizing the head to expose the entire throat. Gently slide the index finger and thumb up and down from the larynx to the thoracic inlet. If a nodule is present, it will "jump" when passing the fingers over it as described above.

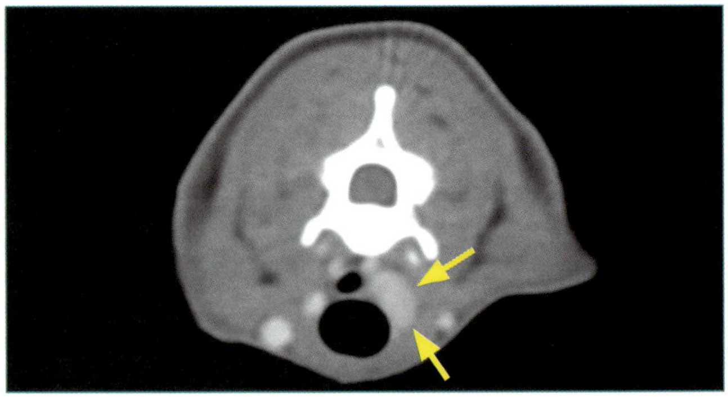

FIGURE 4. Computed tomography image showing a unilateral left thyroid adenoma (arrows). Image courtesy of Pedro Esteve, Diagnosfera.

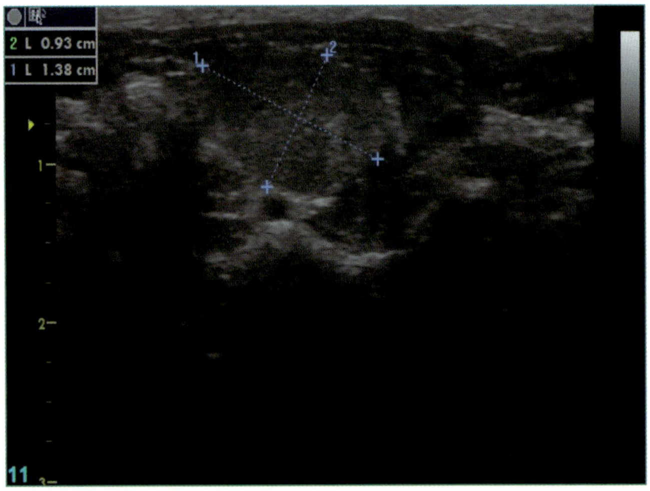

FIGURE 3. Transverse plane ultrasound image of the thyroid gland in a cat. The width is greatly increased in two measurements (0.9 and 1.4 cm), compatible with a thyroid adenoma (normal width, 0.2–0.25 cm). Image courtesy of Alejandro Casasús.

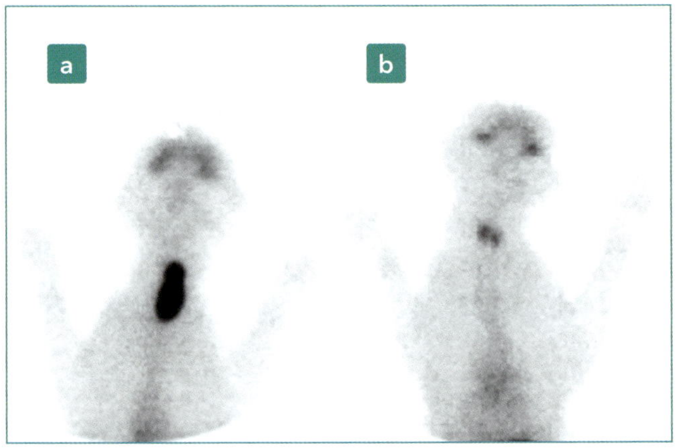

FIGURE 5. Scintigraphy of a cat (a) before and (b) after radioactive iodine treatment. The thyroid gland:salivary gland ratio, which was very high (reflecting hyperfunctionality of the adenoma), appears normalized (1.25; normal range, 0.5–1.5). This image confirms that the thyroid adenoma has been destroyed, leaving an appropriate accumulation of normal thyroid tissue. Image courtesy of Pilar Xifra, Iodocat.

Preoperative and postoperative considerations

If left untreated, hyperthyroidism ultimately leads to metabolic and cardiac deterioration, and consequent death of the patient. Although surgery is one of the most effective curative treatments for feline hyperthyroidism, there are several modalities currently used to treat this disease. While the use of iodine-free diets has become increasingly common in recent years, the results obtained are not very promising. Treatments based on thioamides (e.g., methimazole, carbimazole) are effective for medium-term control of the clinical signs of the disease. These are inexpensive treatments, but do not target the hormone-producing tumor, and therefore the disease progresses and typically recurs.

Currently, radioactive iodine–based treatment is considered the most effective cure for hyperthyroidism. Disadvantages of this treatment include high cost and a limited availability of the necessary equipment. The patient must be isolated in the hospital for 5–7 days after treatment to avoid radioactive contamination.

Thyroidectomy is an effective curative alternative for feline hyperthyroidism. Once the patient has been diagnosed, cardiac and metabolic function should be evaluated to establish the feasibility of performing anesthesia. Cats with advanced kidney disease or severe cardiomyopathy are not candidates for surgical treatment. Regardless, even hyperthyroid patients in a good health condition should start treatment with methimazole or carbimazole 2–3 weeks before the intervention until their TT_4 levels normalize. If they do not tolerate thioamide medication, a cardioselective beta-blocker (atenolol, 6.25–12.5 mg/cat every 24 hours) can be administered to control hypertension and tachycardia.

Once this objective has been achieved, blood pressure and kidney disease values must be reassessed.

> Adequate treatment of a hyperthyroid patient can often result in a **worsening of one stage** according to the IRIS (International Renal Interest Society) guidelines on the diagnosis and assessment of renal disease in small animals.

Potassium (K^+) levels are closely monitored and supplementation provided to normalize the concentration prior to surgery: one study found that approximately 30% of hyperthyroid cats were hypokalemic prior to surgery. Blood calcium levels should also be analyzed before and, above all, after the intervention in anticipation of possible surgical damage to the vascularization of the external parathyroid glands. This can happen more frequently in cases of bilateral thyroidectomy (see below).

During the intervention and in the immediate postoperative period, the patient is provided with a heat source, as these patients often have a low proportion of body fat. The cat should be hospitalized for 24–72 hours until complete recovery from anesthesia and normalization of potassium, calcium, and renal parameters are confirmed.

Thyroidectomy for the treatment of feline hyperthyroidism

Several surgical techniques for the removal of tumorous thyroid tissue have been described. The most frequently used is the **modified extracapsular technique**. Only in cases in which the size or distribution of the thyroid tumor prevents location of the parathyroid glands (especially the cranial gland, which is almost always clearly visible) is the **modified intracapsular technique** used.

In both cases, the same approach is used (Fig. 6).

- **Patient positioning:** the cat is placed in dorsal recumbency with the forelimbs fixed in a caudal direction. The head is extended as far as possible and secured with a band of adhesive tape into which both maxillary canines are embedded. The cervical region is raised a few centimeters by placing a rolled towel beneath the nape of the neck.
- **Surgical field:** the entire neck is shaved, from the base of the tongue to beyond the manubrium of the sternum.
- **Technique**
  1. An incision is made along the midline, from the larynx to about 2 cm before the manubrium of the sternum. The incision should be wide because the thyroid lobes, as they increase in size, can move caudally along the trachea. The fibers of the sphincter muscle of the neck are incised along the midline and the paired bellies of the sternocephalicus muscles are also separated along the midline

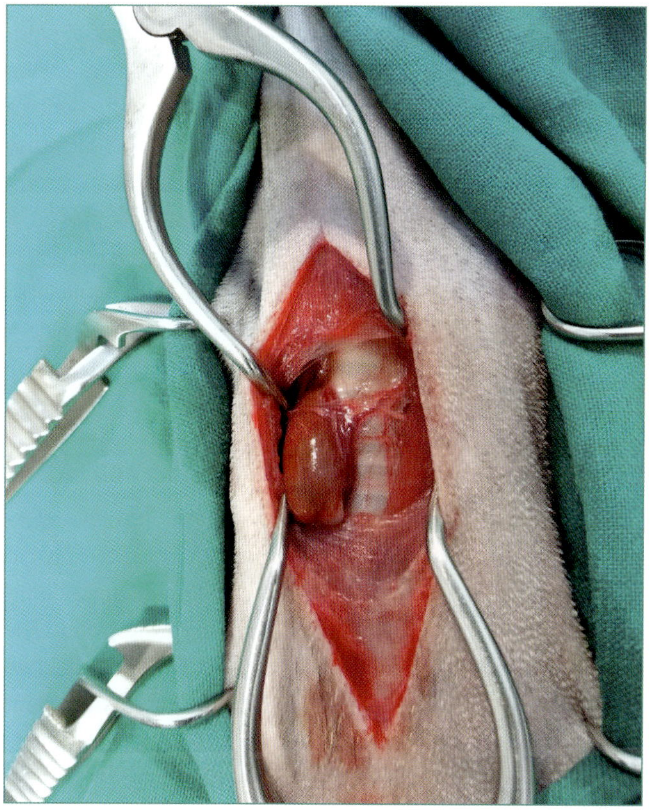

FIGURE 6. Appearance of a thyroid adenoma after dissection of the adjacent muscles and fasciae. The number of vessels is often increased and their anatomical distribution can vary slightly.

(they are joined from the middle of the neck, caudally). Below both structures are the sternohyoid muscles, which are paired and joined at the median raphe. A second incision is made above this raphe to expose the tracheal fascia and the entire surgical field in which we will work.

2. After dissection of the sternohyoid and sternothyroid muscles (immediately dorsolateral), both thyroid lobes and the surrounding structures are visible. It is useful to immobilize both muscles with Gelpi or Weitlaner self-retaining retractors to obtain a wide surgical field. The next, vitally important step is to **locate the recurrent laryngeal nerves** before beginning surgery: the **right nerve** is usually found within the peritracheal fascia, lateral to the trachea and dorsomedial to the sternothyroid muscle; the **left nerve** is located between the dorsolateral aspect of the trachea and the ventral aspect of the esophagus. It is not uncommon for these nerves to be displaced from their anatomical location by the thyroid tumor. The carotid sheath can be found on the dorsal side of the peritracheal groove (carotid artery + vagosympathetic trunk + internal jugular vein). The next structures that we must locate are the external parathyroid glands, especially if we are to perform a bilateral thyroidectomy. If they are well located and easy to dissect while respecting their vascularization, modified extracapsular thyroidectomy will be the technique of choice. Conversely, if the parathyroid glands are not visible or the parathyroid vascularization is not distinguishable from the thyroid one, modified intracapsular thyroidectomy is advisable.
3. **Modified extracapsular thyroidectomy** (Fig. 7) is the most commonly used technique. First, it is necessary to locate the external parathyroid gland (the easiest of the two to locate) and its associated vasculature, if the thyroidectomy will be bilateral. An incision is made in the thyroid capsule around the parathyroid gland, creating a circular cut of about 300° about 2 mm from the gland. The remaining 60° coincides with the thyroid capsule attached to the parathyroid vessels. This way, a **parathyroid peninsula** is created in the thyroid capsule. The cut is made using a no. 11 scalpel blade or needle cautery electrode. The approach should always involve the use of a toothless Bishop-Harmon microsurgery forceps or Adson forceps to minimize trauma. Surgical loupes (×2.5) can be very helpful. To dissect the adenomatous thyroid tissue from the portion of the incised capsule, sterile swabs moistened with saline solution are used (Figs. 8–10).
4. Once the entire peninsula has been dissected, the cranial thyroid artery is located and ligated with 5-0 absorbable monofilament suture material. Ligation is performed about 5 mm from the parathyroid branches, respecting their connection with the common carotid artery. The entire thyroid gland and its capsule are dissected from the tracheal fascia, the caudal thyroid vessels (vein and artery, if present) ligated, and the tumor removed.
5. **Modified intracapsular thyroidectomy** (Fig. 11): this is the alternative technique used in cases in which neither of the parathyroid glands can be located within the tumor gland, or when the vascularization is not clearly differentiated. This method requires more time and much more precise handling of the tissues, and is associated with a greater likelihood of recurrence, since it is easy to leave remnants of adenomatous thyroid tissue after dissection. The technique begins by longitudinally incising the thyroid capsule along its ventral aspect. Next, ×2.5 loupes are used and the tissues handled atraumatically using toothless DeBakey or Adson forceps. The thyroid tissue is dissected from the capsule using blunt dissection (Stevens tenotomy scissors are the author's preference) and saline-moistened swabs. This dissected parenchyma will include the internal parathyroid gland. Once the entire capsule has been dissected, the intervention can be completed. However, it is worth examining whether, by removing the tumor, the cranial thyroid artery can be better visualized. If so, it can be ligated with 5-0 absorbable monofilament suture material, always respecting the integrity of the arterial branches of the external parathyroid gland. In this way we can continue with the modification of this technique and remove most of the empty thyroid capsule, leaving only an islet around the parathyroid gland. This modification of the intracapsular thyroidectomy minimizes the possibility of leaving remnants of adenoma and subsequent disease recurrence.
6. The incision is closed by apposition of the tissue planes of the sternohyoid and sternocephalic muscles using 3-0 absorbable suture material and subsequent intradermal suturing of the skin wound.

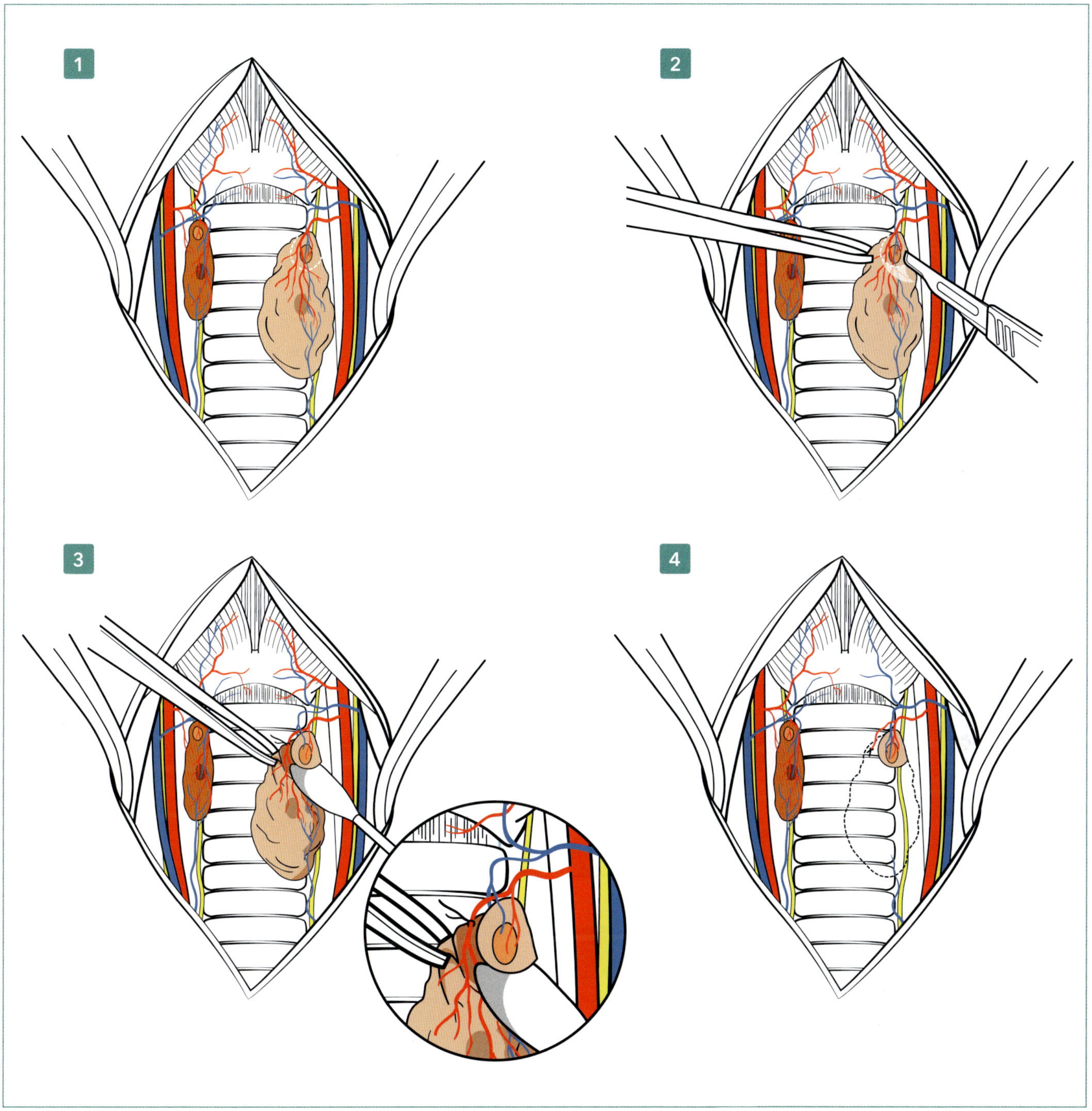

FIGURE 7. Technique for modified extracapsular thyroidectomy.

1. After locating the external parathyroid gland and its vascularization, the thyroid capsule is incised around the parathyroid gland, making a 300° circular incision 2 mm away from the gland, sparing the parathyroid vessels. This creates a parathyroid peninsula in the thyroid capsule.
2. The incision is made using a no. 11 scalpel blade or needle cautery electrode. Tissue handling must be atraumatic, assisted with the use of ×2.5 surgical loupes.
3. The adenomatous thyroid tissue of the incised portion of the capsule is dissected using sterile swabs moistened with saline solution. Once the entire peninsula has been dissected, the cranial thyroid artery is ligated about 5 mm from the parathyroid branches, respecting their connection with the common carotid artery.
4. The entire thyroid gland and its capsule are dissected from the tracheal fascia, the caudal thyroid vessels (if present) are ligated, and the tumor is removed.

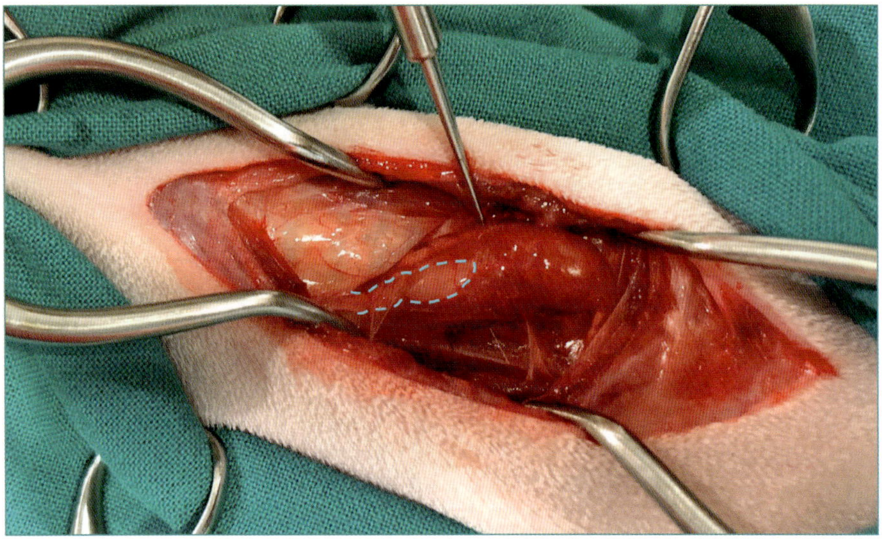

FIGURE 8. Start of the modified extracapsular thyroidectomy technique: the dashed blue line indicates the location of the parathyroid peninsula.

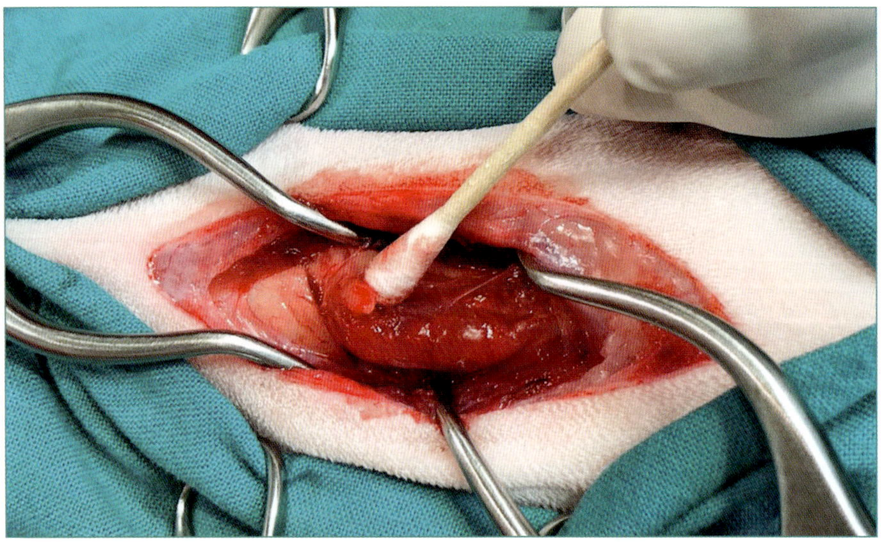

FIGURE 9. Once a semicircular incision of about 300° around the parathyroid gland has been created, respecting the associated vascularization, the adjacent thyroid tissue is dissected, in this case using a sterile swab.

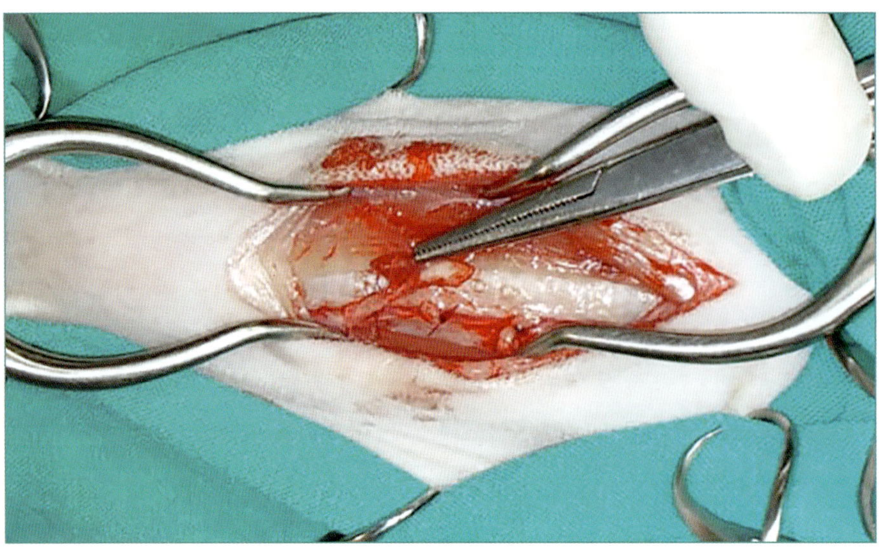

FIGURE 10. Once the technique is finished, the cranial thyroid artery and the caudal thyroid artery (if present) will have been ligated, the thyroid gland dissected together with its capsule, and gland and capsule extracted. The image shows how the parathyroid gland is attached by its artery to the common carotid artery.

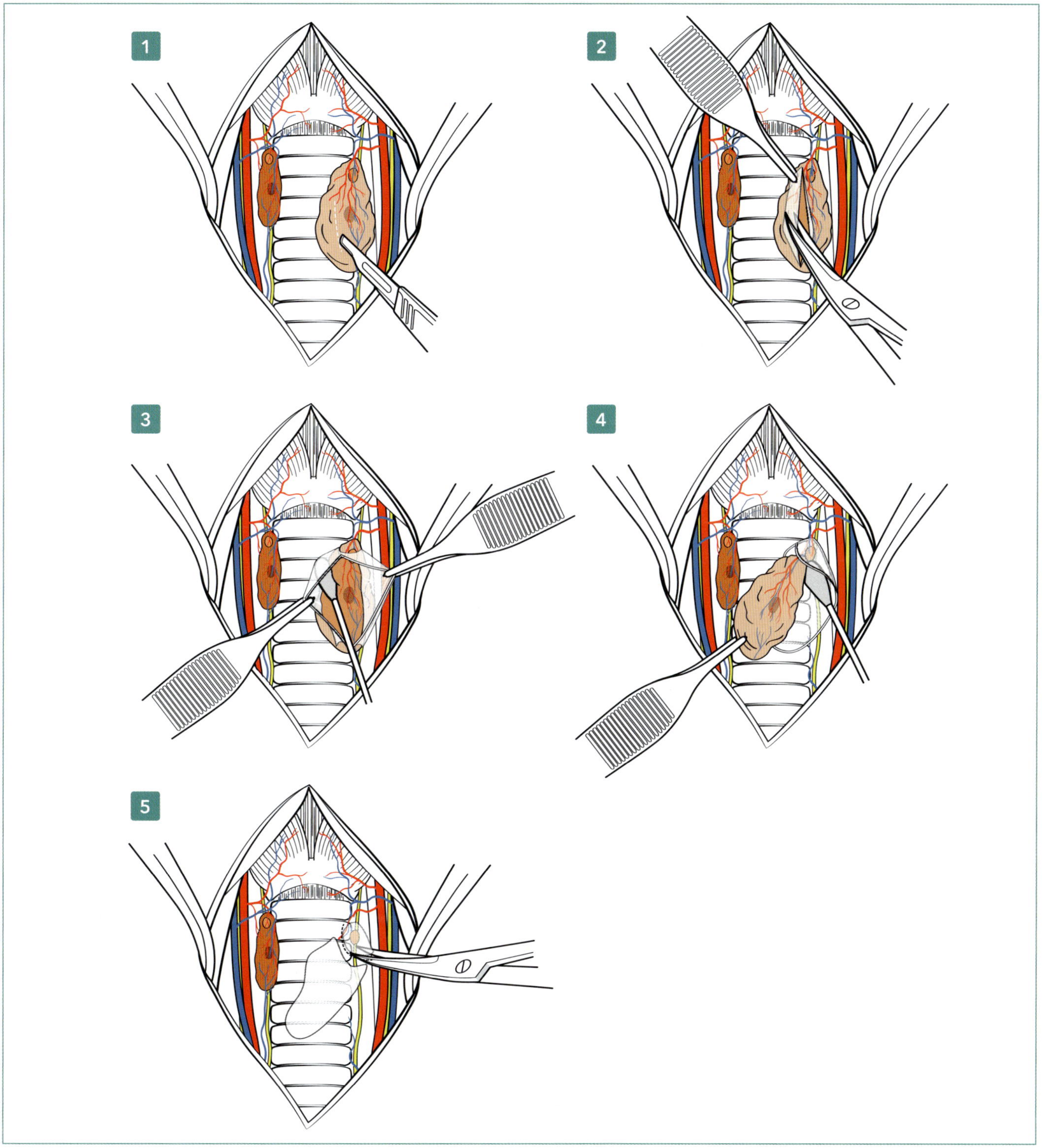

FIGURE 11. Technique for modified intracapsular thyroidectomy.

1. The thyroid capsule is incised longitudinally along its ventral aspect.
2. Using an atraumatic approach, with the aid of ×2.5 surgical loupes, the thyroid tissue is dissected from the capsule by blunt dissection (Stevens tenotomy scissors).
3. For dissection, swabs moistened with saline can also be used. The dissected parenchyma will include the internal parathyroid gland.
4. Once the entire capsule has been dissected, it is advisable to examine whether the cranial thyroid artery can be better visualized after removing the tumor. If so, the artery is ligated respecting the integrity of the arterial branches of the external parathyroid gland.
5. This way, most of the empty thyroid capsule can be removed, leaving only an islet around the parathyroid gland.

Complications

The most common complication is hypocalcemia, especially in cases of bilateral thyroidectomy in which the vascularization of the external parathyroid glands has been damaged. This happens 2–5 days after the intervention, and is characterized by muscle spasms, facial itching, panting, and seizures. It should be treated with intravenous 10% calcium gluconate (0.25–1.5 ml/kg administered slowly over 10–20 minutes until effect is observed). The calcium concentration should be subsequently assessed and treatment with oral calcium and vitamin D continued until, several weeks later, the parathyroid tissue revascularizes and its function is restored.

Cases of postsurgical laryngeal paralysis have been described, either due to careless dissection of the thyroid gland or incorrect placement of the retractors. Only in severe cases is lateralization of the arytenoid cartilage necessary.

Hyperthyroidism recurrence is described in 5%–10% of patients, even in cases of bilateral thyroidectomy. Possible causes include the presence of undetected ectopic thyroid tissue or remnants of thyroid tissue due to the resection technique used (more frequent in cases of intracapsular thyroidectomy). In these cases, radioactive iodine therapy should be considered.

Hypothyroidism is a rare complication, even in cases of bilateral thyroidectomy. If it does occur, it is usually transient and does not require thyroxine supplementation in the medium term.

Bibliography

Birchard SJ. Thyroidectomy in dogs and cats. In: Bojrab MJ (ed.). *Current Techniques in Small Animal Surgery*, 4th ed. Baltimore: Williams & Wilkins, 1998; pp. 498–503.

Birchard SJ. Thyroidectomy in the cat. *Clin Tech Small Anim Pract*, 2006; 21(1):29–33.

Borgatti Jeffreys A, Waters DJ. Chapter 6 Endocrine System. In: Hudson LC, Hamilton WP (eds.). *Atlas of Feline Anatomy for Veterinarians*, 2nd ed. Jackson (WY): Teton Newmedia, 2010; pp. 129–136.

Flanders JA. Hyperthyroidism treatment: surgical thyroidectomy. In: Feldman EC, Fracassi F, Peterson ME (eds.). *Feline Endocrinology*, 1st ed. Milano: Edra, 2019; pp. 211–226.

Flanders JA. Surgical options for the treatment of hyperthyroidism in the cat. *J Feline Med Surg*, 1999; 1(3):127–134.

Harvey AM, Hibbert A, Barrett EL et al. Scintigraphic findings in 120 hyperthyroid cats. *J Feline Med Surg*, 2009; 11(2):96–106.

Kikumori T, Imai T, Tanaka Y et al. Parathyroid autotransplantation with total thyroidectomy for thyroid carcinoma: long-term follow-up of grafted parathyroid function. *Surgery*, 1999; 125(5):504–508.

Naan EC, Kirpensteijn J, Kooistra HS, Peeters ME. Results of thyroidectomy in 101 cats with hyperthyroidism. *Vet Surg*, 2006; 35(3):287–293.

Padgett S. Feline thyroid surgery. *Vet Clin North Am Small Anim Pract*, 2002; 32(4):851–859.

Padgett SL, Tobias KM, Leathers CW, Wardrop KJ. Efficacy of parathyroid gland autotransplantation in maintaining serum calcium concentrations after bilateral thyroparathyroidectomy in cats. *J Am Anim Hosp Assoc*, 1998; 34(3):219–224.

Radlinsky MG. Thyroid surgery in dogs and cats. *Vet Clin North Am Small Anim Pract*, 2007; 37(4):789–798.

Trepanier LA. Pharmacologic management in feline hyperthyroidism. *Vet Clin North Am Small Anim Pract*, 2007; 37(4):775–788.

Wisner ER, Nyland TG. Ultrasonography of the thyroid and parathyroid glands. *Vet Clin North Am Small Anim Pract*, 1998; 28(4):973–991.

4

ABDOMINAL SURGERY

FELINE ABDOMINAL CAVITY. HERNIAS 20

Alberto Barneto and Llibertat Real

Introduction

The **abdomen** is the cavity between a cat's **thorax** and its **pelvis**. Its interior is lined by the **peritoneum**, a serous membrane that itself forms a parallel cavity. It is composed of a layer of flat mesothelial cells over a basement membrane. The mesothelial cells of the peritoneum produce a surfactant that acts as a lubricant and facilitates mobility of the abdominal contents. The basement membrane is made up of fibroelastic tissue that contains macrophages, mast cells, lymphocytes and glycosylated proteins over a network of elastic fibers. This membrane is not present in diaphragm, omentum and mesentery areas, leading to spaces between the mesothelial cells. These mesothelial cells are in direct contact with lymphatic channels, which absorb fluids and material, especially in the diaphragm.

The peritoneum is divided into:

- **Parietal peritoneum:** covers the abdominal wall and the diaphragm.
- **Visceral peritoneum:** contains the stomach, liver, intestines, spleen, uterus and ovaries (in females), part of the bladder, as well as numerous lymph nodes and a complex network of blood vessels, lymph vessels and nerves.

Also found in the abdomen is the **retroperitoneal space**, which contains the organs that rest on the abdominal wall or the pelvic cavity and which are only covered by peritoneum on one surface. These are the kidneys, ureters, adrenal glands, the aorta and its major branches, most of the vena cava, the sublumbar lymph nodes (external and internal iliac node and coccygeal node), prostate (in males), most of the rectum, the urethra, the vagina (in females) and variable parts of the bladder.

Highly important for the surgeon, the abdomen also contains the **epiploon or omentum**, a mesenteric structure that lies between the stomach and the intestines (Fig. 1). It is composed of:

- **Greater omentum:** comprises the visceral and parietal layers. Each of these layers, in turn, is composed of two peritoneal sheets. Between these sheets is a complex network of blood and lymphatic vessels surrounded by adipose tissue, giving them a mesh-like appearance. The visceral layer of the greater omentum originates with the transverse mesocolon from the dorsal abdominal wall and extends caudally, covering the ventrolateral aspect of the small intestine. At the pelvic inlet, it folds back on itself to form the parietal layer of the greater omentum, which is adjacent to the ventrolateral abdominal wall, continues cranially and inserts on the greater curvature of the stomach. The potential space between the visceral and parietal layers of the omentum is called the omental bursa. The left lobe of the pancreas is found between the sheets of the visceral layer of the greater omentum, adjacent to the dorsal aspect of the stomach, and the spleen is found between the sheets of the parietal layer of the greater omentum.
- **Lesser omentum:** the stomach is located between the two layers of the greater omentum, which converge at the lesser curvature of the stomach to form the lesser omentum.

The crucial function of the omentum is to protect the cavity from infection and inflammation. It also encourages healing since it promotes angiogenesis, improves immune function and acts to drain the accumulation of fluid in the tissues. It helps isolate and seal the source of an infection by forming omental adhesions. Present on it are aggregates of cells known as milky spots, which are a source of neutrophils, macrophages and lymphocytes. These milky spots are an important component of this protective function. In medical practice, the omentum is used autologously for wound drainage (e.g., abscesses in the abdominal cavity), as an adjuvant for healing around sutures in enterotomies, and even for drainage in flaps outside the abdominal cavity. The only limitation of these uses is that the availability of omentum depends on its distance from the wound.

Another organ located in the abdominal cavity is the **mesentery**. All the abdominal digestive organs lie on or in it. It consists of a set of tissues that maintain the digestive organs in their place, seamlessly arranged among other systems found in the

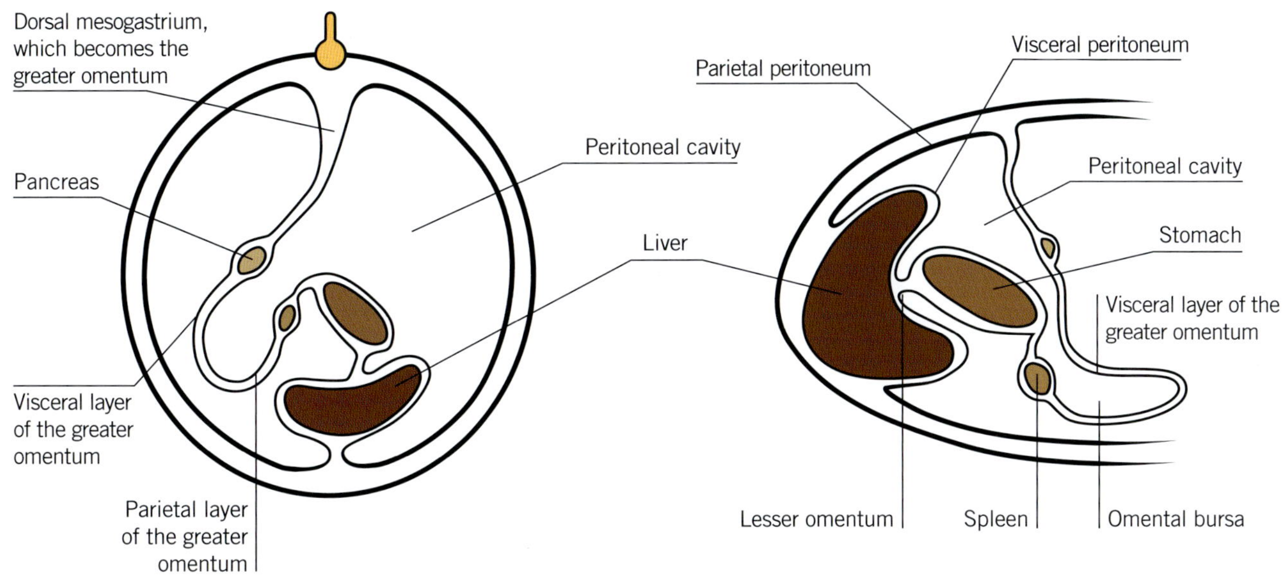

FIGURE 1. Relationship between the peritoneum and some structures of the abdominal cavity over the course of development.

abdomen. It continues uninterrupted from the esophagogastric junction to the anorectal junction. Its function is protective, activating an immune response when faced with bacterial translocation. More and more importance is being attributed to it in human medicine due to this immune response. Changes in its immune regulation is closely associated with Crohn's disease.

From a surgical perspective, detailed knowledge of all the structures of the abdominal cavity is very important, given that we may have to access it for a wide range of reasons using various approaches.

Anatomy of the abdominal cavity

The **vertebral column** and the **psoas muscles** (group of sublumbar muscles) form the dorsal boundary of the abdominal cavity. The **diaphragm** makes up the cranial boundary, the **abdominal walls** make up the lateral and ventral sides, and the pelvis constitutes its caudal wall.

The **diaphragm** (Fig. 2) projects over the abdominal cavity in the shape of a dome. It is made up of an **external muscular part**, which, in contrast to the abdominal wall, is only composed of one layer (which makes it weaker). This muscular portion of the diaphragm consists of a lumbar part, a costal part on each side, and a sternal part (attached to the sternum). The lumbar part, in turn, is composed of the right and left **diaphragmatic crura**, the right crus being larger than the left. The costal and sternal parts measure 2–3 mm in thickness, while the medial zone of the lumbar part measures 3–4 mm. Viewed from the abdominal cavity, the diaphragmatic crura are in the shape of two triangles. Fibers radiate from the muscular part of the diaphragm (lumbar and costal) towards the **central tendon**, which is relatively small in cats. The costal part of the diaphragm is attached to the internal surface of the last ribs, and the dome of the diaphragm originates in the caudal region of the thoracic cavity. There are three natural openings:

- **The esophageal hiatus**, through which the esophagus, vagal trunks, and esophageal vessels pass.
- **The caval hiatus**, through which the caudal vena cava passes.
- **The aortic hiatus**, through which the aorta, the thoracic duct, and the azygos and hemiazygos veins pass.

Dorsal to the diaphragm and ventral to the psoas muscles are also two linear openings on each side. Only a fascia separates thorax from abdomen in these openings. The splanchnic nerves and the sympathetic trunks enter the abdominal cavity through them. In this area, conditions affecting one cavity can pass into the other, without there being any tears in the diaphragm. Ligaments connect the stomach and the liver to the peritoneum, which covers the abdominal aspect of the diaphragm.

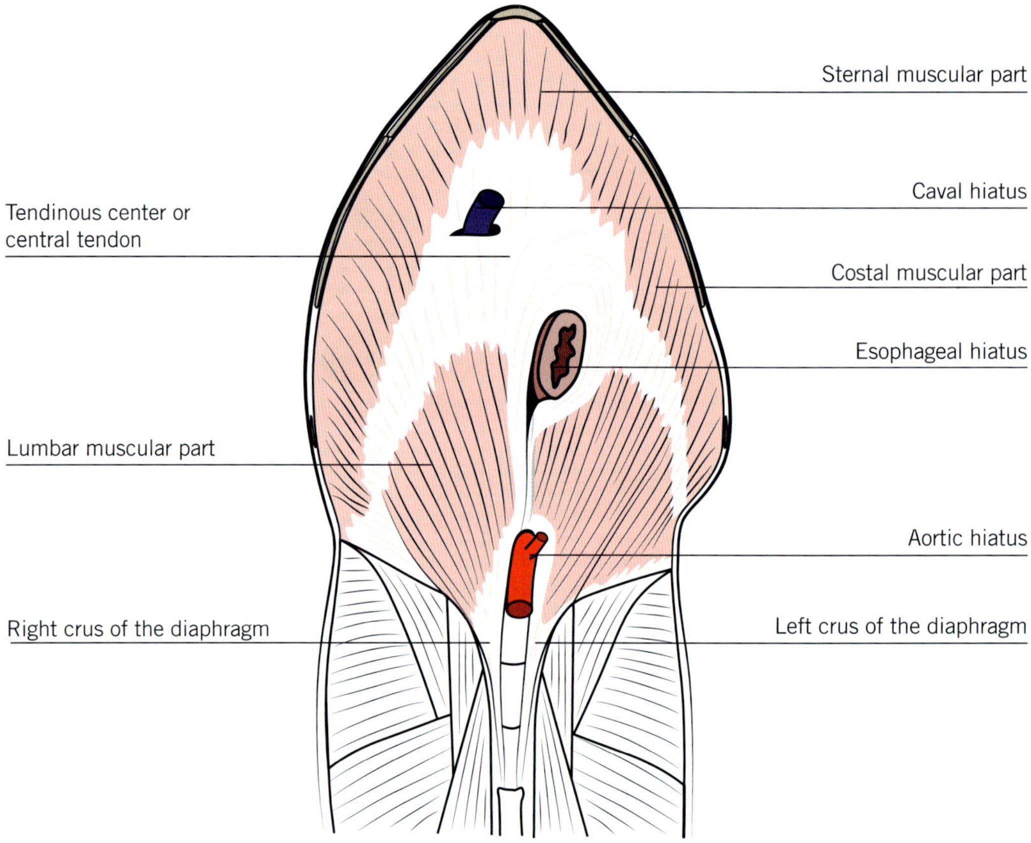

FIGURE 2. Structure of the diaphragm.

The **abdominal walls** delimit the abdominal cavity laterally and ventrally. They support most of the weight of the viscera. They are composed of the abdominal muscles, which are arranged in three layers superimposed upon each other and with their muscle fibers in contrasting orientation (Fig. 3):

- The **external oblique muscle** (fibers in a caudoventral direction) also covers a significant portion of the costal arch.
- The **internal oblique muscle** (fibers in a cranioventral direction) originates mainly in the coxal tuberosity and its caudal margin is free.
- The **transverse abdominal muscle** (fibers in a dorsoventral direction) originates on the internal surface of the last ribs and the transverse processes of the lumbar vertebrae.
- The **rectus abdominis muscle** (fibers in a craniocaudal direction) also covers the caudal portion of the sternum and its associated costal cartilage.

The attachment of the aponeuroses of the abdominal muscles at the ventral midline gives rise to the **linea alba**, which is also associated with the umbilicus, although this is often difficult to see in cats. It is a 3–4 mm wide fibrous and avascular tissue. It is excessively wide in some cats due to a birth defect. The rectus abdominis muscle is situated on either side of the linea alba. It extends from the xiphoid process to the pubis.

Adjacent to the groin in both males and females, the caudoventral abdominal wall presents two discontinuous zones: the **deep and superficial inguinal rings**. A vaginal process or ring has not been found in female cats, although there is one in female dogs. The tunica vaginalis, testicles (in males), external pudendal vessels, genitofemoral nerve, and adipose tissue pass through the inguinal rings:

- The **deep inguinal ring** is formed medially by the rectus abdominis muscle, cranially by the caudal margin of the internal oblique muscle, and caudally by the inguinal ligament. The latter runs from the coxal tuberosity to the pubis, is triangular in shape, and is made up of connective tissue.
- The **superficial inguinal ring** is an elliptical opening in the caudal aponeurosis of the external oblique muscle.

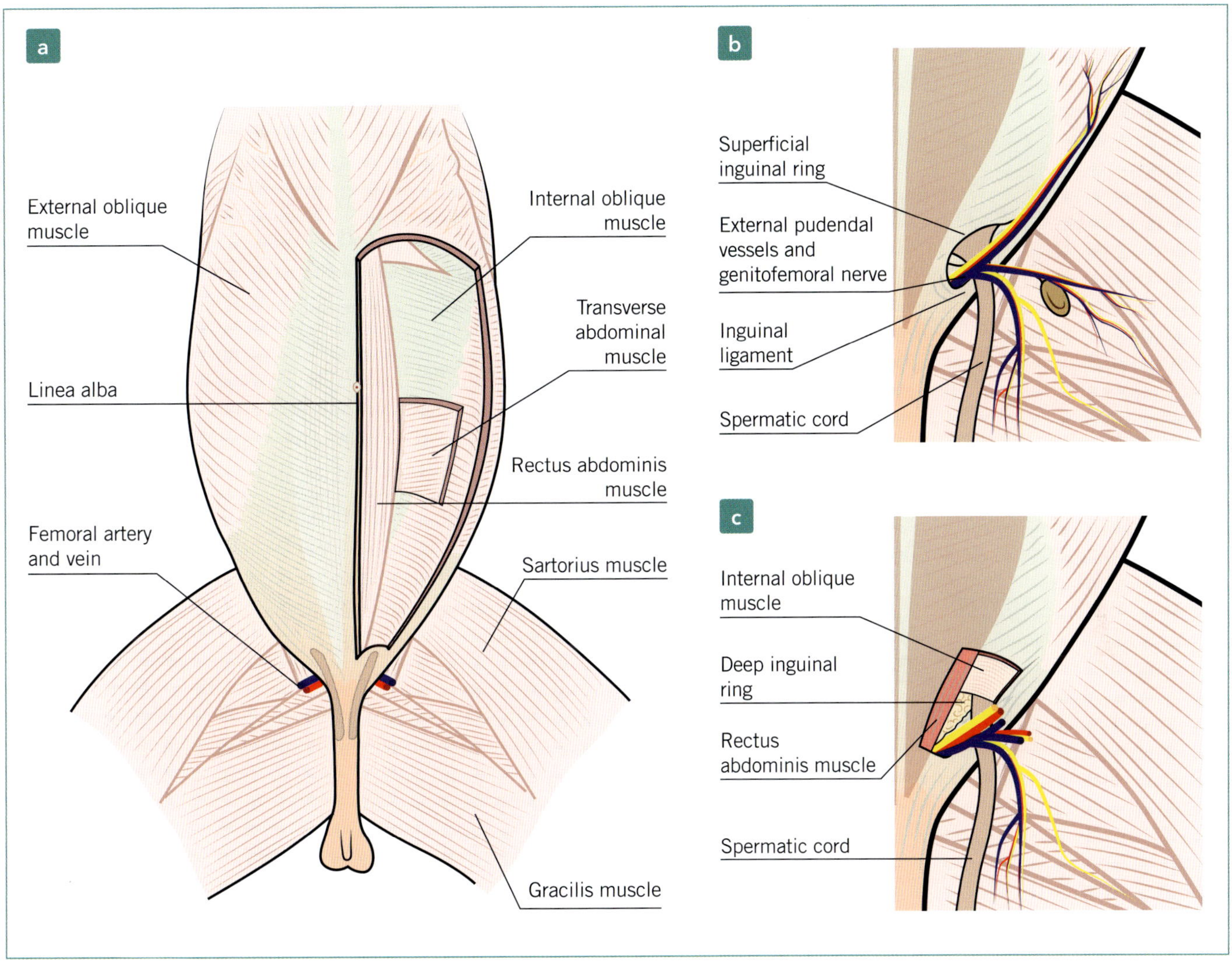

FIGURE 3. (a) Structures that make up the abdominal walls in cats. (b) Superficial inguinal ring. (c) Deep inguinal ring.

Surgical diseases of the abdomen

Exploratory laparotomy

This is not a disease per se, but a surgical technique for the diagnosis and treatment of different pathologies inside the abdominal cavity.

The definitive diagnostic test that will help us decide whether to perform an exploratory laparotomy is an ultrasound. The patient's medical history, a physical examination and laboratory tests will also support our diagnosis. We can perform ultrasounds at regularly scheduled intervals if we suspect cats may have an abdominal neoplasm (Fig. 4), chronic digestive conditions, or kidney conditions that require a biopsy for accurate diagnosis, or we can perform an emergency ultrasound. In the latter case, we can observe the sudden onset of clinical signs associated with the abdominal cavity, such as vomiting, pain on palpation, abdominal rigidity, etc. These signs may or may not be caused by trauma.

An exploratory laparotomy should be performed when there is a suspected digestive perforation, a tear in the urinary or genital tract, pyometra, bacterial peritonitis (or peritonitis for which there is no explanation), or puncture wounds in the abdomen, among many other reasons. It is not always an easy decision to anesthetize a very sick cat for a surgical intervention, but the presence of free abdominal fluid compatible with urine or bile, a cytology indicative of infection of the cavity, or bleeding for which we have no explanation are indications for a laparotomy. For those cats with non-specific abdominal clinical signs that decompensate quickly and progressively, despite having been medically stabilized,

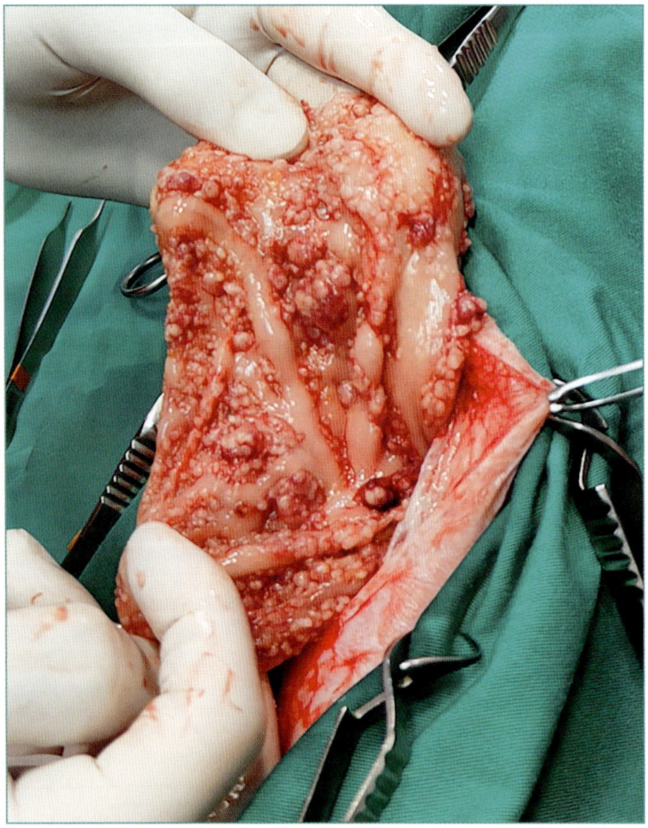

FIGURE 4. Mesenteric carcinoma in a female cat.

exploratory laparotomy is indicated, even if laboratory and imaging tests are not completely conclusive.

Surgical technique

- **Patient positioning:** dorsal recumbency.
- **Surgical field:** the abdomen is explored via a ventral incision. The length of this incision may vary, depending on the underlying disease. If the entire abdominal cavity must be explored, it may originate as far as the xiphoid process and end as far as the pubis. When we perform an emergency celiotomy due to an acute condition, we should surgically prepare the caudal thoracic region and the inguinal region, in addition to the entire abdominal surface. It may be necessary to examine the thorax or pelvic cavity.
- **Technique**
  1. An incision is made in the skin of the ventral midline; the incision length depends on the intervention, as explained above. The incision is continued through the subcutaneous tissues until reaching the rectus abdominis muscle fascia. The linea alba is identified. Any subcutaneous vessels that bleed excessively may be ligated if necessary.
  2. An assistant applies traction to the muscular fascia in an upward direction with baby Allis forceps, forming a tent so the surgeon can make an incision with the scalpel in the linea alba. Any adhesions to the abdominal wall are checked for. Using baby Metzenbaum scissors, the incision is widened cranially and caudally until reaching the edges of the cutaneous incision.
  3. Two surgical maneuvers used during abdominal exploration to help visualize and work in areas of difficult access are as follows:
     - **Duodenal maneuver:** used to visualize the right kidney and its vascularization. Consists of using the mesoduodenum as a natural retractor to contain the intestines and stomach. After locating the duodenum, it is lifted, along with its mesentery, from its position in the right epigastrium, upwards and to the left, taking care not to injure the right pancreatic lobe (Fig. 5).
     - **Colonic maneuver:** in this case the mesentery of the descending colon is used as a retractor (and sometimes the spleen can be included) to be able to visualize the left retroperitoneal space and all of the sublumbar canal (left ureter and kidney with all their vascularization and retroperitoneal lymph nodes) (Fig. 6).
  4. We should note that if a lavage of the abdominal cavity is needed after the surgery (severe ascites, surgical contamination, excessive bleeding), all of the fluid must be removed with gauze dressings or with a surgical aspirator. This prevents disruption of neutrophil activity due to dilution. The solution used for lavage should always be warm and preferably buffered.
  5. Once the intervention or examination is complete, the incision is closed with a simple continuous suture (an interrupted pattern is also possible) using 3-0 or 2-0 absorbable monofilament or absorbable braided (slow-absorbing polyglactin 910). The needle is suitably anchored in the rectus abdominis muscle fascia and the full thickness of the rectus abdominis muscle is taken to prevent or minimize the risk of dehiscence. The suture should be made tight without strangling the muscle. The stitches are made at 3–4 mm intervals and 4 knots are made at each end. If the incision is paramedial, only the rectus abdominis muscle fascia is taken, avoiding the peritoneum or muscle fibers. Next, an inverting Lembert suture (or inverting Cushing suture) is applied with the same material and method. Finally, whenever possible the skin is closed with

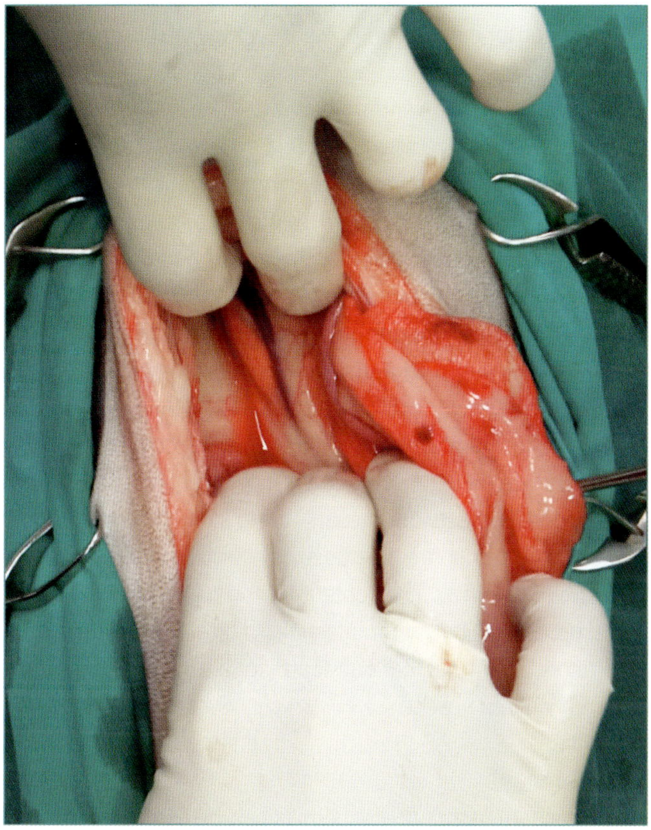

FIGURE 5. Duodenal maneuver.

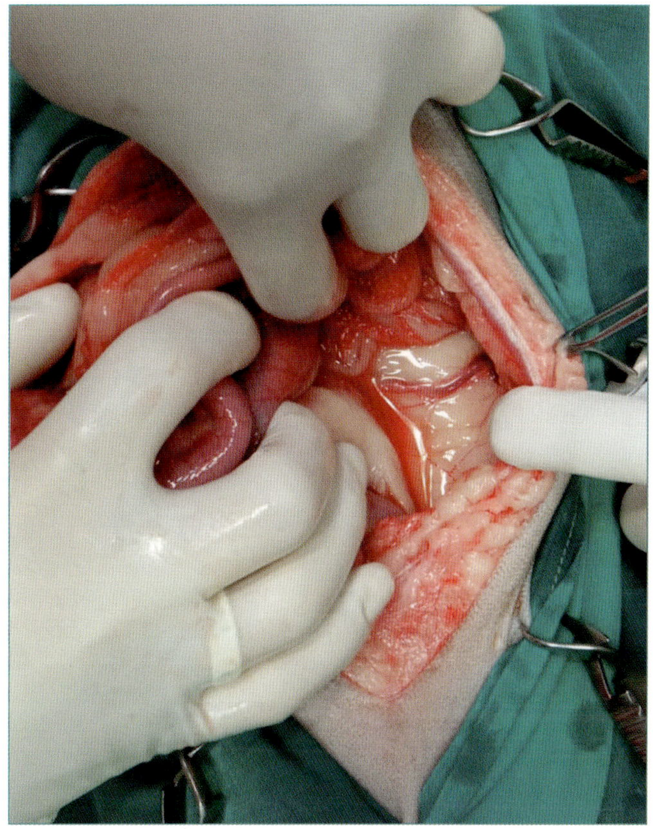

FIGURE 6. Colonic maneuver.

an intradermal suture using 3-0 absorbable monofilament to facilitate postoperative recovery and avoid the need for an Elizabethan collar, which is very stressful for cats. For very large incisions, a continuous or interrupted suture with 3-0 nonabsorbable material is required.

Key point: each stitch to close the abdominal cavity should include the muscular fascia of the abdominal wall. Only this way do we avoid dehiscence during postoperative recovery.

Postoperative complications

Issues that can arise after a laparotomy are:

- Suture dehiscence: associated with an inadequate preoperative assessment of the patient, severe immunosuppression, poor suture technique, or a postoperative infection.
- Accidental incision of the spleen or bladder due to excessive pressure or incorrect technique when accessing the abdominal cavity.
- Retained gauze in the abdominal cavity (especially small pieces) due to not accounting for the number of gauze pads at the beginning of the surgery.
- Intra-abdominal bleeding after invasive techniques performed on viscera, such as biopsies.

Hernias in the abdominal cavity

A **hernia** is the partial or complete protrusion of an organ through a defect in the wall of an anatomical cavity where it is normally situated.

Depending on the origin of the issue, hernias can be:

- **Congenital:** the defect in the wall originates in a malformation of muscle or connective tissue.
- **Acquired:** the defect is caused by a tear of a natural orifice or the wall structure itself. In this case, the origin is usually traumatic. In cats, this is often caused by falls from heights, vehicle accidents, or animal bites. Clinical signs can appear several days or even weeks after the accident.

The **hernial ring or defect** is the opening through which the herniated organ or material passes. The hernial sac is usually made up of a fine pouch of serosa that surrounds the contents of the hernia (e.g., in the abdomen, it would be the peritoneum). There may be additional layers of tissue in the hernial sac (muscle, subcutaneous tissue, skin) depending on the location of the hernia.

The clinical presentation of hernias varies depending on the contents of the hernial sac:

- **Reducible hernia:** there are no adhesions between the contents and adjacent structures, allowing them to easily be returned to their original cavity.
- **Irreducible hernia**: repositioning is not easy due to adhesions, and breaking them is required.
- **Incarcerated hernia:** when structural adhesions between the herniated organ tissue and surrounding tissue come to alter the functionality of the herniated organ. Tends to involve chronicity and may impact the decision on whether or not surgical reduction is desirable.
- **Strangulated hernia:** vascular supply of the contents inside the hernia is compromised by torsion, compression or narrowing of the hernial ring. Usually results in an emergency situation both if we want to recover functionality of the affected organ and because it could put the animal's life in danger.

It is important to note that traumatic hernias in cats are caused by falls from heights, vehicle accidents, or dog bites. Clinical signs can sometimes appear days or weeks after the accident.

Peritoneal-diaphragmatic hernias

Any defect in the diaphragm muscle, whether congenital or acquired (traumatic), can cause one or several abdominal organs to pass into the thoracic cavity, resulting in the lungs, the heart, or both, lacking the space they need to exercise their functions. Three situations have been described:

- **Congenital pleuroperitoneal hernia (CPPH):** very rare, only a few confirmed cases. Can affect any diaphragm zone. The herniated organs (especially the liver) directly occupy the pleural space, and thus exert pressure on the lung. Causes dyspnea to varying degrees, depending on the size of the herniated sac.
- **Acquired pleuroperitoneal hernia (APPH):** traumatic origin in most cases. A heavy impact to the abdominal area results in an abrupt increase in pressure on the diaphragm, and it breaks. Most common are unilateral tears to the intercostal muscles in the ventral diaphragm under the esophageal hiatus. Tears of the sternal muscle and radial tears may also occur. The most frequently herniated organs in tears of the right diaphragm are the liver, small intestine, and pancreas. If the tear is on the left side, the most frequently herniated organs are the stomach, spleen, and small intestine.
- **Congenital peritoneopericardial diaphragmatic hernia (CPPDH):** caused by a developmental alteration in the pleural and peritoneal cavities, which do not separate and fuse to the pericardium, dorsally to the xiphoid process. The three cavities are joined through an orifice, and sometimes other congenital defects are present at the same time, such as in the distal sternebrae (pectus excavatum) or in the linea alba (umbilical hernia). The contents of the hernia tend to be liver tissue, abdominal fat, or intestine. Clinical signs may be respiratory (dyspnea), cardiac (cardiac tamponade), digestive, or, very often, absent.

Clinical signs

All peritoneal–diaphragmatic hernias can be **asymptomatic** (up to 50% of the cases and more often in congenital hernias). In traumatic hernias, clinical signs associated with the hernia can appear days or weeks after the accident.

A respiratory clinical sign that can be observed is **dyspnea**, caused by:

- Direct pulmonary compression by herniated organs (Fig. 7).
- Pleural effusion (transudate) due to venous congestion of the herniated organs.
- Pneumothorax caused directly by lung contusion or indirectly as a result of fractured ribs.

The herniated organs can also present clinical signs such as **congestion** due to vascular compression:

- Liver: obstructive jaundice.
- Stomach: gastric dilatation–volvulus syndrome.
- Intestine: signs of intestinal obstruction associated with ischemia and necrosis.

Cardiac clinical signs such as tachycardia, panting, positive jugular pulse and weak femoral pulse are due to **cardiac tamponade** resulting from an excess volume of abdominal organs inside the pericardium. This occurs more frequently in congenital peritoneopericardial diaphragmatic hernia.

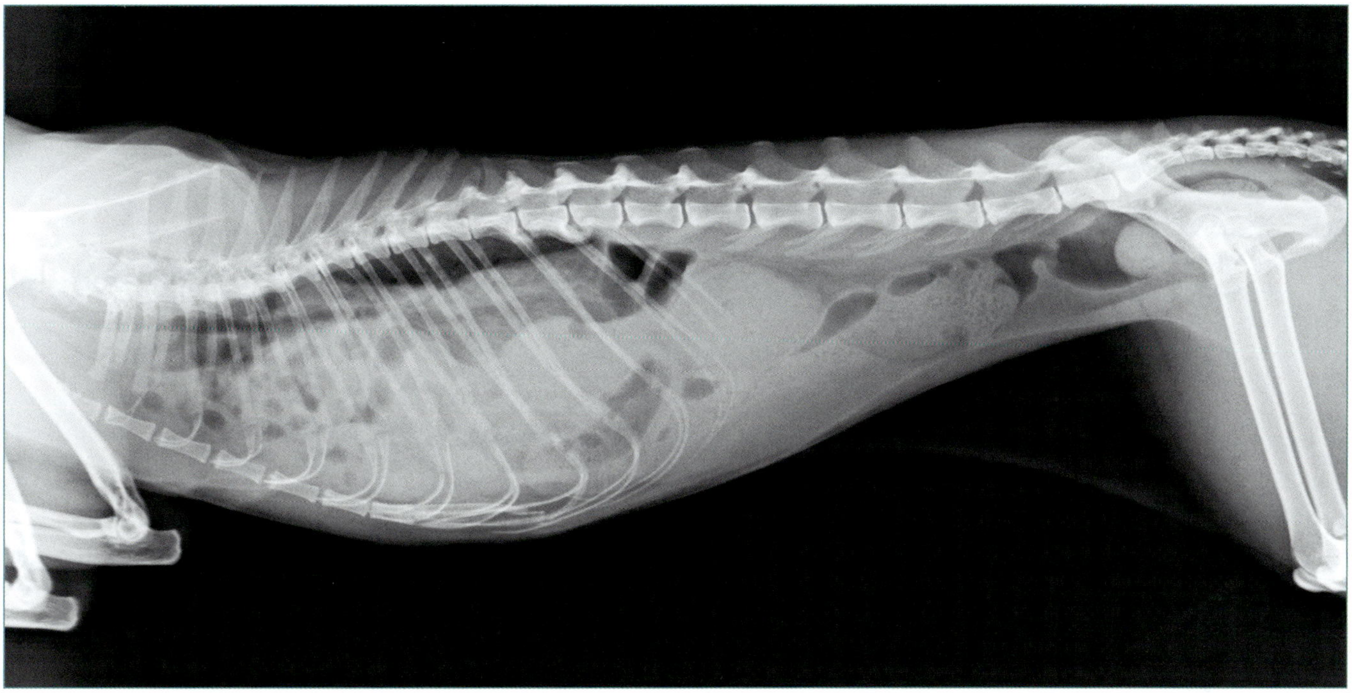

FIGURE 7. X-ray of a patient with peritoneopericardial diaphragmatic hernia. The liver, intestine, and part of the stomach are present in the hernial sac.

The following is heard on thoracic auscultation:

- An increase of borborygmus in the pleural cavity.
- Muffled heart and lung sounds.
- Cardiac sounds that are out of place due to displacement of the heart.

Diagnosis

The diagnosis of hernias in the abdominal cavity is based on the patient's clinical examination and the results of diagnostic imaging tests (Table 1).

Preoperative considerations

Preoperative management of the patient involves:

- Pain control with pure opioids, keeping in mind that respiratory depression may occur. Sometimes local anesthesia is additionally used in intercostal spaces or traumatized areas.
- Intensive fluid therapy.
- The cat must be kept in absolute rest and given oxygen.
- Thoracentesis should be planned if pneumothorax or pleural effusion must be mitigated.
- After stabilizing the patient, the effectiveness of the process must be evaluated in the first 12 hours. If a deterioration of vital signs is observed despite intensive care, if there is evidence of bleeding due to organ damage, or if the stomach

How to take a positive-contrast peritoneography?

This technique is used to verify the presence of communication between the abdominal and thoracic cavities when other imaging techniques are not conclusive. The only limitation is the chronic presence of omentum or some other organ blocking the opening of the defect, which could stop the passage of contrast agent and give a false negative.

The cat is anesthetized for the procedure and placed in dorsal recumbency. The umbilical area is shaved and disinfected. A syringe with 2 ml/kg of contrast medium, tempered to 77°F (25°C), is prepared (intravenous iopamidol, 300 mg/ml) along with a short 23-gauge needle. The injection site is 1 cm to the right of the umbilicus. Prior to this, the abdomen is palpated to avoid the bladder and spleen. After the needle is inserted, aspiration is applied to ensure that a visceral organ has not been punctured. The contrast agent is injected, and the abdomen is gently shaken so that it is distributed well. After waiting for 2–5 minutes, an X-ray of the abdomen and thorax is taken. If the contrast agent has passed into the thorax, the diagnosis of diaphragmatic hernia is confirmed.

TABLE 1. Diagnostic approach to peritoneal-diaphragmatic hernias in cats			
Diagnostic test	**Congenital pleuroperitoneal hernia**	**Acquired (traumatic) pleuroperitoneal hernia**	**Congenital peritoneopericardial diaphragmatic hernia**
Clinical signs (see text for more information)	Very often without clinical signs, or with signs associated with herniated organs.	Frequent respiratory clinical signs, associated with trauma and herniated organs.	Often without clinical signs, and if there are any, they are due to cardiac tamponade and herniated organs.
Plain thoracic radiography	■ Loss of diaphragmatic contour in any area. ■ Accumulation of gas in the thorax. ■ Cardiac and pulmonary shadows displaced cranially or dorsally. ■ Pleural effusion (radiography must repeated after draining to improve diagnosis).	■ Loss of diaphragmatic contour in any area. ■ Accumulation of gas in the thorax. ■ Cardiac and pulmonary shadows displaced cranially or dorsally. ■ Pleural effusion (radiography must repeated after draining to improve diagnosis). ■ Signs of thoracic trauma: pulmonary contusion, broken ribs.	■ Ventrodorsal projection: loss of contour only in the dome of the diaphragm. ■ Cardiomegaly. ■ Accumulation of gas only in the pericardium. ■ Sometimes associated with pectus excavatum (malformation of the sternum).
Plain abdominal radiography	■ Cranial displacement of the gastric axis. ■ Abdomen "empty" of certain organs (liver, intestine, spleen, stomach).	■ Cranial displacement of the gastric axis. ■ Abdomen "empty" of certain organs (liver, intestine, spleen, stomach).	The same signs as in other hernias, but less evident (smaller volume of herniated organs).
Contrast radiography of the abdomen	This is the test of choice if we suspect that the stomach or intestine are in the thorax.	This is the test of choice if we suspect that the stomach or intestine are in the thorax.	This is the test of choice if we suspect that the stomach or intestine are in the pericardium.
Positive-contrast peritoneography (see p. 191)	To verify whether there is communication between the abdominal and thoracic cavities when other techniques are not conclusive.	To verify whether there is communication between the abdominal and thoracic cavities when other techniques are not conclusive.	To verify whether there is communication between the abdominal and thoracic cavities when other techniques are not conclusive.
Ultrasound	■ Helpful when there is pleural effusion and organs in the thorax. ■ The diaphragm is difficult to evaluate with ultrasound.	■ The presence of pleural effusion is more common. ■ The diaphragm is difficult to evaluate with ultrasound.	■ Good test to diagnose the contents of the pericardium (Fig. 8). ■ The diaphragm is difficult to evaluate with ultrasound.
Computed tomography	Good technique to identify the presence of abdominal viscera inside the thorax.	Good technique to identify the presence of abdominal viscera inside the thorax.	Good technique to identify the presence of abdominal viscera inside the pericardium.

is detected inside the hernial sac, with the consequent risk of gastric dilatation–volvulus syndrome, **an emergency intervention to resolve the hernia is obligatory**, even though these cases entail a higher mortality rate (33%).

- If possible, the patient should be shaved and preoxygenated as quickly as possible before anesthetizing.
- Intravenous induction is preferred, and intubation should be done quickly.
- Once intubated, intermittent positive pressure ventilation is initiated (automatic ventilators are used rarely in feline medicine due to the difficulty of properly regulating pressure on the pulmonary tissue and the increased risk of edema).
- The patient is placed in dorsal recumbency with the thorax somewhat higher than the abdomen to decrease the pressure exerted by the herniated organs on the lungs and the heart, until the reduction of the hernia.
- The time between anesthetic induction and the reduction of the hernia should be as short as possible.

The decision whether or not to operate a diaphragmatic hernia depends on several factors: surgery is not recommended if the patient is asymptomatic and the hernia is congenital, unless the patient's clinical condition worsens for reasons associated with the congenital defect (strangulated herniated organ, vascular compromise that causes effusion, progressive pulmonary compression). Ideally, if the cat is symptomatic, and a diaphragmatic hernia has been diagnosed, the defect should be repaired after the patient has been stabilized for 24–48 hours.

Surgical technique

- **Patient positioning:** dorsal recumbency.
- **Surgical field:** the distal half of the thoracic cavity and the entire abdominal area are shaved and disinfected.
- **Approach:** a midline incision is made in the linea alba, from the xiphoid process to the distal umbilicus, sufficient to examine the entire abdominal cavity and the full surface of the diaphragm (there may be more than one tear). Gauze pads moistened with warm saline solution are used to demarcate the surgical field around the diaphragm.

  In general, the approach via lateral thoracotomy is not advisable, as it requires knowing the exact location of the lesion in advance and it does not enable full examination of the abdomen.

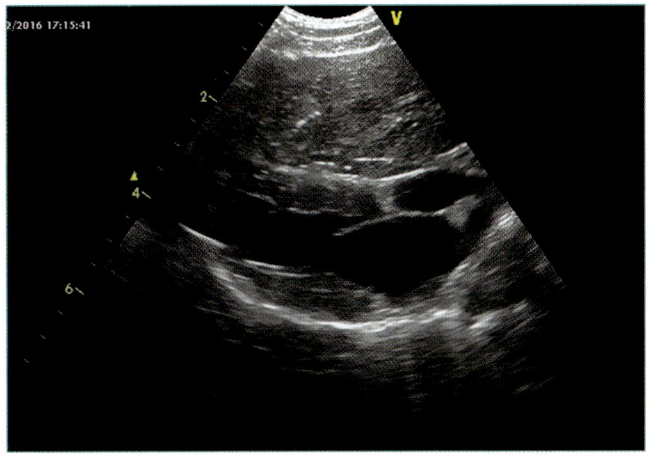

FIGURE 8. Ultrasound of a patient with peritoneopericardial diaphragmatic hernia. A piece of hepatic parenchyma is visible in the pericardium.

- **Technique**
  1. The first step is to examine the herniated organs and evaluate whether they are viable. If they are strangulated and necrotic or if their blood supply is highly compromised (cyanosis, hemorrhagic effusion, thrombosed vessels), they must be quickly excised or resected without releasing any toxins or pro-inflammatory factors into general circulation. If they are viable, they are repositioned in the abdominal cavity. If there are adhesions, they can be resolved by slightly opening the tear to facilitate examination of the thoracic cavity.

> Key point: when the abdominal cavity is opened and work is begun on the torn diaphragm, an anesthesiologist must initiate intermittent positive pressure ventilation.

  2. **Closure of the diaphragm defect:** the most frequent tear affects the muscle and is located in the ventral area. Before proceeding to wound closure, we can place a chest drain through the defect. This is inserted through a subcutaneous tunnel near an intercostal space, using the surgical field itself. Taking advantage of our view of the thoracic cavity, we situate the end of the fenestrated drain tube in the ventral area. This drain will help eliminate any remaining pneumothorax after the hernia is sutured, especially in cases in which we are unable to achieve an airtight seal.

3. The type of suture used is always 2-0 or 3-0 monofilament. The option to use absorbable or nonabsorbable material is largely up to the surgeon, although nonabsorbable material tends to be used with larger defects. In general, continuous sutures are used, always starting at the most dorsal point (the furthest from the surgical field) and continuing in the ventral direction. U-stitches can also be used, especially when closing paracostal areas of the diaphragm. It is important to always include diaphragmatic fascia to make the suture more secure.

   We are faced with several possible scenarios when designing the suture pattern:

- **Radial tears:** simple continuous suture pattern, from the dorsal to the ventral area (Fig. 9a).
- **Paracostal tears:** in this case, a simple continuous pattern is used to close the edge of the lesion around the rib. U-stitches can also be used around the rib (Fig. 9b).
- **Combined radial and paracostal tears:** first one or several initial stitches are applied for approximation and paracostal anchoring of the sections of tissue. Next, closure is effectuated with one or more continuous sutures (Fig. 9c).

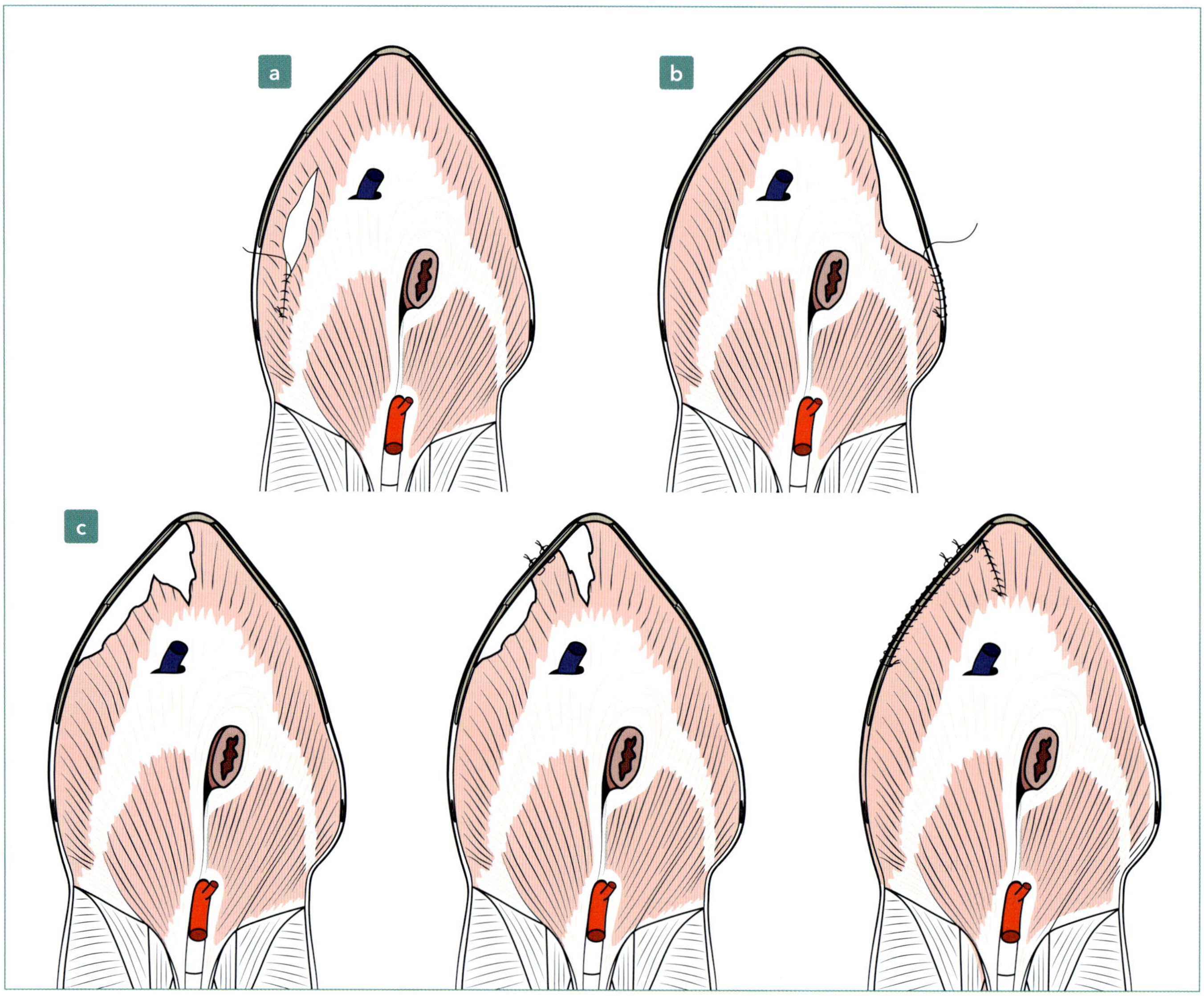

FIGURE 9. Suture patterns for radial, paracostal and combined tears. (a) Radial tear, with closure via continuous suture. (b) Paracostal tear, with closure via continuous suture around the rib. (c) Combined radial and paracostal tear, paracostal anchoring with U-stitches and radial and paracostal continuous sutures.

- **Congenital defects:** there is not enough muscle tissue to effectuate the closure in these cases. This is resolved through two paracostal incisions in the diaphragm, one on each side of the defect (Fig. 10). This prevents excessive tension on the muscle and suture after the repair, which would increase the risk of dehiscence. Once the defect is corrected with a continuous suture, the paracostal incisions are closed with U-stitches around the rib and sternum. Sometimes, the area of insertion of the sutures from the diaphragm to the abdominal wall must be displaced distally in order to compensate for the congenital lack of muscle.
- **Very large congenital defects:** in this case the use of polypropylene mesh is justified. To correct the defect, this mesh is sutured with polypropylene U-stitches to the walls of the diaphragm. Prior to this, the mesh should be lined with a double layer of greater omentum (thoracic and abdominal aspects of the implant) to prevent the mesh from scraping against the lung and abdominal organs (Fig. 11).

Once the defect/tear is sutured, the next step is to drain the pneumothorax as much as possible. This can easily be done with the help of a syringe attached to a three-way stopcock and a 20-gauge needle that goes through the diaphragm and empties out the air while an assistant promotes ventilation with gentle positive pressure. Once barely any air is coming out, the pneumothorax is resolved, and the needle is withdrawn from the diaphragm. If a chest drain has been placed, it will continue operating over the next few hours after surgery, connected to a three-way stopcock. The average amount of time to keep these devices inside cats is 12 hours if we wish to avoid the associated pain and respiratory depression. Another device used as a chest drain in cats is a 14-gauge J catheter.

Postoperative care

Analgesia with pure opiates is mandatory during the first week. The patient should be monitored for **dyspnea**, which could be caused by pneumothorax, pleural effusion, reexpansion pulmonary edema, or dehiscence of the diaphragm suture. The patient should rest for at least a week, until the diaphragm suture becomes strong enough for the cat to return to a normal level of activity.

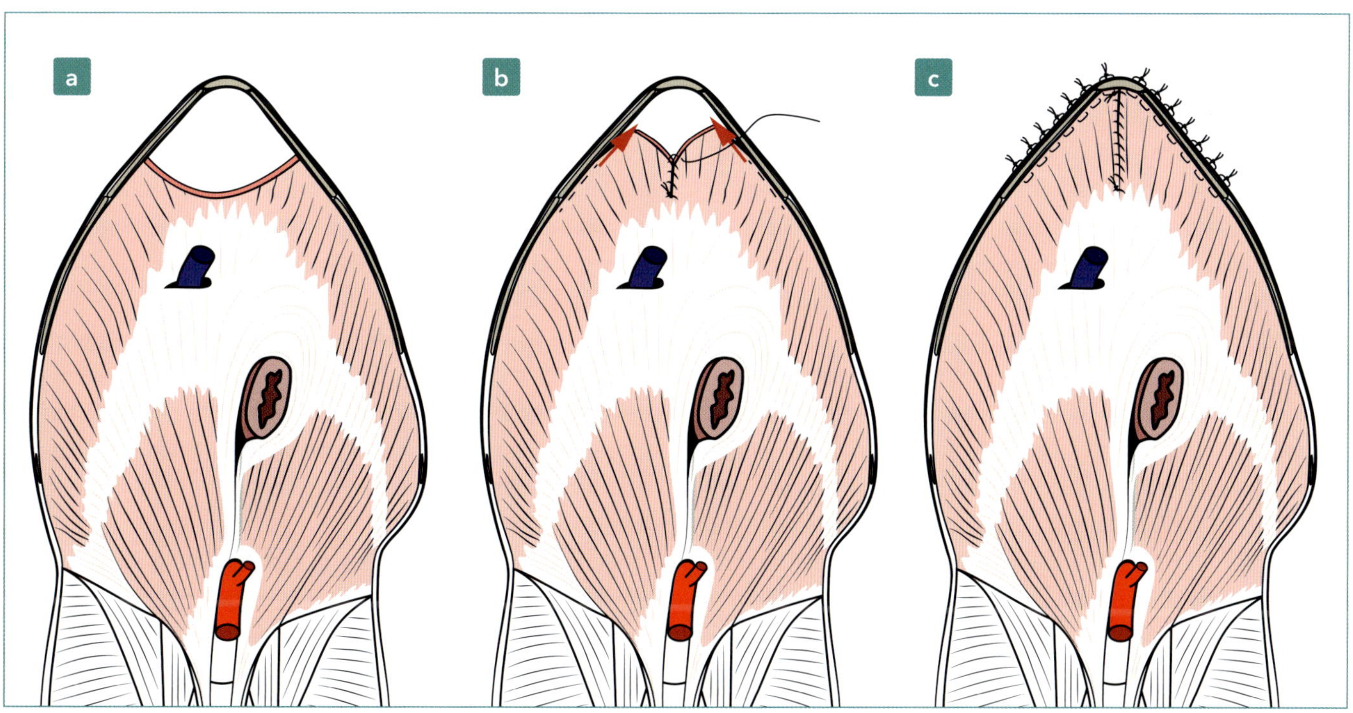

FIGURE 10. (a) Congenital defects. (b) The lack of muscular tissue needed to effectuate the closure is resolved via paracostal incisions in the diaphragm on each side of the defect. (c) Once the defect is corrected with a continuous suture, the paracostal incisions are closed with U-stitches around the rib and sternum.

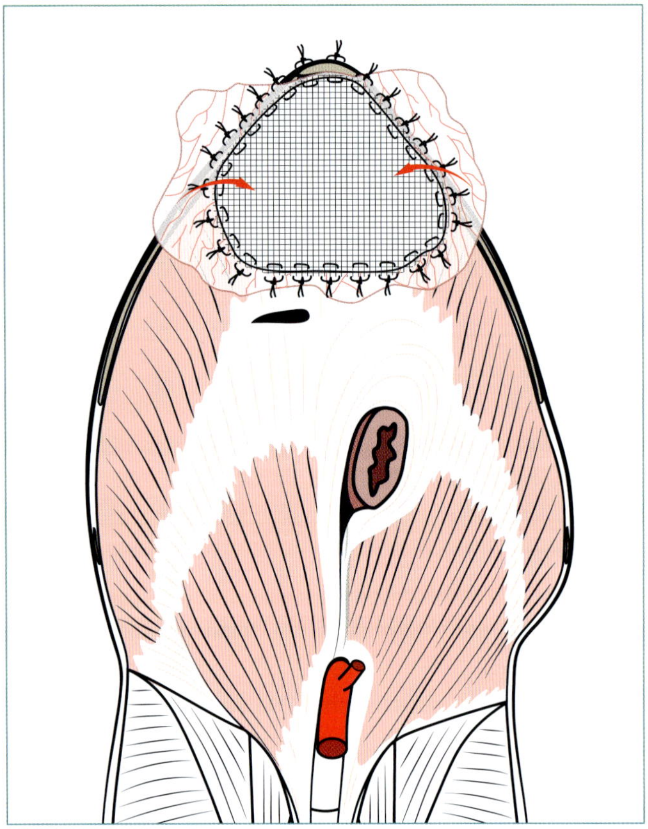

FIGURE 11. Closure of large congenital defects: use of a polypropylene mesh covered with omentum and sutured with U-stitches to the diaphragm walls.

Complications

Published data suggest a mortality rate of 14% in peritoneopericardial diaphragmatic hernia surgery. In cases of traumatic hernia, the rate drops to only 8%. The majority of these deaths occur in the first 24 hours after surgery. The principal cause of death in patients with surgically resolved diaphragmatic hernia is reexpansion pulmonary edema. To avoid this, positive pressure ventilation must be monitored the entire time while under anesthesia. Another complication that has been described is elevated intra-abdominal pressure as a consequence of the lack of space for the herniated organs, along with an inability of the abdominal walls to adequately distend. This occurs more often in cases of congenital hernia. The associated risks are suture dehiscence and dyspnea caused by restricted diaphragm mobility. To avoid this, a preventive splenectomy or partial hepatectomy can be effectuated.

Inguinal hernias

The double pillar structure of the prepubic tendon (called the **external oblique abdominal aponeurosis** in cats) as well as the very narrow and taut femoral and inguinal canals mean that this type of hernia is not very common in cats. Case studies in the literature are due to traumas or very large congenital defects of the wall (see the following sections), and they do not exclusively involve these two natural orifices.

Umbilical hernias

Real umbilical hernias occur rarely in cats (0.15% according to studies). They are always congenital and result from defects in the closure of abdominal muscle folds during fetal development. They should not be confused with **cranial abdominal hernias**, which are defects of the wall associated with peritoneopericardial hernias. Nor should they be confused with **omphaloceles**, which consist of a complete agenesis of the abdominal midline and the skin, causing congenital evisceration.

The technique used to resolve umbilical hernias consists of dissecting the hernial sac of its adhesions until the hernial ring is revealed. A cut is made around the ring to debride the edges of the wound so that it subsequently heals safely. The usual suture used for abdominal closure is then effectuated.

Abdominal wall hernias and ruptures

The majority of abdominal hernias in cats occur after blunt trauma to the caudomedial wall or the paracostal region (areas of osseous insertion of the pelvis and the ribs, respectively). Other possible origins of abdominal hernias are iatrogenic; due to suture dehiscence, either as a result of careless technique or poor choice of suture materials; or as a result of defects of the abdominal wall in cats with cutaneous asthenia. In such cases, the linea alba is very wide and weak. Therefore, any sutures should include well formed muscle fascia, which sometimes means that a large part of the weakened fascia must be cut before repairing the surgical wound (Fig. 12).

Agenesis of the abdominal wall is due to congenital defects in the formation of one or several abdominal muscles, either partially or completely. If the defect is limited to one area, the cat may survive and present abdominal hernia. Such cases can be associated with cutaneous asthenia due to a defect in the structure of the connective tissue.

Resolution always consists of reconstructing the damaged muscle along with its anchors. The earlier the diagnosis and intervention is done, the more effective the results. When the damage is very severe, in very chronic cases or if the defect is congenital and very extensive, the use of polypropylene mesh to repair the defect is mandatory (Fig. 13).

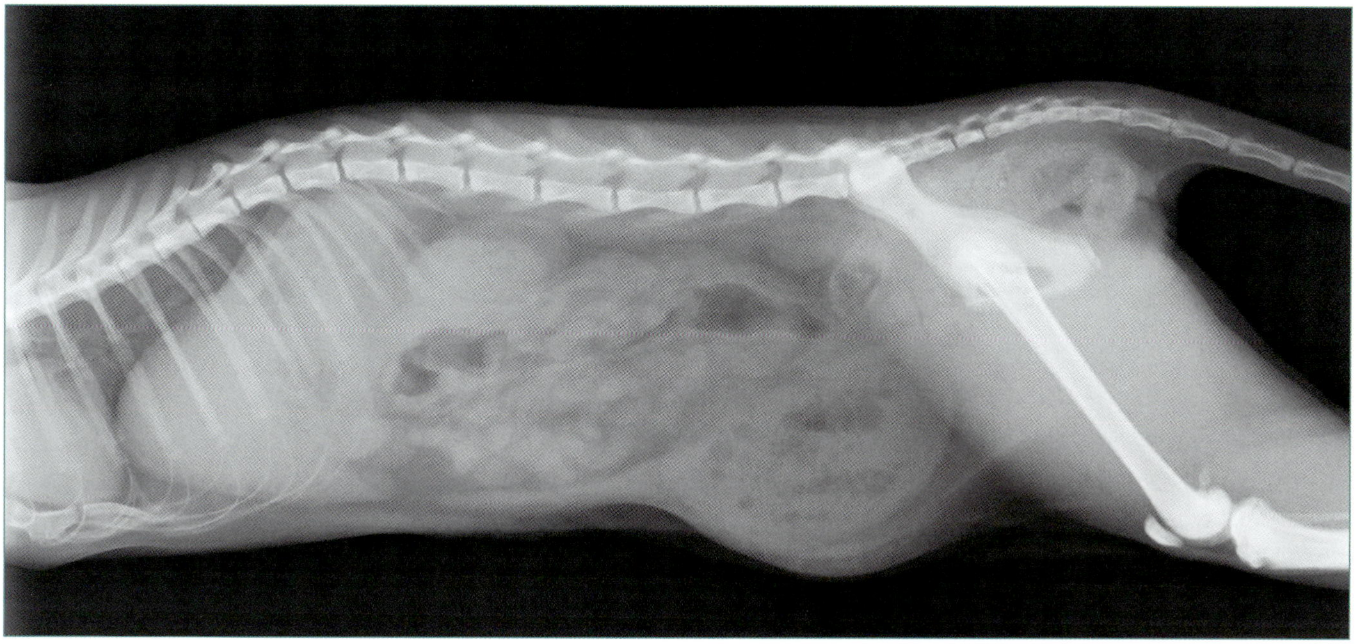

FIGURE 12. Rupture of the abdominal wall in a cat with cutaneous asthenia and congenital perineal hernia. Greater omentum lodged in the subcutaneous space following dehiscence of the surgical wound 2 days after performing an ovariohysterectomy.

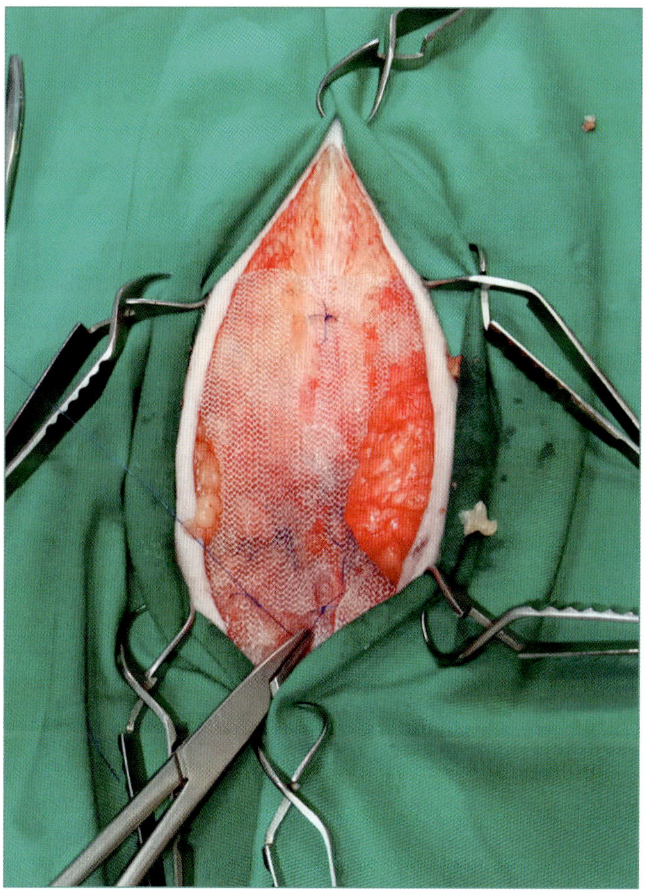

FIGURE 13. Placement of a polypropylene mesh to resolve a bilateral prepubic tendon tear in a cat. The disinsertion was very large and required the help of mesh to ensure the proper reconstruction of the insertions in the pubis.

Bibliography

Bellah JR. Diafragma. In: Bojrab JM (ed.). *Técnicas actuales en cirugía de pequeños animales*, 4th ed. Buenos Aires: Intermédica, 2001; pp. 289–298.

Benitah N, Matousek JL, Barnes RF et al. Diaphragmatic and perineal hernias associated with cutaneous asthenia in a cat. *J Am Vet Med Assoc*, 2004; 224(5):706–709, 698.

Boothe HW, Slater MR, Hobson HP et al. Exploratory celiotomy in 200 nontraumatized dogs and cats. *Vet Surg*, 1992; 21(6):452–457.

Burton C, White R. Surgical approach to a ruptured diaphragm in the cat. *In Pract*, 1997; 19:298–305.

Cariou MP, Shihab N, Kenny P, Baines SJ. Surgical management of an incidentally diagnosed true pleuroperitoneal hernia in a cat. *J Feline Med Surg*, 2009; 11(10):873–877.

Clugston RD, Greer JJ. Diaphragm development and congenital diaphragmatic hernia. *Semin Pediatr Surg*, 2007; 16(2):94–100.

Charlesworth TM, Moores AL. Post-trauma inguinal seroma formation in the cat. *J Small Anim Pract*, 2012; 53(5):301–303.

Coffey JC, O'Leary DP. The mesentery: structure, function, and role in disease. *Lancet Gastroenterol Hepatol*, 2016; 1(3):238–247.

Formaggini L, Schmidt K, De Lorenzi D. Gastric dilatation-volvulus associated with diaphragmatic hernia in three cats: clinical presentation, surgical treatment and presumptive aetiology. *J Feline Med Surg*, 2008; 10(2):198–201.

Fossum TW. Surgery of the lower respiratory system: pleural cavity and diaphragm. In: Fossum TW (ed.). *Small Animal Surgery*. St Louis, MO: Mosby Elsevier, 2007; pp. 896–929.

Larson MM. Imaging the thorax. Diaphragm. In: Holland M, Hudson J (eds.). *Feline Diagnostic Imaging*. Hoboken, New Jersey: Wiley Blackwell, 2020; pp. 315–322.

Liptak JM, Bissett SA, Allan GS et al. Hepatic cysts incarcerated in a peritoneopericardial diaphragmatic hernia. *J Feline Med Surg*, 2002; 4(2):123–125.

Parry A. Positive contrast peritoneography in the diagnosis of pleuroperitoneal diaphragmatic hernia in a cat. *J Feline Med Surg*, 2010; 12(2):141–143.

Pratschke KM. Abdominal wall hernias and ruptures. In: Langley-Hobbs SJ, Demetriou JL, Ladlow JF (eds.). *Feline Soft Tissue and General Surgery*. London: Elsevier Saunders, 2014; pp. 269–280.

Reimer SB, Kyles AE, Filipowicz DE, Gregory CR. Long-term outcome of cats treated conservatively or surgically for peritoneopericardial diaphagmatic hernia: 66 cases (1987–2002). *J Am Vet Med Assoc*, 2004; 224(5):728–732.

Reina Rodriguez FS, Buckley CT, Milgram J, Kirby BM. Biomechanical properties of feline ventral abdominal wall and celiotomy closure techniques. *Vet Surg*, 2018; 47(2):193–203.

Schmiedt CW, Tobias KM, Stevenson MA. Traumatic diaphragmatic hernia in cats: 34 cases (1991–2001). *J Am Vet Med Assoc*, 2003; 222(9):1237–1240.

Sieck GC, Roy RR, Powell P et al. Muscle fiber type distribution and architecture of the cat diaphragm. *J Appl Physiol Respir Environ Exerc Physiol*, 1983; 55(5):1386–1392.

Spattini G, Rossi F, Vignoli M, Lamb CR. Use of ultrasound to diagnose diaphragmatic rupture in dogs and cats. *Vet Radiol Ultrasound*, 2003; 44(2):226–230.

Stampley AR, Waldron DR. Reexpansion pulmonary edema after surgery to repair a diaphragmatic hernia in a cat. *J Am Vet Med Assoc*, 1993; 203(12):1699–1701.

Williams J, Leveille R, Myer CW. Imaging modalities used to confirm diaphragmatic hernia in small animals. *Comp Cont Ed Pract Vet*, 1998; 20(11):1199–1209.

Worth AJ, Machon RG. Traumatic diaphrragmatic herniation: pathophysiology and management. *Comp Cont Educ Pract Vet*, 2005; 27(3):178–191.

Yool DA. Diaphragm. In: Langley-Hobbs SJ, Demetriou JL, Ladlow JF (eds.). *Feline Soft Tissue and General Surgery*. London: Elsevier Saunders, 2014; pp. 521–530.

GASTRIC FOREIGN BODIES AND TUMORS 21

Alberto Barneto

Surgical anatomy

Past the esophagus, the digestive tube widens to form the stomach, where food accumulates and digestion begins. In cats, the stomach is situated in the cranial portion of the abdomen. Covered in part by the concave region of the liver, it has a characteristic J shape when viewed during a laparotomy in the ventrodorsal position.

The stomach consists of several anatomical zones (Fig. 1):

- **Cardia:** located below the liver, near the esophageal hiatus of the diaphragm.
- **Fundus:** dome shaped and situated directly dorsal to and past the cardia.
- **Body or corpus:** the largest part of the organ, from the fundus to the narrowing at the pyloric antrum. Its function, along with the fundus, is to mix food with gastric juices for the purpose of digestion.
- **Pyloric region:** here the stomach's shape and direction changes. It gradually narrows cranioventrally and towards the right, adapting itself to the lesser curvature. Its function is to transfer food through the pylorus into the intestine for further digestion.

The widening of the digestive tube at the stomach gives it two well differentiated curves:

- **Greater curvature:** touches the left abdominal wall and extends caudoventrally. When the stomach is full, this is the most mobile part, occupying even more space caudoventrally.
- **Lesser curvature:** oriented toward the right side of the craniodorsal region of the abdomen. It remains in place even when the stomach is filled to capacity.

Gastric vascularization proceeds in its entirety from one of the principal branches of the aorta, the **celiac artery**, which in turn gives rise to three branches:

- The **hepatic artery**, along with others branches, gives rise to the arteries that irrigate the right side of the greater curvature (**right gastroepiploic artery**) and the lesser curvature (**right gastric artery**).
- The **left gastric artery**, which supplies blood to the left part of the lesser curvature, the fundus, cardia, and the distal part of the esophagus.
- The **splenic artery**, which gives rise to the **left gastroepiploic artery**, which irrigates the left part of the greater curvature of the stomach via its two branches.

All these arteries branch off at regular intervals, spreading out over the gastric walls. The venous tree collects blood and carries it through the gastroduodenal and splenic veins to the hepatic portal vein, where the liver processes the absorbed nutrients.

Gastric innervation belongs to the autonomic nervous system. These nerves begin from branches of the **vagus nerve** and others originating in the celiac and cranial mesenteric ganglia.

The stomach wall consists of four layers:

- **Mucosa:** its surface comprises numerous longitudinal folds, especially in the corpus and fundus regions. Histologically it is composed of a simple columnar epithelium, characteristic of the digestive tube, with numerous glands. The mucosal glands of the cardia and pylorus regions produce protective mucus. The gastric glands of the corpus and fundus segregate the hydrochloric acid and enzymes of the gastric juice.
- **Submucosa:** supports the mucosa, giving it elasticity and strength to enable mucosal displacement by movements in the muscular layer.
- **Tunica muscularis:** fibers are distributed as typical in the digestive system, externally longitudinal and internally circular, and another internal layer in the stomach has oblique fibers. The longitudinal and oblique fibers are found in the

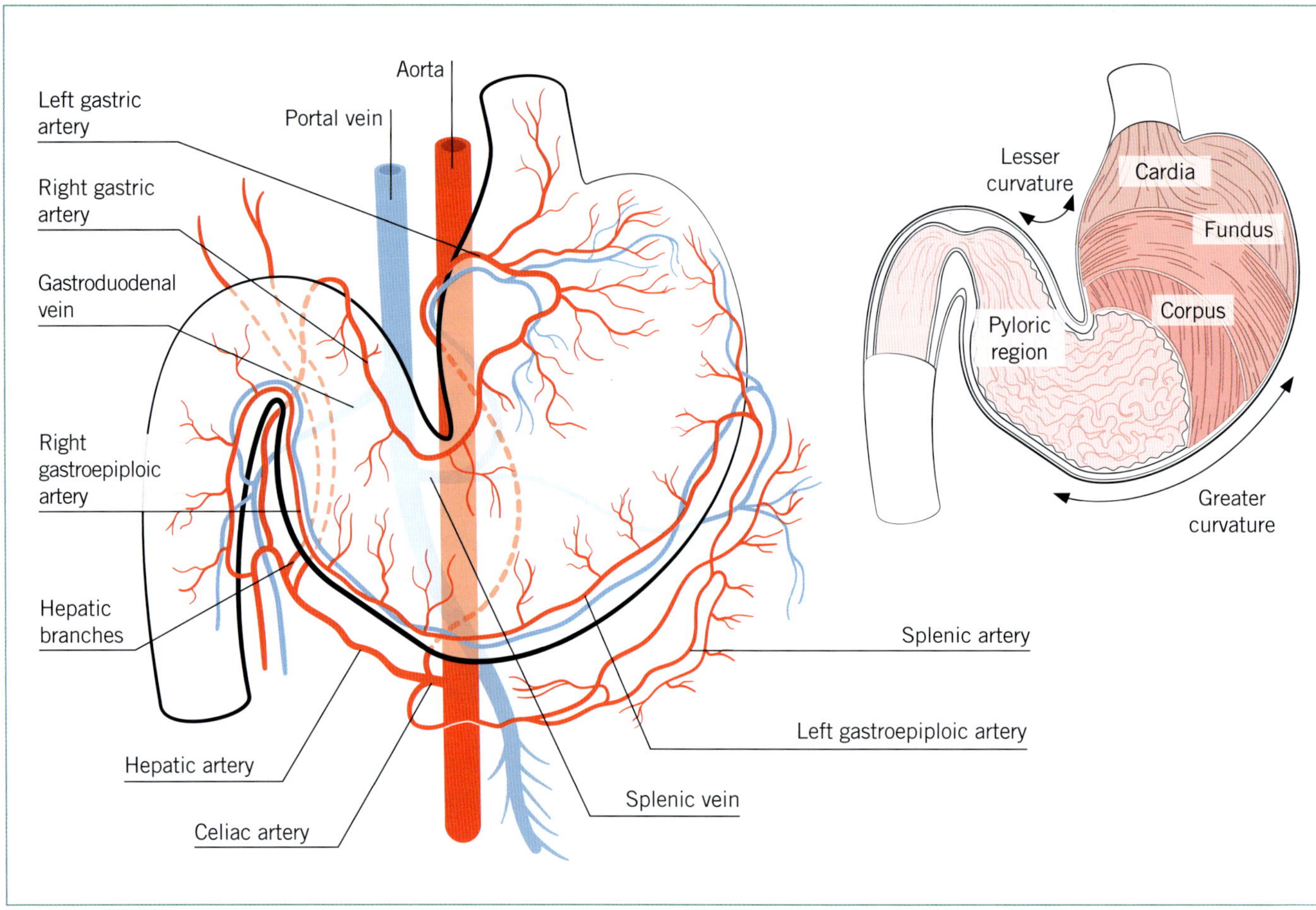

FIGURE 1. Structure and vascularization of the stomach.

corpus and fundus, while the circular fibers are mostly concentrated in the pyloric antrum.

- **Serosa:** the outermost layer continues with the visceral peritoneum, giving rise to several folds (ligaments) that attach the stomach to the spleen, liver and duodenum.

Surgical diseases of the stomach in cats

The following gastric conditions and techniques may involve surgical intervention:

- **Extraction of foreign bodies:** cats, especially young cats, play with many different objects in order to develop their

Omentum or epiploon

Fold of peritoneum made up of two sheets, joins the stomach to its adjacent organs (also see Ch. 20 "Feline abdominal cavity. Hernias"). There are two omentums:

- The shorter **lesser omentum** attaches the liver to the lesser curvature of the stomach and duodenum.
- The **greater omentum**, is in turn, made up of two more layers and extends to form a kind of fine sheet with infiltrated fat that covers the intestines. It begins in the greater curvature of the stomach from where it opens, and extends for over half a square meter, finally inserting in the transverse colon.

The omentum houses the main vessels that supply all these abdominal organs, and it itself is highly vascularized. This enables the repair and recovery of any small lesion in the walls of adjacent abdominal organs.

hunting instinct. Compared to dogs, the hyoid apparatus has less mobility in cats. Therefore, when cats bring objects (or hunted food) to the center of their mouths, they tend to swallow them automatically. If the objects are elongated (threads, cords) they can cause obstruction of the stomach and intestine (see Ch. 22) (Fig. 2).

- **Gastric biopsies:** in inflammatory diseases, biopsies of the mucosa and submucosa are usually taken with the help of gastroscopy. Nevertheless, if the diagnosis is a mass on the gastric wall, it usually affects the submucosa, and the endoscopy biopsy forceps may not go deep enough to obtain a representative sample. Therefore, it is more realistic to use a surgical approach and perform an incisional or excisional biopsy.
- **Technique to place a gastrotomy tube:** these long-lasting tubes allow fast feeding (see Ch. 3). Although techniques have been described to place these tubes endoscopically, modern feeding tubes in the shape of a mushroom are implanted via a small gastrotomy, and are sutured to the wall of the stomach (tobacco-pouch suture) and abdomen (gastropexy). These gastrotomy tubes can be used for up to several months. The area must be protected with a dressing or a shirt.
- **Gastric ulcers and perforations:** ulcerative gastritis is diagnosed through gastroscopy, which enables biopsies to be taken to learn the cause. If there is a perforation (chronic ulcers, improper use of NSAIDs, parasites, mast cell tumors, etc.), the perforated area of the wall is removed surgically.
- **Pyloric stenosis:** when pyloric stenosis does not respond to medical treatment, several pyloroplasty techniques have been described to widen the opening of the exit of the stomach. These cases are very rare in cats (tumors or corrective surgery for perforated ulcers near the pylorus).
- **Esophageal invagination:** invagination of the stomach inside the esophageal lumen has been described in very few cases in cats, and it is always associated with chronic vomiting and megaesophagus. Good results have been obtained with the combined technique of reduction of the invagination, fixation of the stomach wall (gastropexy) and placement of a gastrotomy tube until the issue has been corrected.
- **Gastric hernias:** gastric or hiatal hernias are defects in the esophageal orifice of the diaphragm, which causes part of the stomach to pass into the thoracic cavity. These hernias are rare in cats, and they may be traumatic or congenital in origin. The most effective technique to resolve this issue consists of dissecting the hernial ring in the diaphragm, repositioning the stomach in the abdominal cavity, and suturing the diaphragm defect, additionally using suture anchors in the serous and muscular layers of the cardia region.
- **Gastric neoplasia:** gastric tumors in cats represent less than 1% of all neoplasms diagnosed in this species. They affect senior cats more often, and the majority of them are malignant. Lymphoblastic lymphoma is the most frequent gastric tumor in cats, although infiltrative lymphocytic lymphoma, adenocarcinoma (mainly in Siamese cats) and plasmocytoma have also been described. The most effective treatment of any mass in the stomach is surgical resection.

> To avoid iatrogenic perforation of the stomach, an endoscopic biopsy of the center of a gastric ulcer should never be taken.

Diagnosis

The most prevalent clinical sign of gastric disease is acute or chronic **vomiting**. This should be distinguished from **regurgitation**, which results from esophageal disease. Vomiting is accompanied by spasmodic movements of the abdominal wall and

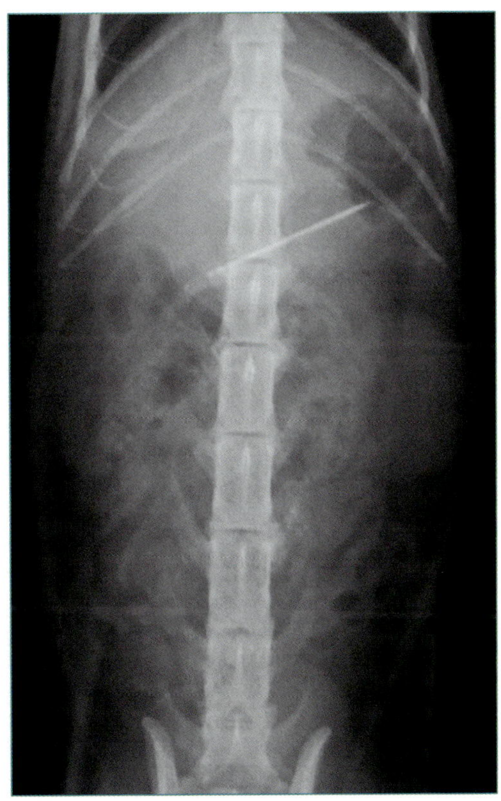

FIGURE 2. Foreign body (sewing needle) visible in an X-ray of the stomach. If the needle has a piece of thread attached, it can become a linear foreign body, with the concomitant complications.

usually contains food, hair, bile reflux, and, in chronic cases or repeated vomiting, blood. Vomiting is not exclusive to stomach disease, although it usually accompanies them. Intestinal, pancreatic, hepatic and renal diseases can also cause vomiting.

Diagnostic imaging techniques should always be used to learn the cause of the gastric disease (Table 1).

Preoperative and postoperative considerations

Things that should be kept in mind before and after surgery:

- Prior tests: especially to evaluate electrolyte abnormalities and correct them before anesthesia. It is worthwhile to find out albumin levels, especially in cases of chronic vomiting and anorexia, to decide whether to institute parenteral-assisted feeding after surgery.
- Gastric surgery is considered a clean–contaminated operation. Therefore, perioperative antibiotic therapy is indicated.
- Over the course of the intervention, an assistant should identify any material that is contaminated and material that is not contaminated.
- When the surgery is over, the assistant must make sure to account for and recover all gauze from the surgical field.

TABLE 1. Diagnostic methods used in different surgical diseases of the stomach

Diagnostic technique	Indications	Observations
Plain radiography	■ Radiopaque foreign bodies (Fig. 2) ■ Tumors of the gastric wall ■ Pyloric stenosis	■ Two projections (LL and VD) to locate foreign bodies. ■ The image is improved if there is some air in the stomach. Masses are visualized as rigid and thickened areas in the wall. ■ Pyloric stenosis may be suspected if the stomach presents a large amount of fluid content (poor emptying), but this test is not very sensitive.
Positive-contrast radiography (barium or iodine)	■ Radiotransparent foreign bodies ■ Gastric perforations ■ Evaluation of gastric emptying ■ Hiatal hernias and invaginations	■ Two projections (LL and VD) to locate foreign bodies. ■ **Iodinated contrast media is always used** if perforation is suspected. ■ Contrast media should be mixed with wet food. ■ Barium contrast adheres better to the mucosa than iodine. As such, it improves sensitivity of the test. ■ A normal cat stomach empties the contrast agent in 60 minutes.
Ultrasound	All gastric diseases	■ Technique of choice for any type of foreign body. ■ If well distended, the layers of the gastric wall can be evaluated. ■ Ideal for the diagnosis of tumors of the wall. Samples may also be taken via ultrasound-guided puncture (Fig. 3). ■ Enables evaluation of alterations of lymph nodes associated with the disease. ■ Enables evaluation of the morphology and functionality of the pylorus (proper emptying, in time and form).
Gastroscopy	■ Any type of foreign body (Fig. 4) ■ Ulcerative or inflammatory conditions that affect the mucosa (Fig. 5)	■ Diagnosis and possible extraction of foreign bodies if they are small, round and are not lodged. ■ Also enables biopsy with forceps, although the full thickness of the wall cannot always be obtained. ■ Often when dealing with tumors of the gastric wall, obtaining diagnostic biopsies through gastroscopy may not be possible.
Computed tomography (CT)	■ Hiatal hernia and invaginations ■ Gastric tumors ■ Foreign bodies	The only limitation is that if the stomach is poorly distended, its wall cannot be adequately evaluated.

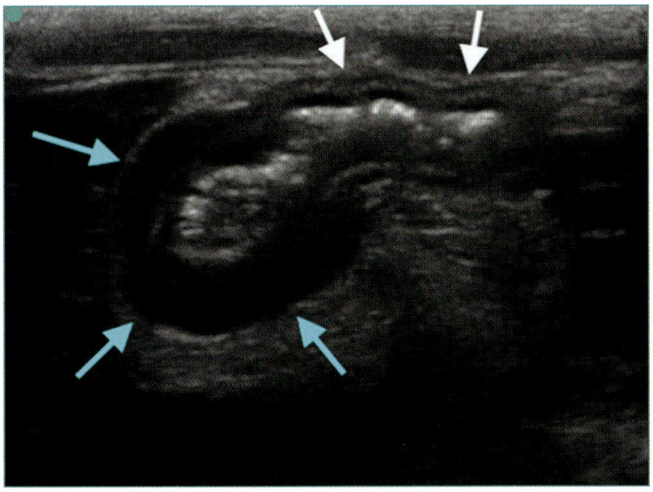

FIGURE 3. Gastric ultrasound of a cat showing severe thickening of a part of the gastric wall, along with loss of wall stratification compatible with a stomach tumor (blue arrows). A normal layered structure is seen in the remainder of the wall (white arrows). Image courtesy of Alejandro Casasús.

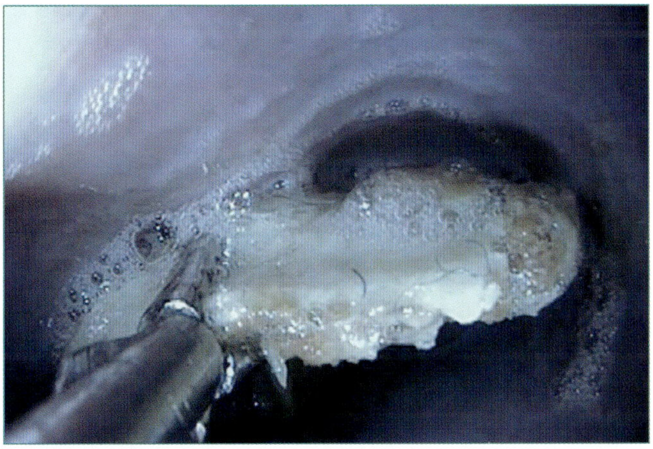

FIGURE 4. Extraction of a foreign body from a cat's stomach using forceps via gastroscopy.

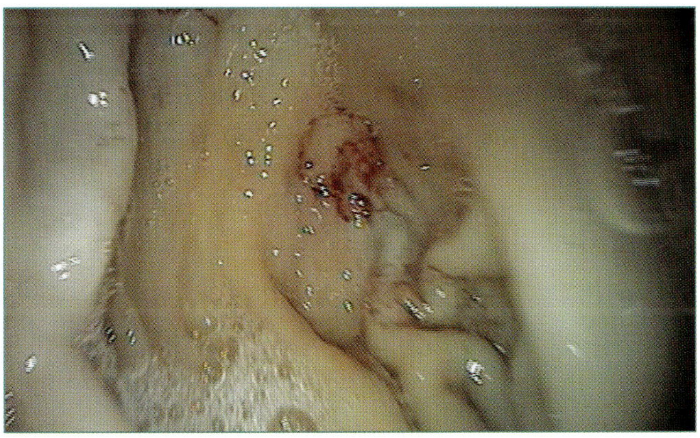

FIGURE 5. Endoscopic image of the stomach of a cat with ulcerative gastritis before taking samples for a biopsy.

- Before closing the gastrotomy incision, the surgeon should put on a new pair of sterile gloves.
- In surgeries associated with peritonitis due to perforations, antibiotic therapy is maintained during the postoperative period, always supported by the results of an antibiogram done on the basis of in situ sampling. In these situations, peritoneal lavage with warm isotonic saline solution is performed before closure of the laparotomy site.

Surgical techniques

Gastrotomy

- **Patient positioning:** dorsal recumbency, with at least the forelimbs held in place and stretched cranially with straps or gauze. Proper head support and endotracheal tube placement must be monitored in this position to avoid kinks.
- **Surgical field:** the entire ventral surface is shaved, from the first intercostal spaces to the genital area, including laterally the axillary and inguinal areas. For better exposure of the surgical field, we can use a Balfour self-retaining retractor. Once the laparotomy has been performed and the stomach held in place with stay sutures (see below), a second surgical field is prepared around the working area (Fig. 6). For this purpose, gauze pads and warm isotonic saline solution is prepared ahead of time. The gauze pads are moistened, the assistant counts them, and they are placed in a complete circle around the area of stomach that will be operated on. This way we can safely have the space we need to work while avoiding spillage of the gastric contents inside the peritoneal cavity.
- **Approach:** through an incision in the linea alba from the xiphoid process to the caudal area of the umbilicus.
- **Technique**
  1. Once the laparotomy is carried out, the location of the stomach is found, just below the hepatic border and anterior to the sheet of greater omentum. The ventral aspect of the stomach is visible, and this is where the gastrotomy is effectuated. An intermediate area between the greater and lesser curvature is found. The wall here has less vascularization. Two stay sutures are placed through almost the full thickness (including the submucosa), with a distance of 10 cm between them. The line that joins them should be parallel to the main axis of the stomach, where the incision is made (Fig. 7.1).

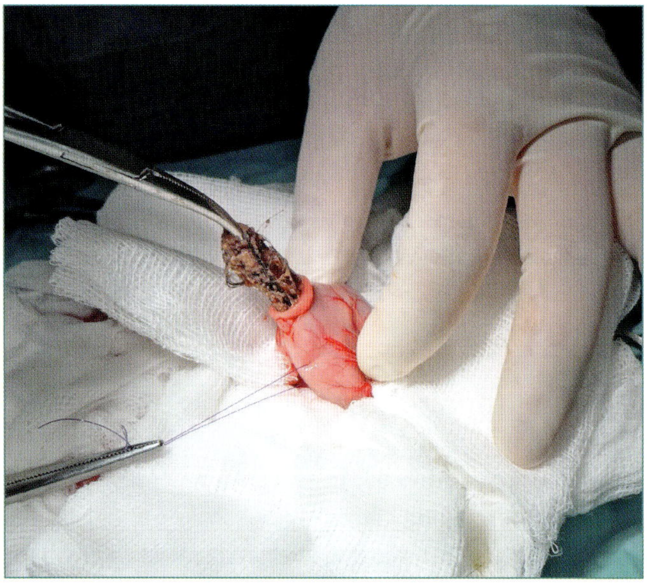

FIGURE 6. Gastrotomy to extract a foreign body (trichobezoar). The position of one of the stay sutures is seen, along with the second surgical field to avoid contamination. Image courtesy of Barcelona feline clinic.

2. The gastric wall is fairly thick and firm. It is common to need two cuts with the scalpel to be able to incise it completely. The first cut reaches the mucosa. Once the required length is cut, the gastric wall is gently pinched with one hand to hold it in place, and the mucosa is cut using the scalpel in the other hand. Once incised, it is preferable to widen the cut in the mucosa with Metzenbaum scissors. This maneuver and the following ones are done with the assistant applying traction to the stay sutures to maintain the opening at a higher plane with respect to the rest of the organ (Fig. 7.2).
3. At this point, the required surgical intervention is performed. If a biopsy is required, a spindle-shaped fragment is cut from the edge of the wound, taking care to obtain the full thickness of the wall. If we need to take a fragment from the interior of the organ, examine the mucosa, or remove a foreign body, enlarging the gastrotomy incision is recommended. This maneuver is facilitated by placing two additional stay sutures, one on each side of the incision at the midpoint of each side of the incision. Not only does this improve visualization inside the stomach, but it also allows us to insert our fingers or an instrument to work in the gastric lumen.
4. If we need to extract a **linear foreign body** whose proximal end is lodged in the pylorus, it is pulled very gently to cut the end, thus freeing the inserted piece that is attempting to advance through the duodenum. To pinpoint the location of this end, it is useful to use a fingertip to direct the cut of the scissors. This minimizes the risk of intestinal perforations associated with these types of foreign bodies.
5. The gastrotomy is always closed with a double layer of sutures. The authors prefer a simple continuous suture for the initial closure of the mucosal layer, and over this, a partial-thickness inverting Cushing suture, including submucosa (Fig. 7.3). Sometimes the gastric mucosa everts towards the outside of the incision, and it must be cut before closing the wound. The advantage of this technique is that bleeding of the mucosa is minimized inside the stomach after the intervention. Another alternative described for closure of the gastrotomy site is to use two inverting sutures. The first Cushing suture includes the submucosa (as described above), but the end of the knot is left long. As soon as this first suture is done, we go back in the other direction without knotting, effectuating an inverting Lembert suture on the serosa. The final stitch of this double suture is made taking advantage of the long end at the beginning of the inverting Cushing. In this technique, the mucosa is not sutured. It heals via secondary intention without further complications. The material used in any of these techniques is 3-0 absorbable monofilament, with an atraumatic needle.

Y-U pyloroplasty

Of all the surgical techniques described in cats to treat functional pyloric stenosis, the most effective is Y-U pyloroplasty. Nevertheless, this is a rarely diagnosed condition in cats that usually responds well to nonsurgical medical treatment. When a gastric tumor or perforated lesion must be removed near the pyloric sphincter, resection can be accompanied by this technique to prevent postoperative stenosis.

The surgery is initiated with a full-thickness Y-shaped incision in the stomach over the pyloric sphincter. The vertical section of the Y is situated over the duodenum, and the two arms over the pyloric antrum. When the simple interrupted sutures are placed, the first stitch joins the vertex of the Y with the end of the incision in the duodenum, with an advancement flap from the pyloric antrum towards the duodenum (the Y-shaped wound becomes U-shaped). This increases the diameter of the pyloric sphincter. The two remaining lines are sutured in a simple interrupted pattern or the usual two-layer suture used for the gastric wall (Fig. 8).

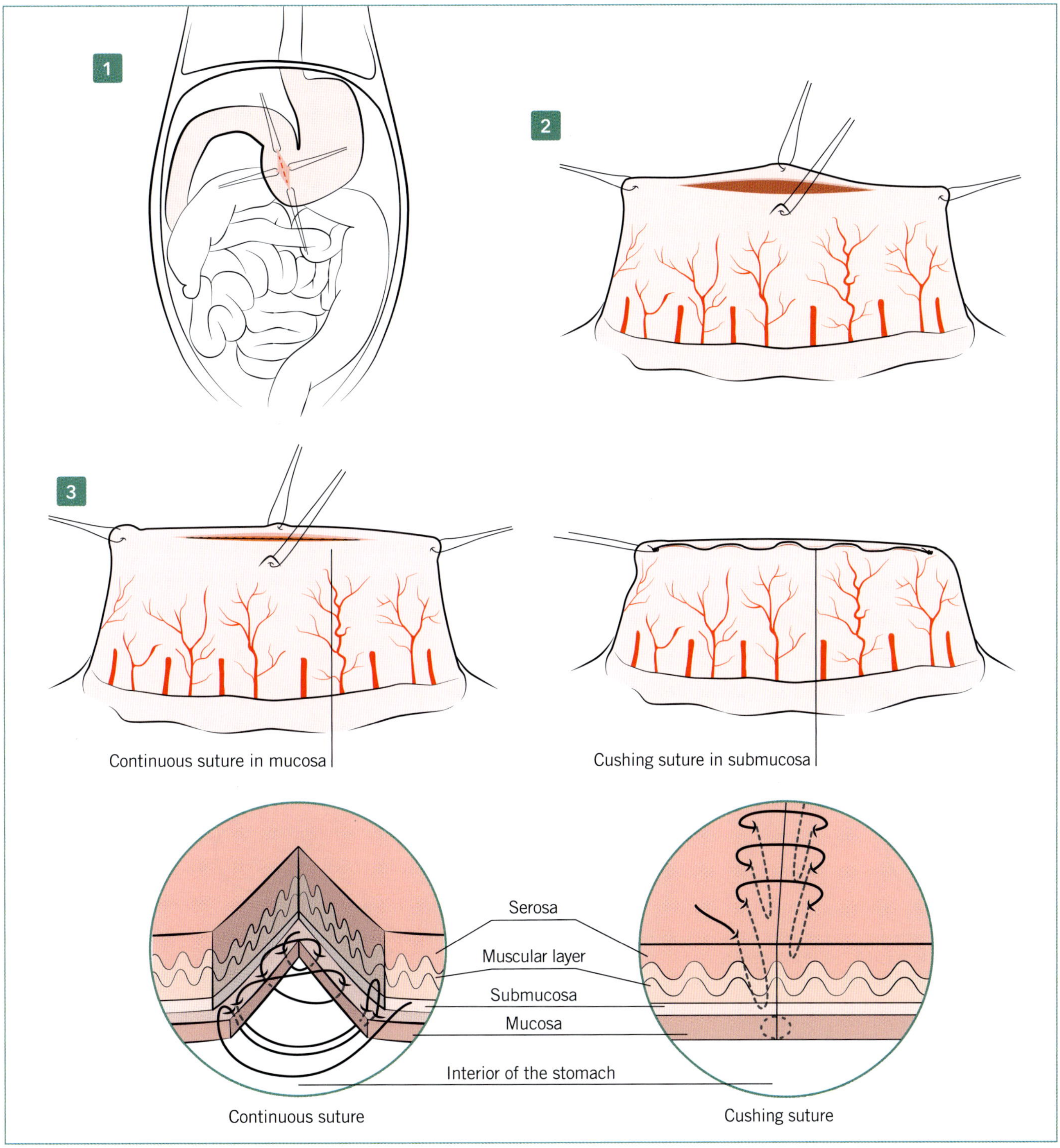

FIGURE 7. Steps in the gastrotomy technique.

1. The incision is made in an intermediary area with little vascularization between the greater and lesser curvatures. Along the main axis of the stomach, where the incision will be made, two stay sutures are placed though almost the full thickness of the wall (including the submucosa) with a distance of 10 cm between them. Two additional stay sutures can be placed, one on each side of the incision to facilitate the approach and handling.
2. Two cuts with the scalpel are usually needed to fully incise the gastric wall. Once incised, the cut in the mucosa is widened with Metzenbaum scissors. This maneuver and the following ones are done with the assistant applying traction to the stay sutures to maintain the opening at a higher plane with respect to the rest of the organ.
3. Once the surgery has concluded, the gastrotomy site is closed with a double layer of suture: the first closure of the mucosa with a simple continuous suture, and over it, a partial-thickness inverting Cushing suture, including submucosa.

Postoperative care

During the patient's postoperative hospital stay:

- The cat's head must be kept elevated to prevent gastro-esophageal reflux.
- Antacids are administered (omeprazole twice per day, or ranitidine to additionally stimulate gastric emptying).
- Food is first given after 12 hours if there is no vomiting and if the patient is no longer sedated. If feeding through a tube, only a quarter ration is given on the first day, slowly increasing the amount on each subsequent day.
- Antiemetics (maropitant) and mucosal protective agents (sucralfate) are administered for 4–8 days, depending on the reason for the surgery.
- Fluid therapy is administered for at least 48 hours.

Complications

Complications associated with gastric surgery include suture dehiscence, bleeding and infections. Dehiscence of gastric sutures occurs much less frequently than in the intestine, since it is done in two layers and the organ walls are very thick. Infection (septic peritonitis) has only been described in cases where there is leakage of gastrotomy tubes due to poor placement technique or chronic gastropexy failure.

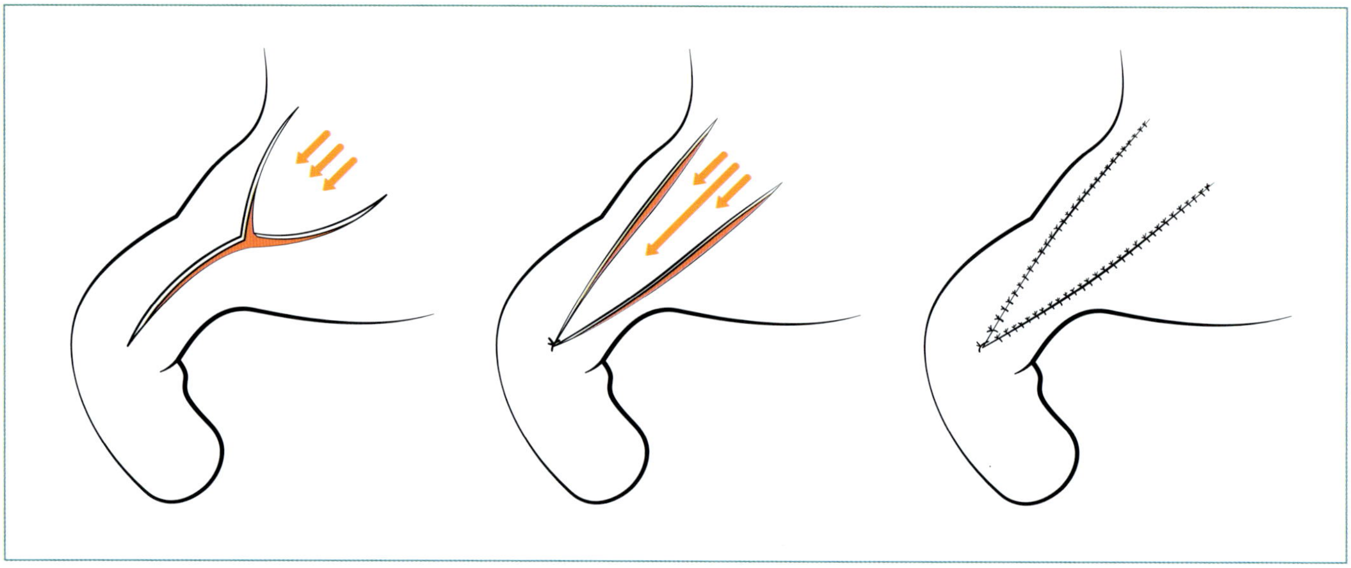

FIGURE 8. Flap and suture in a Y-U pyloroplasty.

Bibliography

Barnes JA. Digestive system. In: Hudson LC, Hamilton WP (eds.). *Atlas of Feline Anatomy for Veterinarians*, 2nd ed. Jackson, WY: Teton Newmedia, 2010; pp. 100–105; 153–170.

Basher AW, Fowler JD. Conservative versus surgical management of gastrointestinal linear foreign bodies in the cat. *Vet Surg*, 1987; 16(2):135–138.

Bebchuk TN. Feline gastrointestinal foreign bodies. *Vet Clin North Am Small Anim Pract*, 2002; 32(4):861–880.

Boysen SR, Tidwell AS, Penninck DG. Ultrasonographic findings in dogs and cats with gastrointestinal perforation. *Vet Radiol Ultrasound*, 2003; 44(5):556–564.

Bright RM, Sackman JE, DeNovo C, Toal C. Hiatal hernia in the dog and cat: a retrospective study of 16 cases. *J Small Anim Pract*, 1990; 31(5):244–250.

Bright RM. Y-U pyloroplasty. In: Bojrab MJ (ed.). *Current Techniques in Small Animal Surgery*, 4th ed. Baltimore, MD: Williams & Wilkins, 1998; pp.194–195.

Cariou MP, Halfacree ZJ, Lee KC, Baines SJ. Successful surgical management of spontaneous gastric perforations in three cats. *J Feline Med Surg*, 2010; 12(1):36–41.

Center SA. Diseases of the gallbladder and biliary tree. In: Guiford WG, Center SA, Strombeck DR et al. (eds.). *Strombeck's Small Animal Gastroenterology*, 3rd ed. Philadelphia: WB Saunders, 1996; p. 860.

Dulisch ML. Gastrotomy. In: Bojrab MJ (ed.). *Current Techniques in Small Animal Surgery*, 4th ed. Baltimore, MD: Williams & Wilkins, 1998; pp. 187–188.

Evans KL, Smeak DD, Biller DS. Gastrointestinal linear foreign bodies in 32 dogs: a retrospective evaluation and feline comparison. *J Am Anim Hosp Assoc*, 1994; 30(5):445–450.

Evans SE, Bonczynski JJ, Broussard JD et al. Comparison of endoscopic and full-thickness biopsy specimens for diagnosis of inflammatory bowel disease and alimentary tract lymphoma in cats. *J Am Vet Med Assoc*, 2006; 229(9):1447–1450.

Forman MA, Steiner JM, Armstrong PJ et al. ACVIM consensus statement on pancreatitis in cats. *J Vet Intern Med*, 2021; 35(2):703–723.

Fossum TS, Rohn DA, Willard MD. Presumptive, iatrogenic gastric outflow obstruction associated with prior gastric surgery. *J Am Anim Hosp Assoc*, 1995; 31(5):391–395.

Gualtieri M, Monzeglio MG, Scanziani E. Gastric neoplasia. *Vet Clin North Am Small Anim Pract*, 1999; 29(2):415–440.

Halfacree ZJ. Stomach. In: Langley-Hobbs SJ, Demetriou JL, Ladlow JF (eds.). *Feline Soft Tissue and General Surgery*, 1st ed. Oxford, UK: Saunders Elsevier, 2014; pp. 301–312.

Hall JA, Washabau RJ. Diagnosis and treatment of gastric motility disorders. *Vet Clin North Am Small Anim Pract*, 1999; 29(2):377–395.

Hall JA. Clinically evaluating gastric disease in dogs and cats. *Vet Med*, 2000; 95(1):450–465.

Hickman MA, Cox SR, Mahabir S et al. Safety, pharmacokinetics and use of the novel NK-1 receptor antagonist maropitant (Cerenia™) for the prevention of emesis and motion sickness in cats. *J Vet Pharmacol Ther*, 2008; 31(3):220–229.

Hudson J. Gastrointestinal disease. In: Holland M, Hudson J (eds.). *Feline Diagnostic Imaging*, 1st ed. Hoboken, NJ: Wiley & Sons, 2020; pp. 347–379.

Hudson J. Normal gastrointestinal anatomy. In: Holland M, Hudson J (eds.). *Feline Diagnostic Imaging*, 1st ed. Hoboken, NJ: Wiley & Sons, 2020; pp. 333–346.

Kleinschmidt S, Nolte I, Hewicker-Trautwein M. Structural and functional components of the feline enteric nervous system. *Anat Histol Embryol*, 2011; 40(6):450–456.

Liptak JM, Hunt GB, Barrs VR et al. Gastroduodenal ulceration in cats: eight cases and a review of the literature. *J Feline Med Surg*, 2002; 4(1):27–42.

Little SE. Diseases of the stomach. In: Little SE (ed.). *The Cat. Clinical Medicine and Management*, 1st ed. St. Louis, MO: Elsevier Saunders, 2012; pp. 450–458.

Marolf AJ, Bachand AM, Sharber J, Twedt DC. Comparison of endoscopy and sonography findings in dogs and cats with histologically confirmed gastric neoplasia. *J Small Anim Pract*, 2015; 56(5):339–344.

McGill SE, Lenard ZM, See AM, Irwin PJ. Nonsurgical treatment of gastroesophageal intussusception in a puppy. *J Am Anim Hosp Assoc*, 2009; 45(4):185–190.

Moore PF, Rodriguez-Bertos A, Kass PH. Feline gastrointestinal lymphoma: mucosal architecture, immunophenotype and molecular clonality. *Vet Pathol*, 2012; 49(4):658–668.

Newell SM, Graham JP, Roberts GD et al. Sonography of the normal feline gastrointestinal tract. *Vet Radiol Ultrasound*, 1999; 40(1):40–43.

Salinardi BJ, Harkin KR, Bulmer BJ, Roush JK. Comparison of complications of percutaneous endoscopic versus surgically placed gastrotomy tubes in 42 dogs and 52 cats. *J Am Anim Hosp Assoc*, 2006; 42(1):51–56.

Tobias K. Gastrotomía (cap. 18). In: Tobias K (ed.). *Manual de cirugía de tejidos blandos en pequeños animales*, 2nd ed. Sant Cugat del Vallès, Barcelona: Multimédica Ediciones Veterinarias, 2019; pp. 93–96.

Trepanier L. Acute vomiting in cats: rational treatment selection. *J Feline Med Surg*, 2010; 12(3):225–230.

van Geffen C, Saunders JH, Vandevelde B et al. Idiopatic megaoesophagus and intermittent gastro-oesophageal intussusception in a cat. *J Small Anim Pract*, 2006; 47(8):471–475.

Washabau RJ. Gastrointestinal mobility disorders and gastrointestinal prokinetic therapy. *Vet Clin North Am Small Anim Pract*, 2003; 33(5):1007–1028.

INTESTINAL FOREIGN BODIES AND TUMORS 22

Anna Calvet

Surgical anatomy

The small intestine is the portion of the digestive system that runs from the exit of the stomach (**pylorus**) to the large intestine (**ileocecal valve**). It is divided into three parts, the **duodenum**, **jejunum** and **ileum**.

The function of the initial part of the small intestine is secretory, while the final section has an absorptive function.

In the initial section of the duodenum, shortly after the exit of the stomach, is the **major duodenal papilla**, into which the **pancreatic duct** and the **common bile duct** or ductus choledochus drain (Fig. 1). In approximately 20% of cases we will also find a **minor duodenal papilla**, into which an **accessory pancreatic duct** drains.

The blood supply comes basically from branches of the **cranial mesenteric artery**, which divides into 12–15 **jejunal arteries**; these anastomose with each other creating arches from which the **vasa recta** emerge (these straight vessels form a vascular network under the serosa and submucosa).

The duodenal branches of the cranial and caudal **pancreaticoduodenal artery** supply the duodenum.

The ileum is supplied by branches of the **ileocolic artery** at the mesenteric border and by antimesenteric ileal branches of the **cecal artery**.

Venous drainage occurs through the **cranial mesenteric vein** that empties into the **portal vein** (Fig. 2).

The lymph nodes are basically located in the root of the mesentery, although we can also find smaller ones closer to the intestine. The hepatic and colic lymph nodes also drain part of the intestinal lymph.

As for innervation, the fibers that reach the mesenteric portion are branches of the **vagus nerve** and the **splanchnic nerve**.

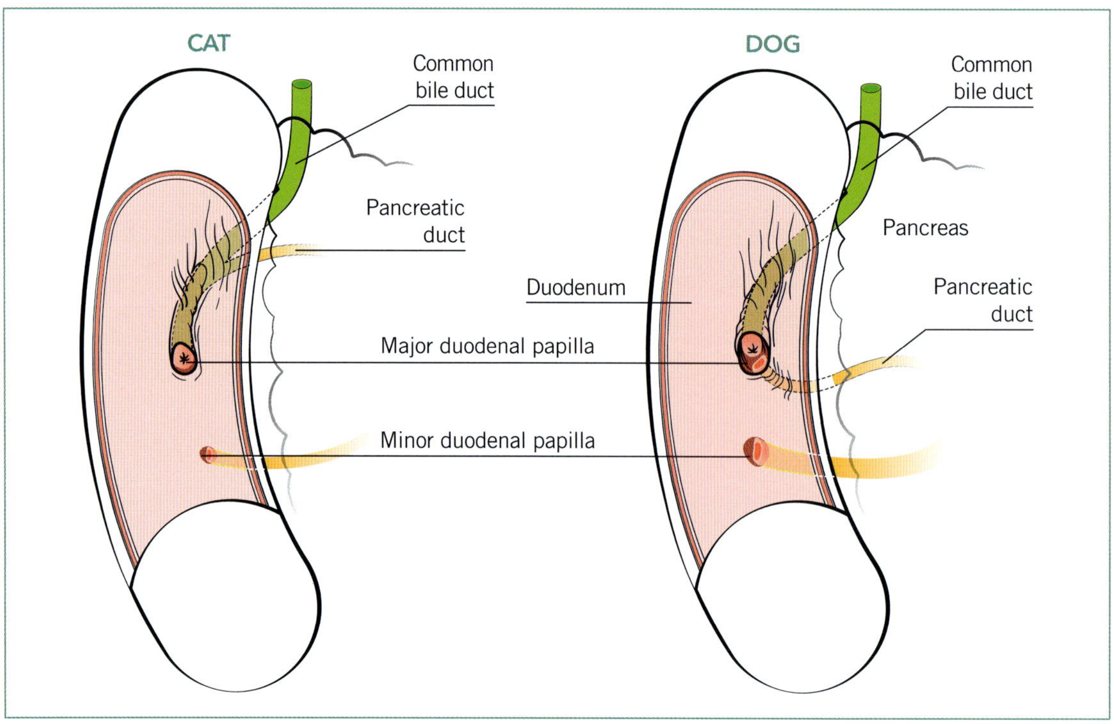

FIGURE 1. In the cat, the pancreatic duct joins the common bile duct before emptying into the duodenum.

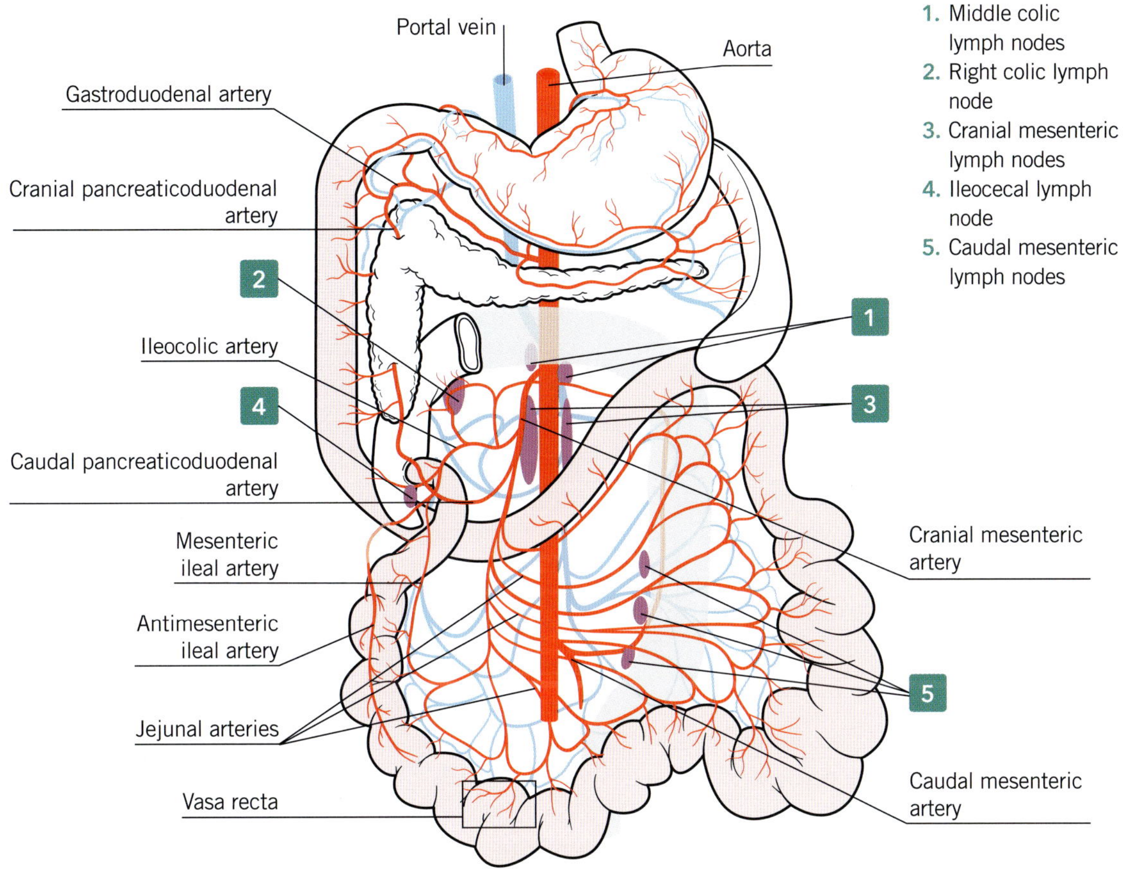

FIGURE 2. Vascularization and lymph nodes of the small intestine.

The intestine is composed of several layers, which from the outermost to the innermost include the (Fig. 3):

- **Serosa:** corresponding to the lining formed by the visceral peritoneum.
- **Muscularis:** formed by two layers, one that is more external, longitudinal, and one that is more internal, circular.
- **Submucosa:** rich in collagen, resistant and a base for suture attachment.
- **Mucosa:** formed by a layer of columnar epithelial cells mixed with a variable amount of **goblet cells**, another kind of columnar cells specialized in mucus secretion (they are present in other epithelia as well, such as the respiratory or reproductive epithelia). The mucosal villi increase the surface area about 15 times.

The small intestine is responsible for pushing the food bolus, starting at its exit from the stomach to the large intestine. Intestinal motility is a combination of peristaltic contractions, which if decreased can lead to paralytic ileus, and segmental

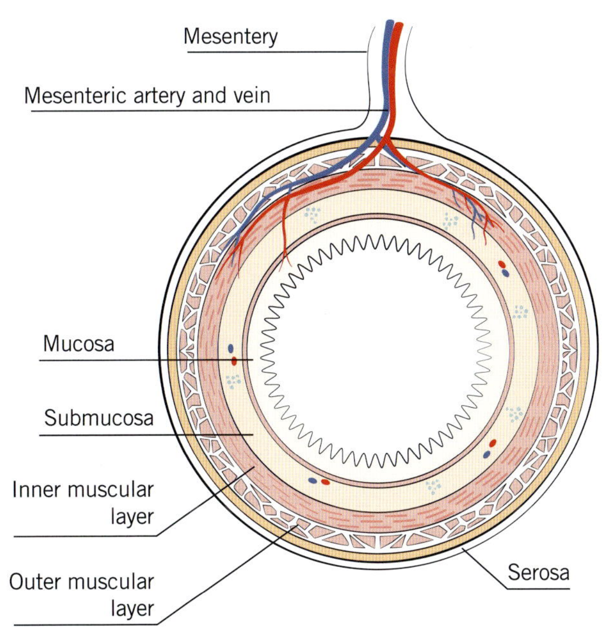

FIGURE 3. Layers of the small intestine.

contractions, which if decreased can lead to diarrhea (this is because segmental contractions are stimulated when the intestine is full, thus slowing the passage of food and causing digestion and absorption to be more effective).

General diagnostic approach to surgical diseases of the intestine

Clinical signs

In a cat with gastrointestinal disease, weight loss and anorexia are as common as vomiting.

> In the case of foreign bodies, we must keep in mind that cats, more so than other species, are prone to the ingestion of linear foreign bodies, so we must always examine under the tongue, where these objects tend to remain anchored.

Given a similar clinical picture, in young kittens we will tend to suspect infectious processes or an obstruction due to the ingestion of a foreign body, while in an adult or older cat a condition of a chronic inflammatory or tumoral origin will be more frequent (although we can never rule out that they have eaten something inadequate).

Pathophysiology of obstruction

Mechanical obstructions of the bowel may have various causes:

- Luminal: lodgement of a foreign body.
- Intramural: neoplasms.
- Extramural: due to adhesions.

Complete intestinal obstruction is characterized by a buildup of fluid and gas. Fluid accumulates due to increased secretion, decreased absorption and lack of drainage. Gas accumulates due to aerophagia and fermentation of contents (Fig. 4).

This fluid and gas accumulation increases intramural and intraluminal pressures. Under normal conditions, these pressures range from 2 to 4 mmHg and at their peaks, corresponding to peristaltic contractions, they rise to 12–25 mmHg. In case of obstruction, lymphatic and capillary stasis occurs starting at 30 mmHg and at 50 mmHg venous drainage is compromised.

Arterial blood supply is generally unaffected, resulting in increased capillary hydrostatic pressure and causing edema in the intestinal wall that may eventually move through the serosa into the abdominal cavity.

Circulatory compromise leads to hypoxia and ischemia. Also, the permeability of the mucosa increases, resulting in bacterial and toxin translocation to the abdominal cavity.

Partial obstructions can have a long course, even weeks. In contrast, complete obstructions, especially proximal obstructions, present more acutely and the cat's condition deteriorates more rapidly (Table 1).

> The small intestine under normal conditions contains very few bacteria, but after only 6 hours of stasis, the number of bacteria in the small intestine increases considerably.

Diagnostic tests

Radiology

In patients with bowel disease, different radiographic findings can be seen on lateral and ventrodorsal abdominal projections (Fig. 5):

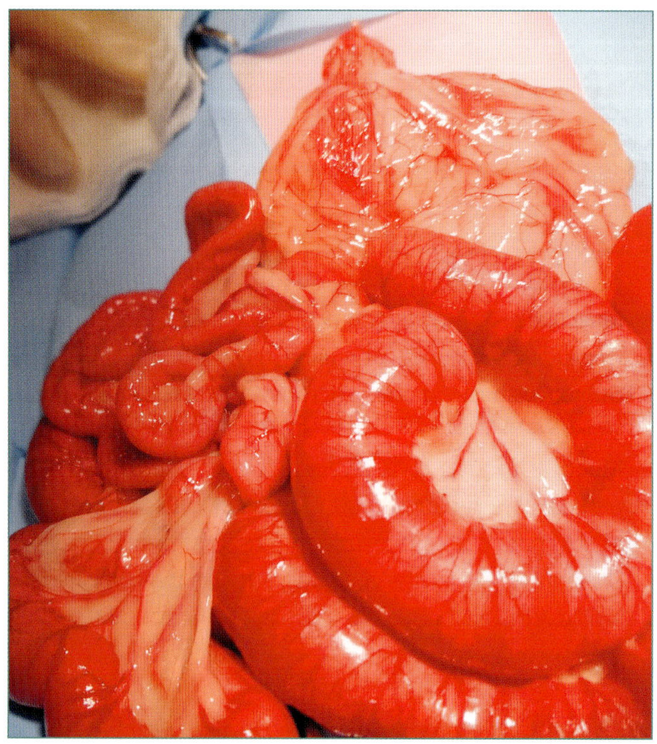

FIGURE 4. This image shows the difference in diameter between the normal and the dilated small intestine (proximal to the obstruction).

TABLE 1. Clinical signs of intestinal obstruction

Obstructed area	Clinical signs
Duodenum	■ Rapid progression ■ Vomiting associated with eating ■ Vomiting of bile ■ Dehydration ■ Abdominal pain
Jejunum	■ Slower progression ■ Vomiting may not occur ■ Diarrhea ■ Dehydration ■ Weight loss ■ Abdominal pain

- Gas-filled intestine.
- Dilated bowel: we can use a quantitative index by calculating the quotient between the maximum diameter of the small intestine and the maximum height of the second lumbar vertebra (L2). The probability of an obstruction if the result is more than 3 is over 70%. A result greater than 2 is indicative of intestinal disease.
- Corrugated bowel, indicative of a linear foreign body.
- Mass effect: displacement of adjacent viscera.
- Radiopaque foreign body.

Contrast X-rays may also be performed if nothing conclusive is observed. Barium sulfate will be used for this purpose, unless an intestinal perforation is suspected, in which case an iodinated contrast agent should be utilized.

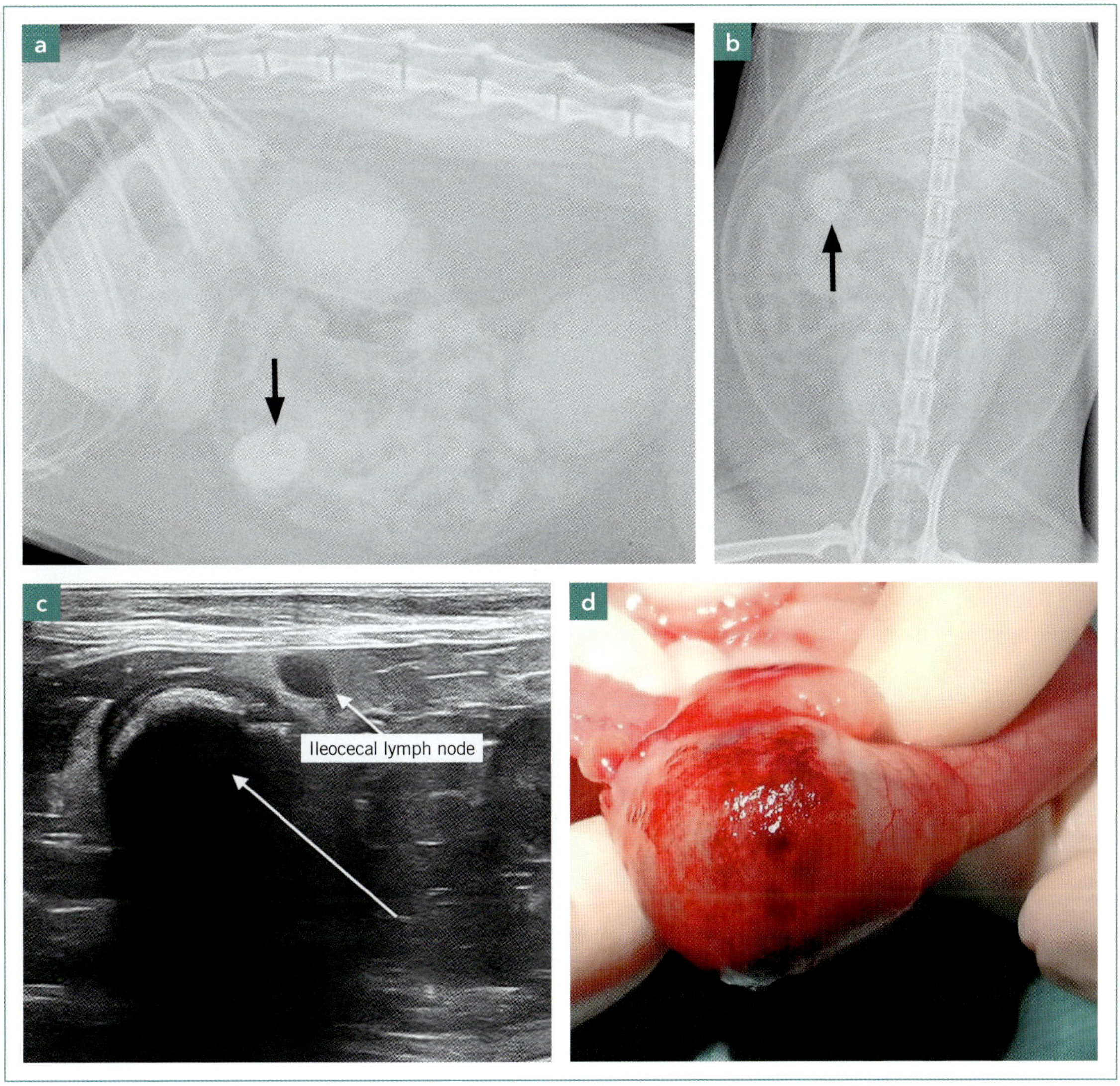

FIGURE 5. (a) Lateral and (b) ventrodorsal X-rays, (c) ultrasound and (d) intraoperative image of a patient with typhlitis. The intraoperative image corresponds to a carcinoma, but X-rays and ultrasound only indicated the site of the lesion due to the presence of impacted feces.

Ultrasound

Ultrasonography provides us with a lot of information on the bowel disease and currently seems to have displaced X-rays, but the combined information from both tests is more helpful.

Thanks to ultrasound we can:

- Observe the intestinal layers, their size, preservation or focal alterations that may exist.
- Detect the specific sign of intussusception (Fig. 6).
- Directly observe a mass, with the ability to perform a fine needle aspiration and guide the diagnosis.
- Evaluate motility.
- Detect linear foreign bodies in a noninvasive manner.
- Observe the effect of obstructions, even if the cause is not detected (Fig. 7).
- Discover enlarged lymph nodes, even if the bowel appearance is within the normal range, which will indicate that we should take samples for biopsy.

Endoscopy

Endoscopy is generally a less invasive option to study the upper intestinal tract. It is preferred for the observation of lesions and the extraction of foreign bodies from the esophagus and stomach. Its limitation, however, is that in the intestine it only reaches as far as the duodenum, and the entire length of the intestine cannot be explored.

Ultrasound in the case of suspected obstruction

When the abdomen of a patient with suspected intestinal obstruction is evaluated ultrasonographically, it is possible to observe a portion of the intestine, the portion proximal to the obstruction, with liquid content and dilated, and the intestine distal to the obstruction, which is normal. Cats with a clinical suspicion, but without clear ultrasound signs, and that are stable, can be hospitalized with intravenous fluid therapy for repeat testing at 6–8 hours. Sometimes fluid content is not seen initially because the cat has not eaten anything in the last 24–48 hours, has vomited and is dehydrated, so once the dehydration is resolved, this ultrasound sign may "appear."

In principle, it is impossible to recover intestinal foreign bodies by endoscopy and for biopsies we must remember that it is not possible to collect full-thickness samples.

Abdominocentesis

It is indicated if peritonitis or peritoneal effusion is suspected. It is performed by means of an ultrasound-guided puncture of four quadrants. If the result is negative or inconclusive, we can try to take a sample a few hours after starting fluid therapy, since many of these patients are in shock at the time of admission.

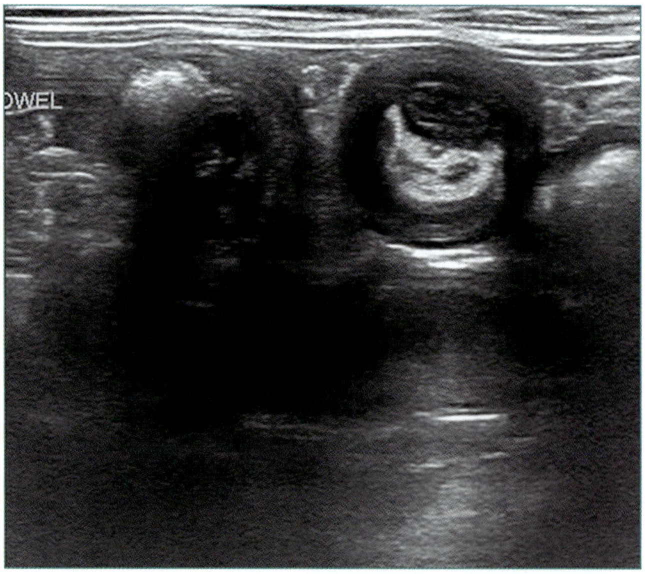

FIGURE 6. Typical ultrasound image of an intussusception: the dilated bowel with its contents is observed, a more echogenic one corresponding to trapped and inflamed mesenteric fat and next to it an image of the bowel trapped in the bowel itself. Eight intestinal layers can be counted.

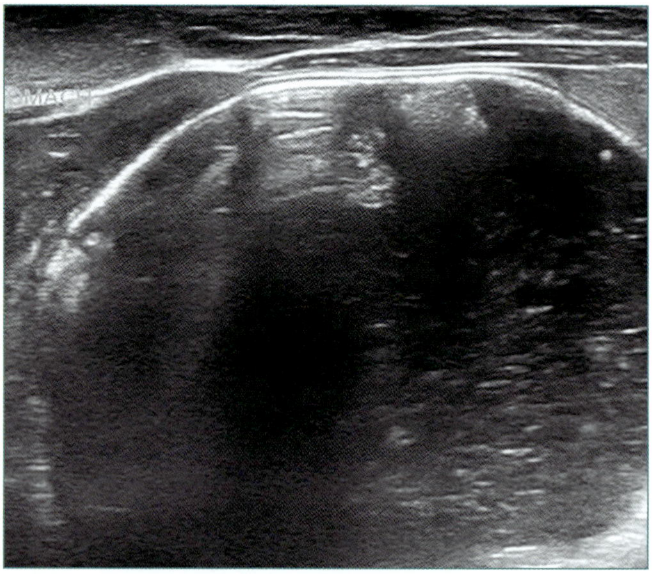

FIGURE 7. Ultrasound of a dilated stomach, filled with liquid contents due to a more distal intestinal obstruction.

The fluid sample obtained should be analyzed and submitted for culture.

It is not unusual, if we submit a pus sample for culture, for the result to be negative, even though we have observed numerous bacteria in the cytology of that same sample. For this reason, it is recommended that an epiploon/omentum or peritoneal biopsy be sent for culture.

Blood testing

Full blood work is important to be able to correct, whenever possible, dehydration and electrolyte disorders before induction of anesthesia.

If the hematocrit is below 20%, we must be prepared with blood products for possible transfusion.

Surgical pathologies of the small intestine

Foreign bodies

Approximately half of the foreign bodies ingested by cats are linear.

Foreign bodies can cause complete or partial obstructions. The clinical signs will vary depending on the type of obstruction and its location, whether more cranial or caudal.

Partial obstructions can sometimes be treated medically with close monitoring of the patient, although it is essential for the patient to continue to ingest some food or for intestinal motility to be maintained and transit not to be prolonged over a long period of time.

Complete proximal obstructions may be detected within 6 hours after ingestion of the foreign body, while more distal complete obstructions may take 24 hours.

Foreign bodies can vary widely: toys, pieces of cloth, plastic, cellophane, olive pits, and even needles (which we must remember can make the complete transit without causing problems, unless they are accompanied by thread) (Fig. 8).

Radiologically, there are radiopaque and radiotransparent foreign bodies. Even if the object is not seen on the X-ray, signs of distension can be seen proximal to the obstruction, which will be accompanied by blood work abnormalities and clinical signs.

In thin cats, the presence of a foreign body can be diagnosed during abdominal palpation.

Linear objects are usually a more complicated process, as they may be anchored under the tongue or in the stomach. Due to intestinal motility, this anchor point will cause the intestine to fold in on itself (Fig. 9).

Initially, linear foreign bodies can be treated by cutting the anchor point, but multiple enterotomies are almost always required for removal (Fig. 10).

Making few cuts, insufficient to fragment the foreign body when gently removing it, may cause ruptures on the mesenteric side of the intestinal wall. Although the prognosis for intestinal surgery is favorable in the cat, when there is intestinal perforation, survival drops to 50%.

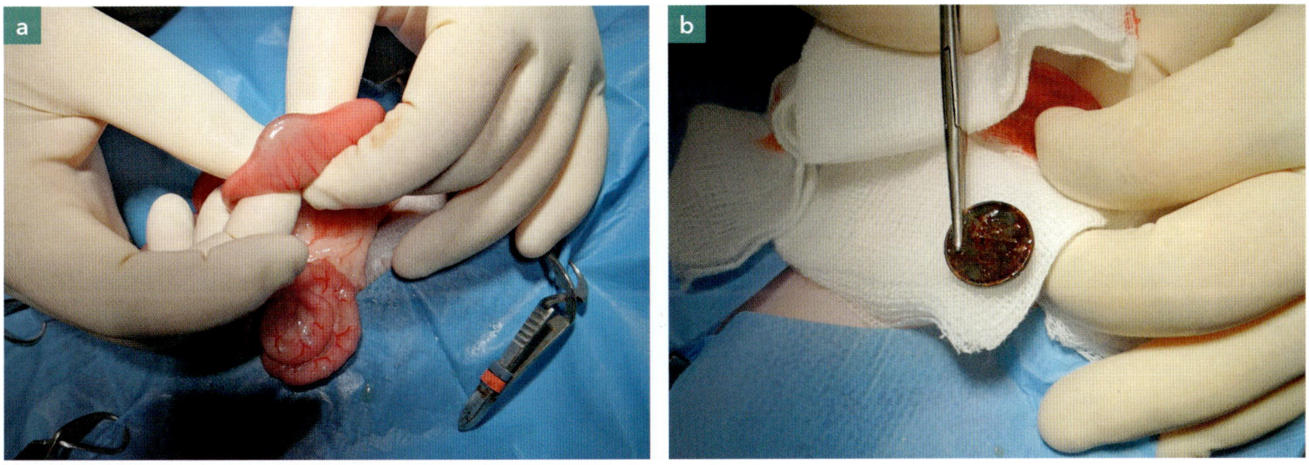

FIGURE 8. (a) Localization and (b) removal of an intestinal foreign body.

In cases that last days, fibrosis may occur, maintaining intestinal plication despite foreign body removal. Enterectomy and anastomosis is required in these patients.

Intussusception

The pathogenesis of intussusception is unknown but, in general, we can say that in cats there are two groups of patients:

- Young cats less than 1 year old with parasitosis.
- Cats older than 6 years with tumor-associated intussusception.

Intussusception has also been diagnosed in cats that have previously undergone abdominal surgery.

All these patients usually present with vomiting, anorexia, lethargy, dehydration and usually poor body condition. The ultrasound diagnosis is clear in these cases.

As for surgical treatment, reduction of the lesion can be attempted, but sometimes an enterectomy is all that can be done (Fig. 11).

The recommendation to perform enteroplication after treating intussusception is controversial, since the complications associated with this procedure are more significant than the recurrence rate reduction achieved.

Mesenteric volvulus

Mesenteric volvulus occurs when the intestine rotates on its mesenteric axis. It is rare in cats, there are few cases described in the literature and in general the prognosis is not good. In the few cases of survival described, acting quickly, stabilizing as much as possible and transfusion (the cats presented with signs

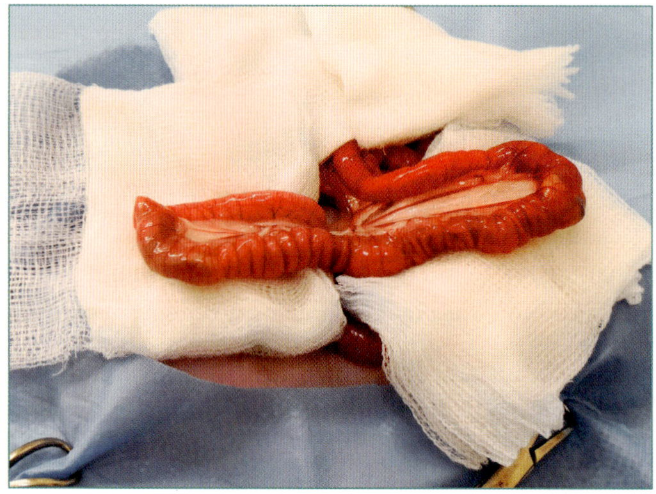

FIGURE 9. Intestinal plication caused by a linear foreign body.

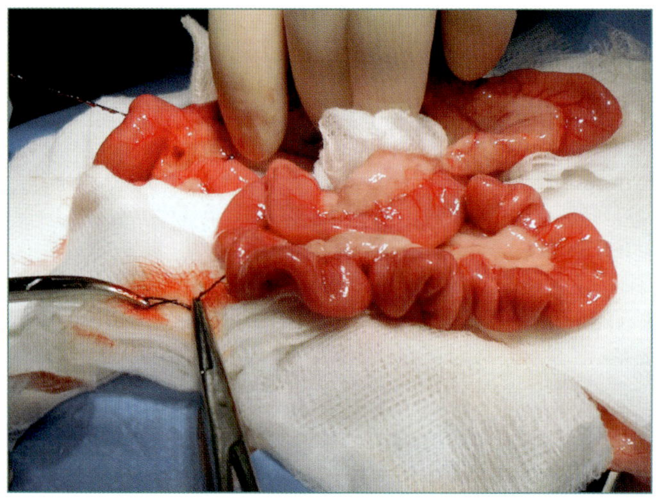

FIGURE 10. Two enterotomies for removal of a linear foreign body. Thread fragments of the linear object can be seen.

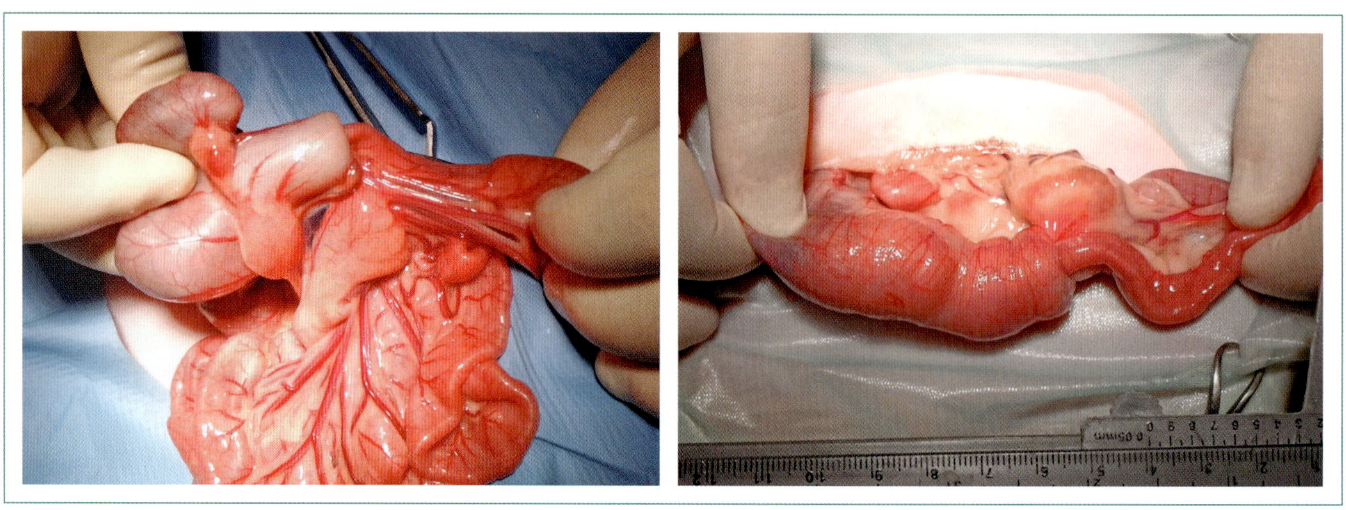

FIGURE 11. Intraoperative images of intussusception.

of acute abdomen and a hematocrit below 10%) may have been the reasons for success.

The onset of clinical signs is acute, cats quickly go into shock. In this case, X-rays are better for diagnosis, since the intestine is distended and filled with gas.

Trauma

Intestinal trauma may be secondary to abdominal injury or suture dehiscence resulting in evisceration. With a rapid response and adequate antibiotic treatment, the evolution can be good.

Occasionally, we may be able to wash out and reintroduce the affected bowel, but it is more likely that the exposed part of the bowel will have to be removed.

Neoplasia

The most frequently diagnosed tumors are lymphoma, adenocarcinoma and mast cell tumors.

Lymphoma may present as a diffuse infiltrative lesion or as a nodular lesion (Fig. 12). Regarding its cellular typology it can be:

- Low-grade lymphoma, one of the most frequent in the cat's digestive tract, also called small cell lymphoma or lymphocytic lymphoma. It usually consists mainly of T cells.
- Intermediate/high-grade lymphoma or lymphoblastic lymphoma, which may be composed of B or T cells.
- Large granular lymphocyte lymphoma, which is actually a subtype consisting mainly of NK (natural killer) T cells.

Intestinal lymphomas can be more or less aggressive. Patients with mucosally circumscribed lymphoma and those with small cell lymphoma can survive more than 2 years with treatment.

> If a nodular lesion is observed, it is advisable to remove it before starting chemotherapy for lymphoma because there is a risk of rupture, since chemotherapy could weaken the intestinal wall.

Intestinal adenocarcinoma usually presents as a segmental, annular lesion and accounts for 25%–30% of intestinal neoplasms. It is more common in older cats (average 10 years old) and in Asian breeds such as Siamese. Persians are predisposed. In 70% of cases it affects the small intestine. There may be metastases in regional lymph nodes.

Treatment is surgical, an enterectomy must be performed with margins of between 5 and 10 cm. Survival ranges between 0 and 24 months.

Intestinal **mast cell tumors** are the third most frequent neoplasms in the small intestine of the cat. Unlike the cutaneous and splenic forms of this tumor, feline intestinal mast cell tumors have an extremely variable biological behavior.

They most commonly affect the distal part of the small intestine or the large intestine. They may be associated with peritoneal effusion and may be nodular or multifocal.

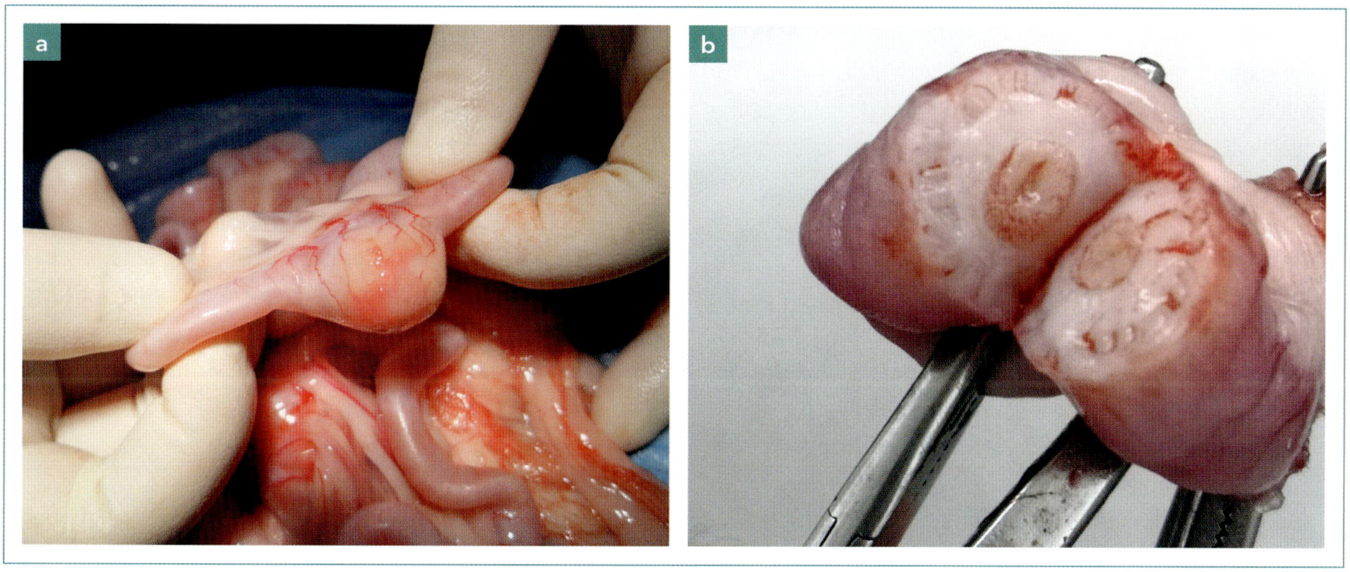

FIGURE 12. (a) Intestinal lymphoma. (b) Open nodule; note the decreased intestinal lumen.

They also tend to affect older cats. Median survival after diagnosis is approximately 1.5 years with treatment (with cortisone or receptor tyrosine kinase inhibitors). In the sclerosing variety of this same tumor, which also has a greater tendency to metastasize, the prognosis is guarded.

Nonneoplastic lesions: polyps and granulomas

Adenomatous polyps are benign lesions, but they can be recurrent if not well removed. They can develop in the most proximal portion of the duodenum, and therefore can sometimes be removed by endoscopy.

The average age at presentation is 12 years old, with a higher incidence in Siamese and Himalayan breeds. Approximately half of all cats present with anemia due to chronic blood loss.

In the course of feline infectious peritonitis (FIP), **granulomas** may form that may be mistaken for neoplasms. They are usually lesions that extend from the intestinal wall, forming a nodule. From an ultrasound and surgical perspective, granulomas are no different from other masses. In these cases, the difference lies in the clinical history, in the blood work findings and, frequently, in the presence of granulomas in other organs, in addition to the lymphadenopathy present in the exploratory laparotomy.

Preoperative and postoperative considerations

Aspects to be taken into account before and after the intervention:

- Intestinal obstructions cause severe acid–base and electrolyte imbalances. Fluid accumulation and dilatation of the intestinal tract proximal to the obstruction is associated with the possibility of hypovolemic shock.
- Whenever possible, as in other surgical cases, stabilization of the patient is extremely important.
- To avoid rhinitis or aspiration pneumonia due to a leakage of contents through the nostrils when sedating the patient, we will keep the patient's head elevated during induction and after intubation we will pass a tube down to the stomach to empty as much content as we can before placing the patient in dorsal recumbency.
- It is important to apply the proper surgical technique with effective and tight tissue apposition to minimize the most frequent complications, which are surgical dehiscence and septic peritonitis.
- It is essential to check motility in the postoperative period, since blood supply to the operated area depends to a large extent on the presence of peristalsis. In this regard, it is recommended to start enteral feeding early (6–8 hours after the intervention in awake and stable patients).
- Healing of the intestine goes through three phases: inflammation, proliferation and maturation. Of these three, the first is the most critical, as dehiscence and breakdown are most likely in the first 72–96 hours.

Surgical techniques

Indications for bowel surgery include:

- Extraction of foreign bodies
- Sampling
- Excision of resectable tumors
- Management of ulcerative lesions

Whichever technique we use, if there is an obstruction and there has been dilatation and an accumulation of gas or fluid in the intestinal section proximal to the obstruction, the first step will be decompression. To this end, we have already discussed how to empty the stomach by inserting a tube during induction. To empty the bowel we can use a 20-gauge needle coupled with a suction system, which can be an automatic aspirator or a system with a tube, a three-way stopcock and a 60 ml syringe.

Intestinal biopsy

Intestinal biopsy is performed by means of a midline laparotomy with cranial extension in order to properly explore the stomach, liver, biliary tract, spleen and pancreas. Normally intestinal biopsy is taken for histopathological analysis to indicate whether it is an inflammatory bowel disease or lymphoma, and to determine the origin in case of diffuse nodular lesions. In any case, it is always advisable to explore the entire abdomen for further lesions and to take lymph node samples.

The technique is described in Chapter 7 "Biopsy techniques and most common uses in feline medicine."

Enterotomy

The main indication for enterotomies is the removal of foreign bodies. In these surgeries the key points are to:

- Determine bowel viability: standard criteria are color, presence of pulse and peristalsis. After decompressing the affected bowel and removing the cause of the obstruction, it is necessary to wait a few minutes since changes in these signs may occur. As a general rule, we will remove any tissue that remains distended and has a grey, bluish or black color and does not bleed when it is cut.
- Determine the presence of possible discontinuities in the intestinal wall that may cause extravasation of intestinal contents and, therefore, cause peritonitis.
- Detect changes that occur in the viability and continuity of the intestine when foreign bodies are removed. This is especially important in linear foreign bodies, since, once removed, if they were very embedded in the mucosa and the intestine was very retracted, by returning it to its usual shape we can detect critical points that were not visible before the intervention.

Technique

1. After performing a laparotomy, the point of obstruction/foreign body is located. We isolate the fragment on which we are going to work and cover the rest of the exposed abdomen with moist sterile gauze.
2. The area is prepared by gently squeezing the intestinal contents in both directions to avoid extravasation. An atraumatic intestinal forceps (Doyen) is placed about 6–10 cm away or an assistant can isolate the area with their fingers.
3. For nonlinear foreign bodies, the next step is to make an incision immediately distal to the foreign body in the healthy bowel area with a no. 11 scalpel blade. The cut should be approximately the length of the diameter of the foreign body on the antimesenteric border.
4. The foreign body is carefully removed and the viability of the tissue and the absence of perforations are evaluated.
5. The bowel is closed with simple interrupted sutures. Depending on the surgeon's preference, enterotomy is also successfully resolved using a continuous suture.

Enterectomy and anastomosis

The indications for this surgery could be summarized as follows:

- Removal of tumors and nonneoplastic masses
- Areas with devitalized bowel
- Nonreducible bowel intussusceptions
- Eviscerated and contaminated bowel

Particularities when the foreign body is linear

First of all, the linear foreign body must be unanchored, either by cutting it under the cat's tongue or by means of a small gastrotomy if the origin is at that point.

Multiple enterotomies will be performed to avoid excessive traction. The greater the number of enterotomies, the greater the risk, but if we apply too much traction to reduce the number of enterotomies, intestinal perforation is even more likely, which is more difficult to control and has a worse prognosis.

Surgery should be performed soon after dislodging the foreign body lodged under the tongue. This is because when the bowel loses the abnormal plication, perforations may become evident and, in such a case, enterectomy of the affected segment should be performed.

Urinary catheter technique

This technique reduces the number of enterotomies required to one or two.

- As always, the first step is to unanchor the foreign body.
- We look for the proximal end of the linear foreign body and we tie or sew it to the tip of a catheter between 8 and 12 Fr in diameter (we can use vinyl urinary catheters or red rubber catheters; we look for them not to be too rigid).
- We introduce the catheter into the intestine and push it, advancing gently, dragging the foreign body with it.
- With a second enterotomy we remove the catheter along with the entire length of the foreign body.
- Longer catheters can be used to reach into the colon and out directly through the anus.

Technique

1. With the cat in dorsal recumbency, a midline laparotomy is performed. The area to be removed is located and isolated from the rest of the abdomen as described in other techniques.
2. There should always be about 2 cm of healthy tissue on both sides of the fragment to be resected.
3. The bowel is gently emptied by squeezing the contents on both sides and Carmalt or Doyen intestinal forceps are placed (Fig. 13.1).
4. We then locate the mesenteric vessels that irrigate the area to be removed and perform a double ligation. It is very important at this point, when we are about to cut, to leave enough mesentery to be able to suture it later without compromising vascularization.
5. When the bowel is resected, it is normal for mucosal eversion to occur and although it can be trimmed, this is not necessary.

> If the lumen of both bowel fragments is very uneven, the smaller diameter fragment should be cut diagonally to increase the area to be sutured.
>
> If the difference is even greater, two triangular flaps can be created.

6. The suture is always started on the mesenteric side, since the presence of fat and vasa recta makes this point the most complicated (Fig. 13.2).
7. We can choose between a simple interrupted suture pattern (in which case it is usually advisable to place the second stitch right in the middle of the suture area, at the antimesenteric midpoint), a continuous suture and later reinforce with simple interrupted sutures if necessary, or we can use the modified Gambee suture, which avoids grasping the entire mucosa to better seal the intestinal lumen. A 4-0 monofilament suture with atraumatic needle is used (Fig. 13.3).
8. We check that the suture is properly sealed with a leak test, injecting saline solution into the sutured bowel to look for leaks.
9. An omentum flap is placed, as with other techniques, and the abdomen is closed in a routine fashion.

Postoperative care

The main complications in intestinal surgery are suture dehiscence and peritonitis.

It is advisable to hospitalize cats for 24 hours after surgery in order to:

- Evaluate and perform correct postoperative pain control.
- Perform an ultrasound check at 24 hours to detect the presence of free fluid or signs of exaggerated swelling at the surgical site, paralytic ileus or obstruction.
- Detect the presence of fever or a leukogram with neutrophilia for closer monitoring of possible septic complications.
- Perform a new abdominal exploration at any sign of peritonitis.

In general, feline bowel surgery has a good prognosis; the complication rate in the absence of peritonitis/dehiscence is 7.2%. In any case, the literature shows that, in general, the rate of dehiscence-associated complications is lower than in dogs and, if they do occur, survival is higher than in the canine species.

Perioperative factors associated with an increased risk of dehiscence are:

- Previous peritonitis.
- Hypoalbuminemia (although less frequent than in dogs).
- Left-shift leukogram.
- Nature of the obstruction (tumors entail less risk than foreign bodies and, of these, there is less risk for simple than for linear ones). The fewer enterotomies, the better.

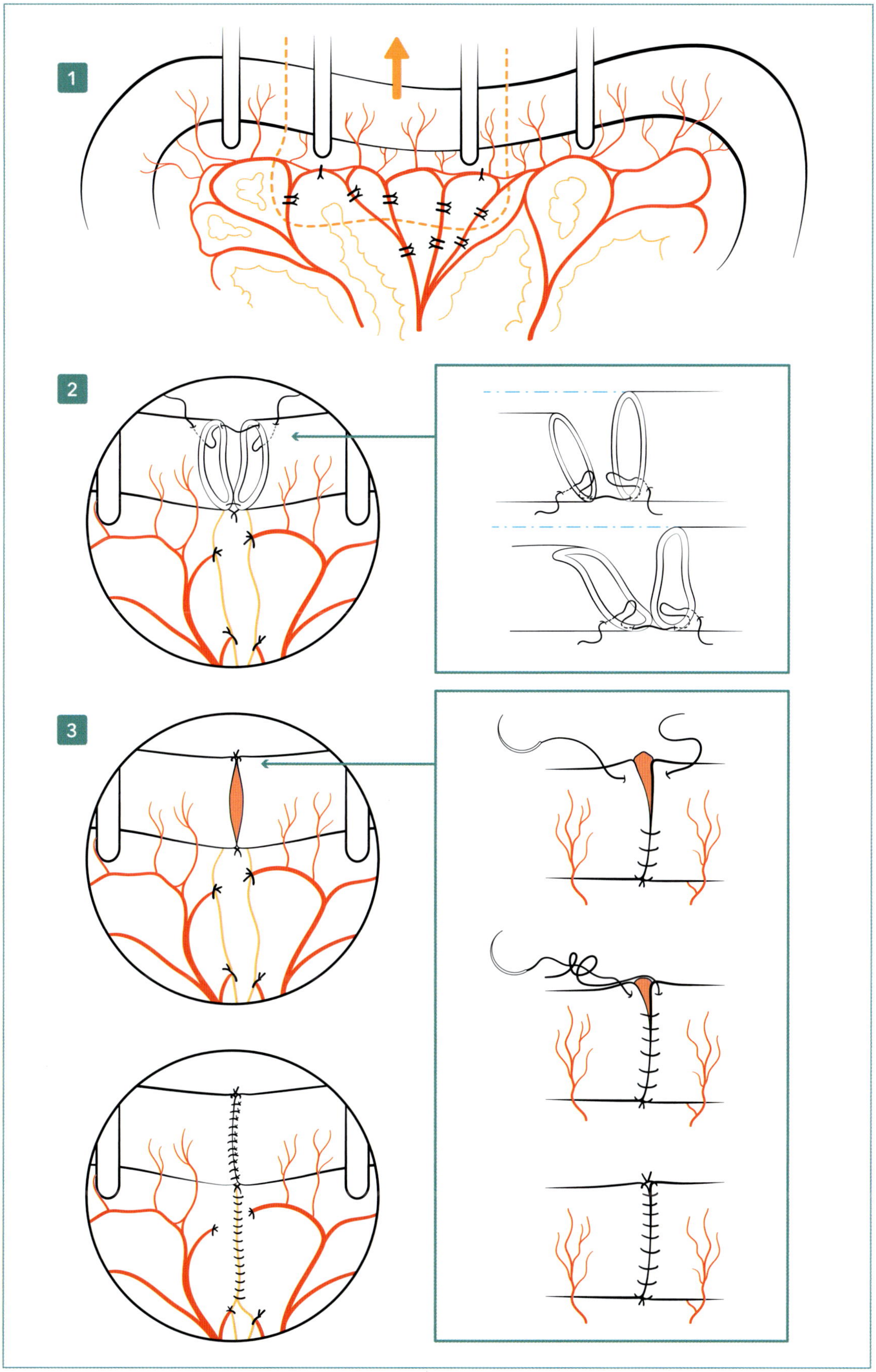

FIGURE 13. Steps of the enterectomy and anastomosis technique.

1. Placement of Doyen intestinal forceps leaving 2 cm of healthy tissue on each side of the planned resection site and on both sides of the mesenteric vessel cutting and ligation areas.
2. After apposition of the fragments, one suture is applied on the mesenteric side and another on the antimesenteric side. The mucosa may protrude through the opening.
3. Closure is continued with simple continuous or interrupted sutures. It is not necessary to trim the mucosa; when adjusting the stitches, a sliding maneuver can be performed to invaginate the mucosa. The mesentery defect must also be sutured.

Short bowel syndrome

We cannot finish without discussing how much intestine we can remove in an enterectomy, since the resection of large portions of small intestine produces maldigestion, malabsorption, diarrhea, bacterial overgrowth and gastric hypersecretion, which is known as short bowel syndrome.

The possibility of developing this syndrome depends on:

- The amount of tissue removed
- The location of the resection
- The time needed for the intestine to adapt

As for localization, in the duodenum and the initial portion of the jejunum resection produces a decrease in the amount of pancreatic enzymes, since the hormones that stimulate their secretion are secreted in the wall of the intestine. On the other hand, if we have to resect the ileocecal valve, we facilitate the entry of bacteria from the large intestine that can overgrow in the small intestine.

Over time, the remaining intestine increases in diameter, increasing the number of villi and, ultimately, it adapts. This adaptation may take a few weeks.

Given that this is a process that is not compensated, it is recommended to administer a low-fat diet, antibiotics that are not well absorbed in the intestine, such as neomycin, and to supplement as needed with pancreatic enzymes, vitamin B, antidiarrheals, medium-chain triglycerides and other dietary supplements.

Bibliography

Adams WM, Sisterman LA, Klauer JM et al. Association of intestinal disorders in cats with findings of abdominal radiography. *J Am Vet Med Assoc*, 2010; 236(8):880–886.

Applewhite AA, Hawthorne JC, Cornell KK. Complications of enteroplication for the prevention of intussusception recurrence in dogs: 35 cases (1989–1999). *J Am Vet Med Assoc*, 2001; 219(10):1415–1418.

de Laforcade AM. Management of septic peritonitis in dogs and cats. World Small Animal Veterinary Association World Congress Proceedings, Geneva, Switzerland, 2010.

Felts JF, Fox PR, Burk RL. Thread and sewing needles as gastrointestinal foreing bodies in the cat: a review of 64 cases. *J Am Vet Med Assoc*, 1984; 184(1):56–59.

Gabor LJ, Canfield PJ, Malik R. Haematological and biochemical findings in cats in Australia with lymphosarcoma. *Aust Vet J*, 2000; 78(7):456–461.

Gorman SC, Freeman LM, Mitchell SL, Chan DL. Extensive small bowel resection in dogs and cats: 20 cases (1998–2004). *J Am Vet Med Assoc*, 2006; 228(3):403–407.

Haider G, Leschnik K, Katic N, Dupré G. Enteroplication in cats with intussusception: a retrospective study (2001–2016). *J Feline Med Surg*, 2019; 21(6):488–494.

Neiger R, Robertson E, Stengel C. Gastrointestinal endoscopy in the cat: diagnostics and therapeutics. *J Feline Med Surg*, 2013; 15(11):993–1005.

Ralphs SC, Jessen CR, Lipowitz AJ. Risk factors for leakage following intestinal anastomosis in dogs and cats: 115 cases (1991–2000). *J Am Vet Med Assoc*, 2003; 223(1):73–77.

Sabattini S, Giantin M, Barbanera A et al. Feline intestinal mast cell tumours: clinicopathological characterisation and KIT mutation analysis. *J Feline Med Surg*, 2016; 18(4):280–289.

PERIANAL SURGERY 23

Anna Calvet

Surgical anatomy

The rectum is the segment of the large intestine that ends at the anus after passing through the pelvic canal. The anatomical landmarks used to determine the colorectal junction (which is difficult to locate) are the pelvic brim, the pelvic inlet, the last lumbar vertebra and the seromuscular penetration point of the cranial rectal artery.

The caudal part of the rectum is held medially by the levator ani muscles and laterally by the coccygeus muscles. The external anal sphincter muscle marks the caudal limit of the rectum. The terminal area is retroperitoneal.

The **cranial rectal artery**, which is the main vascular supply, is a branch of the **caudal mesenteric artery**. There is also a **middle rectal artery** (a branch of the internal pudendal artery, itself a branch of the internal iliac artery) and a **caudal rectal artery** (which comes either from the caudal branch of the middle sacral artery or from the internal pudendal branch, although its contribution is insignificant).

The lymphatic vessels of the anal canal and rectum drain cranially into the medial iliac lymph node.

The anal sphincter surrounds the caudal part of the rectum and anal canal to control defecation. It consists of two bands, a cranial smooth muscle band lining the anal canal and a caudal striated muscle band, which is mainly responsible for fecal continence. The openings of the anal sacs are located between the two portions of the sphincter.

The innervation of the sphincter is composed of parasympathetic branches that have an inhibitory effect and originate from the **pelvic nerve**, whose roots emerge from vertebrae S1–S3. The sympathetic input comes from the motor fibers of the **hypogastric nerves**. A single voluntary nerve reaches the external anal sphincter from the caudal rectal branches of the pudendal nerves. The blood supply comes from the **perineal arteries**.

> Fecal incontinence occurs if the last 1.5 cm of the terminal part of the rectum is removed or if more than 4 cm is resected, if the nerves have been damaged or if more than half of the external anal sphincter is deformed.

Anal and perianal surgical diseases

The following is a summary of the lesions affecting the anus, including the anal sacs, which may require surgery:

- Anal atresia
- Incomplete anogenital closure
- Anal sac disease
- Perianal fistula
- Anal stenosis
- Rectal prolapse
- Perianal gland adenoma (very rare in cats): related to androgenic stimulus and responds to castration
- Trauma

Anal atresia

Congenital anorectal diseases are rarely observed in small animals, the most common of which is anal atresia or atresia ani (Fig. 1). The actual incidence is difficult to determine, as most animals die or are euthanized.

Kittens affected by this congenital abnormality present with tenesmus and constipation during the first weeks of life. There are four types of anal atresia (Table 1).

In the case of rectovaginal fistulas (type IV) it is normal for the kitten to show no clinical signs while it is on a liquid diet. Diagnosis is made by meticulous examination, and positive-contrast X-rays are very helpful.

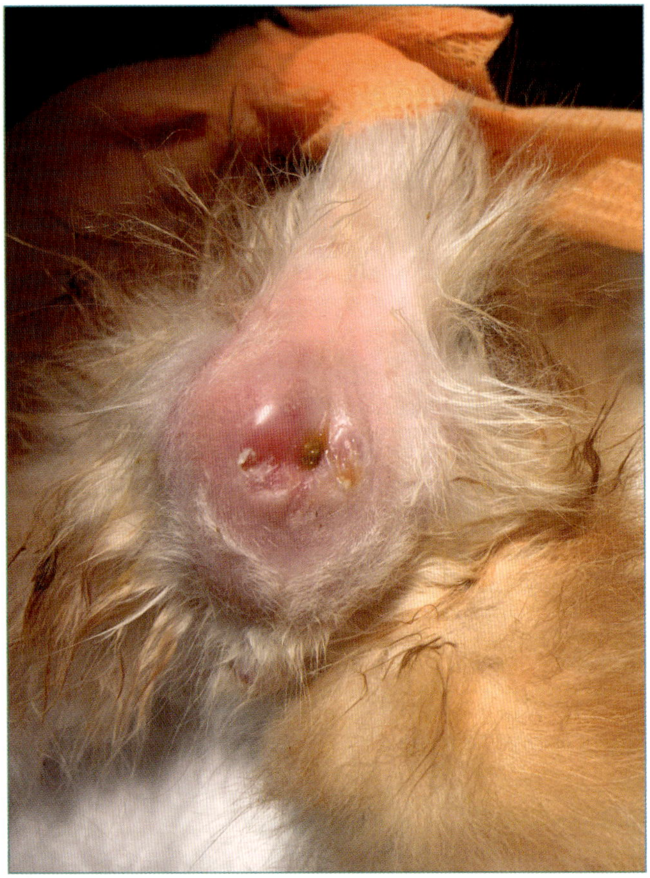

FIGURE 1. Seven week old kitten with imperforation of the anus. Dilatation of the rectum is due to impaction of intestinal contents.

The solution is always surgical, although this varies depending on the type, but in all cases it is aimed at redirecting the stool towards the natural opening.

Incomplete anogenital closure

It is caused by a failure of the embryonic cloaca to close, creating a communication between the anus and the vagina or urethra. Clinical signs are fecal and urinary incontinence. Both complications can remain postoperatively.

Surgical resolution can be attempted, although the risk of dehiscence due to infection is significant.

In males, the penile tissue is often insufficient for closure. Therefore, in addition to ventral closure of the anus, we must perform a perineal urethrostomy (see Ch. 27).

Anal sac disease

Anal sacs may present various conditions:

- Fecal impaction (retention)
- Sacculitis
- Abscesses
- Tumor/adenocarcinoma

Anal sac diseases are rare in cats, but they are always associated with some degree of obstruction of the anal sac duct. Their etiology is not clear, but the following have been described as perpetuating factors of these conditions:

- Abnormal stool consistency (too hard or too liquid)
- Any diet that prevents adequate stool consistency
- Poor sphincter muscle tone
- Inactivity
- Obesity
- Generalized seborrhea
- Recent estrus
- Genetic predisposition

TABLE 1. Types and characteristics of anal atresia

Type	Characteristics
Type I	Imperforate anus (persistence of the anal membrane).
Type II	Imperforate anus and rectum ending in a blind pouch in a portion more cranial to the anus.
Type III	The anus and the terminal portion may develop normally. However, there is a loss of continuity of the rectum separating it into a cranial and caudal portion. The cranial portion of the rectum ends as a blind sac cranial to the pelvic canal.
Type IV	More common in females. It is characterized by a communication between the rectum and the urogenital tract (with the dorsal wall of the vagina or the urethra in males) due to a lack of fusion of the sinovaginal bulbs, which generates an opening in the ventral wall of the rectum that generally ends in a blind sac.

Initially, medical treatment may be undertaken, but in the event of recurrence, a sacculectomy should be performed.

Perianal fistulas

In cats these fistulas are almost always secondary to an anal gland problem or a communication with the rectum (Figs. 2 and 3). This is not the case in dogs, especially in German Shepherds, in which fistulous lesions are not necessarily related to the anal sacs or intestine and respond to immunosuppressive treatment.

Anal stenosis

Tenesmus, hematochezia, dyschezia and the presence of flattened stools are the clinical signs of this problem. It is a process secondary to trauma, neoplasia or surgery.

Treatment consists of dilating the stenosis. If it is zonal, we can try surgical excision. In extreme cases, radical surgery may be the best option because, even with the risk of causing fecal incontinence, the patient's quality of life is greatly improved (Figs. 4–6).

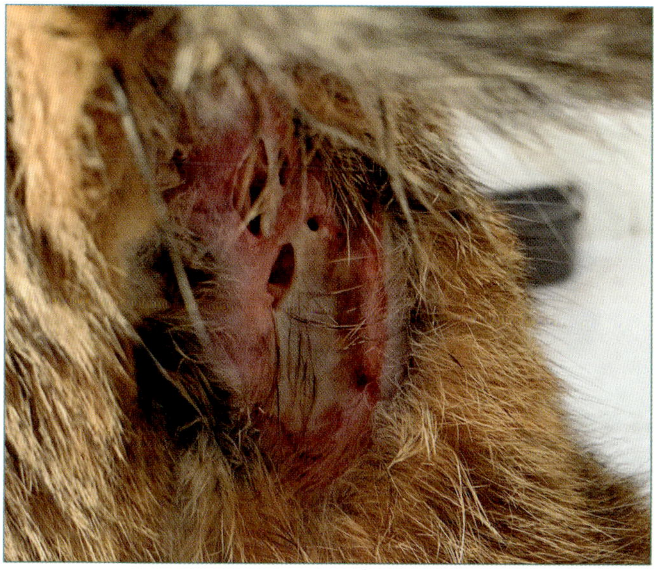

FIGURE 2. A 5-year-old female cat with a perianal fistula affecting the posterior part of the limb.

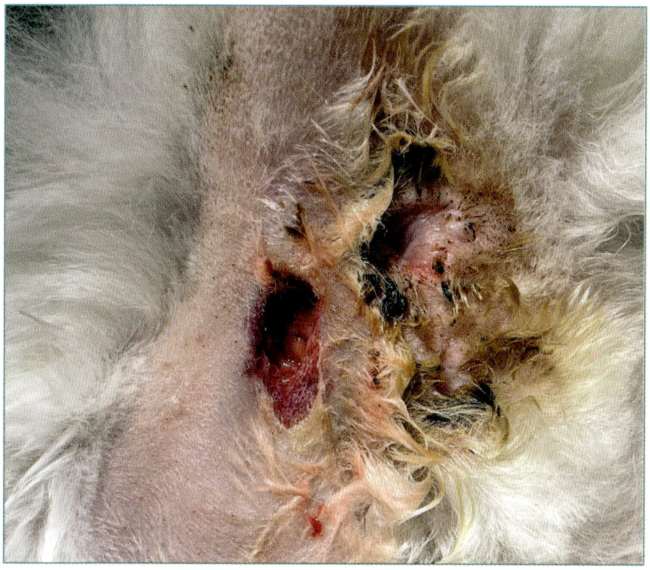

FIGURE 3. Another case of perianal fistula once cleaned and shaved.

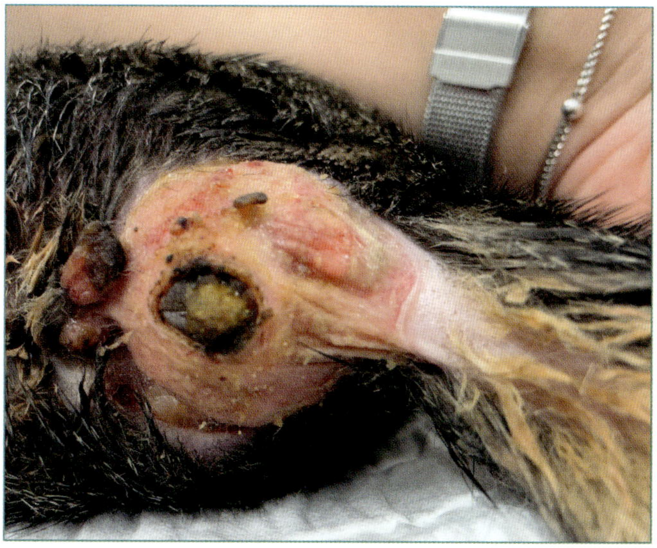

FIGURE 4. Anal stenosis in a cat secondary to eschar produced by a burn.

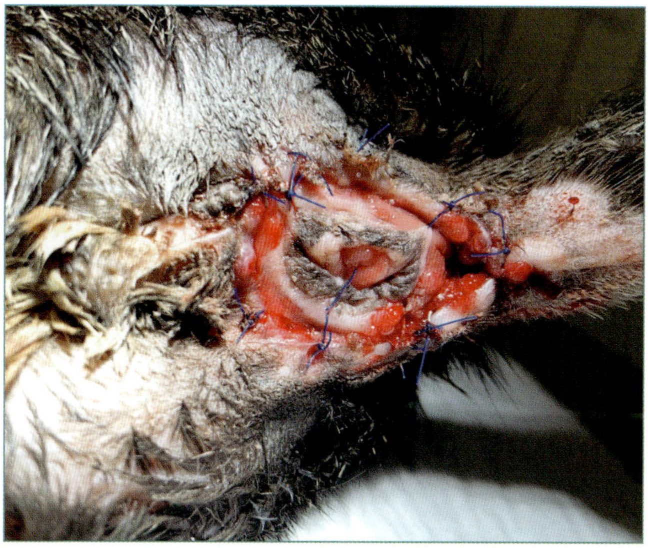

FIGURE 5. Wound created after breaking the fibrous ring and removing scar tissue during the surgical resolution process.

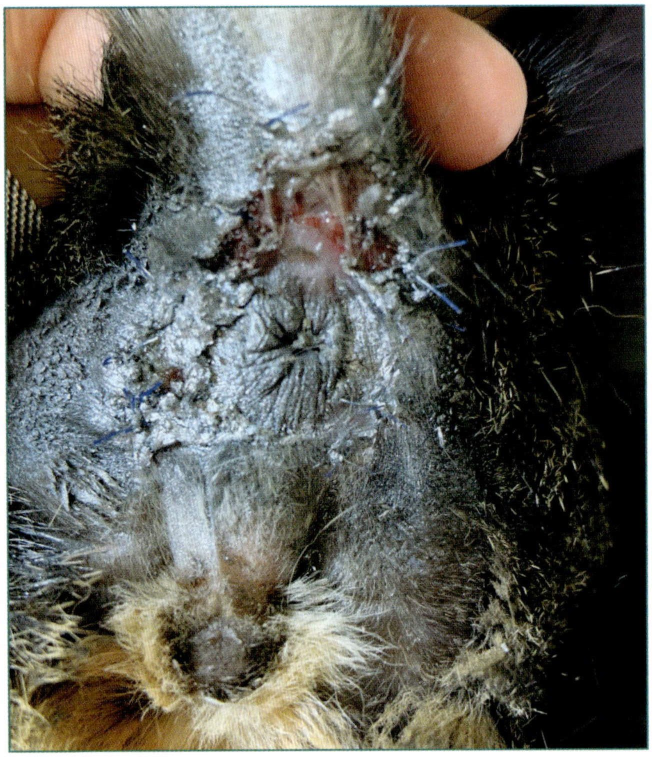

FIGURE 6. Appearance of the anal area during the last dressing change.

Anal/rectal prolapse

Prolapse of more or less of the rectum through the anal opening (Fig. 7) is a process that is observed relatively frequently in cats due to profuse parasite-associated diarrhea that causes continuous tenesmus, especially in young kittens; also in processes with a more neurological component or related to pain from spinal injuries or old hip fractures that narrow the pelvic canal. In this case, they are associated with hard and bulky stools.

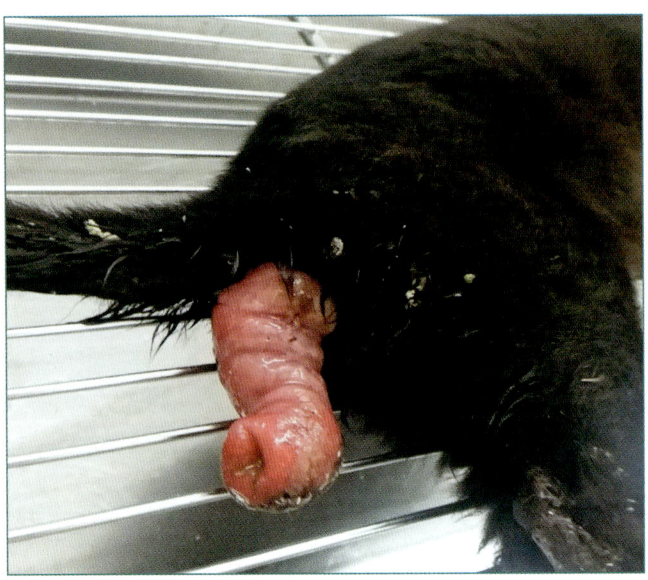

FIGURE 7. Cat with rectal prolapse.

Rectal prolapse has also been related, as in the case of intussusception, to the presence of intestinal tumors.

Initial management consists of reintroduction and the placement of a tobacco pouch suture around the anus for 3–4 days. Occasionally, it may be necessary to combine this with other surgical procedures, which are explained in the following section.

Surgical techniques

The use of antibiotics is recommended in surgeries that in any way involve the manipulation of the large intestine. Likewise, in the postoperative period it will be necessary to be very attentive to signs of infection. However, there is a great difference between rectal surgery and colon surgery, since in the latter there is a risk of peritonitis, which is clearly a more serious complication.

Reconstruction of the anus in anal atresia

To perform this technique (Fig. 8):

1. With the cat in dorsal recumbency, the entire perianal area is aseptically prepared and the tail is tucked cranially, so that it is not in the way.
2. The imperforate membrane/skin is incised by making a cross-shaped cut and bluntly dissecting under the skin in search of the anal sphincter.
3. Using Allis forceps, the blind end of the rectum is grasped, a transverse incision is made in the tissue and suturing of the rectum to the skin is started.
4. The first sutures are ideally placed as a guide at the four cardinal points and then stitches continue to be placed 2–3 mm apart. For this purpose, a 4-0 absorbable suture that takes time to degrade, such as PDS, or a nonabsorbable monofilament such as nylon is used (Figs. 9 and 10).
5. If there is a rectovaginal junction, an episiotomy is initially performed, extending between the two openings. The rectum and the vagina are identified and reconstructed separately (Figs. 11 and 12).
6. The area is well cleaned with abundant saline solution and chlorhexidine or hypochlorous acid and closed in layers.

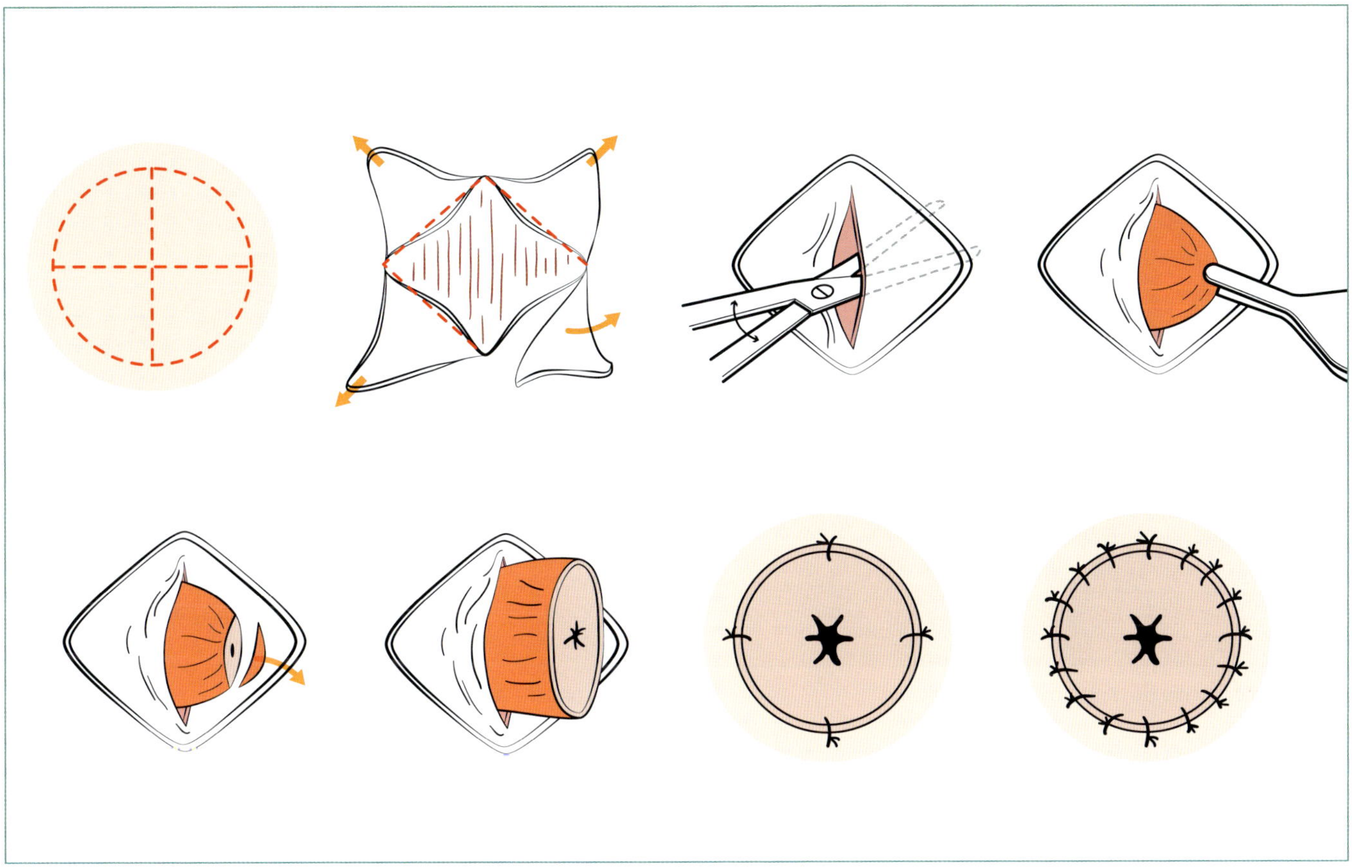

FIGURE 8. Steps of the technique for reconstruction of the anus in anal atresia.

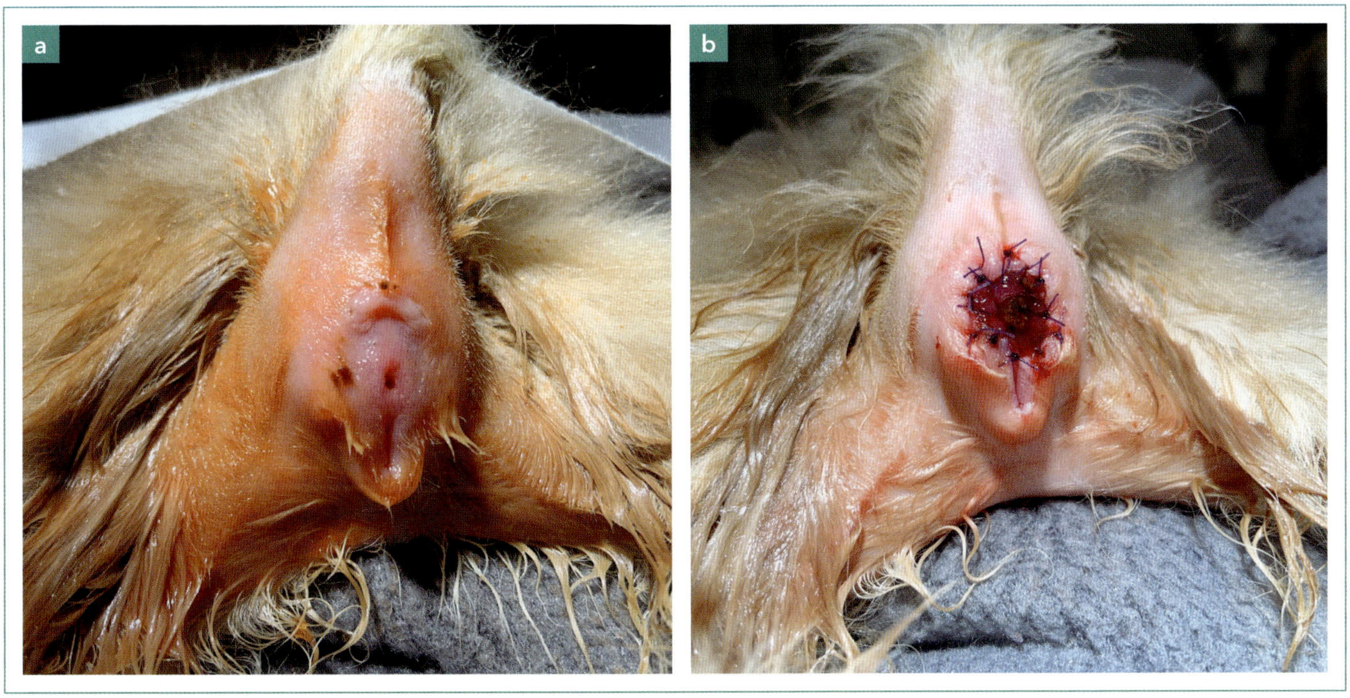

FIGURE 9. (a) Female kitten with imperforate anus. (b) Appearance after anal reconstruction surgery.

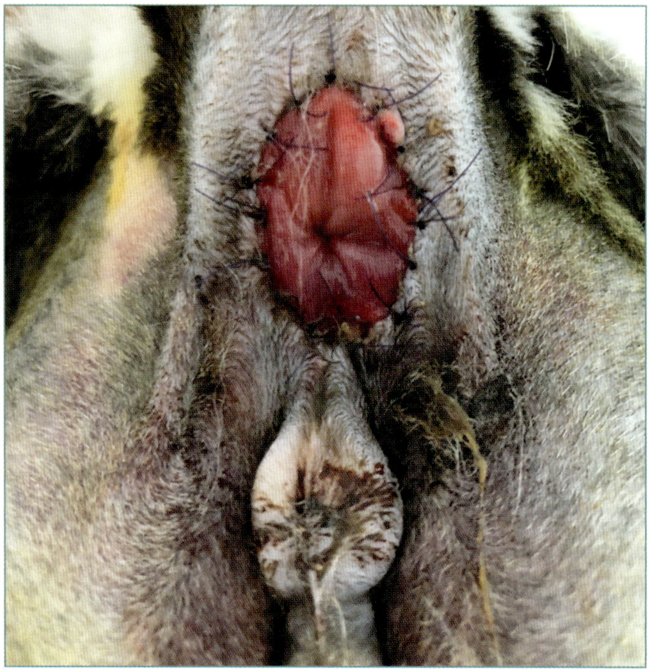

FIGURE 10. Another example of anal reconstruction.

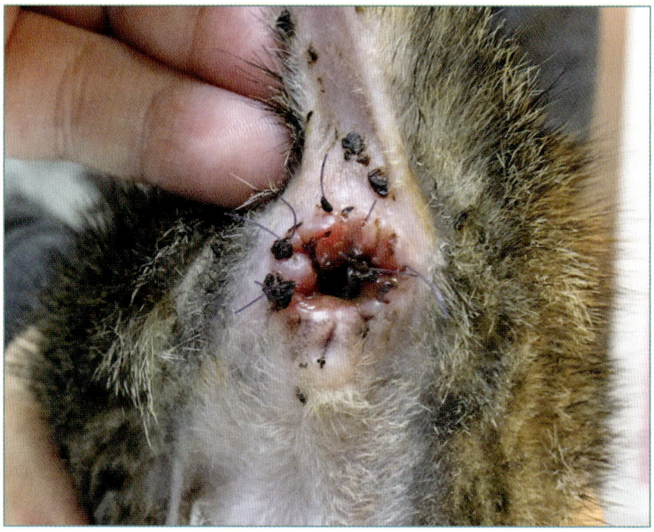

FIGURE 12. Postoperative checkup of a 5-week-old female cat weighing 350 g with an imperforate anus. In this case there was also rectovaginal communication. In such small kittens there is hardly any space between the anal opening and the vagina. In this patient it was only possible to place two stitches to close the defects, one in the rectum and the other in the vaginal vestibule.

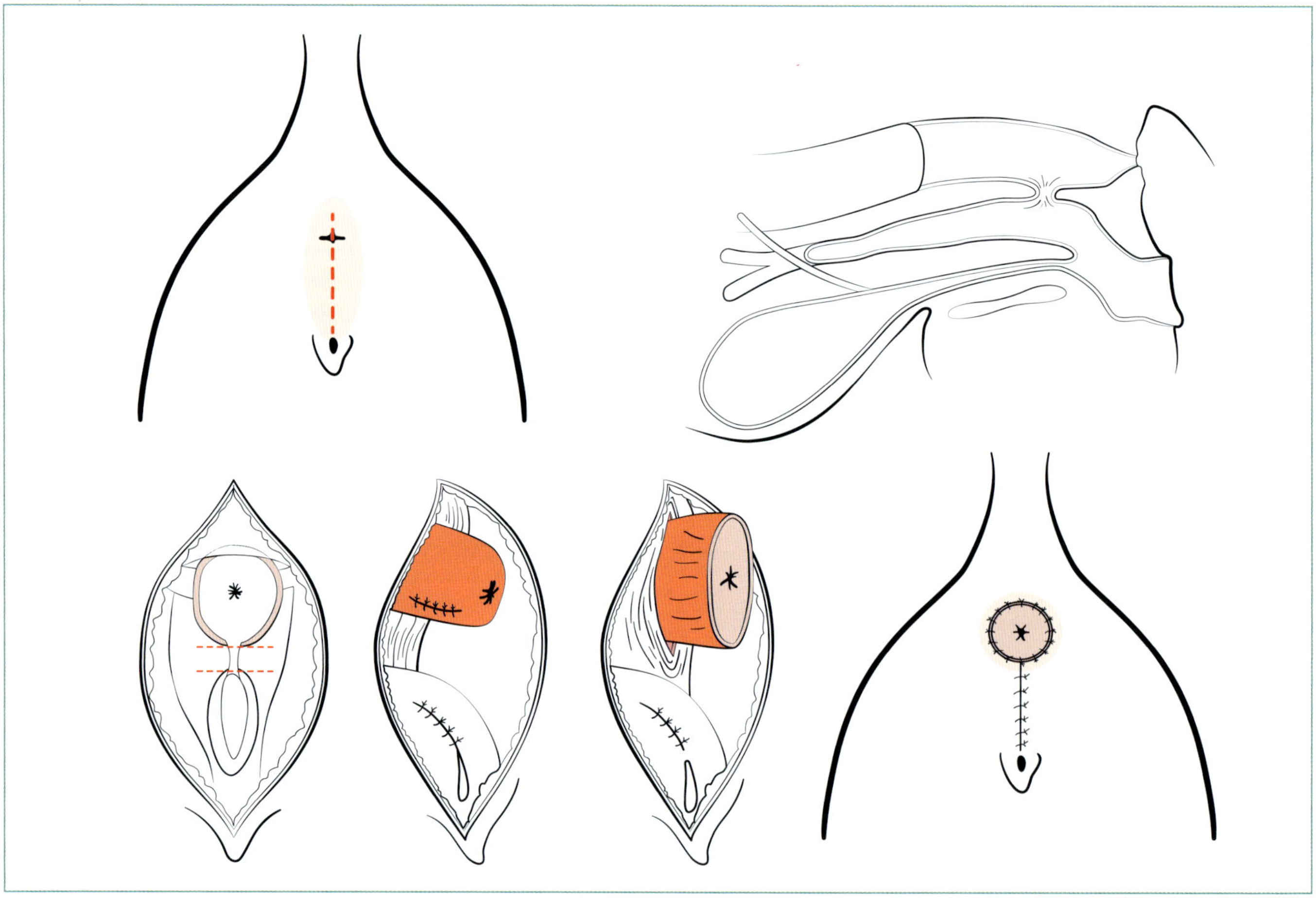

FIGURE 11. Steps of the technique to reconstruct the anus when there is also a rectovaginal fistula.

Postoperative considerations for anal reconstruction

In rectal/anal surgery, the main disadvantages to overcome are infection and patient discomfort, for this:

- The use of an Elizabethan collar is recommended to prevent them from touching the area, although in the authors' experience kittens do not usually do this very much.
- Provide adequate analgesic control.
- Clean the area daily. It is ideal to use warm water and neutral soap (soapy sponges are very useful) and wipe with a damp cloth to rinse.
- Achieve a stool consistency of 4/7 (Bristol scale of fecal consistency modified for cats); aim for a stool that is formed but moist to minimize pain during defecation and excessive tension on the stitches.

It is normal for there to be some initial degree of incontinence, but this problem usually resolves. In any case, we must warn caregivers that it may last for several weeks. A longer postoperative hospital stay (7–10 days) may be advisable.

Treatment of rectal prolapse

After sedating the cat, the prolapsed rectum is cleaned with saline solution to assess its viability. If viable, it is carefully reintroduced.

> To manipulate the rectum without damaging the mucosa, the use of ultrasound gel is very helpful.

Once the rectum has been reintroduced, a tobacco pouch suture is placed around the anus to prevent it from prolapsing again (Fig. 13). This suture is performed with nonabsorbable thread such as 2-0 or 3-0 nylon, depending on the size of the patient.

We should leave a sufficient opening so that the cat can defecate normally, and a soft diet with a variable amount of laxatives is introduced so that feces are formed but soft (4/7 consistency).

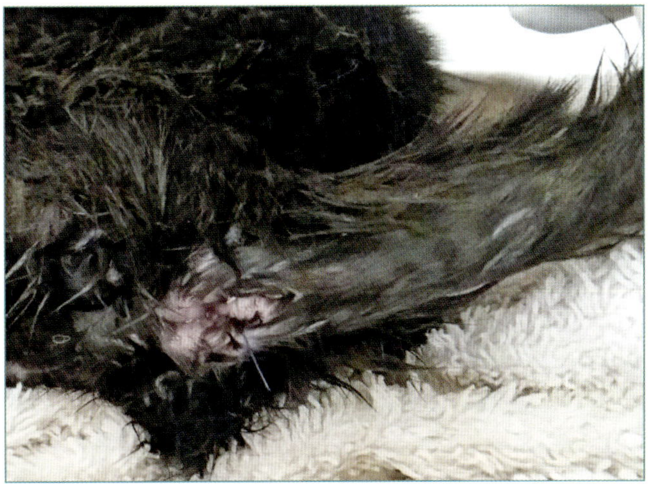

FIGURE 13. Patient in Figure 7 with reintroduced rectum and a tobacco pouch suture.

> To tighten the tobacco pouch suture while leaving a sufficient opening for the patient to defecate, we can use a well-lubricated 5 ml syringe or urine collection tube. In kittens we can use a catheter or a smaller syringe.

Colopexy

In the event of recurrence, it is advisable to perform a colopexy:

1. With the cat in dorsal recumbency, a midline laparotomy is performed.
2. The colon should be fixed to the abdominal wall about 2 or 3 cm from the linea alba, ensuring that the position of the colon is adequate, without tension. There are two possible techniques for colopexy, incisional and nonincisional:
   - In incisional colopexy, we make an incision in the abdominal wall and another in the serosa of the colon on its antimesenteric border. We then suture each edge of the abdominal wall wound to its corresponding edge in the intestine (Fig. 14).
   - In nonincisional colopexy, we place a continuous suture or 5–6 simple interrupted stitches between the antimesenteric border of the colon and the abdominal wall.

> Regardless of the technique used, it is essential to ensure that the sutures include the submucosal layer of the colon to resist tension, avoiding penetration into the intestinal lumen.

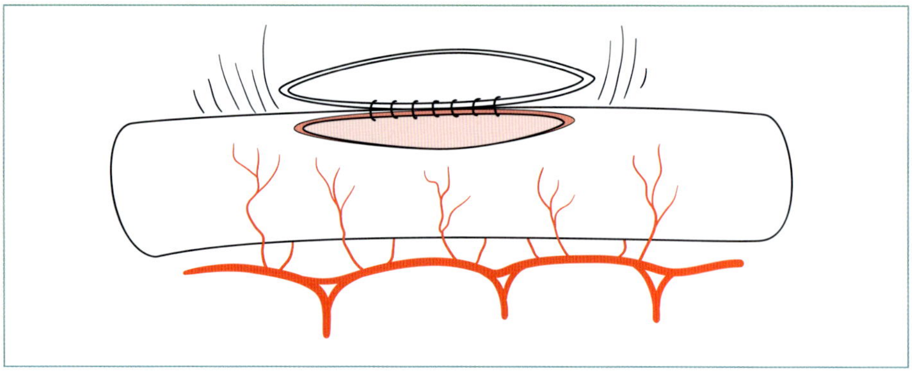

FIGURE 14. Suture in incisional colopexy.

3. The suture used can be nonabsorbable monofilament.
4. The colopexy site is covered with omentum before completing the surgery with routine closure of the abdominal wall.

> If the prolapsed tissue is severely damaged, it should be resected and sutured before reintroduction.

Anal sacculectomy

When there are recurrences of inflammatory problems of the anal sacs or in the case of tumors, a sacculectomy may be performed. There are several techniques described, which can be classified as open or closed.

Open technique

To perform it (Fig. 15):

1. The patient is placed in sternal recumbency and the tail is elevated and held in place with a gauze bandage, a cord or adhesive tape.
2. After emptying the perianal glands, a tomcat urinary catheter is introduced through the outflow orifice and the glands are flushed with a dilute chlorhexidine solution.
3. With the help of a blunt-tipped needle 1 or 2 mm in diameter to serve as a guide, we incise the skin with a no. 11 scalpel blade (the guide needle is introduced through the same orifice through which we previously passed the catheter).

> Perianal glands are typically located between the external and internal anal sphincter, at approximately 4 and 8 o'clock on an imaginary clock drawn on the anus.

4. The incision is made on the ventral aspect of the gland and, for its dissection, we are guided by the grayish color of the mucosa.
5. We can gently grasp and pull the gland with mosquito forceps while with curved Metzenbaum scissors we stick to the wall of the gland and carefully dissect it, minimizing the chances of damaging the sphincter.
6. The ligature is placed at the level of the perianal gland duct.
7. After removal, the tissue is closed in layers.
8. It can be finished with an intradermal suture using 3-0 or 4-0 absorbable monofilament.

Closed technique

We will follow the same initial steps as in the open technique but, instead of using a guide needle, we will locate the gland by dissection of the surrounding tissue.

There are kits with a material that can be introduced into the gland, filling it to make it easier to remove. This product hardens and facilitates gland localization and dissection.

> A special note: it is important to point out that in cats that have experienced the formation and rupture of gland abscesses on several occasions, it is very probable that the scenario in the operating room will be different from that described in the techniques, since the integrity of the gland is lost and the scar tissue that forms during the healing process of the fistulas makes it very difficult to identify what is and what is not glandular tissue.

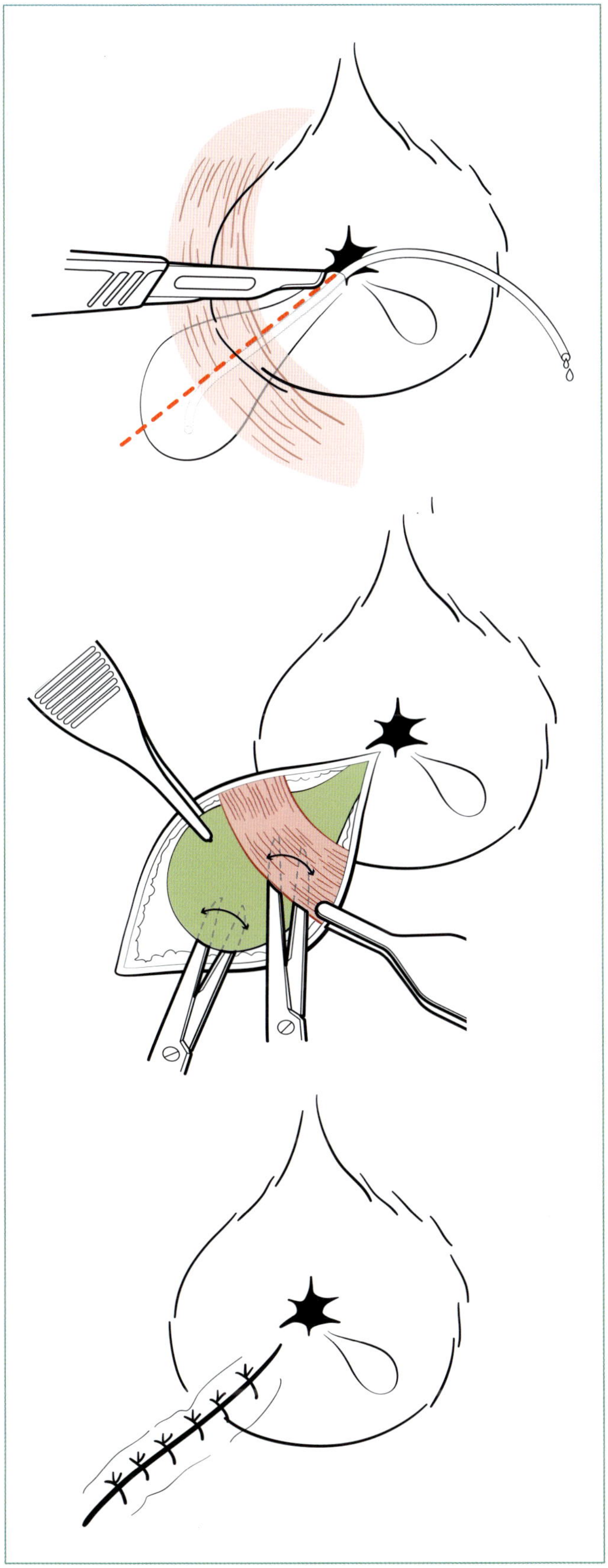

FIGURE 15. Anal sacculectomy using the open technique.

Complications and postoperative care

The main complications of anal and perianal surgery are tenesmus, incontinence and suture dehiscence.

In these cases, postoperative care includes:

- An Elizabethan collar should always be placed to prevent self-injury.
- We should recommend a diet rich in fiber and consider the use of mild laxatives to give the stool an adequate texture during the first days after surgery, in order to facilitate bowel movements.
- A nonsteroidal anti-inflammatory drug will be administered during the first week to reduce pain and inflammation, and an analgesic such as buprenorphine will be administered for the first 2 or 3 days.
- Daily cleaning of the area with soapy sponges may be recommended. Mild soap and warm water are usually less irritating than cleansing wipes.

Bibliography

Aronson L. Rectum and anus. In: Slatter DH (ed.). *Textbook of Small Animal Surgery*, 3rd ed. Philadelphia, PA: WB Saunders, 2003; pp. 682–708.

Fransson BA. Rectocutaneous fistulas. *Compend Contin Educ Vet*, 2008; 30(4):224–227.

Rahal SC, Vicente CS, Mortari AC et al. Rectovaginal fistula with anal atresia in 5 dogs. *Can Vet J*, 2007; 48(8):827–830.

Suess RP Jr, Martin RA, Moon ML, Dallman MJ. Rectovaginal fistula with atresia in three kittens. *Cornell Vet*, 1992; 82(2):141–153.

White RN. Large intestine, rectum and anus. In: Langley-Hobbs SJ, Demetriou JL, Ladlow JF (eds.). *Feline Soft Tissue and General Surgery*, 1st ed. Oxford, UK: Saunders Elsevier, 2014.

SPLENECTOMY 24

Anna Calvet

Surgical anatomy

The spleen is located in the craniodorsal abdomen, on the left side. It is not always immediately visible when performing a midline laparotomy.

The external structure of the spleen consists of a **head** located cranially to the cranial pole of the left kidney, with a relatively fixed position, and a **body** and **tail**, which form the rest of the organ and have a more variable position.

Internally the structure of the spleen is organized into the **red pulp**, formed by macrophages and granulocytes that line vascular structures and whose role is phagocytosis, and the **white pulp**, formed by periarterial lymph nodes and germinal centers that act as an immune organ.

We can summarize the basic functions of the spleen as follows:

- It is a reservoir of blood (it can contain 10%–20% of erythrocytes and up to 30% of platelets).
- It filters the blood and removes parasites, bacteria, nuclear remnants (Howell–Jolly bodies) and denatured hemoglobin (Heinz bodies), and recycles nondeformable red blood cells, whether because they have wall problems or are old, damaged or abnormal for other reasons.
- It performs hematopoiesis if necessary (less frequent than in dogs), since in the cat the spleen stops performing hematopoiesis at birth.
- It is part of the immune system.

> Cats have a unique nonsinusoidal internal circulation that decreases the susceptibility of the spleen to hyperplasia and hematoma formation, and also allows the release of more erythrocytes with Heinz bodies, which are normal in circulating blood.

For surgical considerations, it is very important to understand how the blood supply to the organ is organized. The **splenic artery** (or gastrosplenic artery) is a branch of the celiac artery. The splenic artery gives off branches to the left lobe of the pancreas. Then, the splenic artery divides into a dorsal and a ventral branch approximately one centimeter from the spleen.

The ventral branch branches into the **left gastroepiploic artery** after dividing into small branches that supply almost the entire body of the spleen. The dorsal branch irrigates the dorsal area of the spleen.

The venous drainage empties into the splenic vein, which drains into the portal vein via the gastrosplenic vein (Fig. 1).

Splenic diseases

We can divide splenic disorders into those of traumatic origin, such as ruptures or lacerations, and torsions on the one hand, and those derived from disease on the other.

Splenic disease is more typical of middle-aged or older cats, with an average age of 12 years, and no differences between sexes.

Splenic pathology usually presents with a nonspecific clinical presentation, although historical findings often include lethargy, vomiting, weight loss and apathy.

Splenomegaly may be identified during a general physical examination of the patient, upon palpation of an abdominal mass, but the most useful test is ultrasound (Fig. 2). The normal feline spleen is homogeneous, with a finer ultrasound texture than that of the liver, and hyperechogenic with respect to the liver and renal cortex.

Ultrasound is sensitive enough to detect lesions, but to obtain a definitive diagnosis we will need to collect samples, since we will not be able to differentiate benign from malignant lesions by appearance alone.

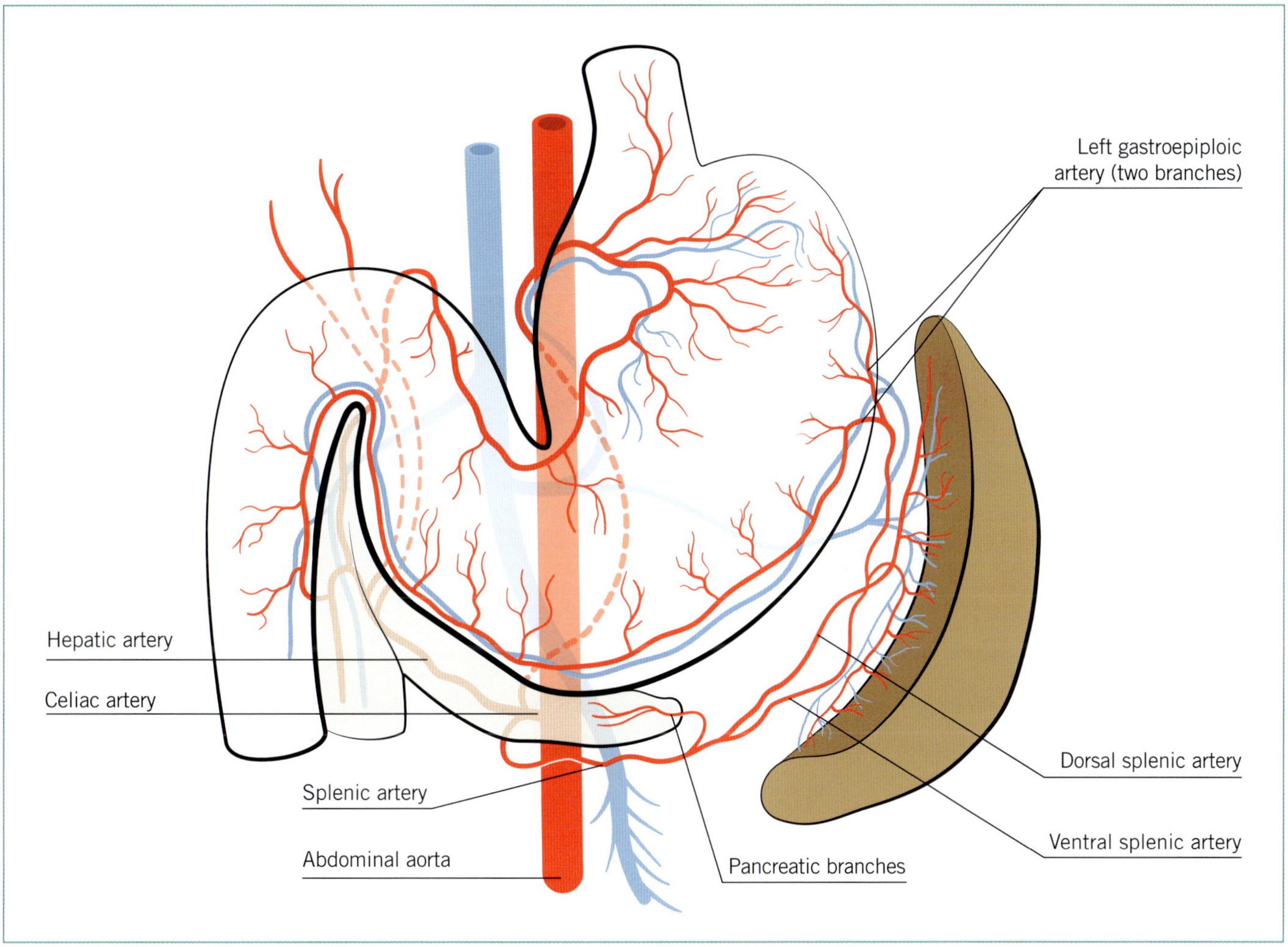

FIGURE 1. Vascularization of the spleen.

Ultrasound-guided fine needle aspiration (using a 22- to 25-gauge needle without a syringe attached, thus minimizing blood contamination of the specimen) is very useful, as many splenic diseases are exfoliative (Fig. 3).

Performing a fine needle aspiration is a relatively simple and inexpensive test, and has been shown to be safe even in the presence of thrombocytopenia or coagulopathy. Special care should be taken to avoid repositioning the needle while it is in the spleen, in order to avoid laceration.

For diffuse diseases of the spleen we can even carefully perform a blind aspiration by immobilizing the spleen under the skin with one hand.

Box 1 shows a summary of splenic lesions.

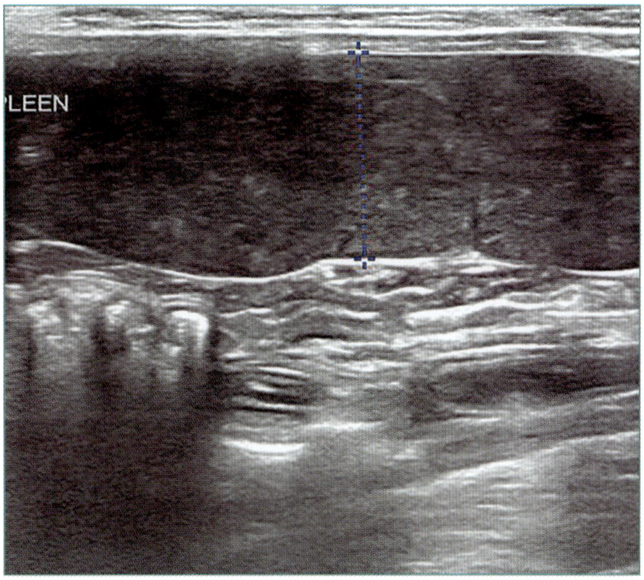

FIGURE 2. Ultrasound showing splenomegaly. The spleen has a coarse appearance.

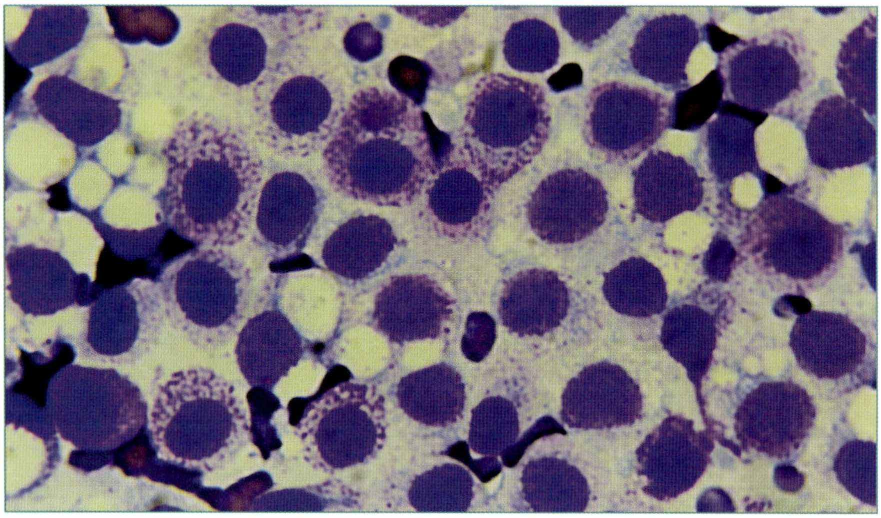

FIGURE 3. Cytology of the sample obtained by puncture of the spleen of the patient in the previous figure: diagnosis of mast cell tumor.

Hemoperitoneum

Most cases of feline hemoperitoneum are traumatic in origin and bleeding is mainly from the liver or spleen. In the case of spontaneous hemoperitoneum, the spleen has been reported as the origin in only 17% of cases, the most common cause being the rupture of a hemangiosarcoma, a rare tumor in cats, but which has malignant behavior.

BOX 1. Main focal and generalized splenic lesions

Causes of focal splenomegaly

Infectious inflammation

- Bacterial abscess

Neoplastic

- Lymphoma
- Hemangiosarcoma
- Hemangioma
- Sarcomas arising from other splenic cell types
- Metastatic lesions

Nonneoplastic

- Myelolipoma
- Nodular lymphoid hyperplasia
- Extramedullary hematopoiesis

Causes of generalized splenomegaly

Infectious

- Bacterial:
  - Mycobacteriosis
  - Salmonellosis
  - Hemoplasmosis
  - Others
- Fungal:
  - Sporotrichosis
  - Histoplasmosis
- Protozoan:
  - Toxoplasmosis
- Viral:
  - Feline leukemia virus
  - Feline immunodeficiency virus
  - Feline infectious peritonitis

Neoplastic

- Mast cell tumor
- Lymphoma
- Multiple myeloma
- Malignant histiocytosis
- Myeloproliferative disorders

Nonneoplastic

- Amyloidosis
- Osmotic fragility
- Extramedullary hematopoiesis
- Pyruvate kinase deficiency
- Noninflammatory hemolysis

Noninfectious inflammation

- Immune-mediated hemolytic anemia
- Hypereosinophilic syndrome
- Lymphocytic–plasmacytic gastroenteritis

Congestive

- Portal hypertension
- Induced by medication (sedation or anesthesia)
- Right-sided heart failure

Splenic torsion

Splenic torsion is rare, but it always requires surgical intervention. Affected cats usually present with abdominal pain, splenomegaly and cardiovascular shock. Sometimes the onset may be more insidious, with anemia, anorexia, vomiting, ascites and neutrophilia.

When torsion occurs, the veins are occluded but not the arteries, so the blood reaches the organ but cannot be evacuated, causing distension of the spleen, sequestration of the blood and finally hemolysis. When thrombosis of the splenic artery occurs, necrosis of the spleen begins, which can secondarily lead to bacterial proliferation.

The surgery to resolve a splenic torsion has a particularity. Namely, it is not a recommended to untwist the splenic pedicle in order to avoid the release of toxins and bacteria into the circulating blood.

Preoperative considerations

First we must decide whether our patient is a candidate for splenectomy, since not all spleen lesions require this approach. Splenectomy should be considered:

- In cases of immune-mediated anemia or thrombocytopenia refractory to treatment.
- In cats with splenic nodules, since, as previously noted, it is difficult to differentiate between benign and malignant lesions.
- In cases of generalized splenomegaly when cytology is positive.
- And finally, in torsions, severe lacerations and ruptures.

Before performing a splenectomy to treat a cat with cytopenia, it is important to ensure that the bone marrow is functioning properly.

The best way to approach a patient requiring splenectomy is to plan how to stabilize the patient prior to surgery. In addition to the imaging tests and cytology/biopsy discussed above, a complete blood test will be needed. We must take into account that, especially in cases in which there is also hemoabdomen, the patient may have low hematocrit values, alterations in lactate concentration and prerenal azotemia due to low circulating volume.

Prior antibiotic therapy is not routinely recommended unless there is strong evidence of a bacterial infection and, in such a case, we will try to administer the most appropriate antibiotics based on the results of culture and antibiogram. In the event that insufficient sample is obtained for culture until after surgery, we can start with the antibiotics recommended in the international guidelines.

Fluid therapy with crystalloids is indicated before surgery. In the case of hemoperitoneum, it is recommended to have ready everything necessary for transfusion in case the need arises.

Surgical techniques

There are two techniques used in the spleen: total splenectomy and partial splenectomy (Fig. 4).

Total splenectomy

To perform this technique:

1. A midline laparotomy is performed, with the cat in dorsal recumbency, after preparing the skin of the abdomen. We extend the incision from the umbilicus to the xiphoid process, obtaining an opening of approximately 10 cm. We must prepare more skin in case it is necessary to extend the incision, since we will have to explore the rest of the abdominal cavity in search of possible metastatic lesions and, if so, take samples for biopsy.
2. The spleen is identified and exteriorized. The organ must be manipulated carefully to avoid lacerations or ruptures that could cause bleeding and seeding of tumor cells in the abdominal cavity.
3. Moist gauze is placed around the opening.
4. We now proceed to look for and ligate the vessels that reach the spleen through the hilum. The simplest technique is to stick to the vessels near the hilum so as not to damage branches that supply the pancreas or the greater curvature of the stomach (this is the time to remember how the splenic vascular supply works). We will make two ligatures in all the perihilar vessels with 3-0 absorbable monofilament suture material and cut between them with scissors or a scalpel blade (Fig. 5).
5. Alternatively, we can make a ligature and hold the vessel at the other end with hemostatic forceps. Other methods of vessel occlusion such as hemostatic clips (hemoclips) or electrothermal vessel-sealing devices are currently also available, which considerably reduce surgical time.
6. After checking to ensure there is no active bleeding, we should check the rest of the organs in case it is necessary to take a sample for biopsy and, finally, the abdomen is closed in a routine manner.

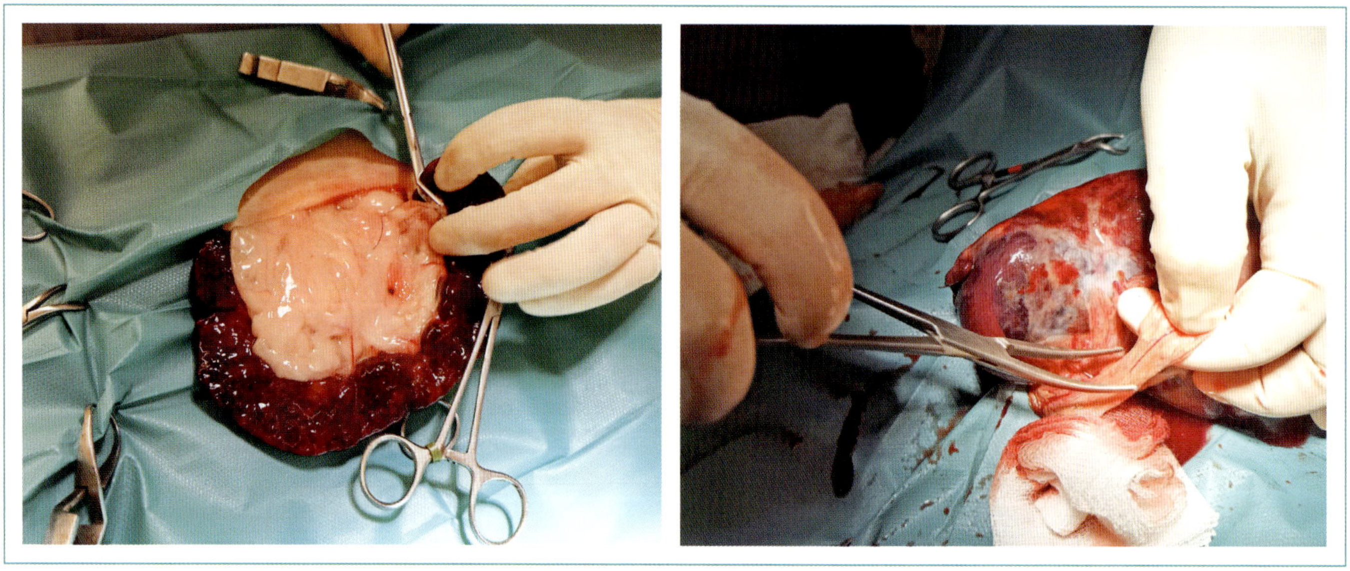

FIGURE 4. Splenectomies will be more or less complicated depending on the underlying problem.

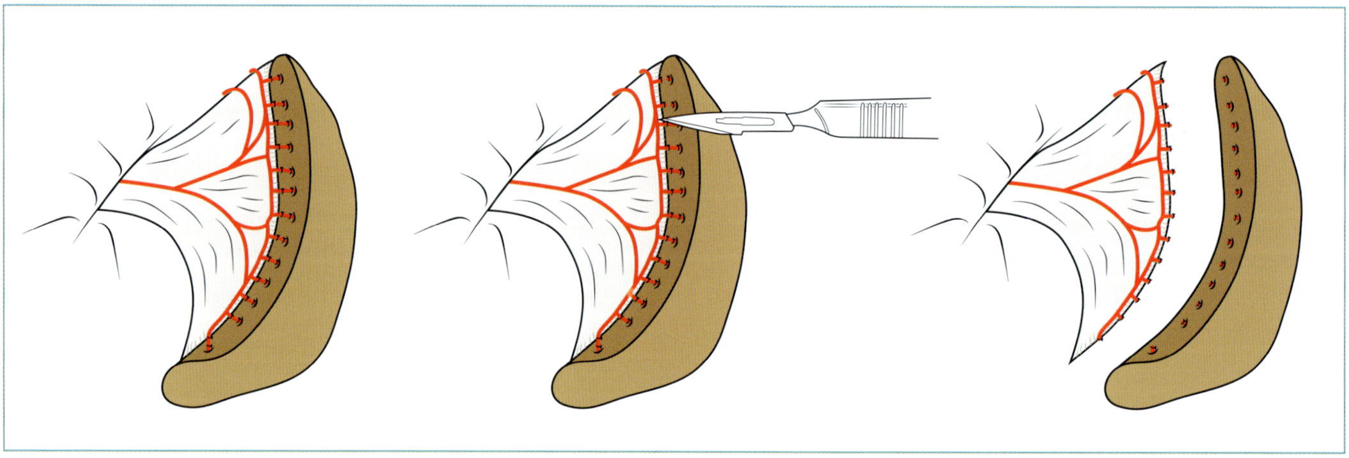

FIGURE 5. Ligation of vessels in total splenectomy.

Partial splenectomy

To excise the affected portion of the spleen:

1. We look for the vessels supplying the abnormal area to be removed and ligate them in the same way described for a total splenectomy.
2. With a thicker suture (0 gauge) we make a circular ligature to surround the area of the spleen to be removed. By tensioning this suture we seek to occlude the pulp vessels (Fig. 6).
3. We must always place the circular suture in healthy tissue, since there should be about 5 mm of healthy tissue between the suture and the cut.
4. It is not necessary to suture the exposed splenic tissue.
5. If required, an omental flap or absorbable collagen sponge can be used to cover it.

Complications and postoperative care

It is recommended that cats that have undergone a splenectomy be kept under observation for 24 hours. During these 24 hours it is not necessary to perform a lot of tests, but it is recommended that a couple of hematocrits and a control abdominal ultrasound be performed.

The most frequent complications are:

- **Hypotension:** due to the loss of volume associated with the removal of the organ. In the absence of further complications, this is usually corrected with fluid therapy.
- **Hemorrhages:** usually caused by suture dehiscence.
- **Reactivation of previous diseases and increased predisposition**: there is a greater predisposition to suffer from previous subclinical infections and hemoparasite infections.

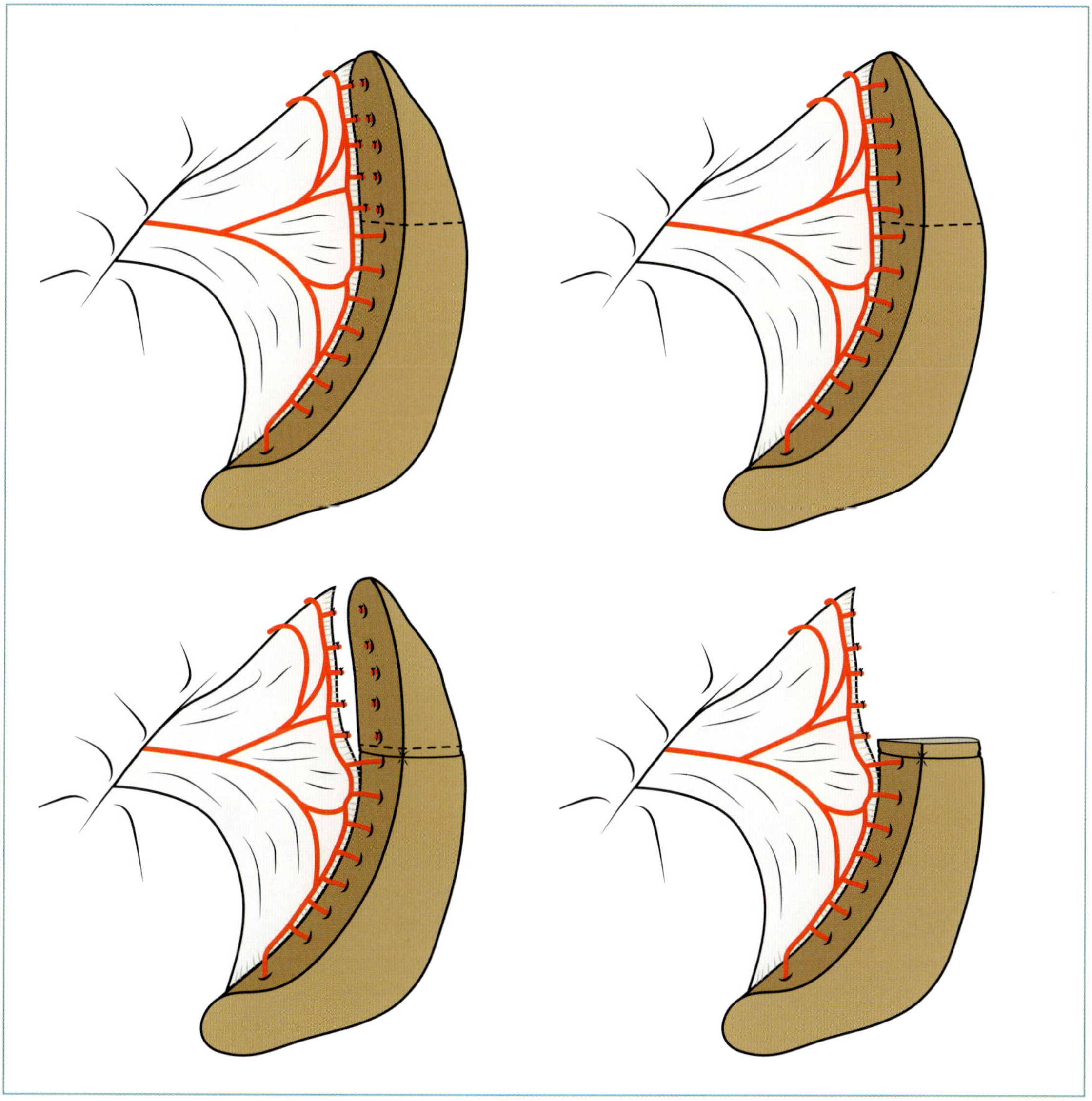

FIGURE 6. Partial splenectomy.

Bibliography

Gordon SSN, McClaran JK, Bergman PJ, Liu SM. Outcome following splenectomy in cats. *J Feline Med Surg*, 2010; 12(4):256–261.

Johannes CM, Henry CJ, Turnquist SE et al. Hemangiosarcoma in cats: 53 cases (1992–2002). *J Am Vet Med Assoc*, 2007; 231(12):1851–1856.

Hanson JA, Papageorges M, Girard E et al. Ultrasonographic appearance of splenic disease in 101 cats. *Vet Radiol Ultrasound*, 2001; 42(5):441–445.

Spangler WL, Culbertson MR. Prevalence and type of splenic disease in cats: 455 cases (1985–1991). *J Am Vet Med Assoc*, 1992; 201(5):773–776.

KIDNEY AND URETER SURGERY 25

Alberto Barneto and Anna Calvet

Surgical anatomy

Anatomy of the kidney

Cats have two kidneys. The right kidney, located in a more cranial position than the left one, is at the level of the L1–L4 vertebrae and is housed in the renal fossa of the caudate lobe of the liver, attached by the hepatorenal ligament. The left kidney is located between the L2–L5 vertebrae. Both organs are retroperitoneal and are situated underneath the sublumbar musculature on either side of the caudal vena cava and the abdominal aorta.

The kidneys are oval shaped, and from their cranial pole to their caudal pole, they measure 3–4.5 cm in healthy cats, although there is wide variability between sterilized and intact animals, males and females, and different breeds.

From the most external to the most internal layer, the kidney is structured as follows (Fig. 1):

- Renal capsule
- Renal cortex
- Corticomedullary junction
- Renal medulla
- Pelvis

The **renal pelvis** collects urine from the **collecting tubules** and directs it towards the **ureter**, which is situated medially in the **renal hilum**. The **renal vein** is also located in the hilum (ventrally), along with the **renal artery** (dorsally) and the nerves.

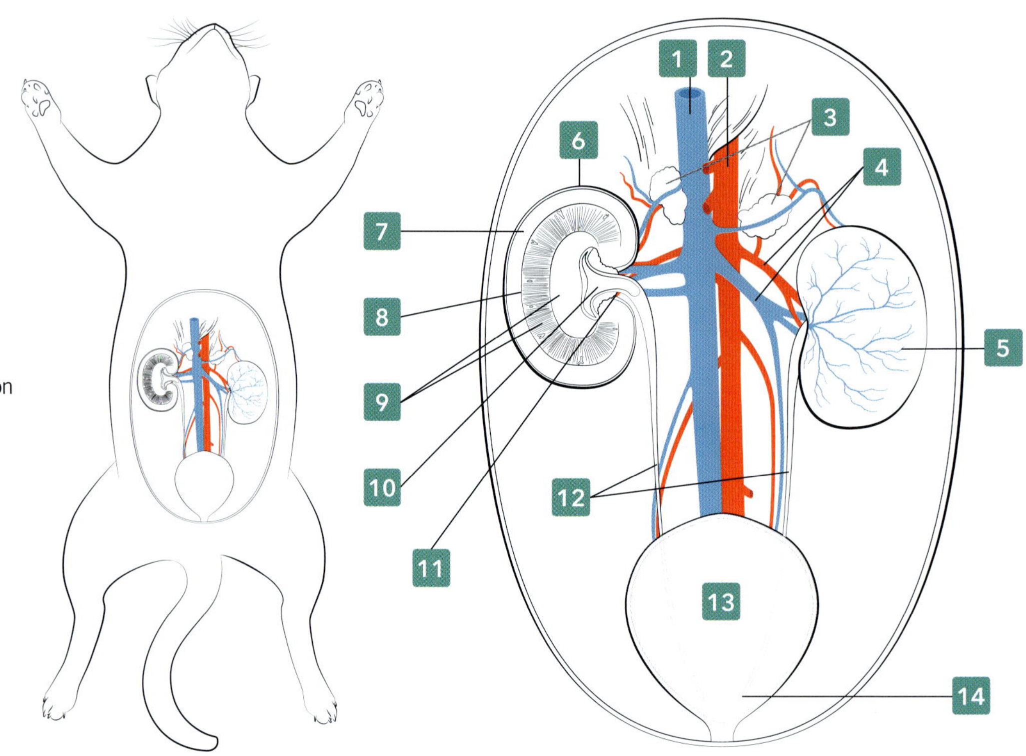

1. Caudal vena cava
2. Abdominal aorta
3. Adrenal glands
4. Renal artery and vein
5. Capsular veins
6. Renal capsule
7. Renal cortex
8. Corticomedullary junction
9. Renal medulla (tubule area and calyces)
10. Pelvis
11. Renal hilum
12. Ureters
13. Urinary bladder
14. Ureteral orifice

FIGURE 1. Anatomy of the feline urinary system

As the aorta is situated to the left of the vena cava, the right renal artery is longer. Multiple renal arteries occur in 10% of cats.

Once the renal artery enters the kidney, it divides into interlobar arteries. These vessels extend along the medulla, forming the arcuate arteries in the corticomedullary junction. Emerging from these arteries are the interlobular arteries, which run in a perpendicular direction towards the renal cortex, where they come to an end, forming the glomerular afferent arterioles. Venous drainage goes in the reverse direction until reaching the renal vein. We may encounter multiple renal veins, more commonly on the right side. This is the opposite of what occurs with multiple renal arteries, which are more often found on the left side.

Both the **capsule** and the **renal parenchyma** are well vascularized. In surgery, this means that any cuts or punctures will bleed profusely.

It is normal to find a large amount of fat tissue surrounding feline kidneys.

Anatomy of the feline ureter

The **ureters** are two tubes with a fibromuscular structure that direct urine from the renal pelvis to the bladder by means of peristaltic contractions. The cranial portion is in the shape of a funnel to attach to the renal hilum. The first two thirds of the ureters run inside the retroperitoneum, while the last third exits into the peritoneal space, maintaining contact with the dorsal wall of the abdomen along their full length. The average width of the feline ureter along the entire middle section is no more than 0.3–0.4 mm. The caudal portion of the duct acquires a characteristic J shape when it attaches to the bladder, with a caudocranial curvature at the point where it penetrates the dorsal wall of the neck of the bladder. The area where the two ureters enter the bladder neck is known as the **bladder trigone**.

The ureters enter the bladder wall at an oblique angle. The gradual filling of the bladder increases the J curvature of the caudal portion of the ureters. After entering the wall, the ureters travel a short distance inside the muscle before opening into the lumen. This tunnel structures allow pressure increases on the **vesicoureteral valves** to close the ureters as the bladder is filled with urine. This stops reflux of urine toward the ureters and kidneys.

The structure of the ureter wall consists of an adventitia, which includes the vascularization, a muscular layer of smooth fibers, a submucosa and a mucosa. The muscular layer, in turn, consists of an inner layer of longitudinal fibers, an intermediate layer of circular fibers, and a superficial layer also made up of longitudinal fibers, more developed near the vesicoureteral valve. When a peristaltic wave originates near the kidney, it runs the full length of the ureter to efficiently advance urine in a caudal direction.

The ureters have multiple sources of vascularization: cranial arterial branches emerge from the renal artery, caudal branches emerge from the vaginal/prostatic artery, and branches of various origins give rise to the **ureteral artery**. The ureteral veins drain blood along the same path as the ureteral arteries.

Innervation of the ureters derives from the sympathetic, parasympathetic and sensory nervous systems. Although the sympathetic system has the most receptors in the ureter, **ureteral peristalsis** has a myogenic origin.

Surgical diseases of the kidney

Nephrolithiasis

Nephroliths that do not cause disease, especially in cats with chronic kidney disease, do not necessarily require surgical extraction. Studies have shown that the presence of calculi in the renal pelvis is not associated with progression of kidney disease or a higher rate of mortality (Figs. 2 and 3). Because nephrolithiasis almost always presents with ureterolithiasis, more information can be found in that section.

Trauma

Given their retroperitoneal location, the kidneys are damaged less often compared to the lower urinary tract. Isolated trauma to a kidney can be difficult to diagnose, as the clinical signs may be nonspecific, so the clinical history should be considered. One of the signs of kidney damage is pain upon palpation of the lumbar area, but this sign in very nonspecific. On the other hand, if hematuria is present, this may guide our diagnosis, although there is no correlation between the severity of the lesion and the amount of blood lost.

Whether or not renal trauma can be repaired depends on its severity. Radiology, ultrasound, and even computed tomography or magnetic resonance studies, along with excretory urography can help us decide whether or not to perform surgery. Conservative treatment may be sufficient for small subcapsular hemorrhages. For more severe lesions, it may be necessary to suture the capsule or cover the defect with a flap of transverse muscle of the abdomen or with omentum. Lesions in the pelvis can be repaired with a nephrostomy tube and placement of an endoprosthesis (stent). But for severe lesions with copious loss of blood or urine, or with the presence of necrotic tissue, a ureteronephrectomy must be performed.

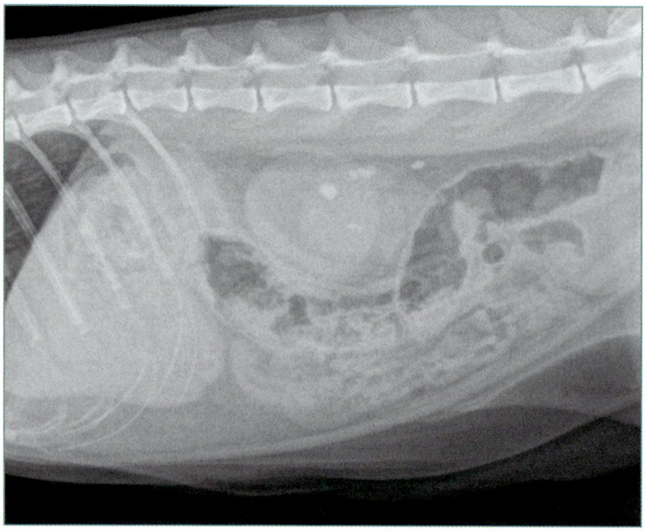

FIGURE 2. Patient with nephroliths and ureteroliths.

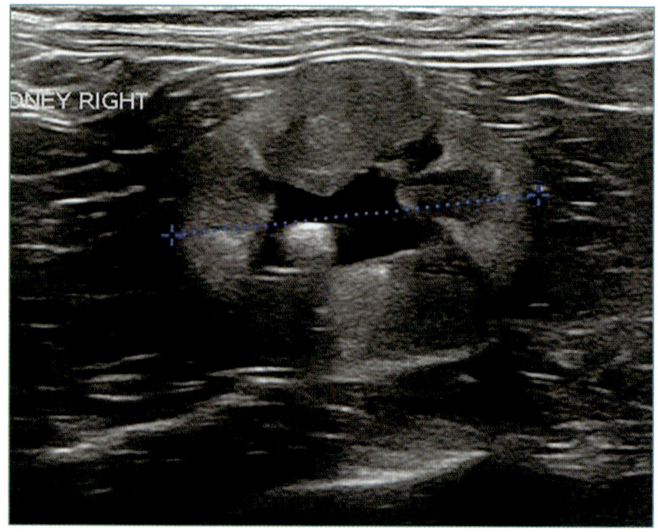

FIGURE 3. Ultrasound of the patient in the previous figure. An intrapelvic urolith is seen.

Neoplasia

Representing 1.6%–2.5% of all neoplasms, renal tumors do not occur frequently. Metastatic lesions are more common than primary lesions, and among these primary lesions, the most frequent are lymphomas, although carcinomas, transitional cell carcinomas, nephroblastomas, and hemangiosarcomas have also been diagnosed. Renal lymphoma is one of the few kidney diseases that can be diagnosed with fine needle puncture–aspiration. This can be done if an ultrasound shows a hypoechoic subcapsular thickening, with a sensitivity of 60.7% and a specificity of 84.6% for renal lymphoma (Fig. 4).

Thoracic ultrasound images and X-rays (three or four projections), or a CT scan if advanced imaging is available, are required for diagnostic evaluation of a renal tumor, to properly plan a surgery and evaluate the presence of other tumors.

Before beginning any surgical treatment, a biochemical profile, urinalysis and a complete blood work is needed to evaluate levels of azotemia, hematuria, proteinuria and any electrolytic abnormalities. Anemia is usually present, as is often the

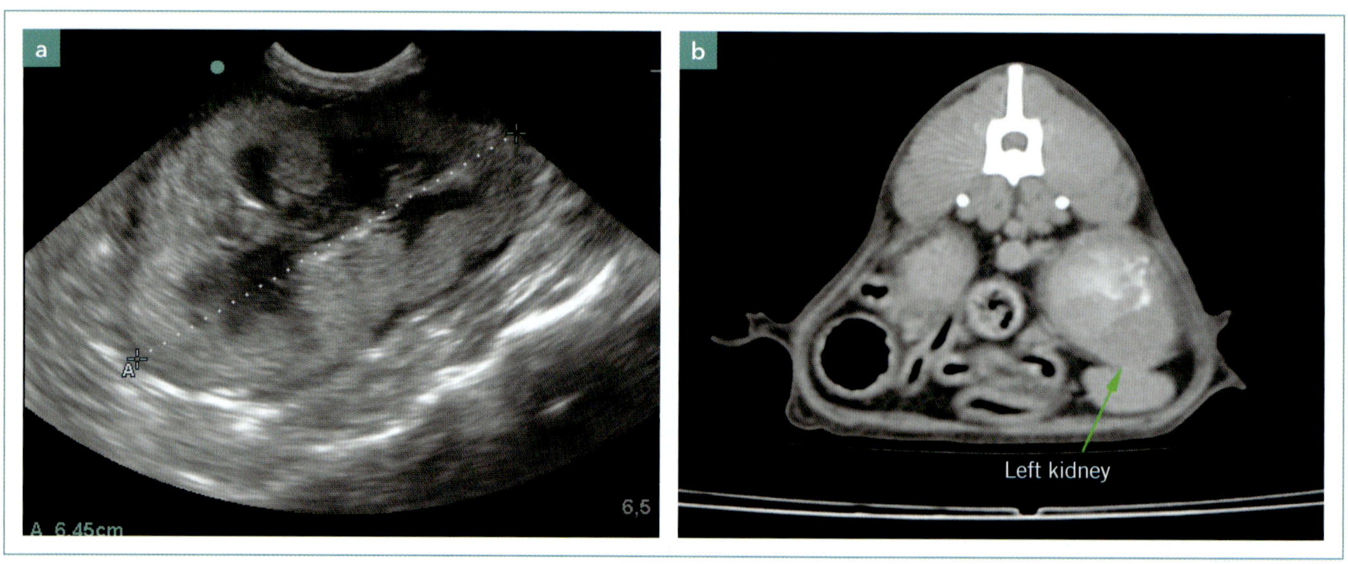

FIGURE 4. (a) Ultrasound of a renal lymphoma. Nephromegaly is observed, along with cortical thickening, increased cortical echogenicity, and a slight presence of subcapsular liquid. Image courtesy of Alejandro Casasús. (b) Computed tomography scan of a left renal carcinoma. Several areas of calcification are seen (white dots). Image courtesy of Diagnosfera.

case in kidney disease, and can be secondary to hematuria, but we should also keep in mind that when there are small erythropoietin-producing kidney tumors, the only change in laboratory analysis is polycythemia/erythropoiesis (Fig. 5).

Renal abscesses

Renal abscesses occur rarely, but they require a nephroureterectomy or a partial nephrectomy if medical treatment fails. In most cases, they are diagnosed secondarily to pyelonephritis that is refractory to treatment, in hydronephrosis complicated by an infection, in cases associated with a tumor, or in cystic kidneys. They can be subcapsular or intrarenal. Patients usually present with lethargy, anorexia, vomiting, pain and leukocytosis. Diagnosis is done via ultrasound and by extracting a sample through puncture–aspiration.

Idiopathic renal hematuria

Idiopathic renal hematuria, or benign essential hematuria, is a rare condition, but it can cause a severe enough loss of blood that removal of the affected kidney is indicated. It is usually a unilateral condition that affects the renal pelvis more often than the parenchyma. Interventional surgery options are very limited due to the size of the feline ureter in comparison to catheters and work channels for minimally invasive surgery. Currently, trying to save as many nephrons as possible it is a given, but the feasibility of ligating one branch of the renal artery versus performing a nephrectomy can only be evaluated with CT angiography in feline patients with this lesion, which is often complicated by clots obstructing the ureter.

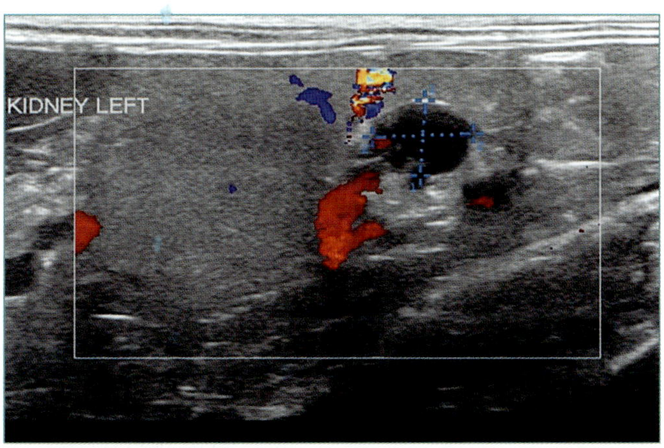

FIGURE 5. Ultrasound of a mass in the kidney. In this case the patient presented with polycythemia.

Surgical diseases of the ureter

Ureterolithiasis

Ureterolithiasis should really be called nephroureterolithiasis, since both organs are always involved. Calculi in the upper urinary tract of cats are almost always made up of calcium oxalate (90%), with an appreciable frequency of calculi comprising dried solidified blood. The latter calculi are difficult to diagnose since they are neither radiopaque nor cast any acoustic shadow in ultrasound. Struvite calculi constitute only 6% of calculi in feline ureters and kidneys.

> In addition to physical obstruction caused by the urolithiasis itself, in 20% of cases the ureter presents scarring and stenosis.

Ureteral calculi cannot be dissolved through dietary changes, as they are not continually bathed in urine. Lithotripsy is not an option for cats, since their ureters are very small organs and iatrogenic injury can easily be caused.

The clinical signs are those of acute renal failure (anorexia, vomiting, weakness, azotemia). Before opting for surgery, we should always try to dislodge the stones and promote their elimination through nonsurgical medical treatment (see below, "Preoperative considerations"). If only one kidney is affected and the other is functioning correctly, the clinical picture may be overlooked. In any case, if the cat is in an oliguric phase, or if there is sepsis, hyperkalemia, marked azotemia or severe hydrophrenosis, the decision to intervene surgically must be made, independently of the presentation of the nephroureterolithiasis.

Ureteral trauma/rupture

Ureteral rupture does not occur frequently. It may be associated with falls from heights, road traffic accidents, gunshots, or iatrogenic causes (accidental ligature in abdominal surgery). It is difficult to diagnose if the loss of urine is in the cranial portion, since the only thing that is seen is a retroperitoneal cyst on ultrasound or CT scan. If it is more caudal, it is associated with peritoneal effusion. Clinical signs are associated with the trauma suffered, along with nonspecific abdominal pain, azotemia and hyperkalemia. Medical treatment includes fluid therapy, dialysis and emergency placement of a nephrostomy tube to stabilize the patient before surgery. Surgical treatment options include repair of the ureter, ureteral reimplantation if the lesion is sufficiently distal, or most commonly, nephroureterectomy.

Ureteral neoplasia

An exclusively ureteral tumor has not been described in cats; it is always associated with kidney or bladder tumors. Clinical signs are nonspecific: anorexia, weight loss and hematuria, which in 66% of cases is due to the presence of a kidney tumor. In the bladder, transitional cell carcinomas that affect the trigone can spread to the ureteral lumen.

Ureteral ectopia

Ureteral ectopia is the abnormal implantation of the opening of the ureters, usually in the urethra, of congenital origin. Unilateral and bilateral cases have been reported, but this pathology is rare in cats (less than 30 described cases). In every case, the predominant clinical sign is urinary incontinence. It is not rare for this condition to present with other congenital abnormalities (hydroureter, hydronephrosis, hypoplasia of the bladder or kidney). If the ureter cannot be reimplanted, the solution is nephroureterectomy.

Diagnosis

Patients with surgical diseases of the kidney and ureter may present with acute or subacute obstructive renal failure. Depending on the pathology, pain may also be a significant clinical sign. If renal failure is part of the clinical picture, anorexia, weight loss, weakness and vomiting may be constant or nearly constant. Lithiasis and tumors may present with hematuria in up to 66% of the cases. Urinary incontinence is associated exclusively with ectopic ureters implanting into the urethra.

Imaging tests are essential to the diagnosis of any kidney and ureter diseases that may require surgery (Table 1)

Preoperative considerations

Patients with bilateral obstructive diseases of the upper urinary tract (or unilateral diseases with a nonfunctioning contralateral kidney) usually present with severe acute metabolic alterations. Prior stabilization of the patient, as much as possible, improves the prognosis and the safety of the anesthesia Treatment varies on a case by case basis:

- If the disease is obstructive, electrolyte and acid–base abnormalities and azotemia are frequent. To correct this, administering a 0.9% NaCl solution (or glucose solution if there is hypernatremia) is safe at an initial dose of 40–60 ml/kg/hour for the first 30 minutes, adjusting the infusion rate depending on the patient's status and response to therapy.
- In case of hyperkalemia, an electrocardiogram is mandatory before anesthesia. Response to therapy must also be monitored.

TABLE 1. Diagnostic tests of surgical diseases of the kidney and ureter in cats

Diagnostic test	Kidney disease	Ureteral disease	Observations
Blood work	■ Neoplasm ■ Nephrolithiasis ■ Renal abscess ■ Trauma ■ Essential hematuria	Bilateral obstructive disease	If the clinical picture is unilateral, and the contralateral kidney is functioning correctly, there may not be alterations.
		Ureteral rupture	Tests show hyperkalemia, azotemia and metabolic acidosis.
Urinalysis	■ Neoplasm ■ Nephrolithiasis ■ Renal abscess ■ Trauma ■ Essential hematuria	Ureterolithiasis	■ Can aid in the diagnosis of a number of pathologies: presence of crystalluria, hematuria, tumor cells or urinary casts. ■ Low sensitivity and specificity.
X-rays	■ Nephrolithiasis ■ Neoplasm ■ Trauma	Radiopaque ureteroliths (oxalate, struvite)	■ Calculi made up of dried solidified blood are radiotransparent and cannot be seen. ■ Very small calculi may not be seen in X-rays.

TABLE 1. Diagnostic tests of surgical diseases of the kidney and ureter in cats

Diagnostic test	Kidney disease	Ureteral disease	Observations
Ultrasound Given its cost–benefit ratio, this is the most recommended test for diseases of the urinary tract	■ Neoplasm ■ Nephrolithiasis ■ Renal abscess ■ Trauma ■ Essential hematuria	■ Any type of ureterolith ■ Ureterocele and ureteral dilatation ■ Parietal fibrosis and stenosis caused by scarring ■ Neoplasm ■ Ectopic ureter	■ Calculi usually generate an acoustic shadow. ■ Higher sensitivity in very small calculi. ■ Congenital ureteroceles and cranial dilatation of obstructive calculi. ■ Ureteral neoplasms are very rare in cats.
Contrast radiography (excretory urography)	■ May be useful in all renal conditions ■ Whenever planning a nephroureterectomy, make sure that the remaining kidney is functioning properly	■ Rupture of the ureter ■ Ureteral functionality	■ Flow of contrast medium into the retroperitoneal space or abdominal cavity, depending on the rupture site. ■ Useful for evaluating functionality and morphology. Helps diagnose stenosis, dilatation and abnormal ureteral insertions.
Computed tomography (Fig. 6)	Can diagnose any of the above pathologies	Can diagnose any of the above pathologies	■ If combined with excretory urography, this is the gold standard for diagnosis of ureteral disease. ■ The limitations are the cost and the fact that sedation is required.
Urocystoscopy	This is the test of choice for idiopathic hematuria: several ureteral jets in each of the vesicoureteral junctions	Ectopic ureter	Aids diagnosis of the type of ureteral ectopia.

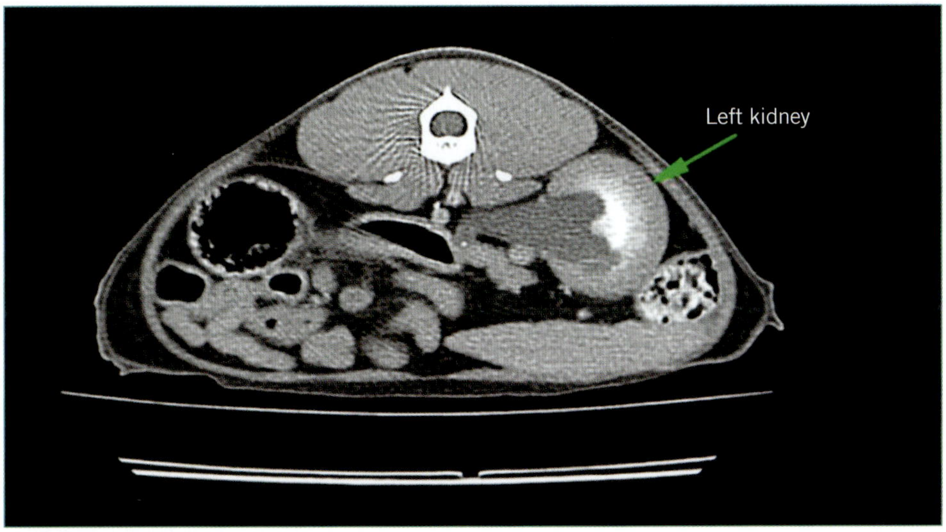

FIGURE 6. Computed tomography scan showing severe dilatation of the left renal pelvis. Image courtesy of Diagnosfera.

How to do an excretory urography

- If using a radiological technique, previous lateral and ventrodorsal X-rays are taken to confirm that the colon is empty, thus avoiding overlaps and artifacts.
- Anesthesia is required to obtain the maximal image quality.
- Intravenous iohexol is used as contrast medium (5 ml of contrast agent at 50% in isotonic saline solution).
- The contrast agent can be administered as a bolus injection (useful for renal parenchymal lesions) or by continuous intravenous infusion (better visualization of contrast in the ureters).

Information that can be obtained with this technique:

- Kidney location, size, morphology and function.
- Leakage of contrast medium into the abdomen or retroperitoneal space.
- Other ureteral transit abnormalities: stenosis, obstructions, morphological abnormalities.
- Abnormal implantation of ureters.

- For distal ureteral ruptures with severe peritoneal effusion, an emergency peritoneal dialysis may be required. The diagnosis can be confirmed by comparing the **blood:ascitic fluid ratio** with respect to the concentration of creatinine or potassium. In ureteral ruptures it is around 1:2 or up to 1:4 in the case of creatinine.
- If there is a single ureterolith that is not very large, attempting to dislodge it with medical treatment is advised before resorting to surgery. The most widely accepted protocol used today includes intensive fluid therapy, analgesics (buprenorphine every 8–12 hours, methadone every 6–8 hours, or even a continuous intravenous infusion of fentanyl or fentanyl with ketamine) and smooth muscle relaxants (prazosin every 12 hours). If both kidneys are affected, or if the second kidney is diseased (big kidney–little kidney syndrome), medical therapy should be attempted for a maximum of 3 days before making the decision to operate (nonsurgical treatment is successful in 17%–20% of cases). If the other kidney is functioning properly, the therapy can be extended for up to 2 weeks, especially if the calculus is monitored and its mobility is confirmed via ultrasound or other imaging tests.
- We should always collect urine by cystocentesis or pyelocentesis for culture and antibiogram beforehand in case there is an associated infection (the frequency of this is up to 25% of cases according to studies).

Surgical techniques for the kidney

Renal biopsy

A renal biopsy can be performed to diagnose the cause of an acute renal disease and in cases with high proteinuria indicating glomerular injury/lesion. The biopsy is taken from the renal cortex, since the medulla is rarely involved and the chance of complications stemming from bleeding and clot formation, which can lead to an obstruction, is higher.

There are three ways to take a renal biopsy sample: percutaneous, ultrasound-guided percutaneous, and via surgery.

Percutaneous biopsy

For this technique:

- The kidney is immobilized, and a 1.5–2 cm incision is made on the skin above the kidney using a no. 11 scalpel blade.
- Blunt dissection is performed until the kidney is found.
- A punch biopsy 3 or 4 mm in diameter is carried out. Depending on the case, it may be worthwhile to take more than one sample. Studies have shown that taking more than one biopsy does not increase the chances of generating a more severe renal lesion.
- Bleeding is inevitable. Simply observe whether it stops in a reasonable amount of time, and close the abdominal defect in layers.

Collagen sponges, such as those used in dentistry, can be used to stop the bleeding of a wound caused by a punch biopsy. A suture made with an atraumatic needle and a 4-0 or 5-0 absorbable monofilament can be used to keep the sponge in place, availing ourselves of the renal capsule and making sure not to exert too much pressure on the stitch. A few drops of medical-grade cyanoacrylate can be used instead of the suture with a similar result.

Ultrasound-guided biopsy

Only a small skin incision is needed to enable us to insert the biopsy needle (tru-cut). To do this:

- The kidney is immobilized.
- The biopsy needle is inserted, taking care to stop before reaching the pelvis. Rather than going in a perpendicular direction, it is worthwhile to take the sample at approximately a 40° angle, or almost parallel to the line of the kidney to avoid penetrating the medulla, as mentioned above (see Fig. 7b of Ch. 7).

Open biopsy

An abdominal approach is required:

- With the cat in dorsal recumbency, a midline approach is used, starting at the umbilicus and extending the incision cranially as far as necessary to expose the kidneys.
- The peritoneum is incised, and the perirenal fat that may be found in this location is carefully dissected (this can be done with curved blunt-tipped Metzenbaum scissors, with sterile swabs, or even with the surgeon's own fingers).
- The biopsy is performed in the desired area of the renal cortex. This can be done with a punch, as described above (preferred technique) or by collecting the sample with the tip of a scalpel (see Fig. 7a of Ch. 7).
- After making sure that there is no bleeding, the peritoneum is first closed with a 3-0 monofilament suture. The abdomen is then closed in layers as per routine.

Variables to consider when choosing the type of biopsy

- **The patient's status:** according to the results of previous tests such as hematocrit, clotting tests, and azotemia levels. The sedation needed for a tru-cut biopsy is less than the anesthesia needed for the other two biopsy techniques, but the risk of being unable to control bleeding is greater.
- **The ability to examine the entire urinary tract:** a laparotomy enables us to expose more of the abdomen and evaluate the ureters and the bladder in case more than one biopsy sample is required.
- **The volume of sample required:** in contrast to punch biopsy samples, specimens taken with a scalpel usually contain more tissue.
- **Postoperative bleeding:** as mentioned above, bleeding is a possible complication. In fact, hematuria is to be expected in the 24–48 hours after a renal biopsy. In addition, monitoring hematocrit and total protein is advised during the 24 hours following the procedure, especially if the cat is not in stable condition. Ultrasound monitoring enables us to check for the presence of retroperitoneal and/or subcapsular fluid and to monitor the quantity.
- Nowadays, renal biopsy and exploration of the abdominal cavity can be done via laparoscopy.

Nephrolithotomy and pyelolithotomy

Both of these techniques aim to eliminate calculi lodged in the renal pelvis. Neither is a first-choice technique, given that nephrolithotomy requires us to stop renal circulation for the duration of the surgery, and pyelolithotomy requires us to work in an area that is impossible to access if not dilated, and difficult to access if it is.

With the emergence of ureteral bypass devices, these are not the techniques of choice in many cases. However, despite modest results, they remain valid techniques.

For a **nephrolithotomy**:

- The kidney is partially dissected from its retroperitoneal position, since the organ is accessed from its lateral, convex side.
- Before cutting, the renal artery and vein are very carefully isolated, since they must be occluded to stop circulation. This is done with a Rummel tourniquet or with vessel loops.

Practical note: small Penrose drains and small pieces of nasal tubing can be used to interrupt renal circulation.

- The kidney is gently held with the surgeon's nondominant hand, using the other hand to cut the lateral part of the kidney lengthwise, through to the pelvis. The tip of a no. 11 scalpel blade is used to start the cut, and the opening of the parenchyma is continued by means of a combined technique of dissection with the scalpel blade and a more blunt dissection using sterile swabs or blunt-tipped scissors to minimize damage to the vessels.

> **Practical note**: if the uroliths are not very large, rather than making an extensive cut, the kidney can initially be accessed with a cut that is smaller but large enough to pass an otoscope head through it, making use of alligator forceps to remove the calculi.

- Once the uroliths have been removed, flushing is performed with saline solution.
- The cut edges of the kidney are brought together, and the capsule is sutured in a simple continuous pattern using polydioxanone or another long-lasting monofilament. Medical-grade cyanoacrylate can be used for reinforcement.
- The tourniquets are released and the surgeon makes sure that there is no active bleeding.
- The kidney is repositioned.
- The peritoneum is closed with a couple of stitches, and the abdomen is sutured as per routine.

For a **pyelolithotomy**:

- To expose the renal pelvis, any adhesions of the pelvis to the peritoneum are gently dissected, along with any perirenal fat found in the area, using swabs, the surgeon's fingers or blunt-tipped Metzenbaum scissors.
- A small incision is made in the pelvis or in the proximal ureter, or both, and the calculi are extracted.

> **Practical note**: a tourniquet can be used to hold the calculi in place (vessel loops proximal and distal to the urolith), since, if there is severe hydronephrosis, the urolith may move to the interior of the kidney when the pelvis is cut, complicating the extraction.

- The suture is begun distally to ensure that the ureter is not obstructed. A 5-0 nonabsorbable monofilament is used to maximally limit the reaction of the pelvis and ureter to the suture material, thus minimizing inflammation. A simple continuous or interrupted pattern can be used.

Nephroureterectomy

To eliminate both the kidney and ureter:

- A midline laparotomy is effectuated.
- To expose the left kidney, the descending colon can be used as a natural retractor for the abdominal viscera. To access the right kidney, the same can be done with the mesoduodenum (colonic and duodenal maneuvers, see Ch. 20).
- The renal artery and vein are isolated via careful dissection of the peritoneal space immediately ventral to the renal hilum.
- Each of the isolated vessels is sutured separately. The sutures should be double, one en bloc and the other transfixing. A 2-0 or 3-0 absorbable suture, such as polydioxanone, can be used.
- Next, the ureter is located and dissected up to the point most proximal to the ureterovesical junction, where a double ligature is also performed (in this case the transfixion suture is not necessary).
- Mosquito forceps are used to grasp underneath the ligatures, the tissue is cut, and the kidney and ureter are extracted.
- The abdomen is closed as per routine.

Partial nephrectomy

This surgery is not advised due to the associated complications. Performing a total nephrectomy is usually simpler, but for the few patients who have a primary tumor located in one renal pole, partial nephrectomy would preserve the maximum amount of healthy renal tissue. This technique is also used for the extraction of subcutaneous ureteral bypass (SUB) devices that no longer work, and which needs to be replaced with another such device or a ureteral stent.

A partial nephrectomy cannot be performed in cats with any type of coagulation disorder. The risk of postoperative bleeding is significant, and this sometimes limits the use of this technique in feline patients.

For this surgery:

- A midline laparotomy is effectuated, and the affected kidney is accessed as described above.
- The capsule of the section of kidney to be eliminated is removed (Fig. 7.1).

- Two thick absorbable sutures (0 or 1-0) are applied with a long straight needle. These sutures are placed at the level of the cut, avoiding damage to the renal vessels or ureter (Fig. 7.2).
- The sutures are knotted such that a double figure-of-eight is traced around the area to be excised (the technique is similar to the overlapping sutures used in liver biopsy) (Fig. 7.3).
- The fragment is cut, and any vessel that bleeds is sutured. It is important to avoid using electrocautery, since it can damage the renal parenchyma too much. The tissue is sutured (Fig. 7.4).
- To prevent the kidney from rotating, the capsule is sutured (Fig. 7.5) and the kidney is anchored to the sublumbar musculature.
- The area of open peritoneum may be reconstructed as much as possible.

Surgical techniques for the ureter

The most frequent ureter surgical procedures performed in cats are those associated with ureteral obstructions, usually caused by one or more calcium oxalate calculi. As mentioned before, this substance cannot dissolve by means of dietary changes. If presenting in combination with progressive and rapid deterioration of renal function, act quickly to achieve patency of the ureter.

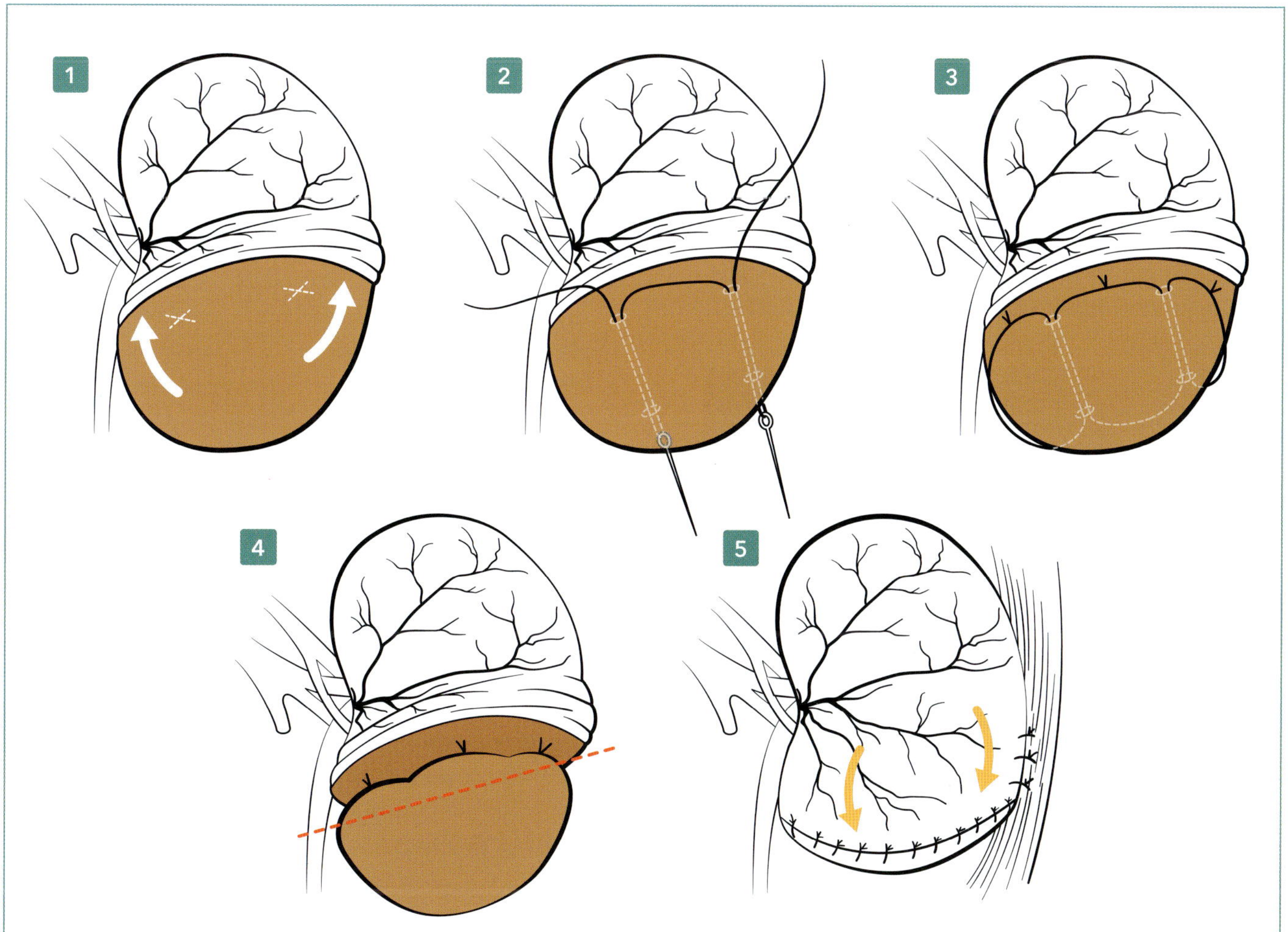

FIGURE 7. Steps for partial nephrectomy.
1. The renal capsule is removed.
2. Two thick sutures are applied with a long straight needle at the level of the cut, avoiding damage to any vessels or the ureters.
3. The sutures are tied around the area in a double figure-of-eight.
4. The fragment is cut, and any vessel that bleeds is sutured.
5. The renal capsule is sutured.

A different case: perinephric pseudocysts

Pseudocysts are defined as such because there is no epithelium that covers them. They are fluid-filled (usually transudate, although cases of pseudocysts containing urine have been described) sacs that surround the kidney (Fig. 8). They can be unilateral or bilateral, and fluid accumulation can be subcapsular or extracapsular.

Feline perinephric pseudocysts usually accompany chronic kidney disease, but the correlation between these two conditions has not been determined.

These cysts can be treated in several different ways:

- Intermittent ultrasound-guided percutaneous drainage
- Capsulectomy or fenestration of the pseudocyst capsule
- Omentalization
- Nephrectomy

Treatment of these cysts has been associated with an improvement in the glomerular filtration rate. Therefore, allowing them to drain into the abdominal cavity is the most compelling treatment.

The entire external capsule can be cut up to 2 cm from the renal hilum. In addition to this, use a continuous suture and apply omentum to the remaining section of capsule.

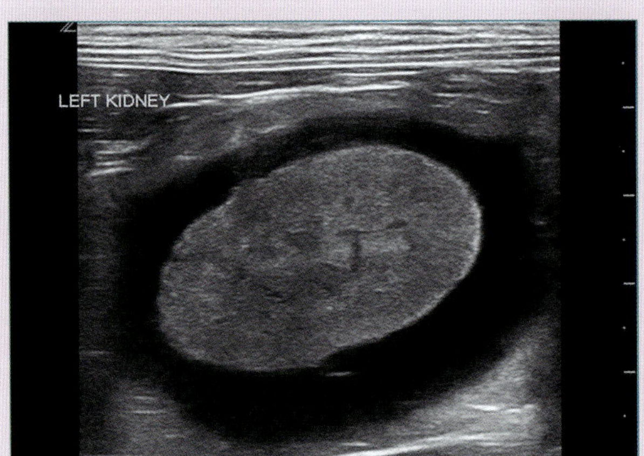

FIGURE 8. Ultrasound of a perinephric pseudocyst in a cat.

A number of techniques, some more successful than others, have been described over the last 30 years to achieve this. The choice of surgical method depends on the surgeon's experience, the particulars of the case, and the availability of materials and devices. In any case, all of these are specialized surgeries that should be performed by experienced surgeons.

Ureterotomy

This is the simplest and most intuitive technique. One or more incisions are made in the ureteral wall to extract the calculi obstructing the ureter. This should only be done by a surgeon specialized in microsurgery, using the proper magnifying equipment (×4 minimum). This technique only provides a 50% improvement over medical treatment.

For this surgery:

- The cat is placed in dorsal recumbency, and a wide incision is made along the midline. Once the location of the calculus has been pinpointed (it appears as a dark shadow through the dilated ureteral wall), the stretch of ureter is isolated with the help of two atraumatic elastic vessel loops (care must be taken not to damage the longitudinal vascularization of the ureteral wall). This demarcates the surgical field, decreases the flow of urine towards the area of intervention, and prevents migration of the ureterolith.
- Using a no. 11 scalpel blade, an incision is made in the dilated area, **cranially to the stenosis or over the calculus if it is lodged in the wall**. To help confirm whether the ureter is patent, and additionally to have a guide, a portion of suture can be passed cranially and caudally to the incision (2-0 or 0 monofilament suture). This suture is removed prior to completion of ureterotomy closure.
- With the help of magnifying lenses, the stoma of the ureter is sutured with interrupted stitches using 8-0 absorbable monofilament. Before placing the two final stitches, the guide suture is removed from the ureteral lumen.
- Upon completion of the technique, excess diuresis of the released kidney is to be expected. Evacuation is aided by the use of an indwelling catheterization system (tomcat catheter).

The most frequent complications described are leakages through the surgical wound and stenosis caused by scarring. Ureterotomy is associated with high rates of recurrence and mortality after surgery.

Ureteral endoprosthesis (stent)

Since 2005, the use of ureteral stents (devices placed in the ureteral lumen to promote the passage of urine through and around them, thus resolving obstruction of the ureter) has given rise to in an improvement in results and prognosis of cats with benign ureteral obstructions treated surgically. Although several techniques have been described to place the stent into the ureteral lumen (e.g., retrograde from the bladder, cystoscopy-guided, via ureterotomy), the most common intervention is **antegrade placement via nephrotomy** (Fig. 9):

- The patient is placed in dorsal recumbency and a surgical field is prepared for a ventral midline laparotomy from the cranial umbilicus down to the prepubic region. A Balfour self-retaining retractor is used to maintain the abdominal cavity open.
- The affected kidney is dissected, separating it from its retroperitoneal anchor. With a blue catheter (22-gauge) the renal capsule is perforated along its greater curvature towards the pelvis. When urine begins to flow out of the catheter, the needle is removed. If fluoroscopy is available, proper positioning of the catheter in the renal pelvis can be verified with an injection of a 1:1 dilution of saline solution and sterile iodinated contrast medium.
- Before introducing the contrast medium, a urine sample is taken for culture.
- A 150 cm long, 0.018 inch (0.45 mm) caliber hydrophilic nitinol guidewire, lubricated with isotonic saline solution, is inserted through the catheter until it reaches the ureter. It is advanced up to and past the stenosis, using combined rotation and forward movements.
- Upon reaching the bladder, a 2–3 mm ventral minicystotomy is done to exteriorize the guidewire. The catheter is removed, leaving the nitinol guidewire, which travels across the renal parenchyma and exits through the cystotomy.
- A 0.034 inch dilation catheter is passed over the guidewire from the kidney across the length of the ureter. If the stenosis makes it difficult to move forward, it can help to hold both ends of the guidewire taut, making it "rigid." To facilitate the forward maneuver of the rigid guidewire–catheter, mosquito forceps are placed in the most cranial end in front of the catheter to serve as a stopper. Once the catheter is extracted, this same technique is used with the polyurethane, multifenestrated double-pigtail stent, which is passed over the guidewire until the cranial end is placed in the renal pelvis (the length can be calculated by measuring beforehand, or preferably, the position is visualized via fluoroscopy).
- Once the renal pigtail stent is properly positioned, the guidewire is extracted by pulling from the end in the bladder. As a precaution, the bladder end of the stent is held with mosquito forceps so that it does not shift out of its proper place. The cystotomy site is closed with an absorbable suture, and the laparotomy site is closed as per routine.
- A closed urinary collection system is left in the bladder for several days.

Compared to cases treated with ureterotomy, this technique improves azotemia levels, as well as the rate of recurrence and survival. However, various complications have been described associated with the use of ureteral stents: stent migration to the bladder, chronic cystitis, feline lower urinary tract disease (FLUTD), and early calcification of the stent, which causes iatrogenic obstruction. For this reason, although some surgeons continue to use ureteral stents, nowadays SUB devices are recommended for the treatment of cats with benign obstructive ureteral disease.

Subcutaneous ureteral bypass (SUB) system

This technique for resolving ureteral obstructions requires the use of a set of devices designed expressly for cats. It basically consists of a urinary bypass from the renal pelvis to the bladder via two catheters attached to a subcutaneous port, thus circumventing the ureteral obstruction. Nowadays, although this surgery requires experience and although it is not exempt from complications, it is the method of choice for treating benign ureteral obstructions. For this surgery:

- With the patient in dorsal recumbency, the abdomen is accessed through the midline from the epigastric region to the prepubic tendon.
- The affected kidney is dissected from its perirenal fat at the caudal pole. Once the greater curvature of the caudal pole is palpated, an 18-gauge catheter is inserted in the direction of the renal pelvis (Fig. 10). When urine comes out through the cone, a sample is taken and sent to the laboratory for culture and antibiogram. The stylet is withdrawn, and the catheter cone is held in place with mosquito forceps. The 0.035 inch, 45 cm long J-tip guidewire is passed approximately 5–8 cm through the catheter for placement into the renal pelvis. The guidewire is held in place with mosquito forceps to stop it from moving as the 18-gauge catheter is removed from inside the renal parenchyma.
- The inside of the 6.5 Fr pigtail nephrostomy catheter is flushed with isotonic saline solution, and it is passed with its metallic straightener over the guidewire, until reaching the renal pelvis (Fig. 11). Once the tip of the catheter is in place, the metallic straightener is withdrawn slightly and the catheter is further advanced into the pelvis. It is very important to withdraw the straightener and the guidewire little by little as the catheter is inserted, so that the catheter can adapt to the pelvic space with its curved shape. Once the entire pigtail end is inserted (the gray radiopaque stripe should enter into the pelvic space), the J-tip guidewire is removed, followed by the metallic straightener. Two strings that protrude

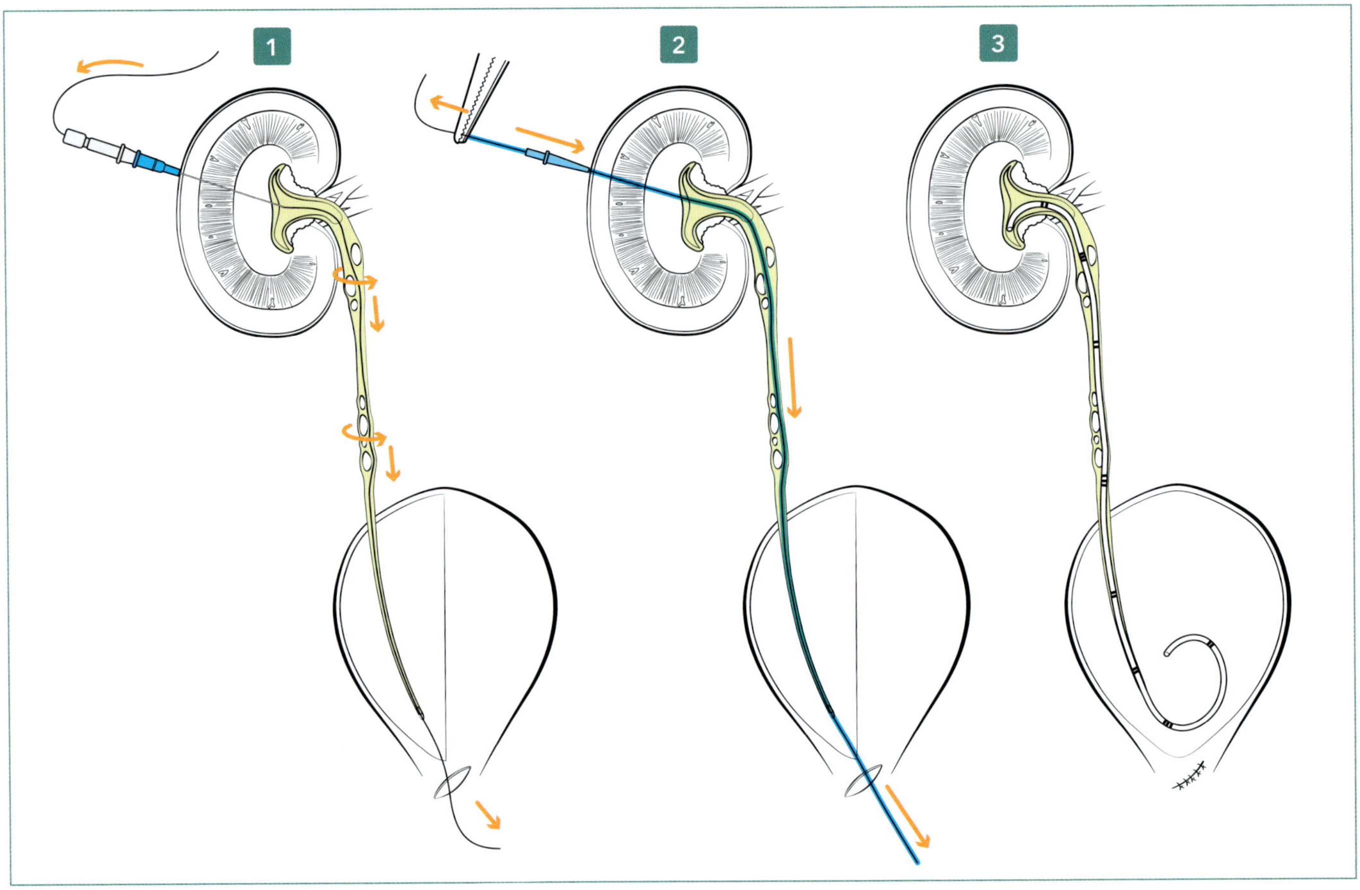

FIGURE 9. Placement of a ureteral stent.
1. Insertion of the hydrophilic nitinol guidewire using rotation and forward movements.
2. Passing the dilation catheter over the guidewire, which is held taut with the help of mosquito forceps.
3. Final placement of the stent inserted over the guidewire from the ventral cystotomy.

from the end of the catheter are pulled tight at this point and grasped with mosquito forceps, which act as a stopper. The curved shape of the end of the catheter is maintained, and as a result, it cannot move from its location. The Dacron cuff is advanced from the center of the catheter until it makes contact with the renal surface. It is glued with a few drops of sterile surgical cyanoacrylate (Fig. 12). After pressing for a few seconds, the catheter is in its proper place in the kidney.

- A nearby area without much vascularization to the side of the bladder apex is chosen. Without closing, a tobacco pouch suture is made on the surface of the bladder wall using 3-0 absorbable monofilament (Fig. 13). In the center of the suture, the bladder wall is perforated with a no. 11 scalpel blade, and the end of the other catheter is inserted with the help of the straightener. The catheter is lubricated beforehand with isotonic saline solution. The curved tip, including the gray radiopaque stripe, is inserted into the bladder, and the tobacco pouch is closed around the catheter. The Dacron cuff is lowered and a few drops of cyanoacrylate are applied to glue the cuff to the surface of the bladder. Once the glue is dry, three stitches are placed between the bladder wall and the Dacron cuff to reinforce the attachment of the catheter and the bladder and to prevent urine leakage (Fig. 14). The straightener is withdrawn and the strings are pulled taut with mosquito forceps, which acts as a stopper, giving the end of the catheter housed in the bladder lumen a curved shape.
- Both catheters are now in place, one in the kidney in a distal direction, and the other in the bladder in a cranial direction.
- Next, the fat from the abdominal wall on the same side as the operated kidney is dissected, leaving a wide area of muscle wall free to receive the subcutaneous port with silicone septum. It is placed 2–3 cm from the edge of the abdominal incision, at about the midpoint between the xyphoid process and the pubis (Fig. 15). The next step is to pass the ends of both catheters through the abdominal wall. Each side of the port is measured, leaving a width of about 3 fingers on each

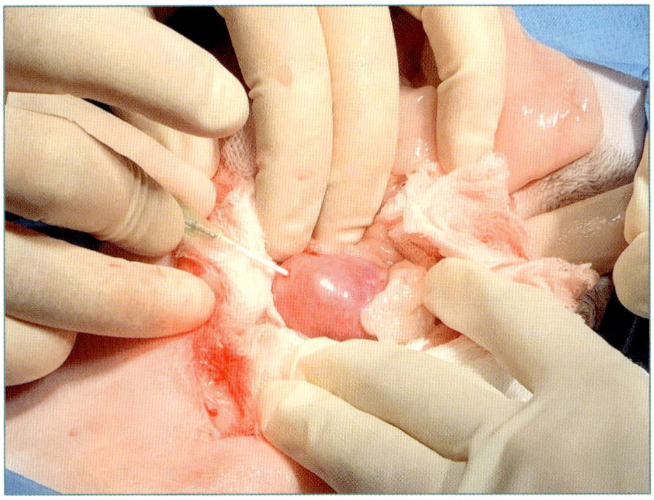

FIGURE 10. Puncture of the caudal pole of the kidney.

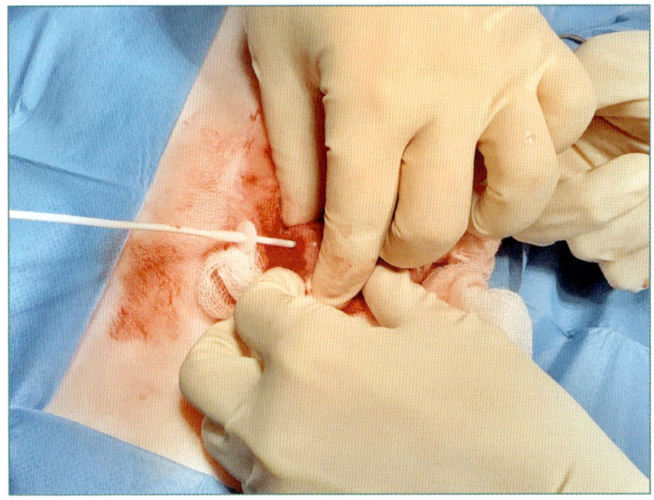

FIGURE 11. Insertion of the nephrostomy tube using the guidewire.

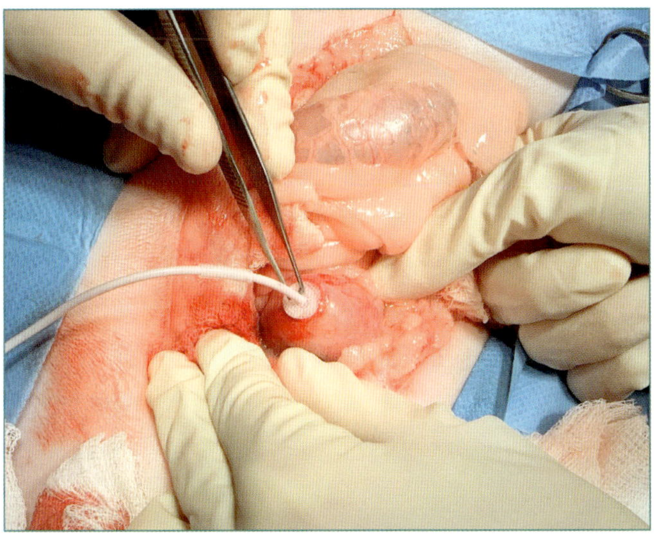

FIGURE 12. The nephrostomy tube is adhered to the kidney with cyanoacrylate thanks to the surface provided by the Dacron cuff.

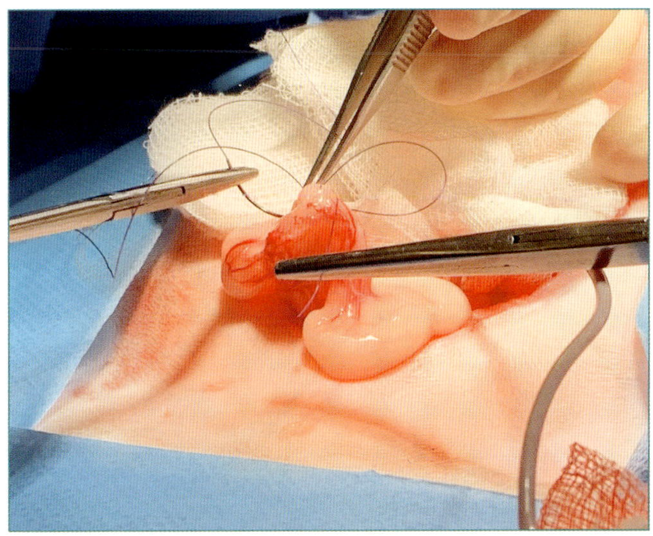

FIGURE 13. The bladder is readied with a tobacco pouch suture, without tightening the knot.

side to make two openings in the abdominal wall (about 9 cm between them) to allow the exit of both catheters (remember: the kidney catheter exits through the caudal opening and the bladder catheter exits through the cranial opening) (Fig. 16). The openings can be made with an electric scalpel or blunt dissection. When the catheters are passed through, care should be taken to keep the sutures on each side taut in order to maintain the pigtail shape.

- Before mounting the catheters in the SUB port, the interior of the port is flushed with isotonic saline solution to confirm its patency. The adequate blue boot is placed over each catheter (the tapered end first). Each catheter is connected to the metallic pin of the port with the following maneuver (Fig. 17): without losing tension in the suture, the pin is pushed approximately halfway into the end of the catheter. The suture is then cut with a no. 11 scalpel blade, using the metallic pin for support, such that when the rest of the catheter is attached to the port, the suture does not protrude, but maintains tension, along with the pigtail shape of the other end of the catheter. The same maneuver is done with the other catheter and the blue boots are placed over the connections to prevent leakage of urine through the port (Fig. 18). To further secure the port, apply a nylon suture to squeeze the blue boots. We once again verify the functionality of the device by aspirating urine with a needle through the silicone port.

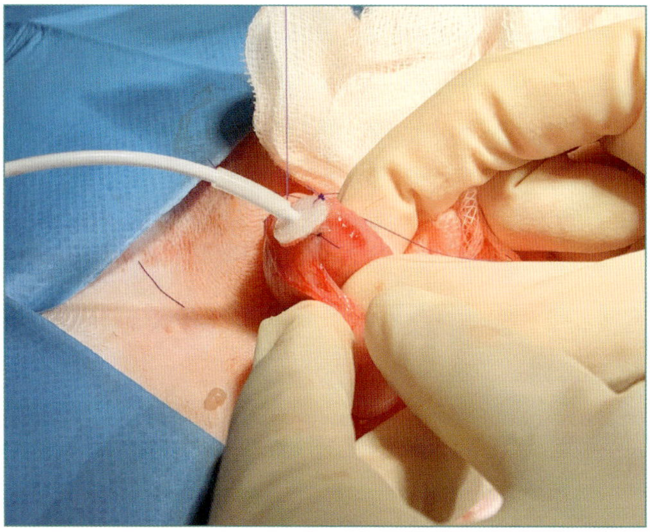

FIGURE 14. Suture of the Dacron cuff to the bladder wall.

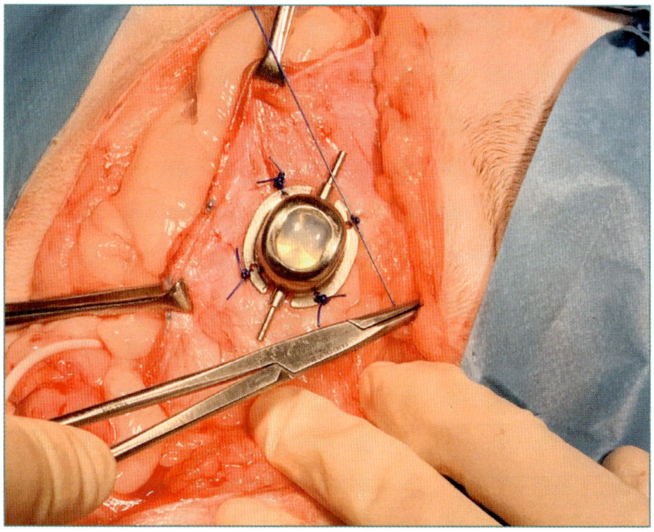

FIGURE 15. Preparation of the subcutaneous port.

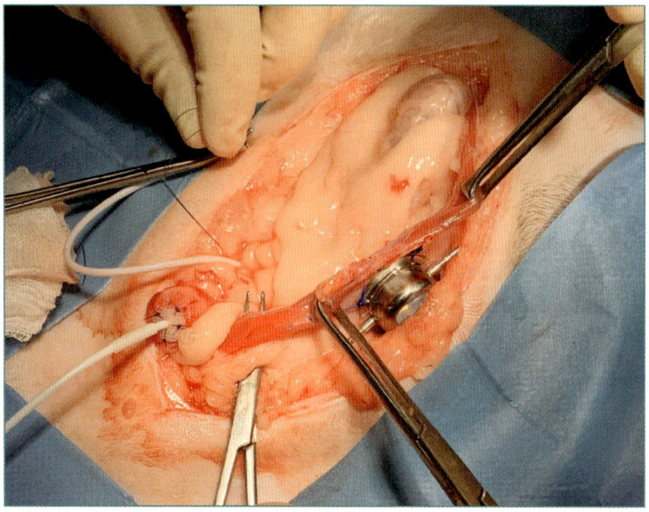

FIGURE 16. To minimize the possibility of kinking that could impede the free flow of urine, about 4 cm is measured between the exit port and the orifice before making the opening through which the tubes are passed

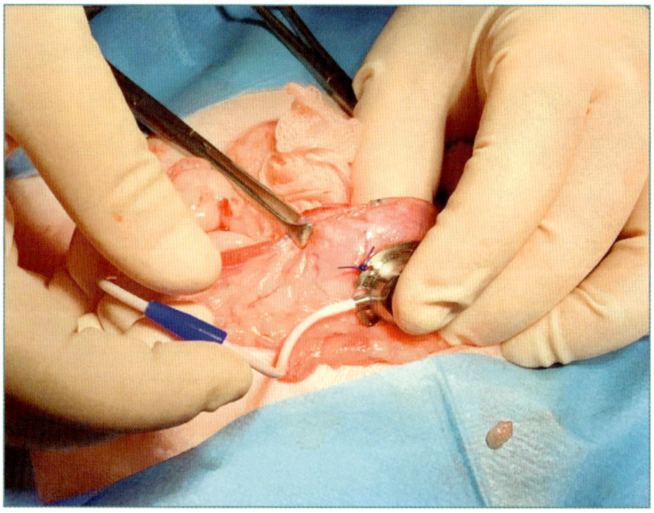

FIGURE 17. The tube is secured to the port.

- Finally, four 3-0 nylon stitches, one through each of the four openings in the base of the port, are used to suture the port to the abdominal wall. The laparotomy site is closed routinely, and the skin is closed with a continuous suture. This technique is more frequently used to resolve unilateral obstruction of one ureter (Fig. 19), but there are ready-made devices for surgery in both obstructed kidneys for use during a single surgical intervention (port with three pins, two for a catheter in each kidney and a third for the single catheter in the bladder) (Fig. 20).

One of the most frequent complications during the lifetime of the SUB device is kinks in the catheters at the entrance of the abdominal wall, with the consequent obstruction to the passing of urine. To avoid this, the device was redesigned, and in its 3.0 version, the subcutaneous port has a single catheter that enters the abdomen and connects to the kidney catheters and the bladder catheter by means of a three-way connector (Fig. 21). Thus, if the catheter has a kink and is occluded, it is easier to change it without having to disconnect any of the other catheters that are essential to the system.

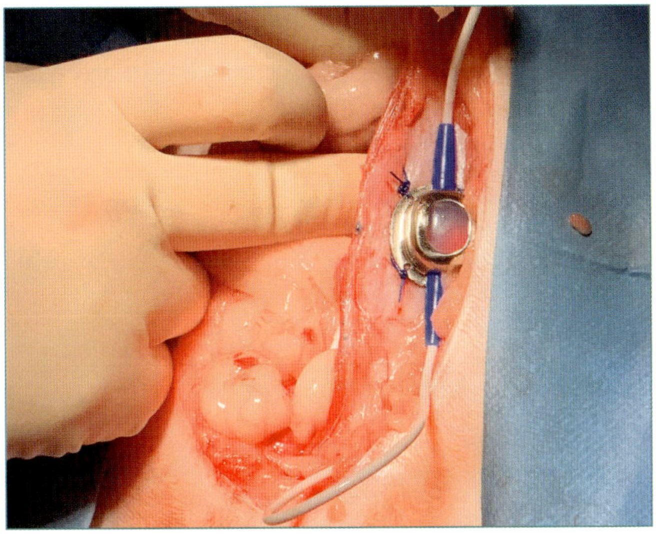

FIGURE 18. Before closure, check that the interior of the port is filling with urine. This is to ensure that no urine leaks through any of the connections.

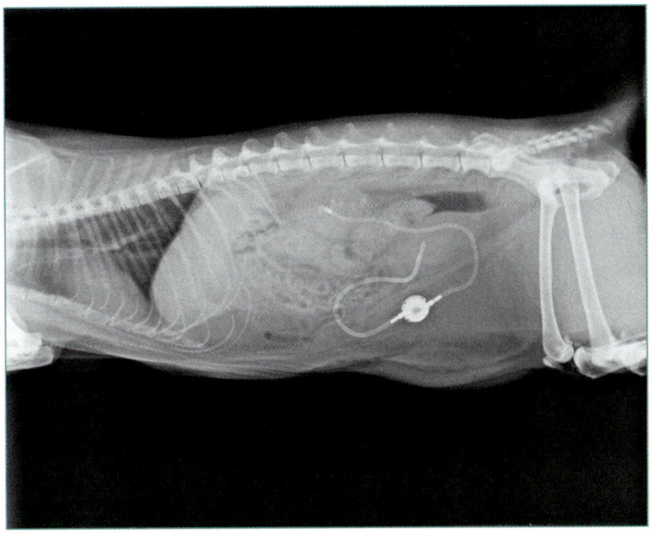

FIGURE 19. X-ray of a subcutaneous ureteral bypass (SUB) system placed in a cat. Both catheters can be seen entering the abdominal wall in a smooth curve without kinks, a key to the proper long-term functioning of the device.

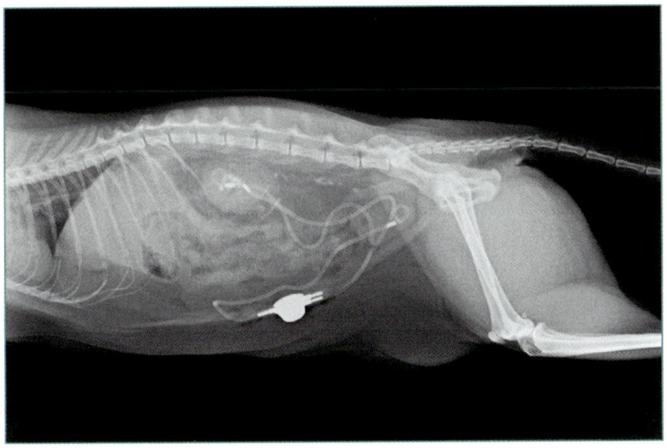

FIGURE 20. X-ray of a double subcutaneous ureteral bypass (SUB) system placed in a cat presenting with bilateral ureteral obstruction. A port with three pins enables a single catheter to be placed in the bladder. This minimizes trauma to the bladder and shortens the duration of surgery.

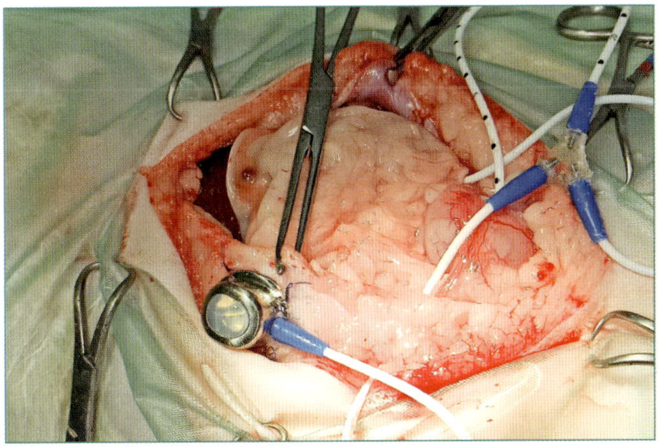

FIGURE 21. Implantation of a 3.0 subcutaneous ureteral bypass (SUB) system. The three-way piece joins the catheter that comes from the subcutaneous port to the kidney catheters and the bladder catheter. Image courtesy of Joaquín Albaladejo and Alicia Miñarro, Aggregata integrative feline medicine / Amigato feline clinic.

Postoperative care

Any surgery of the upper urinary tract requires good postoperative monitoring. There is no single concrete set of recommendations for all patients. While following the required basic checks, postoperative care is individualized.

Things to monitor:

- Urine production (urine flow rate): keep in mind that many patients experience postobstructive diuresis. This requires strict monitoring of the amount of fluids given and the concentration of electrolytes (ionogram).
- Leakage: look for the presence of free fluid around surgical sites in postoperative ultrasounds. Keep in mind that this fluid can be urine or blood.
- Hematocrit monitoring.
- Evaluation of kidney function and electrolytes.
- Pain control.
- Feeding: quickly resuming enteral feeding usually goes hand in hand with a good recovery. Most pathologies that affect

the kidneys and ureters cause anorexia, whether due to pain, azotemia, infection or a combination of these things. To avoid this, an esophagostomy tube can be placed during the same intervention. If it ends up not being necessary, it can be removed within a few days, but if there is anorexia, it ensures adequate caloric intake.

Bibliography

Berent A, Weisse C. Idiopathic renal hematuria/benign essential renal hematuria (chapter 59). In: Monnet E (ed.). *Small Animal Soft Tissue Surgery*. Wiley, 2012; pp. 615–622.

Berent AC, Weisse CW, Todd K, Bagley DH. Technical and clinical outcomes of ureteral stenting in cats for the treatment of benign ureteral obstruction: 2006–2010. *J Am Vet Med Assoc*, 2014; 244(5):559–576.

Culp WT, Palm CA, Hsueh C et al. Outcome in cats with benign ureteral obstructions treated by means of ureteral stenting versus ureterotomy. *J Am Vet Med Assoc*, 2016; 249(11):1292–1300.

DiBartola SP, Westropp J. Perinephric pseudocysts. In: August JR (ed.), *Consultations in Feline Internal Medicine*, vol. 3. Philadelphia, PA: WB Saunders, 1997; pp. 341–344.

Hill TP, Odesnik BJ. Omentalisation of perinephric pseudocysts in a cat. *J Small Anim Pract*, 2000; 41(3):115–118.

Kyles AE, Hardie EM, Wooden BG et al. Management and outcome of cats with ureteral calculi: 153 cases (1984–2002). *J Am Vet Med Assoc*, 2005; 226(6):937–944.

Lulich JP, Berent AC, Adams LG et al. ACVIM small animal consensus recommendations on the treatment and prevention of uroliths in dogs and cats. *J Vet Intern Med*, 2016; 30(5):1564–1574.

Marais J. Cortical microvasculature of the feline kidney. *Acta Anat*, 1987; 130(2):127–131.

Nicoli S. Uréter. In: Nicoli S (ed.). *Cirugía urológica del perro y del gato*. Zaragoza, Spain: Edra, 2020; pp. 63–116.

Ross SJ, Osborne CA, Lekcharoensuk C et al. A case-control study of the effects of nephrolithiasis in cats with chronic kidney disease. *J Am Vet Med Assoc*, 2007; 230(12):1854–1859.

Valdés-Martínez A, Cianciolo R, Mai W. Association between renal hypoechoic subcapsular thickening and lymphosarcoma in cats. *Vet Radiol Ultrasound*, 2007; 48(4):357–360.

Westropp JL, Ruby AL, Bailiff NL et al. Dried solidified blood calculi in the urinary tract of cats. *J Vet Intern Med*, 2006; 20(4):828–834.

BLADDER SURGERY 26

Alberto Barneto

Surgical anatomy

The urinary bladder is the receptacle that collects urine produced previously by the kidneys and transported to it through the two ureters. It is an ovoid-shaped sac having highly distensible walls situated in the caudoventral part of the abdomen, under the descending colon.

> Specifically in the feline species, the bladder can always be palpated in the abdominal position, cranially to the pubis.

When filled to repletion, it can reach the umbilicus. Situated dorsal to the bladder are the vasa deferentia (in males) or the body of the uterus (in intact females) (Fig. 1).

The bladder is held in the peritoneal space by three ligaments or serous folds:

- **Two lateral folds** that in females are the continuation of the broad ligaments of the uterus.
- **A ventrocranial fold** from the abdominal wall called the urachus, which is a vestige of the umbilical cord.

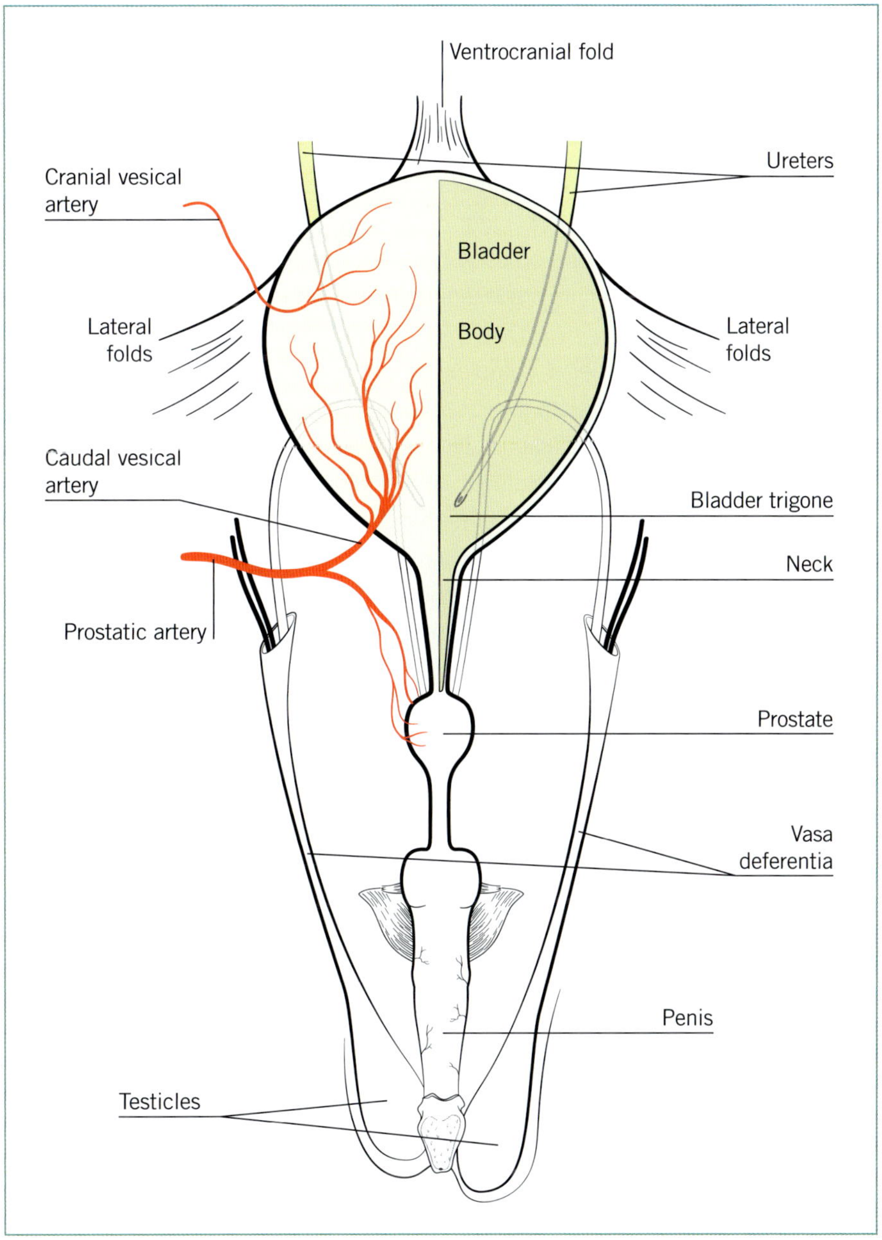

FIGURE 1. Anatomy and vascularization of the urinary bladder in cats (males).

From an anatomical perspective, the urinary bladder is divided into three defined zones:

- The **body** occupies nearly all the volume of the organ. When empty, the cranial part becomes more pointed, forming an **apex**. The structure is more fibrous in this area, and the urachus inserts here.
- The **neck** is at the exit of the bladder on the way to the urethra.
- The **trigone** is situated on the dorsocaudal aspect of the bladder and includes three structures: the insertion of the two ureteral orifices and the urethral orifice.

Blood supply to the bladder originates in the pudendal artery, from which the vaginal or prostatic arteries derive (in females and males, respectively). In the bladder neck, they give rise to the two **vesical arteries**, one on each side. These arteries branch off and supply the entire organ, anastomosing with the contralateral vessels.

Innervation of the bladder is complex: on the one hand, the autonomous nervous system exercises sympathetic control, keeping the smooth muscle sphincter contracted (via the **hypogastric nerve**), and parasympathetic control to empty the organ (via the **pelvic nerve**). On the other hand, the somatic nervous system innervates the voluntary component of urination by means of the **pudendal nerves** (control of the external sphincter). All these nerves enter the organ through the bladder neck.

The bladder wall is structured in four layers:

- The **mucosa** is made up of a highly elastic transitional epithelium, which forms irregular folds when the organ empties.
- The **submucosa** is the support structure, composed of loose connective tissue and collagen.
- The **muscular layer** is structured in multiple, interlaced smooth muscle fibers of various size.
- The **serosa** is a fine layer of fibrous connective tissue that continues with the peritoneum.

Surgical diseases of the feline bladder

The following bladder conditions and techniques may require surgical intervention.

- **Vesical calculi:** this is the most frequently occurring surgical pathology of the bladder in cats. The calculi are most commonly made up of **calcium oxalate** (small, dark brown calculi, sometimes faceted, affecting both the upper urinary tract and the bladder) or **struvite** (magnesium ammonium phosphate, not associated with urinary infection in cats), each of which occurs with a frequency of over 40% (source: Minnesota Urolith Center). The clinical signs of vesical calculi are dysuria, hematuria, strangury, and sometimes almost none. Urinalysis may show signs of cystitis (inflammatory cells, red blood cells, pH alterations, and rarely bacteriuria), but **there may be no crystalluria** in the sediment from recently collected urine. Proper diagnosis always requires the help of imaging techniques (Fig. 2).
- **Trauma (bladder rupture):** often associated with falls from heights or motor vehicle accidents, although iatrogenic cases also exist, resulting from excessive pressure on the bladder or traumatic catheterization. Bladder rupture is not always accompanied by dysuria or inability to palpate the bladder. However, uroperitoneum is always present, and to detect it, creatinine and potassium (K^+) levels are compared in serum and peritoneal fluid. Confirmation is then obtained by means of a positive-contrast urography, which conclusively demonstrates the existence of a leak. Repair is always effectuated surgically, but the traumatized animal should first be stabilized.
- **Neoplasms:** these are rare in cats, but the majority are epithelial in origin and malignant (carcinomas). They usually affect geriatric cats. In most cases, they do not involve the bladder trigone and are not metastatic. Clinical signs mimic those of infectious cystitis or calculi. Hematuria is observed especially often. Neoplasms can be diagnosed via ultrasound or endoscopy (Fig. 3). Fine needle aspiration should not be used to diagnose bladder tumors due to the risk of seeding malignant tumor cells along the needle tract. Cystotomy or endoscopy can be safely used, however, to obtain a sample. Only those neoplasms that do not affect the bladder trigone or neck can be treated by surgical removal.
- **Persistent urachus (urachal diverticulum):** the urachus inserts in the vesical apex during fetal development. The function of this canal is to eliminate waste from the bladder to the amniotic sac (its scar becomes the navel). When the canal, or part of it, remains patent after birth, this is called persistent urachus. Accumulating in a diverticulum of variable length, retained urine can cause infection. It is suspected in any case of chronic cystitis without a clear cause, and diagnosis is made through positive-contrast urography. The most effective solution is surgical closure of the patent urachus and removal of the urachal remnants.

- **Ectopic ureters:** ureteral ectopia occurs when one or both ureters drain in a different place than the vesical trigone (usually distal to it). They can drain directly outside of the trigone, in the urethra or in the vaginal vestibule (extramural ureters). They may also attach to the bladder at the correct position but have a section inside the bladder or urethral wall and drain in an anomalous place (intramural ureters). Both cases are resolved surgically. For intramural ureters, the wall is cut with laser under endoscopic guidance. For extramural ureters, the ureter is reimplanted in its correct location. Extramural ureteral ectopia is more common in cats.

- **Cystostomy tubes:** placement of cystostomy tubes for bypassing urine is a temporary solution in cases of trauma, urethral obstruction, inflammation or stenosis, until it becomes possible to restore normal patency to the urinary bladder. They can be kept in place without secondary infections for 7–14 days, although cases of placement of permanent tubes that were employed for a prolonged period without complications in patients with neurogenic dysfunction of the bladder (atonic bladder) have been described. In protracted cases, the Foley catheter should be replaced every 6 months, along with a new bladder stoma (Fig. 4).

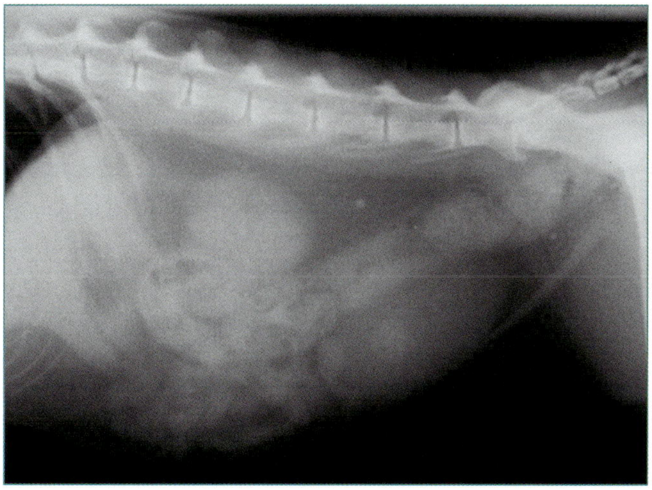

FIGURE 2. X-ray of a cat with multiple bladder calculi. Calcification in the kidneys, a ureteral calculus, and several calculi in the pelvic urethra are also visible. Image courtesy of Valleaguado veterinary clinic.

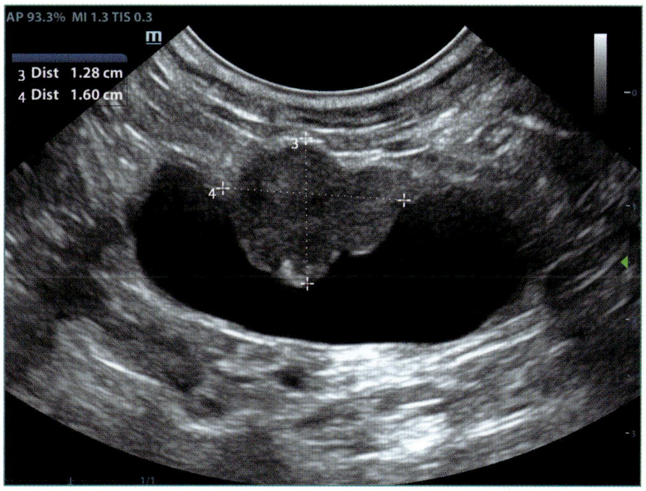

FIGURE 3. Ultrasound image of a bladder tumor in a 15-year-old female cat. The clinical signs were hematuria and dysuria.

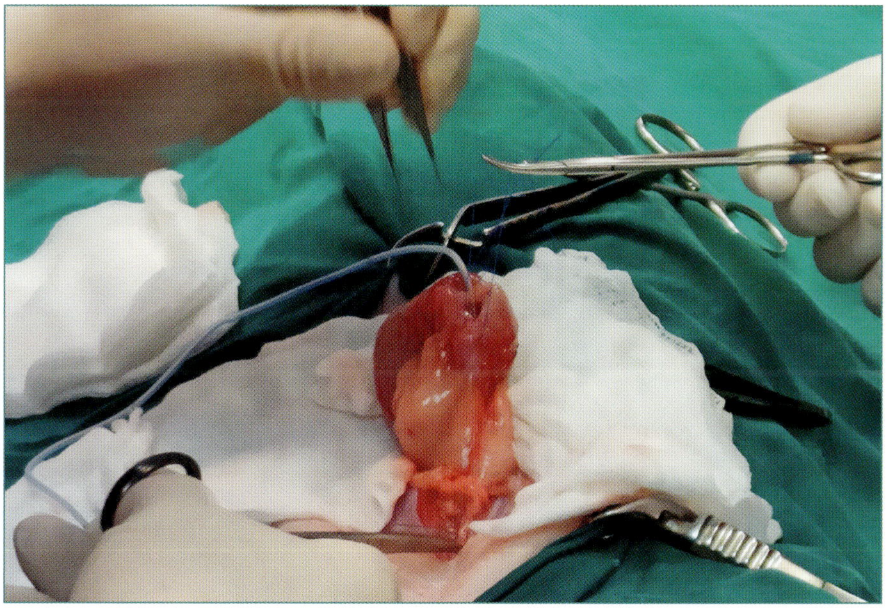

FIGURE 4. Placement of a cystostomy tube. A stoma is made and surrounded by a tobacco pouch suture. A silicone Foley catheter is placed through the stoma.

Diagnosis

Along with a medical history and patient examination, urinalysis and diagnostic imaging (Table 1) are needed to identify the bladder disease.

TABLE 1. Diagnostic tests and their use in different surgical pathologies of the bladder in cats

Diagnostic test	Results/indications	Observations
Urinalysis	Findings indicative of cystitis: hematuria, inflammatory cells, crystalluria, bacteriuria	Should always be done, but rarely provides an etiological diagnosis
Plain radiography	Observation of radiopaque objects (struvite and oxalate calculi)	Can be complemented with pneumocystography (air is the contrast medium, 8 ml/kg BW) for a better visualization of the calculi and wall irregularities
Positive-contrast radiography (8 ml/kg BW via urethral catheter) (Fig. 5)	Excellent technique for diagnosing: ■ Bladder rupture ■ Wall masses (neoplasms) due to defects in filling ■ Urachal diverticula	Double-contrast cystography (half positive-contrast medium, half air, in that order) enables visualization of radiotransparent calculi
Positive-contrast urography	All of the above, plus ectopic ureters	■ X-rays should be taken 15 minutes after administering the contrast agent to see the abnormal insertion ■ Always obtain two radiological projections ■ Diagnosis is improved if coupled with computed tomography
Ultrasound (Fig. 6)	■ Calculi ■ Bladder neoplasm ■ Bladder rupture (urine leakage is seen in the pelvic area)	Experienced ultrasonographers are able to detect urachal diverticula and ectopic ureters
Cystoscopy (more feasible for females than for males due to the urethral caliber)	■ Calculi ■ Bladder rupture ■ Neoplasm ■ Ectopic ureter	■ The rupture is not always visible, depending on the defect and the associated signs in the bladder mucosa ■ Enables visualization and biopsy ■ Enables visualization of an abnormal stoma and its location

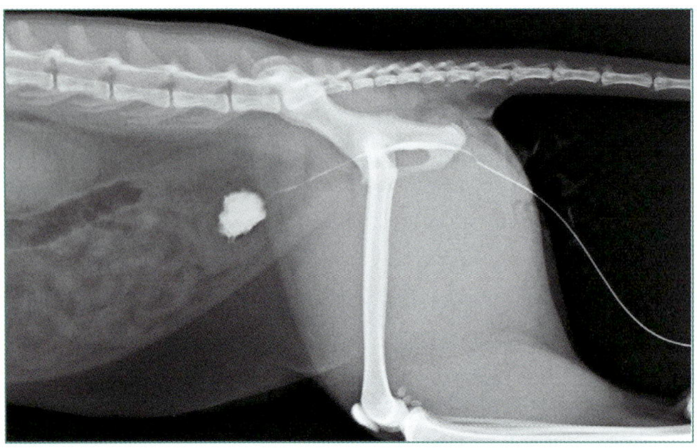

FIGURE 5. X-ray of a cat after positive-contrast cystography. This technique enables better visualization of the bladder walls. In this case, the bladder wall is thickened as a result of chronic cystitis.

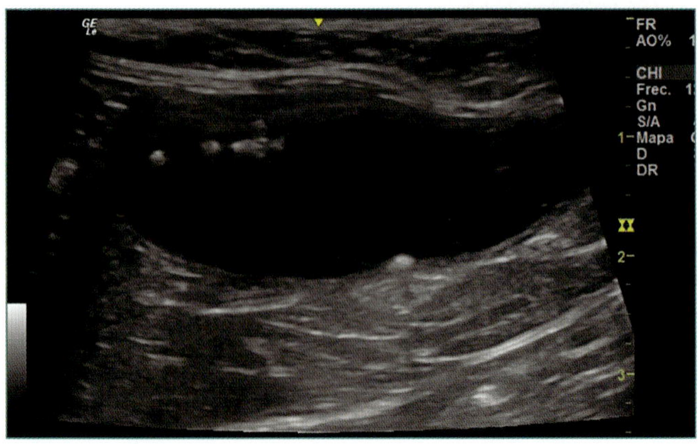

FIGURE 6. Ultrasound image of cystitis with calculi in a cat. Although most of the time the calculi are mobile, paradoxically they are sometimes located on the dorsal and ventral walls of the bladder at the same time. In this case, this is due to the presence of fibrin, which causes the calculi to adhere to the walls.

Preoperative and postoperative considerations

Before performing bladder surgery, a complete analysis of renal function should be effectuated, along with an imaging study (X-rays, ultrasound and/or computed tomography), for assessment of the scope and location of the issue, as well as the possible presence of concomitant pathologies.

A urine culture is often required to be able to treat any infection associated with the bladder disease. If it has not previously been done, a urine sample should be obtained via cystocentesis before performing a cystotomy (Fig. 7). Next, the bladder is further emptied before opening it in order to minimize contamination with urine.

In addition to avoiding urine leakage, a second surgical field made up of gauze dressings moistened with isotonic saline should be placed around the bladder. The gauze is replaced as needed during the intervention as it becomes contaminated with urine or flushing fluids.

Once the bladder is open, do not handle the mucosa more than necessary to avoid causing edema. Also, do not place gauze in contact with the mucosa. If their use is essential, moisten the gauze with warm isotonic saline solution.

It is highly useful, especially when extracting multiple bladder calculi, to place a catheter in the urethra before preparing the surgical field, keeping it there during the surgery in case a retrograde flushing must be done to help eliminate calculi from the bladder neck.

The bladder is sutured with absorbable monofilament suture material, using a nontransfixing Cushing continuous pattern (Fig. 8). This lowers the risk of leaving debris on the mucosa that may act as a nidus for calculus formation (in one study, such debris was the origin of 4% of urinary stones). The bladder heals and recovers full function in 21 days.

If the incision is very large or if the bladder trauma is severe, the bladder can remain catheterized and connected to a closed collection system (tomcat catheter) for 2–3 days.

As with other hollow organs, to access the interior of the bladder, transfixion stay sutures are placed at the two ends of the incision. The advantage of this is that trauma is minimized while handling the wall, and contamination of the surgical field with urine is avoided.

It is very important to obtain the results of the urine culture, the analysis of the composition of the calculi and the anatomopathological study of the samples taken in order to treat the case medically and avoid recurrence.

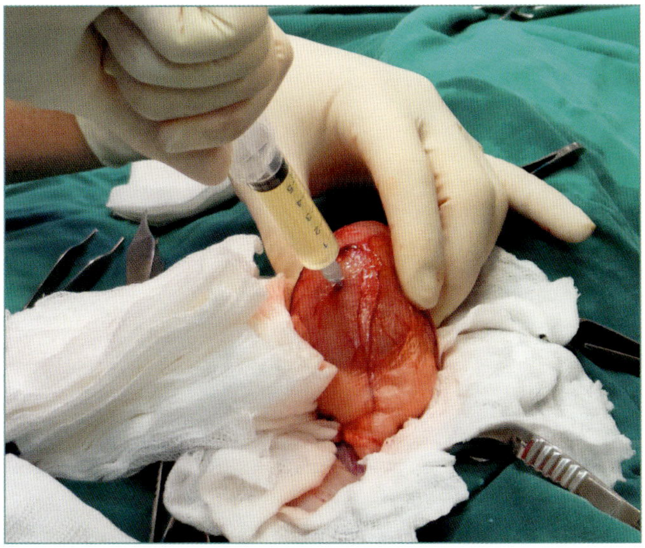

FIGURE 7. Intraoperative sample collection by cystocentesis in a case complicated by bacterial cystitis caused by multiresistant bacteria. Before opening the bladder, an uncontaminated sample was taken for culture and antibiogram.

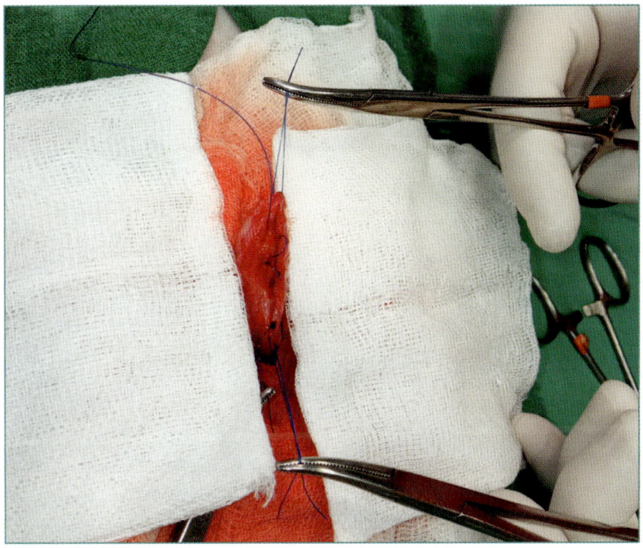

FIGURE 8. As the assistant gently applies traction to the stay sutures, a single-layer suture is placed using a Cushing inverting pattern, taking care not to penetrate into the bladder lumen.

Surgical techniques

Cystotomy/cystectomy

For this technique:

1. A laparotomy is performed on the caudal linea alba (the larger the bladder, the closer to the umbilicus).
2. After exposing the bladder, a second sterile surgical field is placed around it with moistened gauze.
3. The bladder is emptied of its contents and any needed samples are taken (through cystocentesis or surgical aspiration) before proceeding to open it. The best area, free of vascularization, is selected according to the intervention to be performed (Fig. 9).
4. The incision is made in the appropriate location, depending on whether it is for a **biopsy** or to remove a **localized tumor** or **urachal diverticulum**. Bladder function can be maintained if no more than 75% of the bladder body is removed. In the case of resectable masses, computed tomography images guide us in the removal of a 1 cm margin around them. This type of tumor should never be touched, given the risk of spreading malignant tumor cells to other locations in the bladder. After removal, the bladder is lavaged and the secondary surgical field is replaced, along with a change of gloves, before proceeding to closure.
5. If the surgery involves **removal of calculi**, the **ventral aspect** is chosen for the incision. It is easier to work in this location, and it provides good visual access to the trigone. The stay sutures are placed previously. The distance between them marks the length of the incision. The bladder wall incision is begun with the tip of a no. 11 scalpel blade and continued with Metzenbaum scissors.
6. Sometimes the surgery requires a larger field of vision of the interior of the bladder. In that case, a couple more stay sutures can be placed, one in the center of each edge of the wound, which the assistant can open as needed (Fig. 10).
7. Calculi can very often be removed using our fingers. With them, the sensitivity during exploration is excellent, and we can reach around 90% of the inside surface of the bladder. If the calculi are large, another instrument that can help is an Allis forceps.
8. If the presentation consists of multiple and small calculi, a small sterile spoon can be used in addition to digital extraction. These spoons do little damage to the mucosa and can effectively reach the trigone area. Once as many calculi as

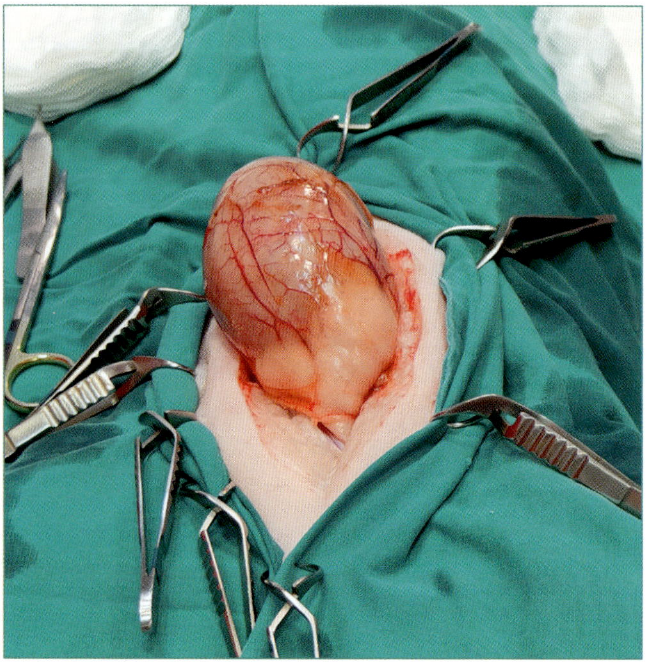

FIGURE 9. Image of an exteriorized bladder after laparotomy. Before setting the second surgical field, the least vascularized area is chosen for cystotomy.

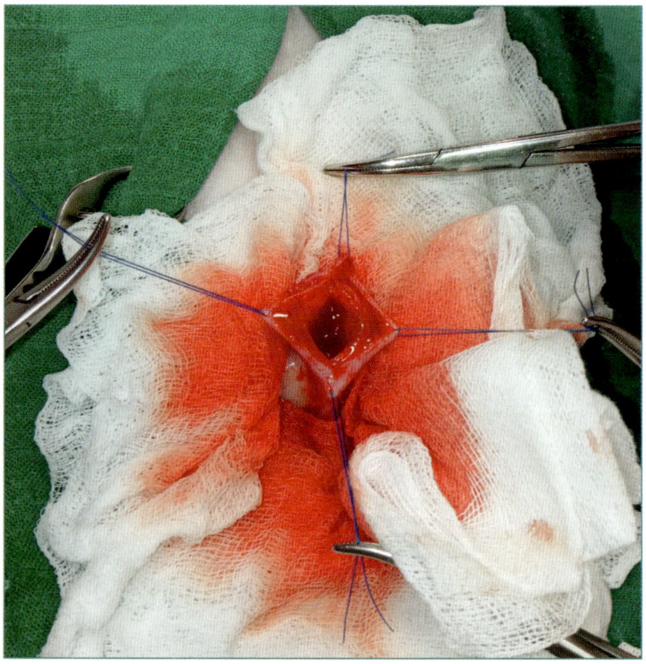

FIGURE 10. Placement of the second surgical field, using gauze moistened with warm sterile saline solution, and four stay sutures for better access to the interior of the bladder.

possible have been removed, the most effective thing to do is retrograde flushing with 10 ml of warm saline solution through the urethral catheter, aided by an assistant. This involves withdrawing the urethral catheter until the tip is in the narrowest area of the urethra. Next, the cystotomy incision is closed almost completely to increase the flow velocity of the saline and move the calculi in an outward direction. The assistant injects the saline quickly, holding the catheter. Any calculi that exit around the second surgical field are collected. Retrograde flushing is repeated as necessary until the surgeon is unable to palpate any calculi inside the bladder. The second surgical field should be changed during the process to avoid contaminating the interior of the abdomen.

> It is very important to carry out all of these processes systematically, making sure not to leave any calculi after the intervention. One study found that calculi debris was left behind 20% of the time after urolith surgery.

9. Before closing the cystotomy site, the interior of the bladder is lavaged with warm saline, and the orifices of the ureters are examined in case any calculus is lodged there (in cats, a large number of bladder calculi originate in the upper urinary tract). If the intervention was to remove a tumor, all used gloves are replaced with new ones before closing the cystotomy incision.
10. The bladder is closed with a simple inverting suture (Cushing) using absorbable monofilament. As mentioned above, the suture should not be transfixing, but it should include the submucosa. If the bladder is ruptured or very traumatized (e.g., in chronic infections, chronic bladder distension), the closure can be effectuated in a double layer: first, the submucosa is sutured with simple interrupted sutures, and subsequently an inverting suture is used for the muscular layer/serosa. After closure, check for any leakage by injecting saline inside the bladder and making sure that it distends sufficiently.

Cystostomy tubes

When the lower urinary tract is obstructed for any reason, temporary cystostomy tubes are placed to enable the bladder to empty until the issue can be resolved. The most frequent indications are:

- Urethral obstruction due to calculi, inflammation or tumors that cannot be remedied with catheterization or medical treatment. The cystostomy tube is kept in place until the underlying cause is resolved.
- Bladder atony with a good short-term prognosis.
- Urethral neoplasm.

For placement, a laparotomy incision is made in the skin above the bladder. Sometimes the incision can be limited to only one portion of the wall, as long as two transfixion stay sutures are placed through the skin and abdominal wall. A tobacco pouch suture is placed on the bladder wall with absorbable material. Next, the bladder wall in the center of the tobacco pouch is incised with a no. 11 scalpel blade, taking care not to cause leakage of urine into the abdominal cavity. An 8 Fr Foley catheter or a mushroom-tipped gastrotomy tube is inserted into the bladder. The tobacco pouch is closed around the device, and the bladder is fixed to the abdominal wall with several cystopexy sutures. After this, the stay sutures are removed and the laparotomy site is closed around the tube. Lastly, the tube is fixed to the skin and protected from any possible trauma or any biting by the patient, leaving easy access to enable emptying of the bladder 2–3 times per day (Fig. 11).

On average, cystostomy tubes are kept in place for 7–14 days, although cases of cats with atonic bladder (neuropathic dysfunction) have been described in which they had them in place for several years. In such cases, replacing the Foley catheter every 6 months is advised, along with surgical reintervention to place it inside a new stoma.

VIDEO

Surgical removal of several calculi (calcium oxalate) in a female cat via cystotomy, using Allis forceps. The use of four stay sutures is seen.

Video courtesy of Lisboa veterinary center

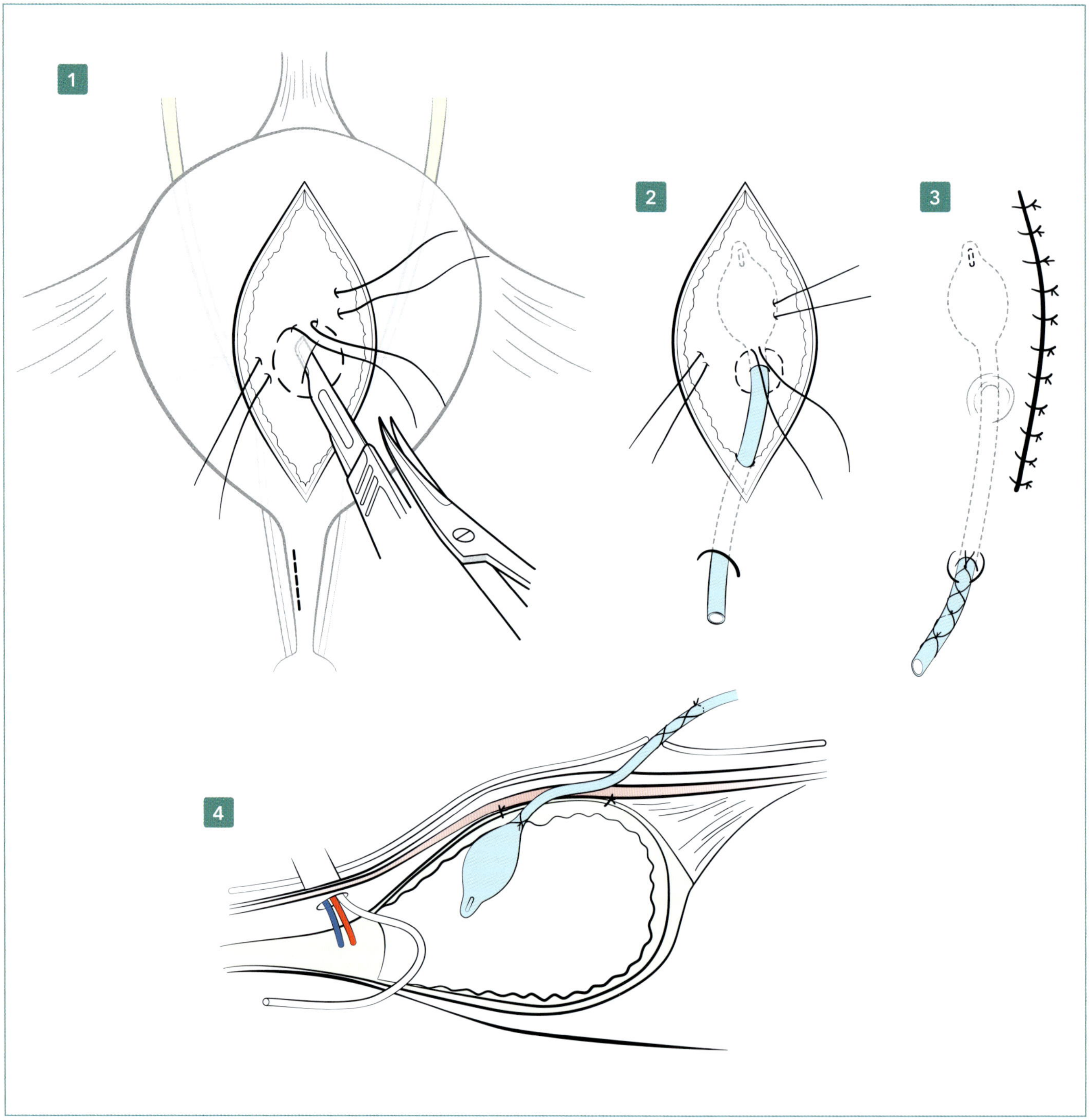

FIGURE 11. Steps for placement of a cystostomy tube.

1. After laparotomy, a tobacco pouch suture is placed on the bladder wall with the help of transfixing stay sutures, and the center is incised with a scalpel blade.
2. An 8 Fr Foley catheter is inserted into the bladder incision.
3. Next, the tobacco pouch is closed around the device, and the bladder is fixed to the abdominal wall with several cystopexy sutures.
4. Lastly, the laparotomy is closed around the catheter, which is fixed to the skin and properly protected.

Complications

Complications of bladder surgery are very much a function of the pathology. Recurrence of calculi is frequent in cases that cannot be medically treated with dietary modifications after the intervention. Metastasis of bladder tumors after removal depends on the nature of the neoplasm and whether it was possible to remove it with sufficient safety margins.

Any intervention, especially those using more delicate sutures (e.g., ureteral reimplantation), can give rise to urine leakage into the peritoneal cavity. If it is not severe, the leak usually resolves after a few days of conservative treatment.

Finally, there have been cases of metastasis caused by seeding of bladder tumor cells (carcinoma, adenocarcinoma) along the needle tract through tissues of the abdominal wall during sample collection via ultrasound-guided puncture. For this reason, this method of taking cytological samples of bladder tumors **is not advised**.

Bibliography

Appel SL, Lefebvre SL, Houston DM et al. Evaluation of risk factors associated with suture-nidus cystoliths in dogs and cats. 176 cases (1999–2006). *J Am Vet Med Assoc*, 2008; 233(12):1889–1895.

Aumann M, Worth LT, Drobatz KJ. Uroperitoneum in cats: 26 cases (1986–1995). *J Am Anim Hosp Assoc*, 1998; 34(4):315–324.

Bommer NX, Hayes AM, Scase TJ, Gunn-Moore DA. Clinical features, survival times and COX-1 and COX-2 expression in cats with transitional cell carcinoma of the urinary bladder treated with meloxicam. *J Feline Med Surg*, 2012; 14(8):527–533.

Cornell KK. Cystotomy, partial cystectomy, and tube cystostomy. *Clin Tech Small Anim Pract*, 2000; 15(1):11–16.

Di Mauro FM, Singh A, Reynolds D et al. Combined use of intravesicular ureteroneocystostomy techniques to correct ureteral ectopia in a male cat. *J Am Anim Hosp Assoc*, 2014; 50(1):71–76.

Eisele JG, Jackson J, Hager D. Ectopic ureterocele in a cat. *J Am Anim Hosp Assoc*, 2005; 41(5):332–335.

Ghantous SN, Crawford J. Double ureters with ureteral ectopia in a domestic shorthair cat. *J Am Anim Hosp Assoc*, 2006; 42(6):462–466.

Gunn-Moore DA. Feline lower urinary tract disease. *J Feline Med Surg*, 2003; 5(2):133–138.

Henry CJ. Management of transitional cell carcinoma. *Vet Clin North Am Small Anim Pract*, 2003; 33(3):597–613.

Langston C, Gisselman K, Palma D, McCue J. Methods of urolith removal. *Compend Contin Educ Vet*, 2010, 32(6):E1–E7.

Laverty PH, Salisbury SK. Surgical management of true patent urachus in a cat. *J Small Anim Pract*, 2002; 43(5):227–229.

Lulich JP, Osborne CA. Changing paradigms in the diagnosis of urolithiasis. *Vet Clin North Am Small Anim Pract*, 2009; 39(1):79–91.

Mason LK, Stone EA, Biery DN et al. Surgery of ectopic ureters—preoperative and postoperative radiographic morphology. *J Am Anim Hosp Assoc*, 1990; 26:73–79.

McLoughlin MA, Chew DJ. Diagnosis and surgical management of ectopic ureters. *Clin Tech Small Anim Pract*, 2000; 15(1):17–24.

McLoughlin MA. Complications of lower urinary tract surgery in small animals. *Vet Clin North Am Small Anim Pract*, 2011; 41(5):889–913.

Nyland TG, Wallack ST, Wisner ER. Needle-tract implantation following us-guided fine-needle aspiration biopsy of transitional cell carcinoma of the bladder, urethra, and prostate. *Vet Radiol Ultrasound*, 2002; 43(1):50–53.

Osborne CA, Lulich JP, Kruger JM et al. Analysis of 451,891 canine uroliths, feline uroliths and feline urethral plugs from 1981 to 2007: perspectives from the Minnesota Urolith Center. *Vet Clin North Am Small Anim Pract,* 2009; 39(1):183–197.

Schwartz PD, Greene RW, Patnaik AK. Urinary bladder tumors in the cat: a review of 27 cases. *J Am Anim Hosp Assoc*, 1985; 21(2):237–245.

Thieman-Mankin KM, Ellison GW, Jeyapaul CJ, Glotfelty-Ortiz CS. Comparison of short-term complication rates between dogs and cats undergoing appositional single-layer or inverting double-layer cystotomy closure: 144 cases (1993–2010). *J Am Vet Med Assoc*, 2012; 240(1):65–68.

Westropp JL, Buffington CA. Lower urinary tract disorders in cats. In: Ettinger SJ, Feldman EC (eds.). *Textbook of Veterinary Internal Medicine*, 7th ed. St. Louis, MO: Elsevier, 2010; pp. 2069–2086.

Wilson HM, Chun R, Larson VS et al. Clinical signs, treatments, and outcome in cats with transitional cell carcinoma of the urinary bladder: 20 cases (1990–2004). *J Am Vet Med Assoc*, 2007; 231(1):101–106.

URETHROSTOMY 27

Alberto Barneto

Surgical anatomy

The urethra is the tube that carries urine from the bladder to the exterior. It extends from the **bladder trigone** to the **external orifice or external meatus**.

The cranial urethra is wider in diameter and contains the **internal urethral sphincter**, formed by smooth muscle. The urethral caliber narrows caudally until it reaches the last third, where the urethra is surrounded by the striated musculature that includes the **external urethral sphincter**. In females, the external meatus empties into the vaginal vestibule; in males, the urethra ends in the **penis**. The penis is protected in its final portion by a skin fold in the form of a pouch, the **prepuce**. The male urethra is longer and its course is divided into several anatomical portions (Fig. 1):

- **Preprostatic urethra:** from the bladder trigone to the **prostate**. It is also called the pelvic urethra. It is the portion with the largest internal diameter.
- **Prostatic urethra:** from the prostate to the **bulbourethral glands**. The urethra narrows and the surrounding muscle fibers change from smooth to striated. The **retractor penis muscle** inserts ventrally.
- **Penile urethra:** from the bulbourethral glands to the external meatus. It is ventrally surrounded by striated musculature and dorsally by profusely vascularized connective tissue (the **corpus cavernosum** of the penis). These two structures form the penis. The **ischiocavernosus** (ventral) and **bulbospongiosus** (dorsal) **muscles** insert externally, immediately caudal to the bulbourethral glands.

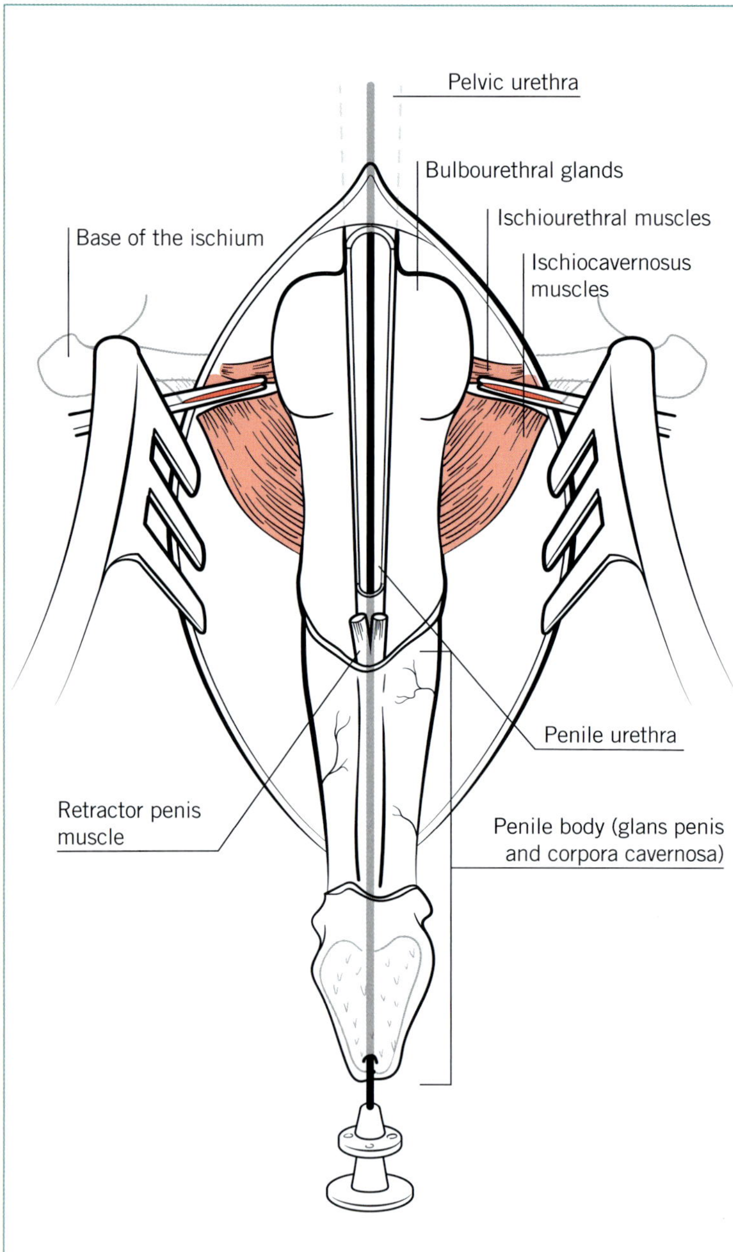

FIGURE 1. Genitourinary surgical anatomy of the male cat.

The preprostatic and prostatic portions of the feline urethra (**pelvic urethra**) have the widest internal diameter.

The vascularization of the female urethra arises from the **vaginal arteries**, which are branches of the urogenital artery. In the male, the internal pudendal artery supplies blood to the prostatic artery, which branches into the **urethral artery** that runs the entire length of the penile urethra.

The external urethral sphincter is innervated by the **pudendal nerve** (segments S1–S3). Another fundamental aspect of micturition lies in the function of the **detrusor muscle of the bladder**, whose contraction, in coordination with the relaxation of the internal urethral sphincter, is governed by the **pelvic nerve** (S1–S3, parasympathetic pathway). The opposite effect, sympathetic stimulation (detrusor muscle relaxation and bladder filling–internal sphincter contraction), is regulated by the **hypogastric nerve** (L2–L5).

Surgical diseases of the feline urethra

The feline species suffers from various pathological processes that require surgical treatment:

- **Feline lower urinary tract disease (FLUTD):** a syndrome that groups together various causes but usually presents with a clinical picture of common signs: pain on urination, dysuria, stranguria, hematuria and, finally, pollakiuria. From there, signs involving other organs appear: vomiting, depression, bradycardia, etc. In advanced cases, the lower urinary tract may be completely obstructed, meaning that the cat comes to the clinic with this clinical picture plus a large, hard and painful bladder (**bladder overdistension**) and **obstructive renal failure** (uremia, hyperkalemia) (Fig. 2). Males that live indoors, are obese, and eat only dry food are predisposed to FLUTD. Different causes for this syndrome have been described:
  - Between 13% and 38% of cats with FLUTD have **urethral stones**. When these are larger than 5 mm, they totally or partially obstruct the cat's urethra. The most frequent stones in cats are composed of **calcium oxalate** (54%) (Fig. 3).
  - **Urinary tract infections (UTI)** are rare (2% of cats under 10 years of age with FLUTD). In cats older than 10 years, the frequency increases to just 3% (10% in some studies, with geographic variations). Despite the described infrequency of UTIs, a urine culture is recommended in all cases of FLUTD, using a sterile collection technique such as cystocentesis.
  - **Urethral plugs** are frequent in cats with FLUTD (20%–50%). They clog but do not severely obstruct, so they are usually well managed with medical treatment.
  - Nearly two out of three cats with FLUTD suffer from **feline idiopathic cystitis (FIC)**, a syndrome of unknown cause associated with stress, neurogenic inflammation and a loss of continuity of the bladder mucosa. Combining medical treatment with environmental management usually successfully resolves these cases without the need for surgery.

  In patients with FLUTD, each cause should always be addressed with medical treatment and interventional techniques to resolve the obstruction. Approximately 30%–50% of cats relapse, and some recurrences may be due to multiple causes in the same cat.

When FLUTD recurrences become frequent (up to four times), a decision should be made whether to perform a perineal urethrostomy.

- **Urethral trauma and ruptures:** although there are cases of severe perineal trauma that require surgical intervention on the urethra, the most frequent causes are iatrogenic, due to inadequate catheterization (Fig. 4).
- **Urethral tumors:** very rare in cats. Transitional cell carcinomas and leiomyomas have been described.
- **Urethrorectal fistulas:** abnormal communications between the urethral lumen and the rectum. Very rare in cats, they are usually associated with congenital anal atresia.
- **Urethral hypoplasia:** a very rare congenital disease in cats. A malformation causes the urethral caliber to be too small, resulting in difficulty in micturition.

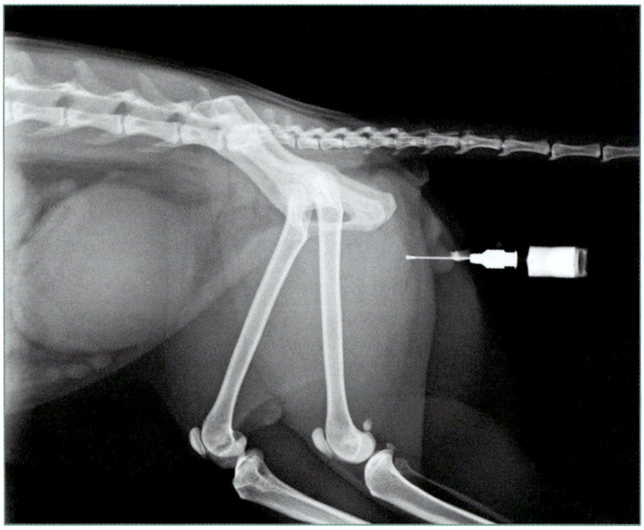

FIGURE 2. Lateral X-ray of an overdistended bladder in a male cat. The urethra has been catheterized to locate the site of obstruction.

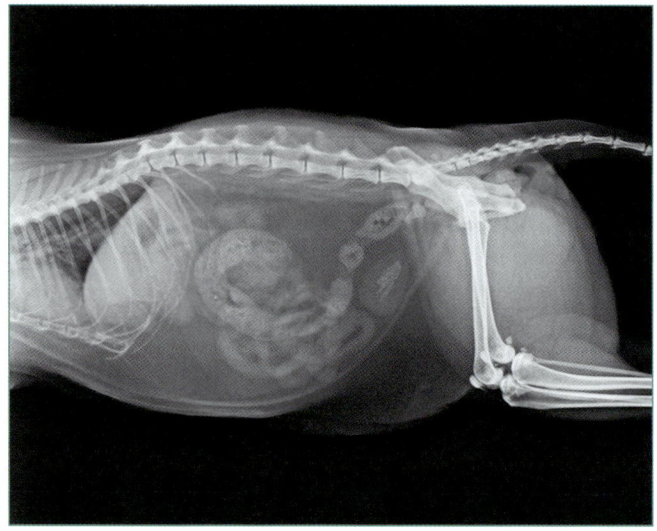

FIGURE 3. Multiple stones in the bladder of a female cat. After surgical extraction and analysis, they were found to be composed of calcium oxalate.

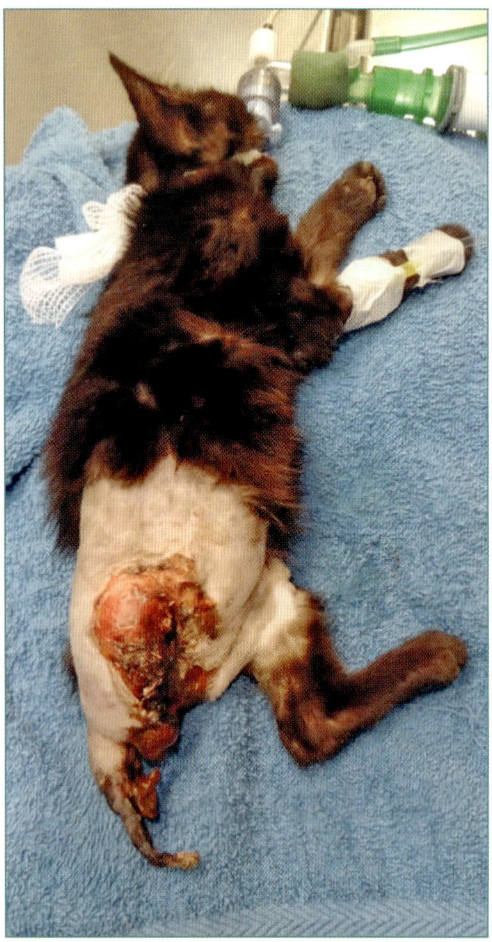

FIGURE 4. Severe perineal injury in a female cat resulting in urethral rupture due to avulsion.

Diagnosis

It is necessary to use imaging techniques (Table 1), in addition to the medical history and the clinical signs, to diagnose urethral alterations and pathologies that may require surgical intervention.

Positive-contrast urethrography technique

- This is the ideal technique for diagnosing urethral ruptures, communications with other organs or lesions in the lumen of the pelvic and penile urethra (Fig. 5).
- Sedation or anesthesia is required.
- The initial patient position is lateral.
- Iodine-based contrast media are preferred.
- Catheterization of the urethra is performed with a silicone catheter or olive-tipped catheter, keeping the orifice of the device as distal as possible.
- Boluses of 5–10 ml of contrast medium are administered and an X-ray is taken after injection.
- Sometimes, when searching for intraurethral lesions, the bladder can be filled with positive contrast prior to the technique to promote counterpressure within the urethra and allow adequate distention with urethrography.

TABLE 1. Diagnostic methods used in the various urethral surgical pathologies

Diagnostic technique	Use (diseases)	Observations
Plain radiography	Radiopaque urethral calculi	■ Always include ALL urinary structures on the film. ■ Not to be confused with the penile bone (os penis).
Positive-contrast urethrography	Urethral ruptures	Contrast medium is seen around the urethra.
	Radiolucent calculi	In cats, dried solidified blood calculi sometimes occur.
	Urethral stenosis and urethral hypoplasia	Difficult to interpret if not very obvious.
	Urethrorectal fistulas	Contrast medium leaks into the colon or rectum, depending on the location of the communication.
	Testing of urethral patency and correct suturing after the surgical intervention	–
Ultrasound	Large urethral calculi	Cast acoustic shadows.
	Urethral obstructions	Even if the obstruction is not visible, signs of obstruction in the bladder, ureters and kidneys can be seen on an ultrasound.
	Urethral neoplasms	Mostly associated with neoplasms in the bladder, in the area of the trigone.
Computed tomography (CT)	In all cases	■ Improves the diagnostic sensitivity of radiography, with or without contrast. ■ Ideal for the diagnosis and exact localization of tumors.

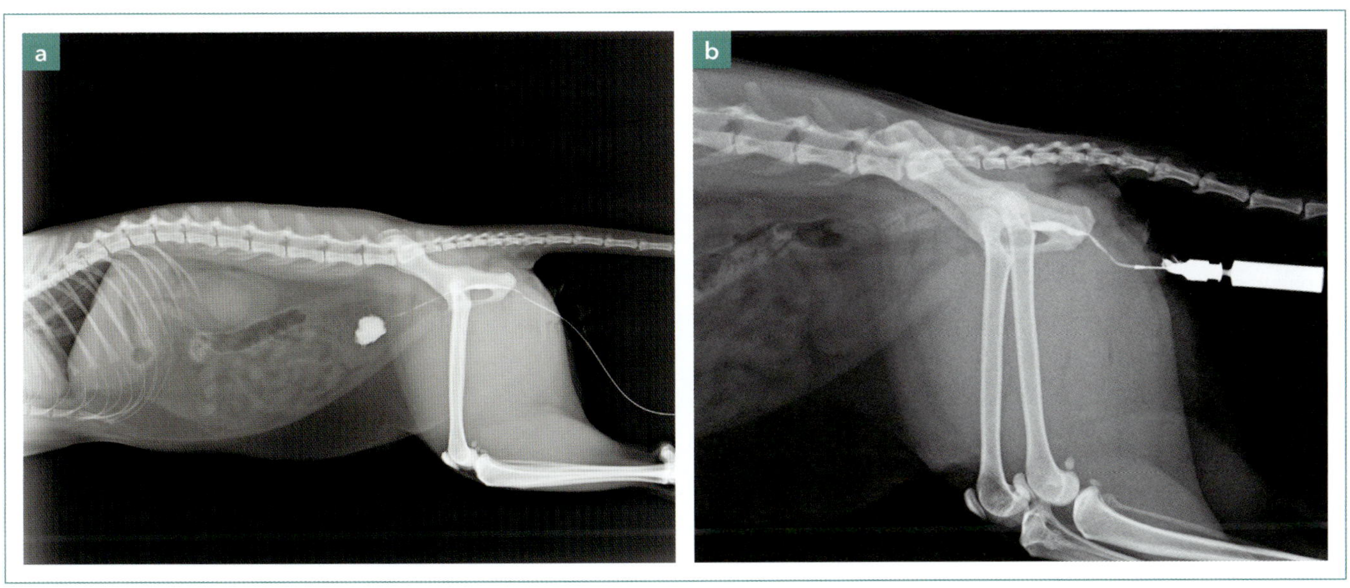

FIGURE 5. Positive-contrast urethrograms. (a) Normal urethrogram. (b) Obstruction to the passage of contrast medium in the pelvic urethra.

Preoperative and postoperative considerations

Aspects to be taken into account before and after the intervention:

- In the preoperative blood analysis, special attention must be paid to azotemia, electrolyte abnormalities and dehydration. Cardiac monitoring should be performed throughout the procedure.
- If catheters are to be used in the procedure, silicone catheters are preferred over polypropylene ones, since they are less traumatic and the consequent risk of iatrogenic urethritis is lower. If the catheter must be kept in place, a closed urine collection system should be used to avoid supervening infections.
- Once the urethra has been dissected and the mucosa exposed, handling the urethra must be done with extreme care. The use of stay sutures or atraumatic Adson forceps is recommended. Controlling heavy bleeding from the corpus cavernosum requires the use of sterile cotton swabs and maintained pressure, or cold saline.
- The urethra heals very quickly; in 7–10 days the sutures can be removed. Use 5-0 gauge absorbable monofilament sutures, always in a simple interrupted pattern.
- Provided the urethral pathology is amenable to surgical intervention, a urinalysis and culture should be performed to rule out a concomitant UTI. Sample sterility is achieved by taking the sample by cystocentesis. If this is impossible due to the urgency of the situation, a urine sample should be obtained intraoperatively and submitted for culture. An amoxicillin or sulfonamide/trimethoprim based broad-spectrum antibiotic therapy is then instituted.
- Perineal urethrostomy offers a high success rate in eliminating clinical signs and has very few complications. Prepubic urethrostomy has more complications in the short term (periurethral dermatitis) and in the long term (urinary incontinence, UTI); however, it improves the patient's life expectancy, as it is a technique used as a last resort due to the severity of its indications.

Surgical techniques

Perineal urethrostomy

- **Patient positioning:** sternal recumbency; forelimbs unrestrained; hind limbs restrained with straps or gauze bandages in a caudal direction and somewhat open. The patient is positioned at the end of the table so that the hind limbs are held outside the table; the stifles are protected with gauze to avoid injury from the table edge. A pillow covered with a soaker is placed under the pelvis to elevate the posterior third and the perineal region. The tail is pulled taut in a cranial direction and secured to the table with two long strips (one on each side) of gauze bandage; the knot over the tail is secured with 2–3 layers of cloth tape to prevent it from slipping.
- **Surgical field:** the entire perineal area, one-third of the base of the tail and half of the hind limbs (thighs) up to the back of the stifles are shaved. The anus is closed with a tobacco pouch suture using 3-0 nylon. A urethral catheter is inserted up to the bladder (if permitted by the patient's pathology); this is helpful in locating the urethra during surgery.
- **Approach:** through an elliptical incision in the perineum encompassing the entire scrotum and prepuce of the patient. If the patient is intact, castration is performed at this stage of the surgery.
- **Technique**
  1. The perineal tissue is dissected with baby Metzenbaum scissors until the penile body is reached, which is then used as an anatomical landmark (Fig. 6.1).
  2. Dissection continues around the corpus cavernosum of the penis. The ventral penile ligament, located on the inferior aspect, is sectioned. The dissection is thus deepened up to the entrance of the pelvic canal (Fig. 6.2).
  3. The ischiourethral and ischiocavernosus muscles are located at their insertion on both sides of the penile body, up to the base of the ischium. They are clamped with straight mosquito forceps near their insertion into the ischium and cut with Stevens tenotomy scissors. By doing so, bleeding is minimized and the ligation of these muscles is not usually necessary. The ischial insertion of these muscles remains clamped (for about 5 minutes) once the penis is freed and then the surgery is continued (Fig. 6.3).
  4. All urethral insertions are freed by blunt and sharp dissection around the penis. The retractor penis muscle (on the dorsal aspect of the pelvic portion of the penile body) is identified and sectioned, and the bulbourethral glands, one on each side of the penile body and immediately cranial to the ischiourethral and ischiocavernosus muscles, are identified and isolated (Fig. 6.4).
  5. Once the surface of the urethra has been cleaned of all adhesions and tissues (on the dorsal aspect of the

penis) and following the guide provided by the urethral catheter placed at the beginning of the surgery, the incision of the urethral wall is started using a no. 11 scalpel blade. It is very important to start at the level of the bulbourethral glands, where the urethral diameter is at its maximum (approximately 2 mm; this is the pelvic portion of the urethra, with no striated muscle around it). If it was impossible to introduce the urethral catheter, now, at the start of the urethrostomy, we can do it, thus delimiting the beginning of the subsequent suture. The dorsal urethrostomy is continued caudally through the entire penile urethra using the scalpel blade or Stevens tenotomy scissors up to approximately the middle of the penile body (Fig. 6.5).

6. It is important at this step to remove the catheter momentarily to check that the diameter of the urethra we have reached is correct. To do so, we should be able to easily introduce the tip of closed Kelly forceps tip or an 8 Fr (2.7 mm) caliber urethral catheter. If this is impossible, the urethra must be further opened in a cranial direction. Once the correct urethral caliber has been verified, the urethra is recatheterized up to the bladder for subsequent suturing (Fig. 6.6).
7. Approximately midway along the penile body (distally), the longitudinal cut of the urethra should curve obliquely around the ventral aspect. In this manner, the distal half of the penile urethra is resected and the distal half of the penis is removed (the pelvic urethra should be kept catheterized to aid in locating the urethral wall when suturing). Thus, the cranial half of the penile urethra is spatulated, leaving the pelvic urethra intact (Fig. 6.7).
8. **Suture:** 5-0 or 6-0 monofilament suture is used, absorbable or nonabsorbable. First two U-stitches for traction unloading are placed to reduce the risk of scar retraction and urethral stoma stenosis. These two stitches (one on each side) are placed with 3-0 nylon entering through the perineal skin, approximately 1–2 cm from each side of the incision, reaching the bulbourethral gland and exiting back through the skin near the entry point of the suture. The authors recommend leaving the suture ends long for removal after 10–15 days. The next suture (the true start of the urethrostomy suture) is at 12 o'clock (on an imaginary clock on the perineum), just at the dorsal apex of the new urethral orifice. It is a horizontal U-stitch (with the knot positioned away from the urethra to avoid scarring and stenosis). As with all stitches from now on, it should **only include the urethral wall and epidermis, and avoid the urethral cavernous tissue and the perineal subcutaneous tissue**. The knot is not tightened yet. The following two stitches are simple interrupted, those corresponding to 11 and 1 o'clock. They are tightened and immediately afterwards the 12 o'clock knot is tightened as well. Subsequently, single interrupted sutures are placed in pairs (10 and 2 o'clock; 9 and 3; 8 and 4, and so on). If the wound in the skin is larger than the spatulated urethra, continue closing with simple interrupted skin sutures (Fig. 6.8).

> Some of the secrets to success in urethral surgery include atraumatic tissue handling, good spatulation of the area of the urethra to be sutured and following the specified order for sutures.

- **Postoperative management**
  - The urethral catheter is removed; some hematuria is normal for the first 24–48 hours. In some cases of severe urethral trauma, urethral catheterization may be maintained for a few days. In this case, closed urine collection systems should be used to avoid supervening infections.
  - The tobacco pouch suture is removed from the anal sphincter.
  - Urethral patency should be regularly checked by palpating the bladder to rule out bladder overdistension. Careful placement of a catheter may be necessary in these cases.
  - Sand bedding should be replaced with strips of absorbent paper to reduce the risk of wound infections.
  - A broad-spectrum antibiotic, anti-inflammatory and analgesic treatment is started.

Modified urethrostomy using preputial mucosa

One of the postoperative complications of conventional perineal urethrostomy is the predisposition to lower UTI. Loss of the distal urethral sphincter and exposure of the urethral mucosa result in an increased risk for UTI. To minimize this risk, a modified urethrostomy technique using preputial mucosa for suturing has been described (Fig. 7).

A triangular-shaped incision is made above the prepuce, respecting the entire preputial structure. The preputial mucosa is dissected around its adhesions to the glans penis. Once the penile end is released, the conventional perineal urethrostomy

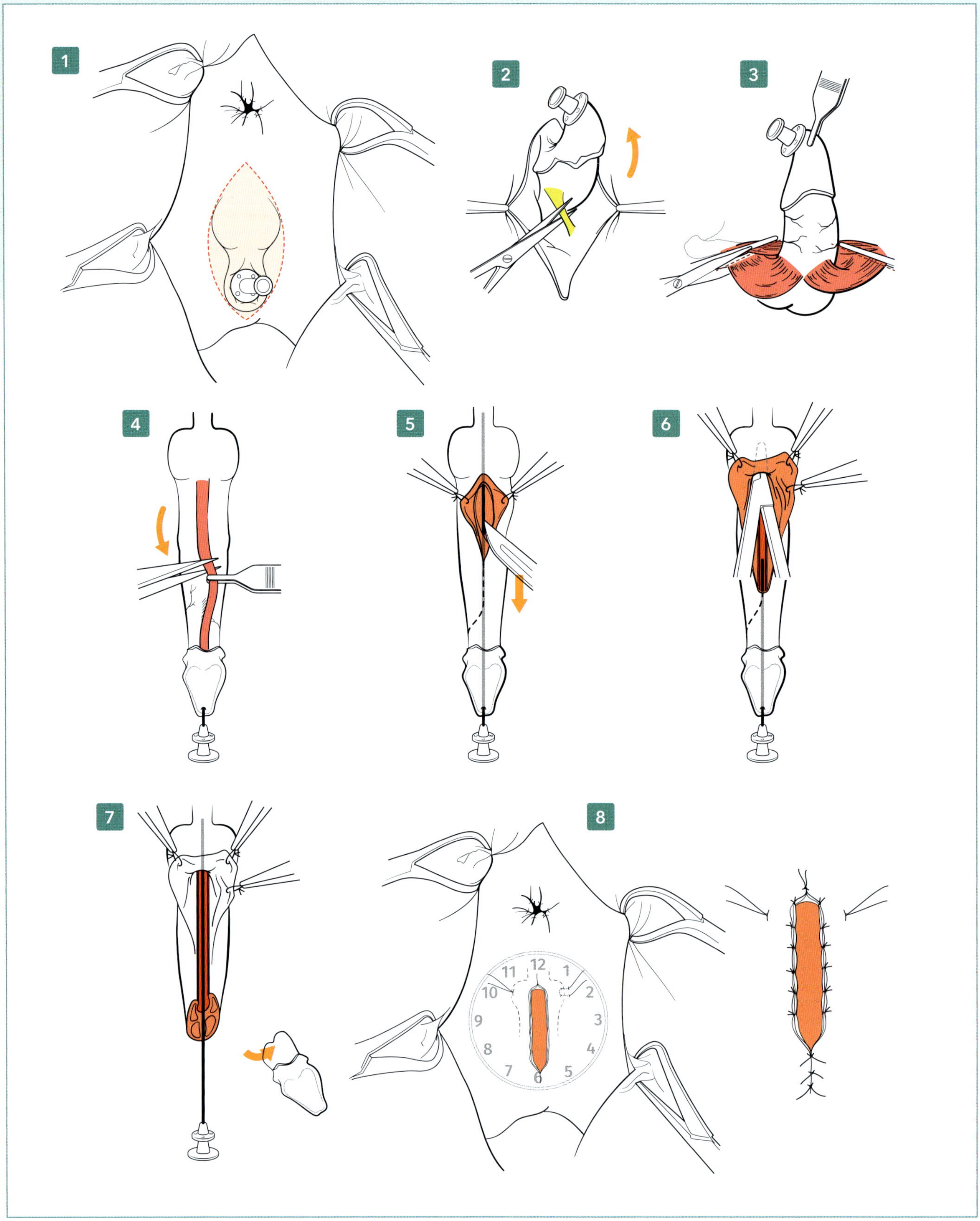
1
2
3
4
5
6
7
8
12
11
1
10
2
9
3
8
4
7
6
5

FIGURE 6. Steps of the surgical technique for performing a perineal urethrostomy in a male cat.

1. Approach for conventional perineal urethrostomy. The anus is closed with a tobacco pouch suture. The initial incision includes the scrotum. Catheterization of the urethra is maintained if possible.
2. The penile body is dissected from all surrounding tissues and the ventral penile ligament is sectioned.
3. The ischial insertions of the ischiourethral and ischiocavernosus muscles are clamped with straight mosquito forceps and the muscles are sectioned caudally to the forceps. The mosquito forceps are left in place for 5 minutes for hemostasis.
4. Dissection is continued up to the bulbourethral glands, and the retractor penis muscle is sectioned on the dorsal aspect.
5. The catheter helps to locate and section the dorsal part of the urethra. Bleeding is controlled with pressure using swabs and cold saline.
6. The catheter is withdrawn slightly to check that the urethral opening is at the correct location, at the level of the bulbourethral glands. For this purpose, the tip of a Kelly forceps or an 8 Fr (2.7 mm) catheter is inserted.
7. The urethrostomy is extended ventrally to about 2–3 cm and the penis is sectioned to about half its length.
8. The suture starts with traction unloading stitches, fixing the bulbourethral glands to the perineal skin. After this, the actual suture is started. The first U-stitch is placed over the apex of the urethral incision, grasping only the skin. All urethral suture stitches are simple interrupted and exclusively include the urethra and epidermis.

technique is performed, including all steps up to spatulation of the urethra. At this point, an incision is made in the ventral wall of the preputial tube. The first suture is placed between the angle of this incision and the ventral apex of the spatulated urethra. The urethral mucosa is sutured to the preputial mucosa, closing both sides with symmetrical stitches. The last stitch joins the most dorsal part of the preputial tube to the dorsal angle of the spatulated urethra, at the level of the bulbourethral glands. Finally, the triangular skin incision is closed with simple interrupted stitches, leaving a straight line.

Prepubic urethrostomy

This is a salvage technique after very severe urethral trauma or serious iatrogenic complications (e.g., perineal urethrostomy with dehiscence, or urethral rupture after traumatic catheterization) (Fig. 8). The key points for the success of this intervention are:

- Performing a laparotomy through the linea alba to the pubis. The authors recommend a cystotomy for antegrade catheterization, from the bladder lumen to the healthy urethral area. This helps to localize and manipulate the urethra during the procedure.

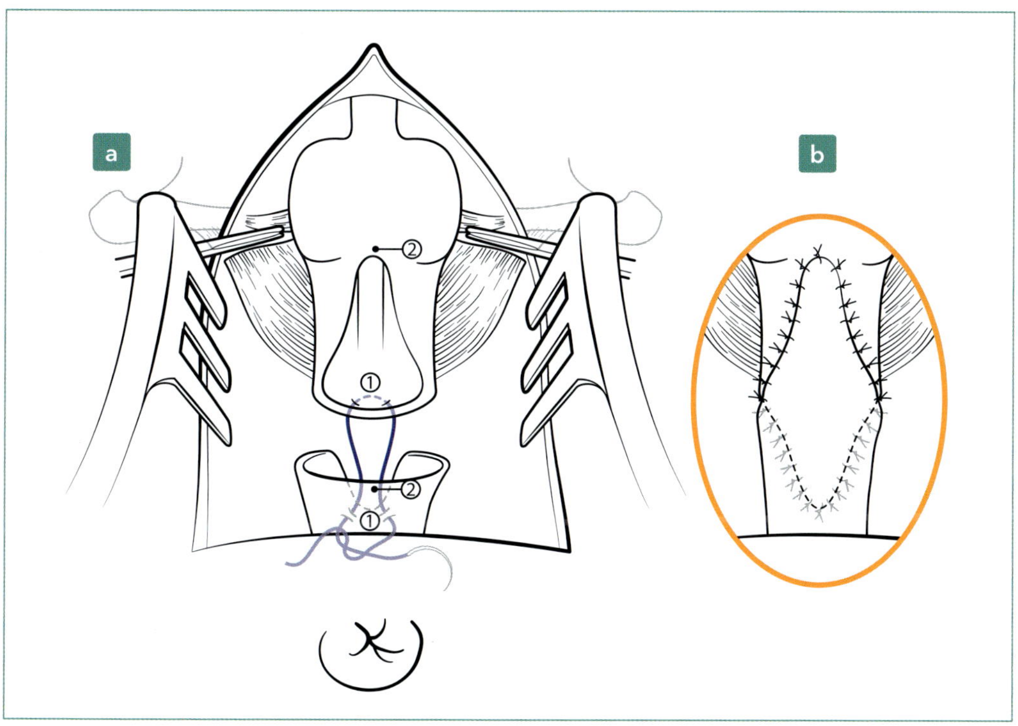

FIGURE 7. Detail of the closure in the modified perineal urethrostomy technique including the prepuce (Yeh and Chin, 2000). (a) The initial incision is made in a triangular shape over the prepuce. After performing the urethrostomy, in the same way as in the conventional technique, the suture is started by joining the ventral apex of the urethra with the most ventral point of the internal mucosa of the preputial sac (1). Both sides of the urethrostomy are sequentially sutured to the preputial mucosa. The last stitch joins the most dorsal points of both structures (2). (b) Completed suture, with all stitches inside the preputial sac.

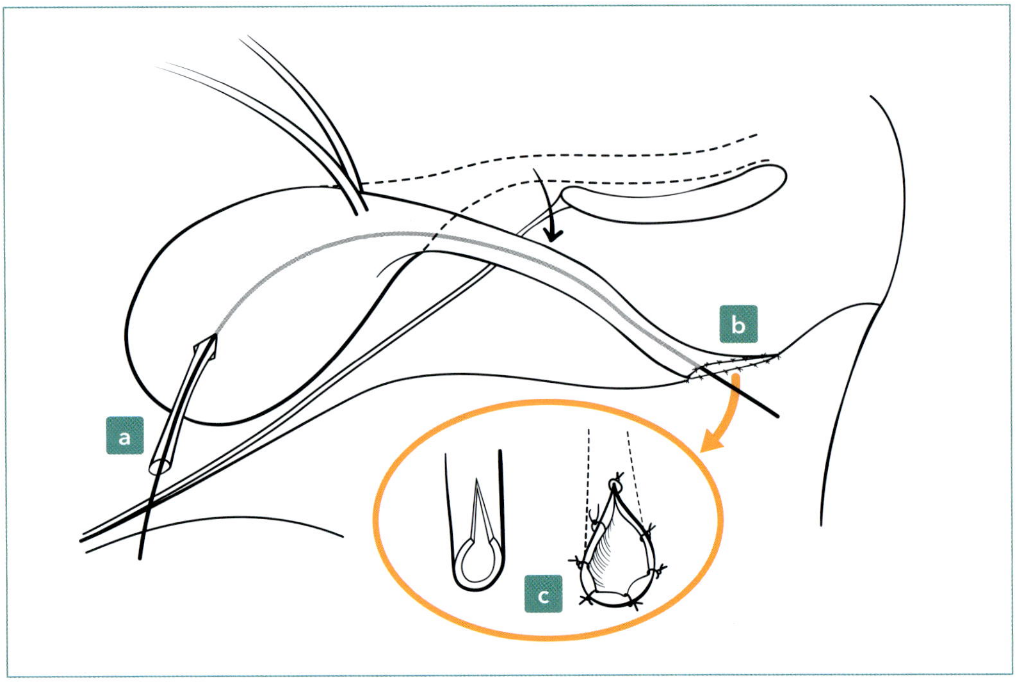

FIGURE 8. Detail of the key points of the prepubic urethrostomy technique. (a) Cystotomy at the cranial vertex made to introduce the urethral catheter that permits anterograde catheterization, making it possible to locate the portion of the urethra where work is to be done. (b) Tunneling of the urethra through a hole in the abdominal wall cranial to the prepubic tendon, on one side of the linea alba. (c) Detail of the technique for the spatulation and suture of the urethral stoma to the skin of the abdomen.

- Leaving sufficient urethral length to maintain the effect of the internal urethral sphincter and avoid scar retraction after surgery.
- Avoiding urethral rotation. Maintaining the urethra catheterized during the procedure helps with this. It may also help to mark the ventral portion with a suture.
- Tunnelling the urethra through an orifice lateral to the laparotomy incision. To do so, a 1–2 cm subcutaneous pathway is made through subcutaneous tissue in the pelvic floor region, and the catheterized urethra is exteriorized through this stoma.
- Sufficiently spatulating the urethra to increase the surface area sutured to the skin and avoid scar retraction. The urethra is sutured to the skin following the same pattern used for the conventional perineal urethrostomy technique. Finally, the catheter is removed and the cystotomy and laparotomy incisions are closed routinely (Fig. 9).

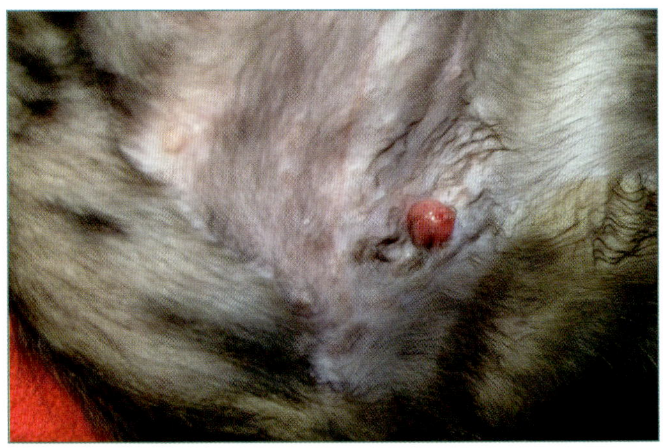

FIGURE 9. Urethral stoma after prepubic urethrostomy in the female cat in Figure 4. One month after surgery, the urethral mucosa is still inflamed, but patency is correct.

Bibliography

Campbell BG. Prepubic urethrostomy and placement of a caudal superficial epigastric flap for treatment of a self-mutilation injury in a serval. *J Am Vet Med Assoc*, 2003; 222(5):628–632.

Corgozinho KB, de Souza HJ, Pereira AN et al. Catheter-induced urethral trauma in cats with urethral obstruction. *J Fel Med Surg*, 2007; 9:481–486.

Cullen WC, Fletcher TF, Bradley WF. Morphometry of the female feline urethra. *J Urol*, 1983; 129:190–192.

Cullen WC, Fletcher TF, Bradley WF. Morphometry of the male feline pelvic urethra. *J Urol*, 1983; 129:186–189.

Gerber B, Boretti FS, Kley S et al. Evaluation of clinical signs and causes of lower urinary tract disease in European cats. *J Small Anim Pract*, 2005; 46:571–577.

Gerber B, Eichenberger S, Reusch CE. Guarded long-term prognosis in male cats with urethral obstruction. *J Fel Med Surg*, 2008; 10:16–23.

Hecht S. Diagnostic imaging of lower urinary tract disease. *Vet Clin North Am Small Anim Pract*, 2015; 45:639–663.

Hostutler RA, Chew DJ, DiBartola SP. Recent concepts in feline lower urinary tract disease. *Vet Clin Small Anim*, 2005; 35:147–170.

Kaul E, Hartmann K, Reese S et al. Recurrence rate and long-term course of cats with feline lower urinary tract disease. *J Fel Med Surg*, 2019; 22:544–556.

Lekcharoensuk C, Lulich JP, Osborne CA et al. Association between patient-related factors and risk of calcium oxalate and magnesium ammonium phosphate urolithiasis in cats. *J Am Vet Med Assoc*, 2000;217:520–525.

Lekcharoensuk C, Osborne CA, Lulich JP. Evaluation of trends in frequency of urethrostomy for treatment of urethral obstruction in cats. *J Am Vet Med Assoc*, 2002; 221(4):502–505.

Lund HS, Eggertsdóttir AV. Recurrent episodes of feline lower urinary tract disease with different causes: possible clinical implications. *J Fel Med Surg*, 2018; 21:590–594.

Nevins JR, Mai W, Thomas E. Associations between ultrasound and clinical findings in 87 cats with urethral obstruction. *Vet Radiol Ultrasound*, 2015; 6:439–447.

Segev G, Livne H, Ranen E, Lavy E. Urethral obstruction in cats: predisposing factors, clinical, clinicopathological characteristics and prognosis. *J Fel Med Surg*, 2011; 13:101–108.

Seneviratne M, Stamenova P, Lee K. Comparison of surgical indications and short- and long-term complications in 56 cats undergoing perineal, transpelvic or prepubic urethrostomy. *J Fel Med Surg*, 2020; 23:477–486.

Wang B, Bhadra N, Grill W. Functional anatomy of the male feline urethra: morphological and physiological correlations. *J Urol*, 1999; 161:208–211.

Westropp LA, Ruby AL, Bailiff NL et al. Dried solidified blood calculi in the urinary tract of cats. *J Vet Intern Med*, 2006; 204:828–834.

Wilson GP, Harrison JW. Perineal urethrostomy in cats. *J Am Vet Med Assoc*, 1971; 159:1789–1793.

Yeh LH, Chin SC. Modified perineal urethrostomy using preputial mucosa in cats. *J Am Vet Med Assoc*, 2000; 216(7):1092–1095.

ORCHIECTOMY AND CRYPTORCHIDISM 28

Anna Calvet

Surgical anatomy

The cat's **prepuce** is short and has a narrow opening that makes externalization of the penis complicated in a conscious animal (Fig. 1).

The **penis** of the cat is ventral to the testicles when not erect. Before reaching puberty, the penis cannot fully extend because of a balanopreputial adhesion that is dependent on androgen secretion. Thus, when the male reaches puberty this fold disappears.

> If the cat is castrated before reaching puberty, this balanopreputial adhesion may persist.

Upon reaching puberty, two-thirds of the length of the feline penis fills with spines, while the tip maintains a smooth appearance. These spines also depend on androgen secretion; therefore, they disappear 5–6 weeks after castration, and if androgens are administered to the cat for any reason, the spines reappear.

Some cats may have penile bone; this is an ossification of the septum between the corpora cavernosa that is about 3–5 mm long and can be seen on X-rays. The appearance of this ossification is age-related, so it is very rare in young cats.

The erectile portion of the penis consists of a corpus spongiosum and two corpora cavernosa surrounding the urethra. It is crossed dorsally by the retractor penis muscle and ventrally by the ventral penile ligament.

The **testes** or **testicles** are located in the scrotum, ventral to the anus. They are separated by a medial septum, which is formed by fibrous connective tissue.

The testicles of the cat consist of the testicular parenchyma, the rete testis (a network of tubules), the mediastinum where the sperm generated in the testicular parenchyma are collected (and which is visualized as a hyperechogenic line on an ultrasound) and the epididymis.

The vas deferens of each testis runs caudally and ventrally after leaving the scrotum and enters the abdominal cavity through the inguinal canal; once in the abdomen, it empties into the urethra at the level of the prostate.

Testicular development

Puberty occurs between 7 and 12 months of age. The testes descend into the scrotal sac before delivery, but it is possible for the testes to move in and out of the abdomen passing through the inguinal canal until reaching puberty.

The testes are surrounded by a layer of parietal peritoneum and a layer of visceral peritoneum, creating a space between them called the vaginal cavity. This communicates with the peritoneal cavity and sometimes may fill with fluid due to certain pathologies, as occurs in the rest of the abdomen. In addition, each testicle is enveloped in another, closely adherent layer called the tunica albuginea, which is fibrous.

With the maturation and growth of the cat, testicular size also increases, which stabilizes starting at 2–3 years of age.

As for accessory glands, cats have two bulbourethral glands and a prostate gland:

- The **prostate gland** consists of two cranial and two caudal lobes that surround the urethra dorsally and laterally. It is located 2–3 cm caudal to the bladder. The prostatic secretion is the major part of the seminal fluid. The prostate is dependent on androgen secretion and atrophies with castration. There are very few prostate pathologies described in the cat (prostatitis, adenocarcinoma).
- The **bulbourethral glands** are located at the base of the penis, near the ischial arch, lateral to the urethra, and measure about 4–5 mm in diameter. Distally to these glands there are two pairs of ischiocavernosus and ischiourethral muscles, which are highly vascularized, while ventrally lies the

pudendal nerve. No pathologies or abnormalities related to the bulbourethral glands have been described in the cat.

Surgical diseases of the male reproductive system

In general, cats suffer few problems related to the genital tract. We could summarize them as intersex conditions, testicular tumors, malformations and cryptorchidism, which, although rare, is by far the problem we will see the most in our day to day practice.

Urethral pathology is common, but due to its complexity it has its own chapter (see Ch. 27).

Surgical procedures of the scrotum and testicles

Congenital disorders are rare and are usually accompanied by abnormalities in other parts of the urogenital tract (Figs. 2–4).

Testicular problems are also rare because most cats are castrated at an early age.

Cryptorchidism

Although infrequent, it is the most prevalent congenital disorder (it represented 1.7% of the cases in one study and 1.3% in another). Even rarer is monorchidism (which according to the same studies had a prevalence of 0.1%).

Cryptorchidism, or retained testis, can be unilateral or bilateral and the testes can be located anywhere along their embryonic pathway from the caudal pole of the kidneys, through the inguinal canal, to the scrotum.

In unilateral cryptorchids, it appears to be more common for the testicle to be retained in the inguinal canal or area (Fig. 5), while in bilateral cryptorchids the testicles are more frequently found intra-abdominally.

The clinical signs are usually related to inappropriate elimination (marking) and strong-smelling urine, even the cat's behavior may be altered by the influence of hormones. On rare occasions, cryptorchidism is related to neoplastic transformation (this is well studied in dogs; a cryptorchid testicle is 17.5 times more likely to develop a tumor, and the same is likely to occur in cats).

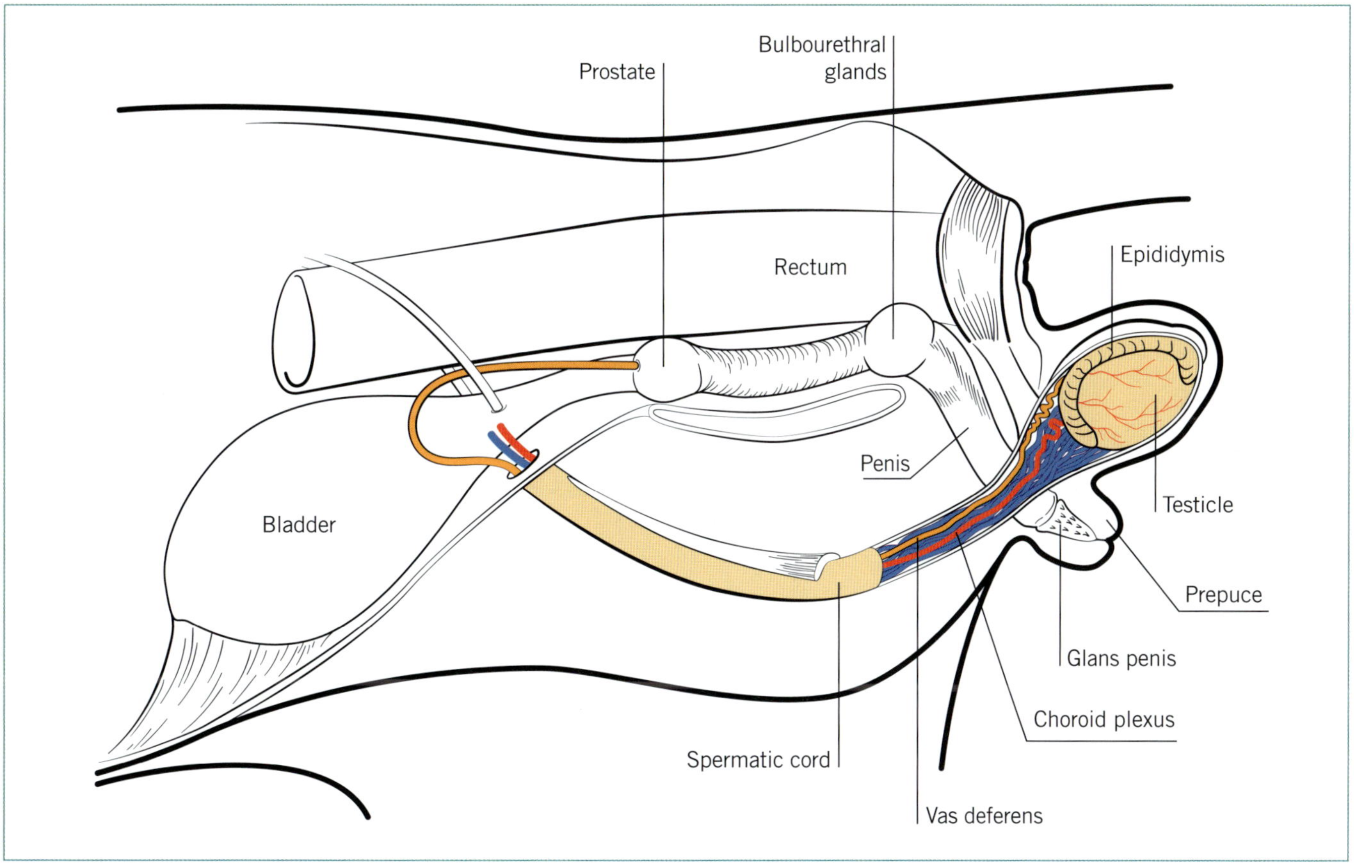

FIGURE 1. Anatomy of the reproductive system of the male cat.

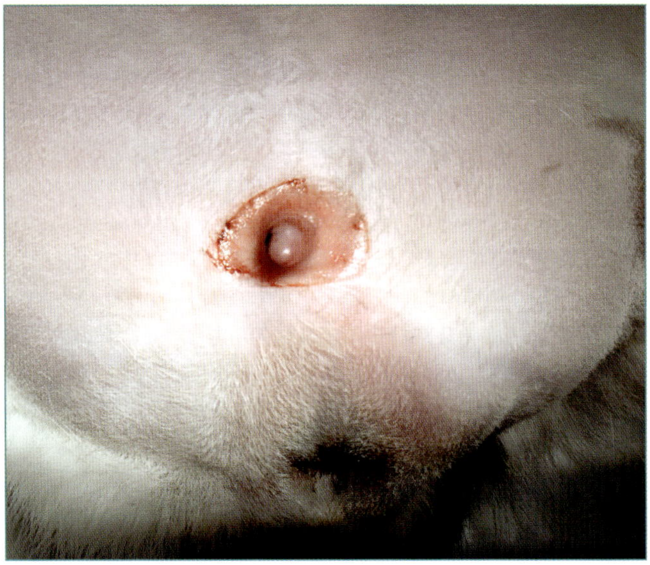

FIGURE 2. Cat with malformation of the prepuce.

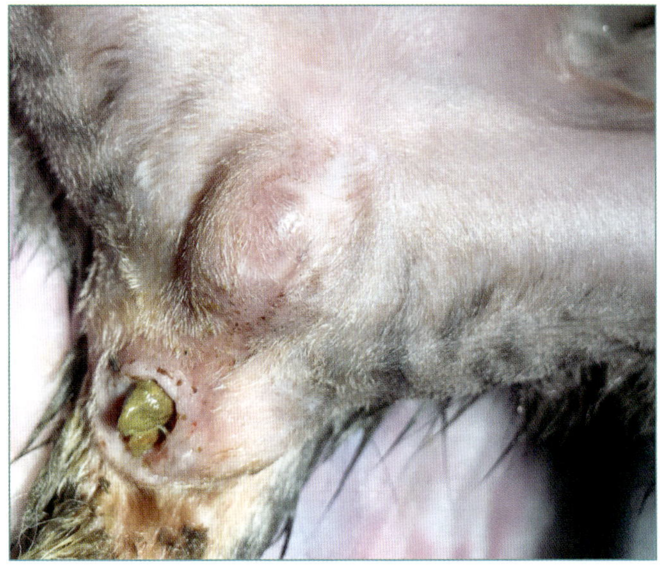

FIGURE 3. Cat with imperforate prepuce.

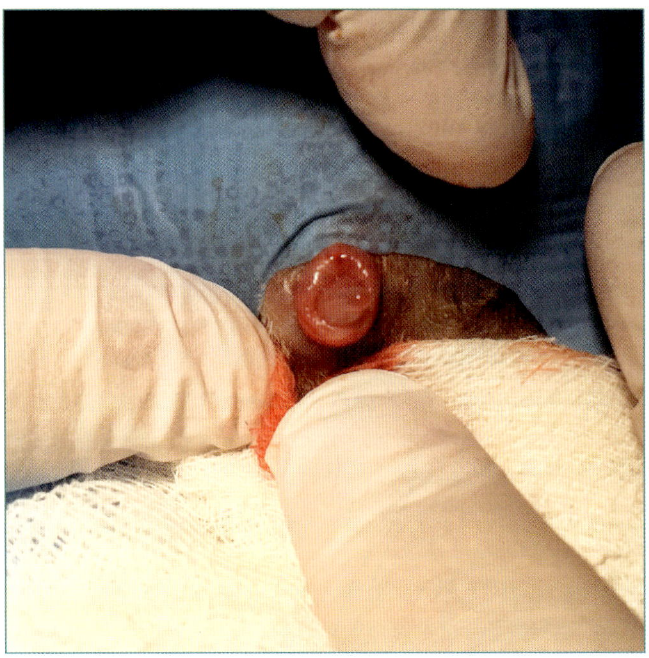

FIGURE 4. Patient in the previous figure once the skin has been incised.

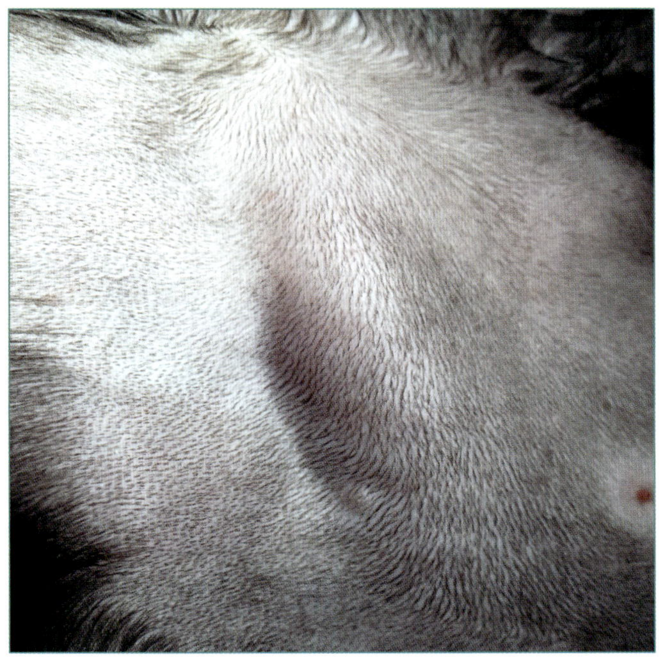

FIGURE 5. In this patient the location of the inguinal testis is clearly visible.

How can we determine if an apparently castrated cat is cryptorchid?

- Hormonal stimulation: testosterone can be measured after injection with human chorionic gonadotropin (hCG). A doubling or quadrupling of testosterone concentration indicates that the animal has testicular tissue and is therefore cryptorchid.
- Palpation and ultrasound: an experienced ultrasonographer can locate the testes among the fat in the inguinal area or abdomen.
- Presence of penile spines: as it depends on hormonal stimulation, it is indicative of the existence of testicular tissue.

Testicular tumors

There are very few cases described in the literature, which complicates the discussion of possible treatments or survival times. Therefore, when a testicular tumor is suspected, we should follow the general guidelines we would apply to any oncologic case:

- Castration (excisional biopsy).
- If there are adhesions, removal of the scrotum along with the testicle.
- Chest X-rays or advanced imaging techniques to rule out pulmonary metastases.
- Examination of the abdomen, either with advanced imaging techniques or with ultrasound, to fully stage the tumor.

Teratomas, Sertoli cell tumors and interstitial cell tumors have been diagnosed, but it can be assumed that malignant transformation of any of the cell types present in the testis could potentially occur.

Surgical procedures of the penis and prepuce

Although rare, hypospadias, phimosis or intersex conditions such as pseudohermaphroditism may be found.

In hypospadias, a failure of the embryonic layers to close leaves a ventral opening in the penile tissue and urethra.

In phimosis, a small preputial orifice prevents externalization of the penis.

In any case, the objective will be to correct the clinical signs, usually of infection, chronic cystitis and all types of discomfort, including dysuria, pollakiuria and stranguria, which are due to inadequate exposure of the urethral tissue or an impediment to normal urine output.

In phimosis procedures, a wider preputial orifice is created; in the other pathologies, urethral function is restored.

Surgical procedures of the prostate

In cats, the prostate is susceptible to prostatitis, prostatic cysts and neoplasms, as in other species, but the castration of most of the cats that come for consultation makes feline prostate pathology anecdotal. Ultrasound is a great ally in these cases.

Surgical techniques

Orchiectomy

Orchiectomy is the removal of the testicles.

> The castration of male cats is important, especially in communities, to avoid unwanted pregnancies, aggressive behavior, fights and marking. In indoor cats, the main reason is to avoid marking and roaming behavior.

Technique

1. The cat is placed in dorsal or lateral recumbency (surgeon's preference), and the scrotum is aseptically prepared.
2. A sterile drape with a small hole in it or a plate with an opening is used to provide a clean surgical field.
3. Between two fingers of our nondominant hand we tighten the testicle against the skin of the scrotum, which is very thin and has hardly any subcutaneous tissue, to make a small incision in a dorsoventral direction (Fig. 6.1).
4. Gently "squeezing" the scrotum, the testicle is exteriorized. Then, the tunica vaginalis is cut (Fig. 6.2).
5. The testicle is separated from its adhesions to the tunica vaginalis; traction can be applied by holding the tunica vaginalis with gauze (Fig. 6.3).
6. The tunica vaginalis may bleed slightly. Hemostatic forceps can be used and left in place during the procedure to obliterate the vessels, which do not need to be ligated (Fig. 6.4).
7. The vas deferens is separated from the blood vessels and cut at the epididymal tail (Fig. 6.4). A simple square knot is tied using the vas deferens and the vessels (Fig. 6.5).
8. An alternative is to tie a knot with the help of mosquito forceps (Figs. 6.6–6.8).

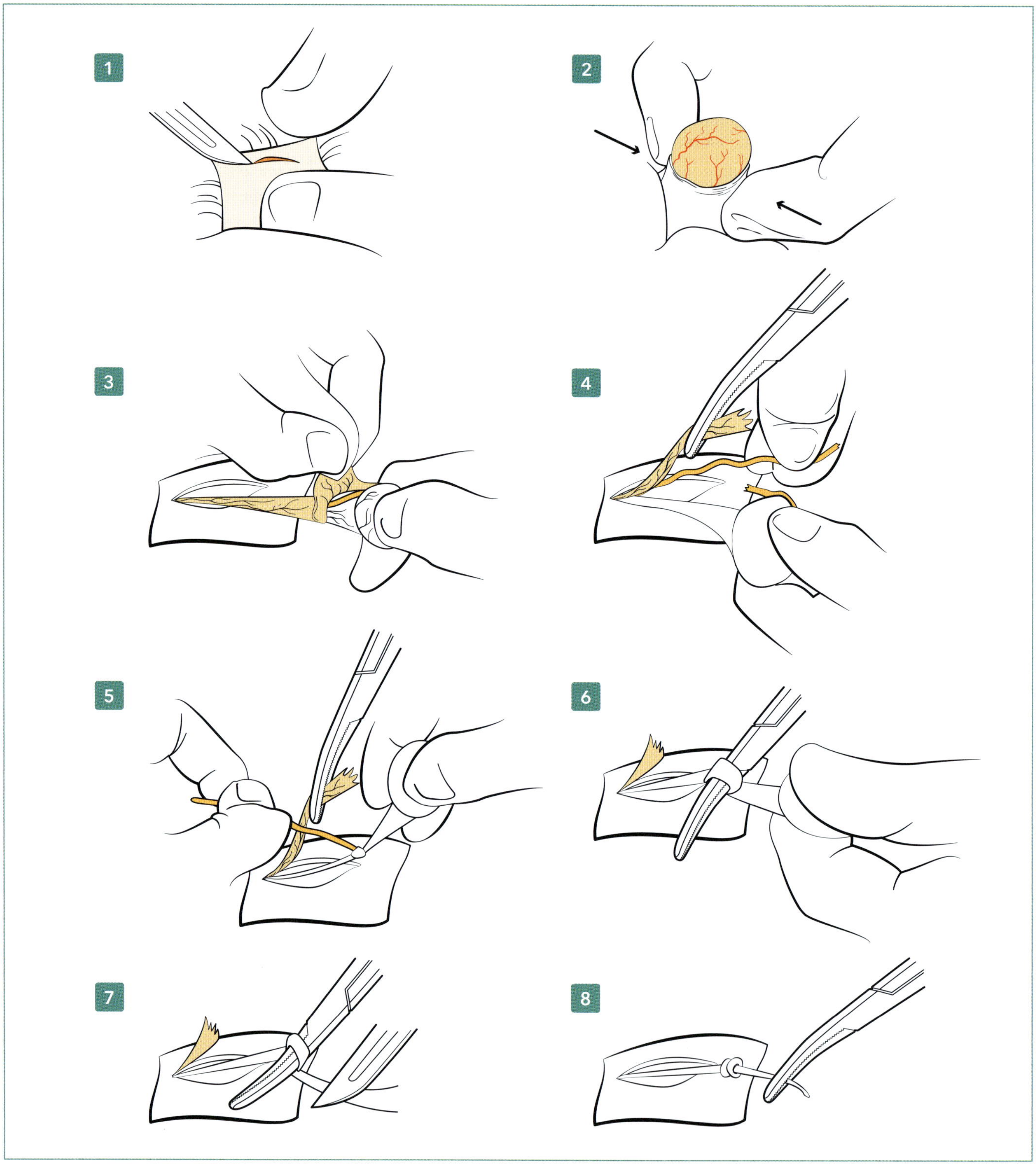

FIGURE 6. Orchiectomy steps.

1. After applying tension to the scrotal skin, it is incised dorsoventrally.
2. The testicle, covered with the tunica vaginalis, is exteriorized.
3. The tunica vaginalis is separated from the testicle.
4. Using hemostatic forceps, the vessels of the tunica vaginalis are obliterated and the vas deferens is separated from the blood vessels and sectioned at the tail of the epididymis.
5. The vas deferens and blood vessels are tied in a knot.
6. The vessels can also be closed by tying them with the help of mosquito forceps.
7. The pedicle is sectioned
8. Final knotting.

9. Another alternative is to perform a mass double-ligation with a 3-0 absorbable suture.
10. Finally, two of the aforementioned techniques can be combined. The forceps clamping the tunica vaginalis are removed.
11. Repeat the process with the other testicle. It can be externalized through a second cut in the scrotum or through the first incision, in which case the fibrous tissue (mediastinum) that separates both testicles and keeps them in their respective scrotal sacs must be cut.
12. The scrotal defect is not sutured.

> For a better recovery and a more comfortable postoperative period for the patient, local anesthesia can be injected into the hilum of the testicle to anesthetize the area before starting the surgery.

Resolution of cryptorchidism

Whether the testicle is retained in the inguinal area or in the abdomen, the patient is positioned in dorsal recumbency and the caudal abdomen is aseptically prepared for the procedure.

Inguinal testicle

Sometimes the presence of the testicle is visible, while other times its location is determined via palpation or ultrasound. In these cases, the skin in that area is incised.

If the testicle is not easily palpable or there is a lot of fat surrounding them:

1. Make a parasagittal incision in the groin and locate the inguinal canal.
2. Follow the vas deferens and testicular vessels and gently pull down on them to find the testicle.
3. It is easier to look for the testicle under the fat in the caudal mammary area than to make an incision over this area, since the fat and local lymph nodes make visibility difficult, obscure the surgical field with small hemorrhages and cause more inflammation in the postoperative period.
4. Once the testicle is located, we tie or ligate the vas deferens and remove the testicle as previously described for castration. The cryptorchid testicle may be smaller and atrophic, making it easier to perform a ligation with suture.
5. The defect is closed in layers. It is important to include the subcutaneous space in the suture to avoid seroma formation.
6. The skin can be closed with an intradermal suture.

Abdominal testicle

In this case, a caudal laparotomy is performed, similar to what is done in a cystotomy, to look for intra-abdominal testicles:

1. The retained testicle is usually located close to the inguinal canal or immediately cranial to the bladder. If the bladder is lifted while shifting the rectum to the left to locate the right testicle and to the right along with the intestines for the left testicle, locating them should not be difficult. The embryonic pathway of the testis runs immediately ventral to the ureters.
2. Once located, proceed as described for orchiectomy.
3. Sometimes only the vas deferens and blood vessels can be located, but not the testicle, which may be lodged between the internal and external inguinal rings or before the inguinal ring, halfway between the abdomen and the groin. In these cases, an incision is made over the groin to gently pull in one direction or the other until the testicle can be released, ligated and removed.
4. Finally, the incisions are closed in layers per routine.

Currently, orchiectomy of abdominal cryptorchids can also be performed laparoscopically.

Complications

Complications are very rare, but can be summarized as:

- Problems associated with anesthesia
- Hemorrhages
- Infections

Hemorrhages can be treated conservatively and only require surgical exploration if they do not stop on their own after applying light pressure on the area. Also, ensure that there are no coagulation problems.

In the authors' experience, infections have only been described in cases in which the basic principles of asepsis and the correct handling of the tissues have been ignored during the application of the surgical technique.

The use of prophylactic antibiotic therapy is not necessary for these surgical procedures.

Bibliography

HART BL, BARRET RE. Effects of castration on fighting, roaming, and urine spraying in adult male cats. *J Am Vet Med Assoc*, 1973; 163(3):290–292.

MILLIS DL, HAUPTMAN JG, JOHNSON CA. Cryptorchidism and monorchism in cats: 25 cases (1980–1989). *J Am Vet Med Assoc*, 1992; 200(8):1128–1130.

PIOLA V, POSCH B, AGHTE P et al. Radiographic characterization of the os penis in the cat. *Vet Radiol Ultrasound*, 2011; 52(3):270–272.

ROOT MV, JOHNSTON SD, JOHNSTON GR, OLSON PN. The effect of prepuberal and postpuberal gonadectomy on penile extrusion and urethral diameter in the domestic cat. *Vet Radiol Ultrasound*, 1996; 37(5):363–366.

OVARIOHYSTERECTOMY, PYOMETRA AND CAESAREAN SECTION 29

Anna Calvet

Surgical anatomy

For all the surgeries described in this chapter, it is essential to understand the anatomy of the female cat's reproductive system.

Ovariohysterectomy and ovariectomy are some of the most common surgical procedures that any general veterinary surgeon performs. In addition to avoiding the attraction of male cats and the inconvenience of sharing a house with a female in heat, these procedures ensure the absence of unwanted pregnancies and provide protection against diseases such as feline mammary tumors (depending on the time at which the procedure is performed) and pathological processes of this organ such as pyometra or uterine torsion. In pregnant females with dystocic deliveries, cesarean section is sometimes necessary (60%–80% of the time according to studies).

The parts that make up the reproductive tract in the female cat include the **ovaries**, **oviducts**, **uterus**, **vagina**, **urogenital sinus** and **vulva** (Fig. 1).

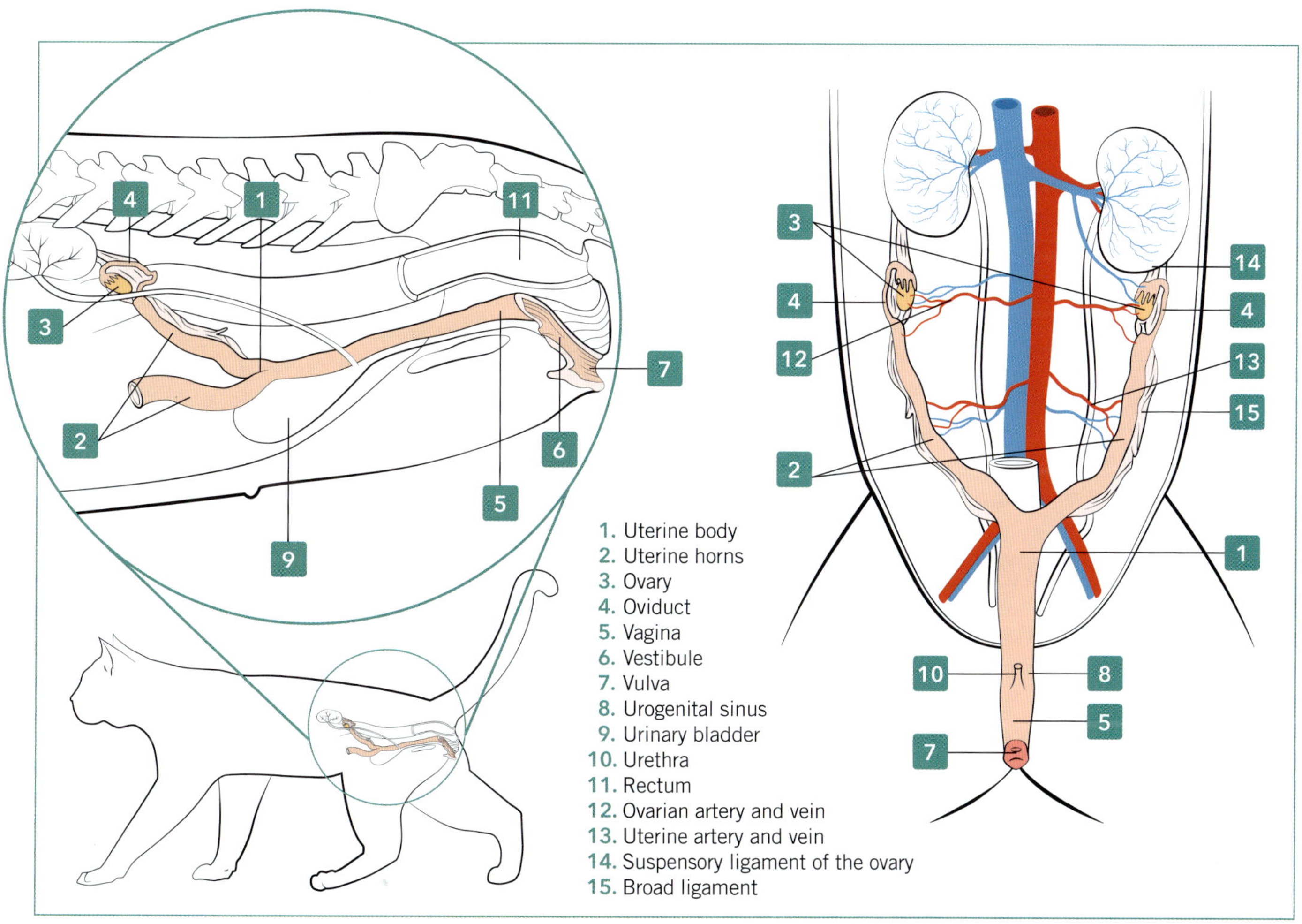

FIGURE 1. Reproductive system anatomy in the female cat.

Female cats have two ovaries measuring approximately 1×0.5 cm (it may be possible to visualize them via ultrasound at the caudal poles of the ipsilateral kidney).

The ovaries are suspended by a portion of the broad ligament called the suspensory ligament of the ovary. There is an **ovarian bursa** that partially covers the ovary and originates from the **mesosalpinx**, which is the portion of the broad ligament that suspends the oviducts (inside of which fertilization of the ovum takes place). The **ovarian ligament** joins the uterine horn to the ovary.

The ovarian blood supply comes through the **ovarian arteries**, which are direct branches of the **aorta**. The **ovarian vein** is responsible for collecting blood from the ovaries, the oviducts and the cranial part of the uterus and diverting it to the caudal vena cava.

Female cats have a short uterine body, about 2 cm long, and two long uterine horns measuring 7–10 cm depending on the cat's sexual maturity, phase of estrous cycle and previous litters. A part of the broad ligament called the mesometrium supports the uterine horns, which unite to form the uterine body that runs ventral to the colon and rectum and dorsal to the bladder. Its blood supply is via the **uterine artery**, which is a branch of the **vaginal artery**. Venous drainage is through the **uterine vein** that empties into the **internal iliac vein**.

Finally, the vagina extends from the pelvic symphysis to the cranial area of the caudal border of the ischial symphysis, where the urethra coming from the urinary bladder opens. The vaginal vestibule or urogenital sinus and the opening to the exterior, the vulva, are located caudally, ventral to the anus.

Lymphatic drainage of the uterus occurs through the lumbar and hypogastric lymph nodes. The vagina and vaginal vestibule drain into the internal iliac lymph nodes, while the vulva drains into the superficial iliac lymph nodes.

Surgical diseases of the ovary

Ovarian pathology is not very prevalent in the feline species. The conditions described below can be found.

Congenital ovarian abnormalities

Ovarian hypoplasia and ovarian agenesis lead to an absence of estrous cycle and infertility. These conditions are not very relevant, as they do not cause complications for the normal development of the patient, and only female cats that are going to be used for breeding will require further analysis.

Ovarian cysts

There are two types of ovarian cysts, and their frequency, in any case, increases with the age of the cat. On one hand, follicular cysts arise from atretic follicles and are associated with a sustained production of estrogens, resulting in prolonged estrus and exaggerated sexual behavior. On the other hand, there are cysts that do not have an ovarian origin, usually remnants of the rete tubules or mesonephric tubules (Fig. 2).

Treatment for female cats with signs of hyperestrogenism may consist of induction of ovulation by administering human chorionic gonadotropin (hCG) or, in a majority of cases, ovariectomy.

Ovarian tumors

Ovarian tumors are classified according to their cellular origin as epithelial, germ cell or sex cord–stromal tumors. The most frequent types are those in the granular layer (with origin in the sex cord stroma), which have the capacity to metastasize. This type of tumor is sometimes associated with hormonal problems; therefore, signs of persistent estrus, cystic endometrial hyperplasia and bilateral symmetrical alopecia are observed.

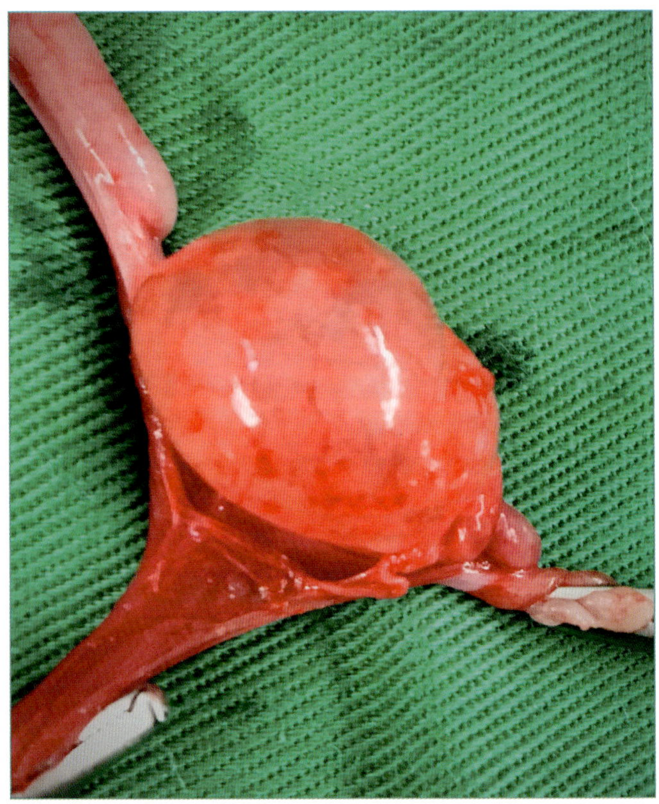

FIGURE 2. Ovarian cyst.

Ovarian remnant syndrome

The most common cause for signs of estrus following ovariectomy or ovariohysterectomy is the presence of ovarian tissue that has regained follicular activity.

There are two theories, the first and most accepted is that this is due to a surgical error. It has been described more in ovariohysterectomies than in ovariectomies (due to the ovary being more visible in the latter) and also in ovariohysterectomies performed from the flank due to poor visualization of the right ovary. In any case, the condition would be related to poor surgical technique, probably with excessive bleeding in the area that prevents a correct visualization of the structures, to entrapment of part of the ovarian tissue with the sutures, or to the accidental fall of part of the ovarian tissue into the abdominal cavity.

The second theory, not entirely proven, is the presence of accessory ovarian tissue that would become functional after removal of the "main" ovary. This tissue would be visualized on different points of the ovarian pedicle in the form of small, whitish spheres, which should be removed if found. Examination of the abdominal cavity is essential. Ovarian remnants are usually located adjacent to the site where pedicle ligation was performed (Fig. 3).

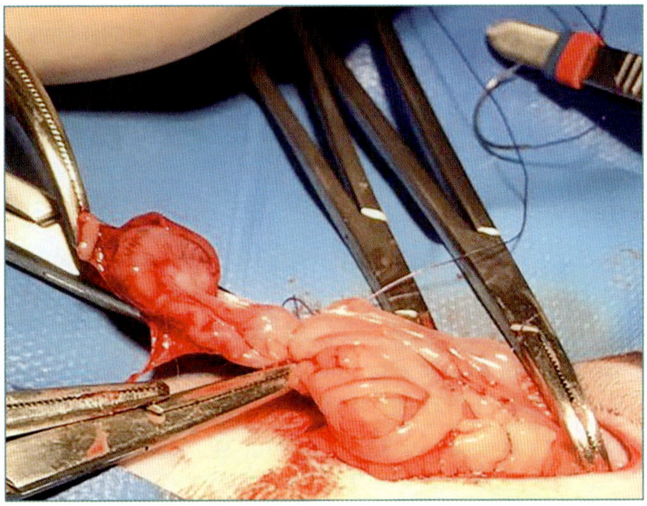

FIGURE 3. Ovarian remnant. In this case part of the ovary had not been removed, as can be seen by the thickened oviduct.

Surgical diseases of the uterus

Congenital uterine abnormalities

We are referring to a single-horned uterus, segmental agenesis of one of the uterine horns or uterine horn hypoplasia. These are usually incidental findings during surgery.

Diagnosis of ovarian remnant syndrome

There are several options available to diagnose this condition:

1. **Ultrasound:** a small cystic structure is found in the caudal aspect of the kidney. In female cats, the ovarian remnants are usually so small that they can be difficult to visualize.
2. **Hormone tests:**
   - Measurement of anti-Mullerian hormone concentration: a positive result is indicative of an ovarian remnant. However, a negative result does not rule it out completely and should be evaluated in conjunction with other tests. The test should be performed at least 9 days after neutering.
   - If the cat is in estrus, 300 IU of hCG is injected and progesterone is measured after 2 weeks.
   - If the cat is in anestrus, a gonadotropin-releasing hormone (GnRH) analog such as buserelin can be administered at a dose of 0.4 µg/kg IM, measuring basal estradiol 2 hours after injection.
3. **Vaginal cytology:** in a female with signs of estrus, it is very useful to perform a vaginal smear, as the presence of numerous cornified epithelial cells is indicative of estrus. This is certainly the simplest and most economical test, although accidental contact with estrogen-containing products, such as those used in human medicine, can interfere with the test results.
4. **Use of GnRH analogs/deslorelin:** on occasion, our patient's caregivers would like to prevent the cat from undergoing further surgeries, and the use of these implants is effective to temporarily control this pathology. Using these as a long-term treatment is not recommended, but they can guide the diagnosis and postpone surgery.

It is important to remember that when a congenital uterine abnormality is identified, evaluation of the ovaries and kidneys is warranted, since ipsilateral renal agenesis is possible, even though the ovaries are usually present.

Uterine tumors

Malignant endometrial adenocarcinoma is the most common uterine tumor. Benign (leiomyoma) and malignant (leiomyosarcoma) myometrial tumors have also been described.

To a lesser extent, other neoplastic lesions such as lymphoma and nonneoplastic lesions such as endometrial polyps or adenomyosis can be found. Adenomyosis is a condition in which the tissue that lines the uterus, the endometrial tissue, forms in the muscular layer of the uterus (myometrium).

Uterine tumors are associated with infertility, vulvar bleeding and masses that may be intra-abdominal or pelvic.

Ovariohysterectomy is the treatment of choice. In patients with adenocarcinoma, its malignancy means that in half of cases metastasis has already occurred at the time of surgery, with life expectancy being 5 months in a retrospective study.

Cystic endometrial hyperplasia and pyometra

Pyometra is the accumulation of pus inside the uterus (Fig. 4). The bacterial pathogens involved are vaginal or anogenital bacteria.

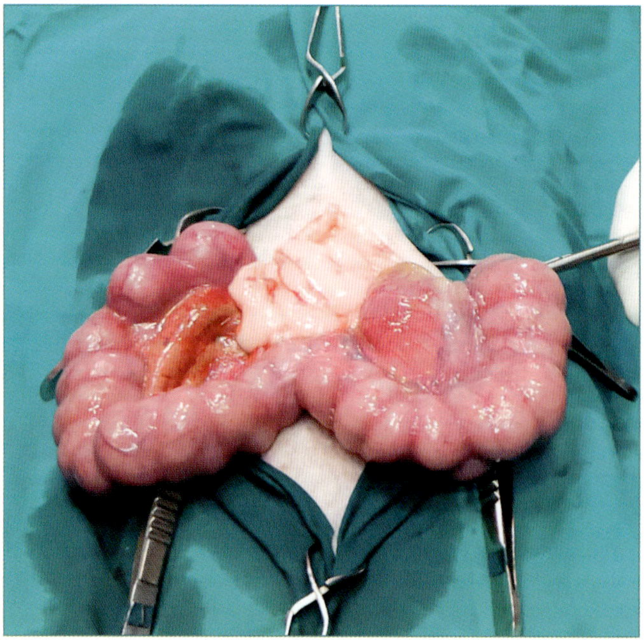

FIGURE 4. Pyometra.

Although initially proposed as a single syndrome, cystic endometrial hyperplasia and pyometra are now considered separate conditions, although endometrial hyperplasia is a risk factor for the development of pyometra (Box 1).

BOX 1. Risk factors for pyometra and associated pathologies

- Middle-aged or older females
- Metaestrus or diestrus phase, approximately 1 month after estrus
- Presence of cystic endometrial hyperplasia
- Hormone therapy with exogenous estrogens
- Subclinical lower urinary tract infections
- Nulliparous females
- Comorbidities such as diabetes or endotoxemia

The pathogenesis of pyometra is probably an interaction between the progesterone-stimulated endometrium, with variations in the presence of sex hormones, and the virulence of the vaginal and/or rectal flora (especially *Escherichia coli*).

Surgical techniques

Midline ovariohysterectomy

A median laparotomy is performed (see Ch. 20). With the cat in dorsal recumbency, the skin of the abdomen is shaved from the xiphoid process to the pubis, including the entire area between the nipples. The bladder can be palpated and emptied, if it is full, to minimize possible damage during surgery and improve the exposure of the uterine body.

Technique

1. The space between the umbilicus and the pubis is divided in three, and a small incision is made in the middle third. The initial incision is 2–2.5 cm long, extending from the skin to the subcutaneous tissue (incising in the midline allows us to enlarge the opening at any time if necessary during the procedure).

> A special note: if this procedure is performed on very young females, less than 12 weeks old, it is better to have a slightly more caudal approach.

2. After finding the linea alba, a pinch is lifted with the help of Adson forceps and a small incision is made with a scalpel. The incision is extended using Metzenbaum scissors.
3. The uterine body is located by moving the urinary bladder or, alternatively, we can look for the left uterine horn, which can be palpated if we move the descending colon medially.
4. The uterine horn is carefully exteriorized with the help of a finger or with an ovariohysterectomy hook. Its route is followed cranially until the ovary is located.
5. The suspensory ligament of the ovary can be gently torn with the fingers, or two hemostatic (mosquito) forceps can be placed before cutting or tearing it. Not removing the forceps that holds the abdominal part of the ligament allows for better visualization of the ovarian pedicle. The discomfort of keeping the ovarian ligament clamped is minimized by instilling a local anesthetic just above it.
6. At this point, it is time to ligate the ovarian pedicle, for which the authors propose four options. The first step is the same in all cases, which is to make a hole in the mesovarium:
   - Two hemostatic forceps are placed approximately 1 cm dorsal to the ovary (Fig. 5.1). A ligature is then placed around the ovarian artery and vein with 3-0 absorbable monofilament. In cats that are older, in estrus or large, it is advisable to place a second ligature. The pedicle is cut with the scalpel or torn between both forceps, and the uterine body with its ovary are completely exteriorized. The second hemostatic forceps is released, the one holding the pedicle in the abdomen, and correct hemostasis is confirmed.
   - Alternatively, three forceps can be placed as is done in female dogs, although in cats this is not usually necessary. In this case the procedure is very similar, but the first suture is placed where the hemostatic forceps farther away from the ovary was. The aim is to take advantage of the vessel obliteration caused by the forceps.
   - With curved mosquito forceps, the vessels of the pedicle are tied in a knot on themselves. This is done just like as in male castration.
   - Finally, other methods of vessel occlusion are available, such as hemostatic clips or electrothermal vessel-sealing devices.
7. The broad and round ligaments are bluntly dissected to exteriorize both uterine horns until the body of the uterus is exposed.

VIDEO

Knotting of the ovarian pedicle

8. As with ovarian pedicles, the cervix is ligated (the same suture material and caliber may be used). A preliminary mass ligation is placed around the cervix and the vessels that run on both sides of the organ. It can be performed directly or with the use of hemostatic forceps (it should be noted that in female cats the uterine tissue can be quite friable, so forceps cut rather than obliterate the tissue; therefore, their use is not recommended) (Fig. 5.2).
9. A second transfixion suture is placed, especially in large cats or those with a very vascularized uterus (Fig. 5.3).
10. A transverse section of the uterus is made, and the uterus and ovaries are removed to check for bleeding. Closing is done in layers.
11. The muscle layer can be sutured in a continuous pattern or in a simple interrupted pattern. The former reduces the amount of suture material present at the surgical site, which reduces postoperative inflammation. Any 2-0 or 3-0 monofilament suture can be used.
12. It is debated whether or not to approximate using a subcutaneous suture. Detractors avoid it because more suture material means more inflammation, more discomfort for the cat and possibly an increased chance of her wanting to touch the wound. Proponents have on their side various studies that prove that the absence of subcutaneous sutures makes it easier for a seroma to develop. As the wound is usually small, a continuous suture or a simple X-stitch to approximate the edges is usually sufficient.
13. The skin can be closed with staples, simple interrupted stitches with nonabsorbable material such as nylon, a continuous suture or the preferred buried continuous intradermal suture.

> To finish the intradermal suture, an Aberdeen knot or a sliding knot, which are well-buried knots, work very well.

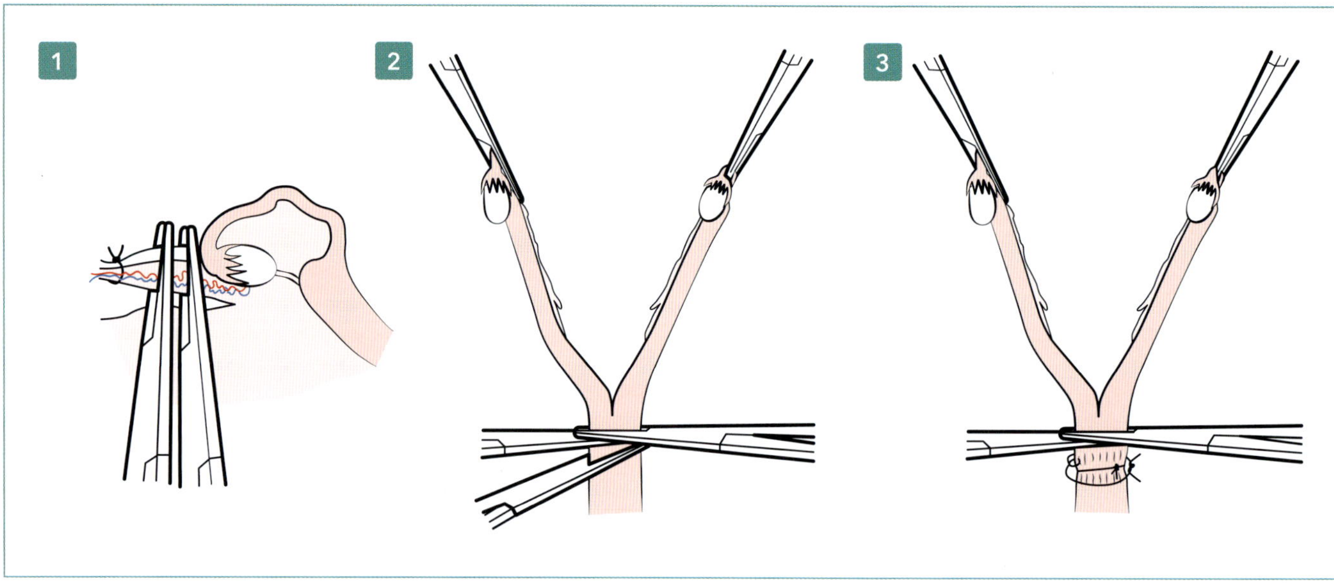

FIGURE 5. Steps of an ovariohysterectomy.
1. Ligation of the ovarian pedicle illustrated with the technique using two hemostatic forceps.
2. Placement of hemostatic forceps to obliterate the body of the uterus.
3. Placement of ligatures on the uterine body before cutting and removing the reproductive tract, ovaries and uterus en bloc.

VIDEO

Intradermal suture and Aberdeen knot

Flank ovariohysterectomy

For this technique, the position of the patient is crucial in order to achieve good access. The cat lies on the right side and the hind limbs are held extended.

Technique

1. The incision site is determined by drawing an equilateral triangle with the iliac wing, the greater trochanter and the incision point as vertices (Fig. 6).
2. The skin, subcutaneous fat and, more deeply, the oblique, rectus and transversus abdominis muscles are incised.
3. The peritoneum is opened and the left uterine horn is located (the cat is in right lateral recumbency).
4. The procedure for the removal and ligation of the ovaries and uterus is essentially the same as in midline ovariohysterectomy.
5. Closing is done by individual muscle layers to give the maximum strength possible.

Ovariectomy

Technique

1. An incision is made closer to the umbilicus or even cranial to the umbilicus for better visualization of both ovaries.
2. After ligating the ovaries, two hemostatic forceps are placed on the proximal part of the uterine horn and suturing is performed in the same way as in the cervix.
3. The closure pattern is the same as for an ovariohysterectomy.

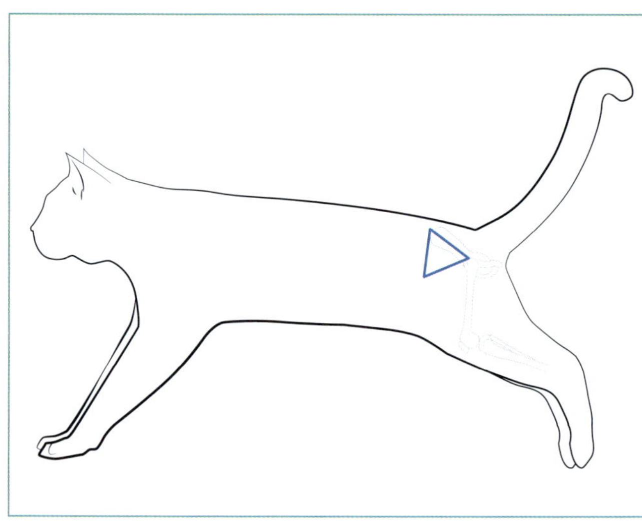

FIGURE 6. Diagram of the incision site, superimposing an equilateral triangle with two of its vertices on the iliac wing and the greater trochanter.

Although it goes beyond the scope of this atlas, it is noteworthy that laparoscopic ovariectomy is currently another surgery that can be relied upon for spaying female cats with very good results.

Technique selection: ovariectomy or ovariohysterectomy?

There has been much discussion over the years about whether it is better to perform midline or flank ovariectomies and ovariohysterectomies, just as it has always been debated whether it is better to perform an ovariectomy or an ovariohysterectomy.

Studies have determined that in flank surgery there is increased acute pain in the immediate postoperative period, while in midline approaches surgical site inflammation is more important over time.

Since there are no significant differences, the recommendation is for each surgeon to find the way of performing the procedure that gives them the most confidence, and with which they obtain the best results.

Regarding the debate between ovariectomy and ovariohysterectomy, the pros of ovariectomy are that it provides effective sterilization, the surgical wound is potentially smaller, visualization of the ovarian pedicles is better, and the risk of complications associated with manipulating the uterus is minimized.

On the other hand, with good technique, ovariohysterectomy is equally effective and the absence of uterus eliminates the possibility of complications if the cat undergoes treatment with exogenous progestogens (although rarely used anymore, they are still available in many countries for the control of dermatitis).

Pyometra as a special case

As previously mentioned, pyometra is among the diseases that affect the uterus and require surgery.

These are the key points that help in the evaluation and diagnosis of this condition in the cat:

- It can be open (50%–86% of cases) or closed.
- Cats with closed pyometra present more clinical signs, such as lethargy, anorexia, polyuria/polydipsia, vomiting, diarrhea, dehydration, abdominal distension and peritonitis.
- In the case of a uterine infection, respiratory rate or temperature may be increased or decreased.
- In up to 25% of cases there is no significant increase in the size of the uterus.
- The laboratory abnormalities caused by pyometra are not pathognomonic, but the results of the complete blood count and biochemical analysis are very helpful in preoperative

Preoperative and postoperative considerations in ovariohysterectomy

Why is sterilization performed and when?

- Population control. An intact female cat can have up to three litters per year.
- It is important that she be spayed before her first estrus. The age varies depending on the breed, weight and even the latitude in which the cat lives. Domestic cats are sensitive to changes in photoperiod and may come into estrus sooner than the 6 months established as a general rule.
- Early sterilization decreases the risk of mammary tumors.
- Having intact females means that from January until the beginning of summer they come into heat every 2 weeks, attracting male cats.
- Intact female cats have increased risk of pyometra.
- Infectious and hereditary diseases in the mother can affect the kittens.

Are there risks?

- Anesthesia entails risk, but this can be minimized with good technique. The combination of drugs used as well as the main complications associated with surgical procedures in cats, such as surgical time, temperature and glycemia, should be taken into account.
- Neutering has not been shown to lead to behavioral changes in female cats.
- Neither have problems in growth or development been demonstrated.

considerations and correlate to the prognosis (findings of azotemia, increased liver enzymes, neutrophilia and hyperglobulinemia).

- Endotoxemia caused by intrauterine bacteria can lead to **endotoxemia-induced cholestasis** (increased alkaline phosphatase, total bilirubin and cholesterol).
- Coagulation disorders may be observed.
- *Escherichia coli* is undoubtedly one of the main causes (80% of cases) of pyometra in cats.
- In 40%–70% of cases there is a concurrent urinary tract infection; therefore, it is advisable at the time of surgery to take a urine sample via cystocentesis for culture.
- Although the definitive solution is surgical, it is advisable to stabilize the patient as much as possible prior to surgery.
- In young cats with nonseptic, open pyometra and in stable cats with breeding potential, medical treatment may be considered.

At present, medical treatment consists of antibiotic therapy and a progesterone receptor blocker (aglepristone) injected subcutaneously on days 1, 2, 7 and repeated on day 14, if necessary. Cooperation by the cat's caretakers is essential, along with good follow-up including physical examination, control ultrasound and blood tests if it is suspected that the cat is not progressing correctly.

Surgical technique in pyometra

The surgical technique in pyometra is basically the same as in ovariohysterectomy, with certain noteworthy differences:

- It is important to make an opening large enough to comfortably access the ovaries and cervix. Likewise, we must ensure that there is enough room to manipulate the tissues, as the walls of the pus-filled uterus may be more fragile.
- Great care must be taken with vascularization, such as in cases involving a pregnant uterus, as the blood vessels of a pus-filled uterus are larger and less elastic.
- The cervical stump does not need to be closed with an inverting suture. The current recommendation is to ensure that it does not bleed; if deemed necessary, it may be covered with omentum.
- In the presence of peritonitis, closing the abdominal cavity with absorbable material is not recommended, as the presence of inflammatory cells does not ensure that suture tension will be maintained for a sufficient time. We can opt for a nonabsorbable monofilament such as nylon; a gauge of 3-0 is usually enough in the cat.

Caesarean section

A cesarean section consists of the removal of kittens by means of a hysterectomy. To maximize the results we should:

- Correctly prepare the mother during the preoperative period.
- Maximize efficiency in the operating room by using good technique, proper anesthesia and correct handling of the kittens.
- Have an adequate postoperative care protocol.

Dystocia

Dystocia or parturition that does not proceed normally is a life-threatening emergency for both the mother and the kittens.

Causes of dystocia can be maternal or fetal (Box 2), and some breeds are more affected (Box 3).

Normal gestation and delivery

The average duration of gestation in the cat is 65 days and, although this interval ranges from 57 to 72 days, 97% of deliveries occur between days 61 and 70.

We can divide parturition into three phases:

1. Uterine contractions and dilation of the cervix.
2. Abdominal contractions that accompany effective uterine contractions and end in the expulsion of the kittens.
3. Expulsion of fetal membranes.

The first phase usually lasts about 2 hours and the second phase, between the birth of the first and the last kitten, about 6 hours (the time between kittens is usually 30 minutes, although 95% of kittens are born within 100 minutes after the preceding kitten). Phases 2 and 3 often overlap.

When to intervene?

A cesarean section is recommended:

- When more than 71 days have passed since mating and there are no signs of parturition.
- If there are strong abdominal contractions for more than 30 minutes, but no kittens are born.
- When there are weak contractions for more than 4 hours without birth taking place.
- If the cat shows signs of discomfort or if at any time during parturition there is abundant bloody discharge.
- If abundant discharge of an inappropriate color, such as blood red, brown or greenish, or having a purulent appearance, occurs before the first kitten is born.

BOX 2. Causes of dystocia

Maternal causes

- Uterine inertia: represents two-thirds of cases of dystocia.
- Uterine torsion (Fig. 7).

Fetal causes

- Malpresentation: this is the most significant fetal cause, 30% of kittens may be delivered rear first (breech).
- Fetal death.
- Malformations.
- Disproportionate size of the kitten relative to the birth canal.

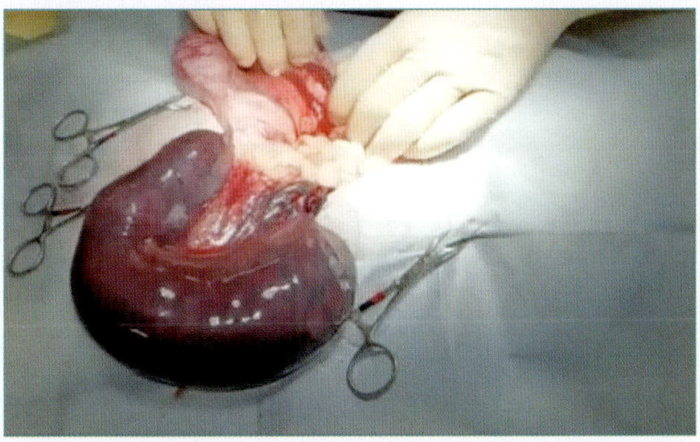

FIGURE 7. Uterine torsion (image extracted from a video).

BOX 3. Breeds at higher risk for dystocia

- British.
- Ragdoll.
- Abyssinian and Somali.
- Oriental breeds.
- Burmese.

- When there are ultrasound signs of fetal distress (normal heart rate >180 bpm; below 150 bpm is considered an emergency). In this case, we must remember that fetal heart rate can be momentarily reduced for 30 seconds to 1 minute by the effect of a uterine contraction, and must be reevaluated after this time.

> In the absence of fetal distress, if the mother is doing well and there is no obstructive dystocia, oxytocin can be administered.

Oxytocin is administered at a dose of 0.1 IU/kg along with intravenous fluids via a slow infusion. A second dose can be administered after 30 minutes. It is not indicated to further increase the number of doses.

Calcium gluconate 10% can also be used, at a dose of 0.2 ml/kg, in a slow intravenous administration while monitoring cardiac function, even though hypocalcemia and hypoglycemia are not common in dystocic cats.

Medical treatment has a success rate of around 30%.

Anesthetic considerations

There is little scientific evidence regarding how to anesthetize a cat for cesarean section, but the goal should be to remove the kittens as quickly as possible to minimize drug exposure.

In general, premedication with opioids is not recommended. Alfaxalone is recommended for induction (based on feasibility studies in puppies), although propofol is a good alternative. Once the kittens have been removed, the mother can be medicated.

Surgical technique in cesarean section

In a cesarean section, **speed** is important to **prevent fetal hypoxia**. The procedure is as follows:

- The surgical field is prepared on the abdomen, from the xiphoid process to the pubis.
- The cat is positioned in dorsal recumbency, if possible tilting the table slightly so that the abdominal contents do not press excessively on the thorax.
- A large incision is made through the linea alba, making sure not to damage the uterus, and the uterine horns are exteriorized.
- A small incision is made with the scalpel in the ventral area of the body of the uterus, in a relatively avascular area in order to minimize bleeding.
- The opening is enlarged slightly with blunt-tipped Metzenbaum scissors until it is sufficiently large to extract the kittens.
- The uterine horns are carefully squeezed until all the fetuses are removed through the opening that has been made.
- Ensure that there are no other kittens left and, whenever possible, carefully traction to remove the placentas together.

- The uterine incision is closed once it has been ascertained that there is nothing left inside the uterus, except for firmly attached placental sacs, which should not be pulled with force due to the risk of causing severe hemorrhaging. For closure, a continuous inverting suture pattern is used, such as a Cushing or Lembert pattern (Fig. 8), using absorbable monofilament such as poliglecaprone or polydioxanone.
- The midline laparotomy is closed routinely. The same technique described in ovariohysterectomy can be used. An intradermal suture is preferred, so that the suture material does not interfere with the kittens as they suckle.

Sometimes the cat's caretakers do not want the cat to have more litters, in which case an ovariohysterectomy can be performed.

It can be performed two ways: either en bloc, with the fetuses still in the uterus, or after the cesarean section has been completed. Kitten survival is decreased in en bloc ovariohysterectomy, but it can be performed when the fetuses are known to be no longer viable.

Postoperative complications and prognosis

Uterine prolapse

Uterine prolapse is rare in cats, but it may occur in the days following parturition in either normal or dystocic cases.

Affected cats may present with little or no discomfort or be severely affected and in shock. Repositioning should only be attempted in cases where the cat is in good health and the uterus has been previously cleaned and aseptically prepared. In all other cases, an ovariohysterectomy should be performed.

Galactostasis and mastitis

Galactostasis and mastitis are usually seen during lactation, although there are cases of mastitis during gestation.

Galactostasis occurs when milk production exceeds demand. The mammary glands are swollen and perhaps painful to the touch, even though the cat is in good health.

Mastitis may present as hot, reddened mammary gland inflammation, and the formation of abscesses in the gland may lead to necrosis; but it may also be subclinical, in which case the warning sign may be the inadequate growth of the suckling kittens.

Galactostasis can be treated with warm cloths and massage, but mastitis requires antibiotic treatment, based on the results of the culture and antibiogram. Always look for a sensitive antibiotic that will cause the least damage to the kittens. In severe cases, it is recommended that natural lactation be stopped.

Postpartum metritis

The cat will show signs of systemic disease, including vaginal discharge, and an ultrasound will show a fluid-filled uterus. In these cases, samples must be taken for culture.

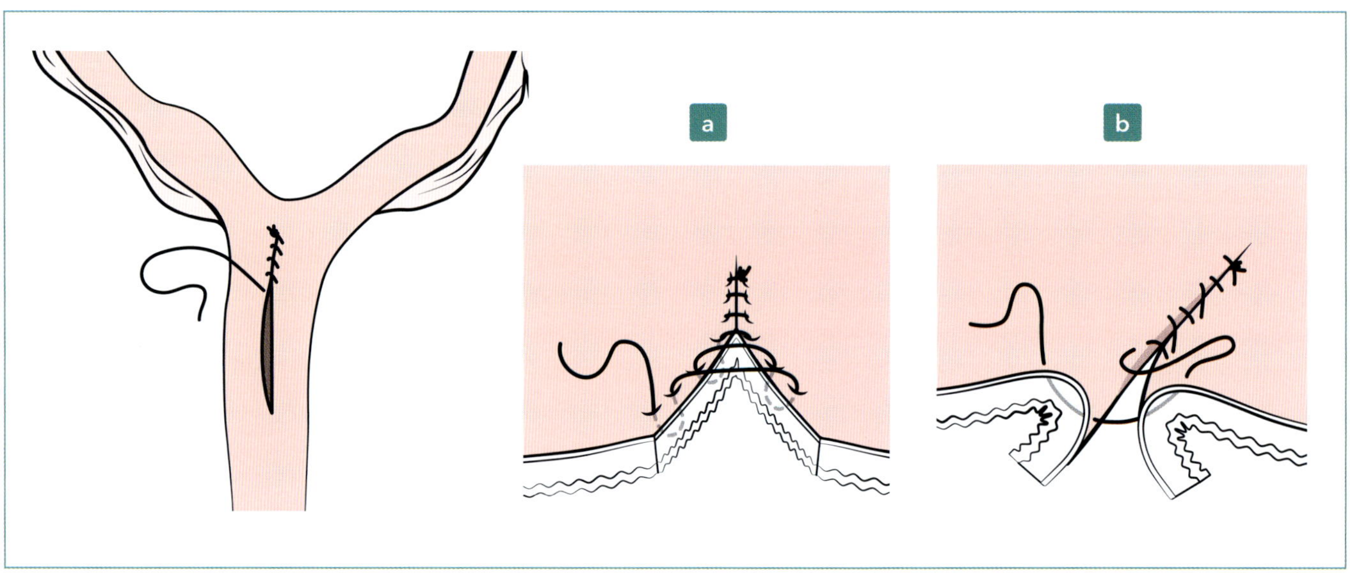

FIGURE 8. Closure of the uterine incision is performed with a continuous inverting (a) Cushing or (b) Lembert pattern.

Kittens born by caesarean section

- The moment a kitten is removed, it is quickly handed over to an assistant for **resuscitation**. The airway should be cleared and fetal membranes should be cleaned off. Fluids can be removed using gentle suction. Gently rubbing the thoracic area with a towel stimulates breathing.
- **Kittens should not be shaken** to mobilize the fluids from the respiratory system. Rather, let gravity take effect or, alternatively, rock them gently with the head and neck well supported.
- **The survival of kittens depends on how quickly they begin to breathe** normally. Breathing can be pharmacologically stimulated with doxapram by placing 1 or 2 drops under the tongue after clearing the airways. Oxygen therapy with a mask can also be administered.
- To **occlude the umbilical artery and vein**, a clamp is placed and left in place for 10 minutes before cutting. If bleeding occurs, suture ligation can be performed.
- **Preventing hypothermia is another important point.** Along with the preparation of the operating room, an incubator should be made available or, failing that, a box with hot water bottles or other devices that allow an environment with a controlled temperature of 30°C–33°C (86°F–91.4°F) to be maintained (Fig. 9).
- When the mother has recovered, she should be reunited with her kittens as soon as possible.

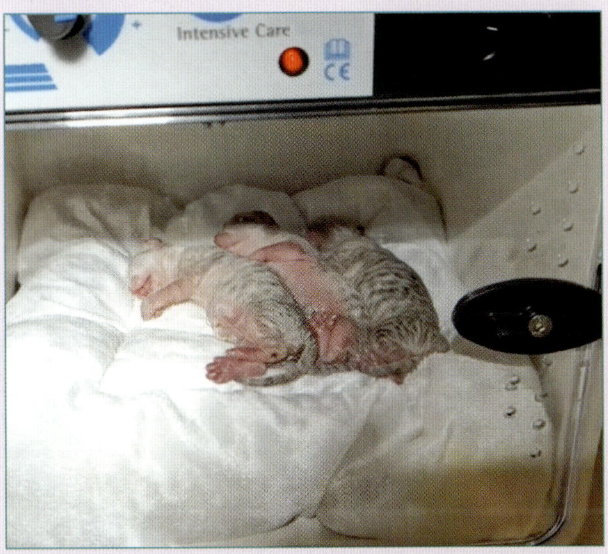

FIGURE 9. Newborn kittens after cesarean section. Placing them in an incubator or intensive care unit, which is a sanitized and disinfected space with controlled temperature and oxygen, improves the chances of success in the kittens' first moments of life.

Hemorrhage

The most significant risk in the postoperative period is suture dehiscence. However, this rarely occurs in internal sutures, provided it has been verified that there is no bleeding upon completion of the surgery. It occurs more frequently with inexperienced surgeons, in obese cats or in very vascularized uteri.

Inadvertent dehiscence of an intra-abdominal suture results in bleeding that can:

- Go unnoticed.
- Result in a slower recovery.
- Cause the patient to present with signs of hypovolemic shock, tachycardia, tachypnea, low hematocrit and free abdominal fluid detectable by ultrasound. In this case, a transfusion and a new intervention will be necessary once the patient has been stabilized.

Inadvertent ligation of the ureter

This is a rare but serious complication. If discovered early in the postoperative period, another intervention can be performed to free the ureter, with a subsequent evaluation of the effect it may have had on renal function. If it goes unnoticed, it results in an increase in renal size and hydronephrosis. It is recommended to implement good postoperative pain control and to perform ultrasound scans in the event excessive pain is observed in relation to the surgery that is not controlled with routine postoperative analgesia.

Stump pyometra

If uterine stump pyometra is diagnosed at some point after surgery, the administration of external progestogens or the possibility of remnant ovarian syndrome should always be considered.

External suture dehiscence

External suture dehiscence may be due to excessive inflammation (reaction to the suture) or excessive licking. In these cases, postoperative NSAID treatment can be continued. If the suture causes too much reaction, it can be removed and the wound closed again with nylon or another nonabsorbable monofilament suture, as they cause less reaction.

Peritonitis

Peritonitis is a possible complication after pyometra or cesarean section surgery.

Adhesions

After a cesarean section, adhesions may occur at surgical sites that could interfere if a repeat surgery is required in the future. To minimize this risk, it is advisable to handle the tissues gently and carefully and to use a proper inverting suture technique in the uterus, so that the inflammatory reaction produced by the suture does not act as a point of union with other tissues.

Bibliography

Davidson J, Black D. Small animal pyometra (chapter 42). In: Aronson LR (ed.). *Small Animal Surgical Emergencies*. Wiley Blackwell, 2015.

Demirel MA, Acar DB. Ovarian remnant syndrome and uterine stump pyometra in three queens. *J Feline Med Surg*, 2012; 14(12):913–918.

DeTora M, McCarthy RJ. Ovariohysterectomy versus ovariectomy for elective sterilization of female dogs and cats: is removal of the uterus necessary? *J Am Vet Med Assoc*, 2011; 239(11):1409–1412.

Holst BS, Axnér E, Öhlund M et al. Dystocia in the cat evaluated using an insurance database. *J Feline Med Surg*, 2017; 19(1):42–47.

Holst BS. Feline breeding and pregnancy management: What is normal and when to intervene. *J Feline Med Surg*, 2022; 24(3):221–231.

McIntyre RL, Levy JK, Roberts JF, Reep RL. Developmental uterine anomalies in cats and dogs undergoing elective ovariohysterectomy. *J Am Vet Med Assoc*, 2010; 237(5):542–546.

Simpson G, England G, Harvey M. *Manual of Small Animal Reproduction and Neonatology*. BSAVA British Small Animal Veterinary Association, 1998.

Swaffield MJ, Molloy SL, Lipscomb VJ. Prospective comparison of perioperative wound and pain score parameters in cats undergoing flank vs midline ovariectomy. *J Feline Med Surg*, 2020; 22(2):168–177.

www.thecatgroup.org.uk

5

TRAUMATOLOGY IN CATS

ASSESSMENT AND INITIAL MANAGEMENT OF POLYTRAUMATIZED CATS 30

Antonio Peña

Most cases of polytraumatized cats involve falls from height, such as from a window or balcony, or road traffic accidents. Other less severe accidents can also cause fractures or joint injuries in cats.

Certain accidents such as falls from height are now less common. This is because cat owners have means at their disposal to avoid these accidents, using various types of screens to make dangerous areas inaccessible to their cats. But other types of accidents, such as vehicle accidents, continue occurring at the same rate. Often, not as much attention is paid to accidents that occur inside the home (cats that jump from furniture or get stuck in radiators).

Initial assessment of polytraumatized cats

The initial assessment of a cat that has suffered trauma should be planned (Fig. 1) and done in advance to enable fast and complete examination and quick intervention if the patient's life is at risk.

Factors that influence the successful treatment of cats with trauma

- Type and extent of the injury
- Organs affected
- Previous condition of the patient and prior pathologies
- Amount of time elapsed between the trauma and the initiation of treatment
- The number of people on the veterinary team and their training
- Equipment available at the veterinary center
- Owner's economic resources

A	Airway
C	Cardiovascular
R	Respiratory: respiratory pattern, effort, auscultation
A	Abdomen
S	Spinal column
H	Head
P	Pelvis; rectal palpation
L	Limbs
A	Arteries and veins; pulses
N	Nerves: neurological examination of limbs

FIGURE 1. Mnemonic device for complete initial examination.

There is no need to interact with the cat during this examination. Upon arrival at the veterinary center, the animal should be observed either inside its carrier or on the examination table. Initially the cat's level of consciousness is determined, along with its respiratory pattern and level of dyspnea (see video). Signs of bleeding or other discharge should be checked for as well. If there is difficulty breathing or poor tissue perfusion, action should be taken immediately to ensure adequate oxygenation and to stop any life-threatening bleeding.

Cats with dyspnea may adopt postures that indicate they are having difficulty breathing. Sometimes they sit without being willing to lie down. They may have their mouths closed, even in the case of severe dyspnea. Other times, they may

VIDEO

Dyspnea in a polytraumatized cat

crouch with all four limbs close together underneath their body, without resting their sternum on the table, breathing with their neck extended and their mouth open, trying to "swallow" air.

Their respiratory pattern should be evaluated, along with the movements of the thoracic wall in relation to the abdominal wall. In some cases, while there may be thoracic movement, it may be such that it does not effectively facilitate adequate ventilation, nonetheless resulting in dyspnea.

Rapid administration of oxygen before carrying out any additional examination is crucial for these patients. It should be as effective as possible without the oxygenation method itself causing additional stress. There are different ways to provide oxygen to the patient: via a mask, by applying oxygen near the nose/mouth or via oxygenation chambers. It may even be necessary to intubate the animal or perform an emergency tracheotomy. Each system has advantages and disadvantages associated with the amount of oxygen that the patient actually breathes in (endotracheal tube > mask > oxygen chamber > source of oxygen near the nose/mouth) as well as the stress involved and the handling required to apply it.

Another system that has been described is to place an Elizabethan collar on the cat, cover almost the entirety of the front part with plastic wrap (approximately 80% of the surface), and administer oxygen inside the makeshift "individual chamber." There are several downsides to this system: the concentration of oxygen inside this chamber never exceeds 75%; heat accumulates inside this chamber, which can be uncomfortable for the cat if used for a long period of time; and the collar itself is difficult to keep on the cat.

Often, it is most effective to place the patient in an oxygen chamber. The cat stays in a controlled, 100% oxygen environment, does not need to be manipulated and can be monitored from outside to evaluate any changes, including any worsening of its condition. There are cages made expressly for this purpose, but a plastic box in which an opening is made for oxygen entry can also be used (Fig. 2). It should be noted that several small accessory openings should be made for carbon dioxide (CO_2) to flow out. A disadvantage to oxygen chambers is that, if accessing the interior is required to perform a procedure on the patient, the chamber loses its oxygen concentration, and it takes some time to regain it. The increase in temperature inside the chamber is also a disadvantage.

If the cat shows no signs of dyspnea or other clinical signs that should be treated immediately, a thorough, prompt and orderly examination should be performed.

To avoid causing or aggravating any irreversible spinal injuries, special attention should be paid to detect injury to the vertebral column before handling the patient. This examination should be done even before initiating oxygen therapy or any other emergency treatment, since such injuries could be fatal.

Any alterations in the alignment of the spine, instability, and crackling sounds should be checked for (Fig. 3). If any of these signs are present, stabilize the position of the cat as much as possible before continuing with other procedures.

The thoracic walls and the sternum are palpated to look for any rib or sternebra fractures. Next, bilateral thoracic auscultation is performed, and normal or abnormal respiratory and cardiac sounds are identified. Mucous membrane color, capillary refill time (CRT) and distal pulse are also evaluated.

The integrity of the abdominal wall should be checked for, and any hematomas, penetrating wounds, and hernias caused by trauma should be ruled out.

If an ultrasound machine is available, it is very useful to examine the thoracic and abdominal cavities, even if the clinician has little ultrasound experience. The protocol used is called TFAST (thoracic focused assessment with sonography for trauma) and AFAST (abdominal focused assessment with sonography for trauma). This procedure is done without restraining or excessively handling the patient, so the cat can remain in a comfortable position. TFAST enables evaluation of the presence of pneumothorax or pleural effusion (Fig. 4), sampling of

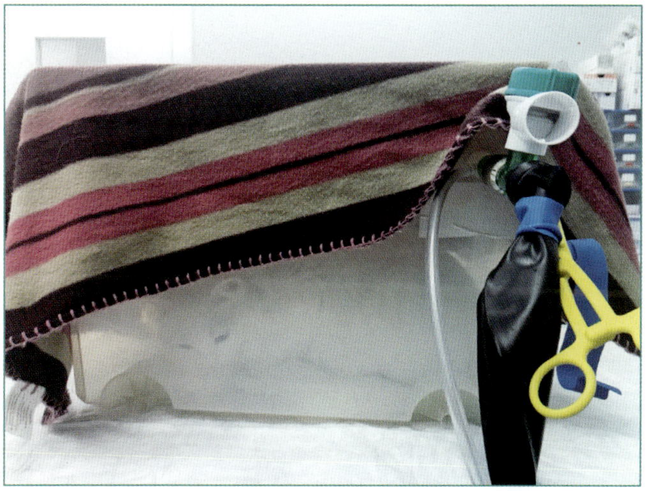

FIGURE 2. Oxygen chamber with a patient inside.

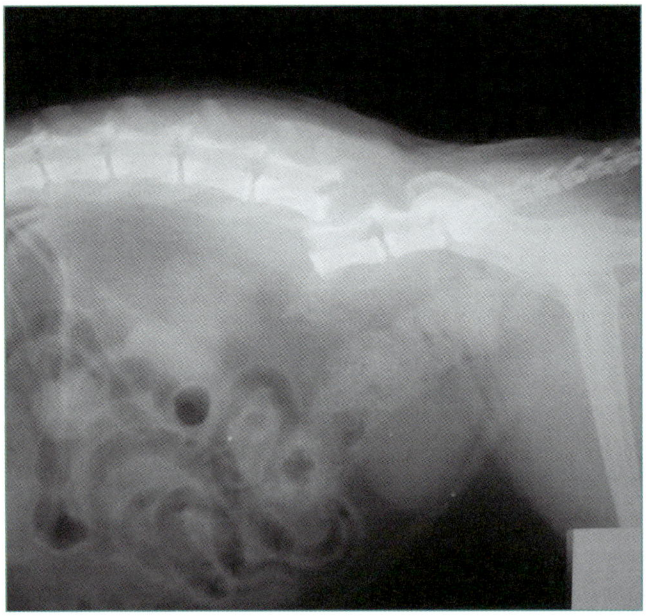

FIGURE 3. Lateral X-ray of a spinal luxation with transection of the spinal cord.

pleural effusion, confirmation of good pulmonary aeration or the presence of liquid in the alveoli. With AFAST, the presence of free abdominal fluid can be confirmed (Fig. 5)—a series of ultrasounds can help evaluate any changes over time—along with the assessment of the integrity of most of the abdominal organs. It also enables basic echocardiography assessment to rule out pericardial effusion, measurement of the cardiac chambers, and evaluation of the myocardium.

Cats that fall from heights may suffer various types of head trauma. Even if they stopped the fall with their limbs, momentum may cause them to hit their head against the ground, producing various bone or soft tissue injuries. In these patients, it is important to consider the following:

- State of consciousness
- Examination of the cranial nerves
- Facial deformities, observation of facial and cranial symmetry
- Nasal or otic discharge
- Integrity of the hard palate
- Improper dental occlusion leading to a suspicion of fractures of the mandible or mandibular symphysis
- Dental fractures
- Traumatic eye injuries

If cranial trauma with increased intracranial pressure is suspected, taking blood samples from the jugular vein should be avoided, since compression of this vein for the blood draw can increase intracranial pressure even more.

In the case of cats with mandibular or maxillary injury that require immediate oxygen therapy, the patient may need emergency procedures such as intubation (sometimes with the help of a guide), tracheotomy, or oxygen administration via a hypodermic needle placed between the tracheal rings (Fig. 6).

In the case of head trauma, especially if mandibular or maxillary fracture is involved, it may be necessary, after the patient has been fully examined, to subsequently place a feeding tube

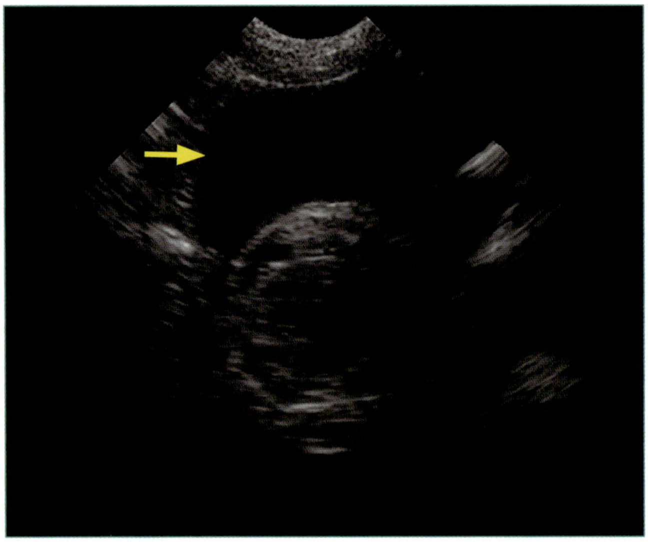

FIGURE 4. Thoracic focused assessment with sonography for trauma (TFAST) showing the presence of pleural effusion.

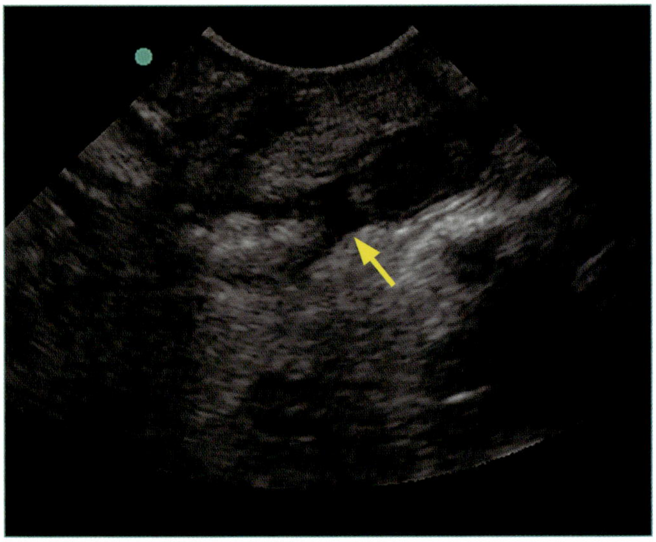

FIGURE 5. Abdominal focused assessment with sonography for trauma (AFAST) showing the presence of free abdominal fluid.

until these fractures have been treated, thus ensuring that the patient receives proper nutrition.

The following step is to palpate the pelvis for asymmetries or possible fractures. Rectal palpation should also be done to examine the final portion of the intestine.

Next, the limbs are examined for any bone abnormalities or pain on palpation of the various bones and joints, as well as any exposure of long bones in the case of open fractures. At the same time, distal pulses are palpated, and a neurological examination of the four limbs is done.

If there are any articular fractures or injuries, the cat's movement should be restricted, and to the extent possible, padded dressings should be applied to reduce pain and minimize fracture fragment mobility.

Complementary tests

After the initial assessment and stabilization of the trauma patient, the following stage involves taking samples and additional testing, as long as the patient's condition allows for it. Some of the samples may have been taken during the initial assessment and stabilization of the cat (abdominal or pleural fluid during ultrasound, urine during spontaneous micturition).

At a minimum, the **laboratory analyses** that should be done are hematocrit, plasma proteins, blood glucose and blood urea. If possible, more extensive tests are done, including complete blood count and serum biochemistry profile, electrolytes, blood gas analysis and coagulation tests. Serum lactate concentration is also useful, as it is indicative of organ perfusion. However, the necessary equipment is not always available for all these tests.

X-rays can involve some risk in the case of cats with dyspnea, since this can be aggravated by placing the patient in lateral or dorsal recumbency. If the cat can be placed in lateral recumbency, a good option is to obtain a radiographic image of the entire body in the same cassette (Fig. 7). Because the width of the thorax is usually very similar to the width of the abdomen in cats, the same radiological technique can be used to obtain a good image of both areas. At a minimum, this radiographic image should encompass from the thoracic inlet to the pelvic outlet. An attempt should also be made to include the forelimbs and hind limbs almost completely. A radiographic image of nearly the entire body can be taken if the animal is small. This X-ray enables general visualization of the thorax and abdomen, identification of any pleural effusion, pneumothorax, the integrity of the urinary bladder, and bone injuries of the spinal column, ribs, sternebrae, pelvis and any limbs that could be included in the radiography.

Once the patient has been fully stabilized, a radiographic examination can be done of specific areas where injuries were seen on the full-body X-ray or where there is a suspected injury.

Pain management for polytraumatized patients

Various analgesics were described in Chapter 2, along with their doses and methods of administration in feline patients. Cats that have suffered trauma should be assumed to have pain from the moment they arrive at the clinic. While the pain may vary depending the nature of the trauma, there is always pain of

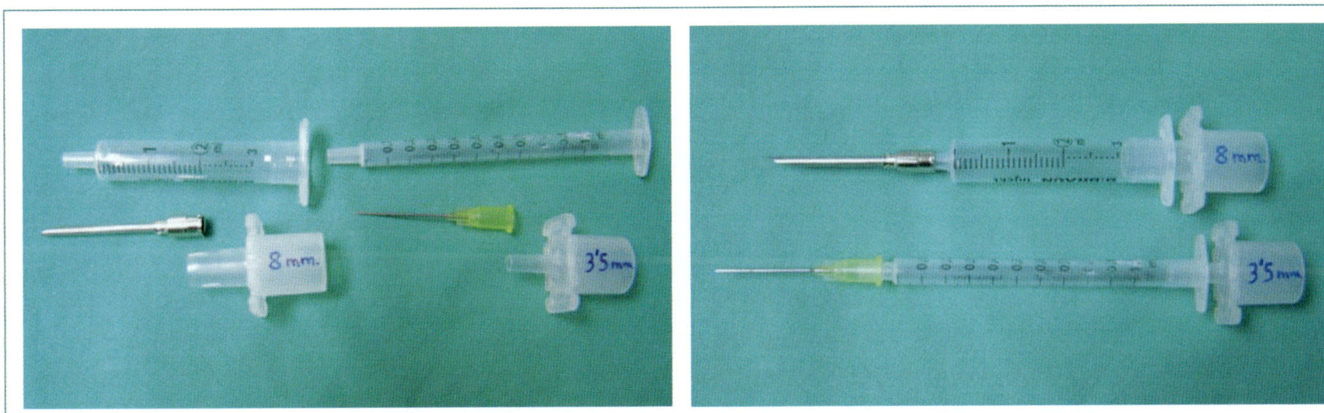

FIGURE 6. Systems for emergency oxygen administration between the tracheal rings, which are connected to a source of oxygen.

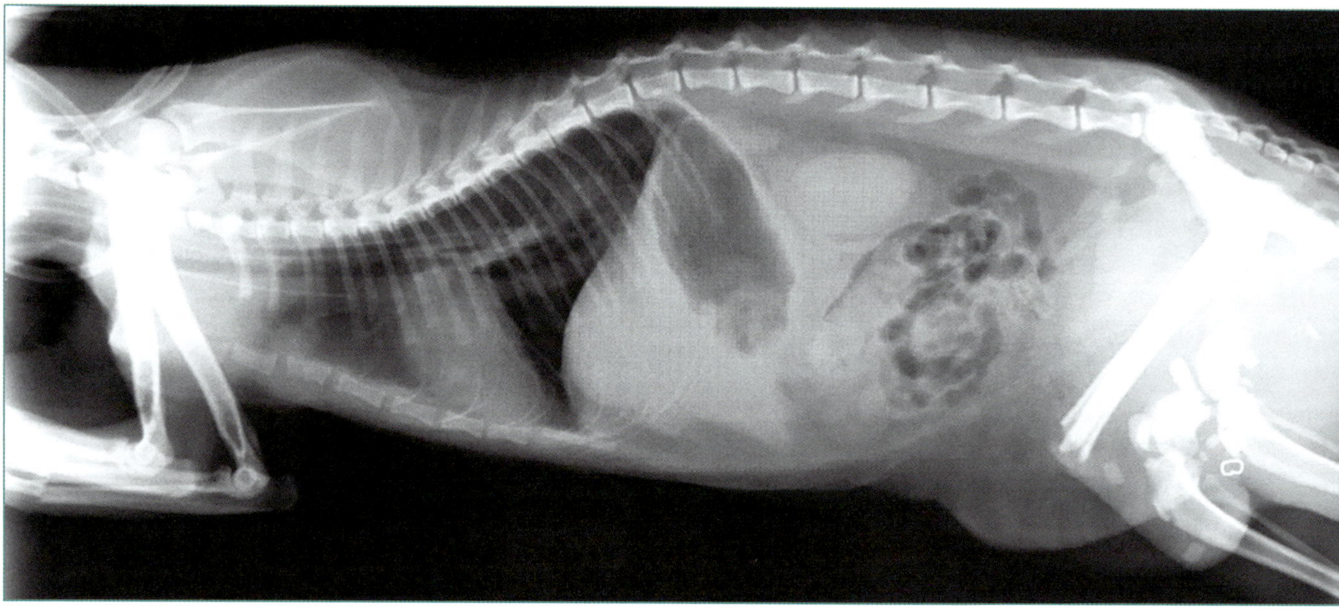

FIGURE 7. Full-body X-ray of a polytraumatized cat. Fracture of the radius, ulna and both femurs are seen.

When is emergency treatment necessary?

- Hemoabdomen with shock
- Evisceration
- Respiration or blood flow compromised by hernia
- Penetrating wounds in the thorax or abdomen

some sort. Therefore, a sufficient amount of analgesia should be applied early on for these patients.

Before administering analgesic drugs, especially opioids, a neurological examination should be done so that the cat's response is not conditioned or diminished by these drugs. But once this examination is finished, and if there are no contraindications, adequate analgesia should be provided so that the patient is as comfortable as possible. This also helps during subsequent examination and assessment procedures, since decreasing the patient's pain makes them more cooperative and willing to be handled.

In addition to analgesic drugs administered parenterally, local anesthetics such as lidocaine, bupivacaine or mepivacaine can be administered in various ways. If there is an open wound, an instillation can be done in the area. These local anesthetic drugs can also be administered via subcutaneous catheters or by epidural anesthesia. Regional anesthetic blocks can also be effectuated.

Initial treatment of fractures

Polytraumatized cats often present fractures in different areas: head, axial skeleton and appendicular skeleton.

In the case of **skull fractures**, the integrity of the hard palate should always be evaluated (see Ch. 13) as well as any fractures of the mandible or separation of the mandibular symphysis. Often in these cases, placement of a feeding tube is indicated until the cat can feed on its own.

Mandibular symphyseal separation is common in cats that fall from heights, as they usually hit their head against the ground as a result of momentum from the fall. In most cases, this injury is easily repaired, if it is not accompanied by any fractures in another part of the mandible.

For patients that only present mandibular symphyseal separation, the technique used to align and fix this separation is cerclage wire behind the canine teeth, circling both hemimandibles (Fig. 8). 0.6–0.8 mm cerclage wire is passed through two 18-gauge hypodermic needles, which serve as guides. These needles are placed at an incision made in the skin of the chin just behind the line of the mandibular incisors. From this area, they go through the tissue until their tips protrude from the oral mucosa, caudal to the two mandibular canines. The cerclage wire enters through the cone of one of the needles, goes past its tip, circles the mandibular rami behind the canines, is inserted into the tip of the other needle, and comes out of the cone. Both ends of the cerclage wire are knotted in a routine fashion, this

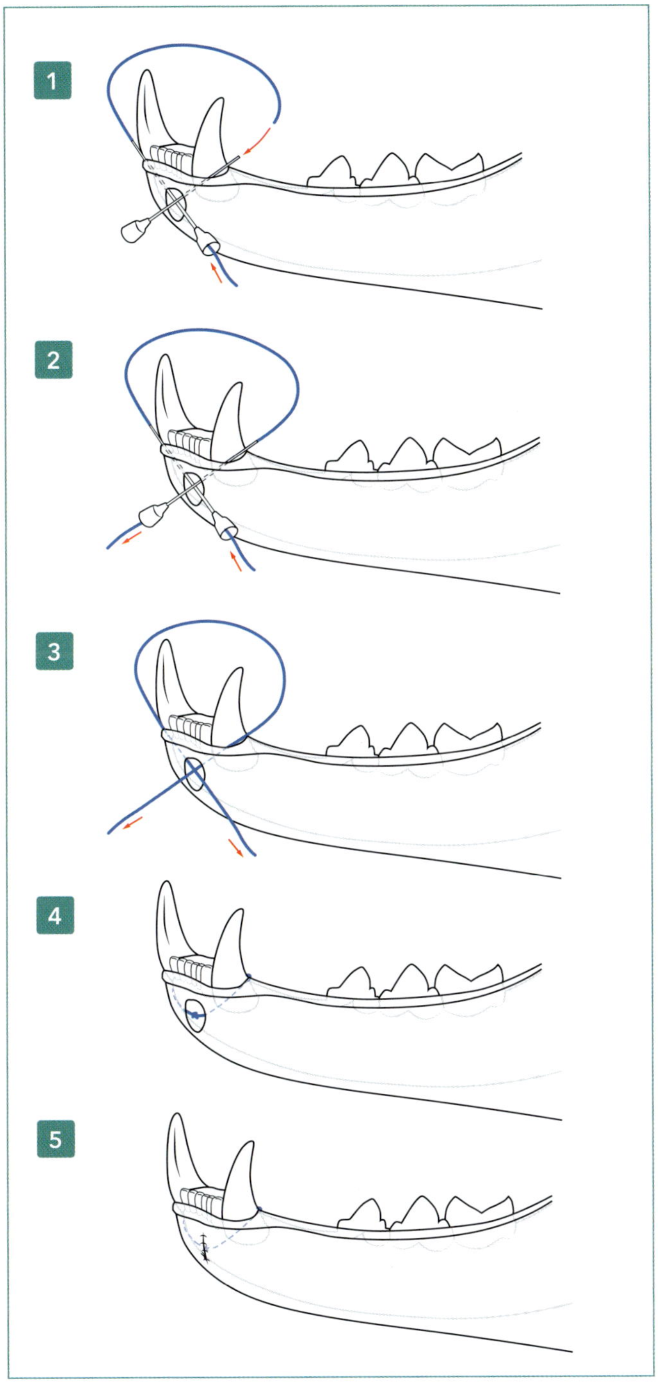

FIGURE 8. Steps for repair of mandibular symphyseal separation via cerclage wire behind the canine teeth.
1. An incision is made in the skin of the chin, into which two 18-gauge hypodermic needles are inserted (they will act as guides). 0.6–0.8 mm cerclage wire is passed through the cone of one of the needles until it protrudes from the tip.
2. After circling the mandibular rami behind the canines, cerclage wire is inserted into the tip of the other needle and extracted through its cone.
3. The hypodermic needles are removed and the ends of the cerclage wire are knotted.
4 & 5. Final result with the cerclage wire knot under the skin incision in the chin, which is sutured in a routine fashion.

knot being underneath the incision of the skin of the chin, which is sutured. This technique produces sufficient stability.

When it is time to tighten the cerclage wire, the incisors must be properly aligned to ensure that the reduction is done properly, they do not overlap, and the dental occlusion is not altered. One possible complication of this cerclage wire is excessive pressure on the canines. This can cause damage to the surrounding mandible and create a bone resorption lesion.

In **fractures or luxation of the spinal column**, it is important to try not to manipulate these areas and to prevent the cat from making movements that could aggravate the injury and the involvement of the spinal cord. If the cat is anxious and is moving excessively, sedation may be needed to prevent further injury. A neurological examination should be done first so that the sedatives do not interfere with the results. The body of these sedated patients should be immobilized on a rigid surface (table, board) (Fig. 9). Care should be taken when shifting their position or carrying out other examinations. The next step is diagnostic imaging via CT scan or X-rays. Emergency surgery is required in some cases to stabilize vertebral luxations or fractures that compromise the integrity of the spinal cord.

In the case of **bone fractures of the limbs**, emergency surgery is seldom required, and it is not a priority when treating the patient. However, these fractures should be initially managed so that subsequent treatment offers the best results possible.

It is important to determine whether there are skin lesions that entail an open fracture, regardless of whether any bone fragments are exposed. Irrigation with isotonic saline solution should be done to clean the wound and the bone fragments. It should then be covered to decrease contamination of the fracture site. In addition to analgesia, if the fracture is deemed contaminated, parenteral antibiotic therapy is administered.

Initial immobilization of limb fractures is aimed at reducing pain and minimizing bone fragment displacement and soft tissue damage near the fracture. Padded dressings are applied to immobilize the fracture area, including the joint proximal and distal to the fracture. Cats usually do not tolerate dressings on their limbs; they try to take them off, and often succeed at doing so. In this case, the patient's movement should be restricted and any handling of the affected area avoided. Sometimes it is necessary to sedate the patient to prevent it from moving too much, especially in the case of uncooperative or aggressive cats.

If cats with limb fractures are aggressive or have had to be sedated or anesthetized, the initial fixation of the fracture can be done with osteosynthesis material, as long as their health status permits this. In this case, an external fixator can be applied to

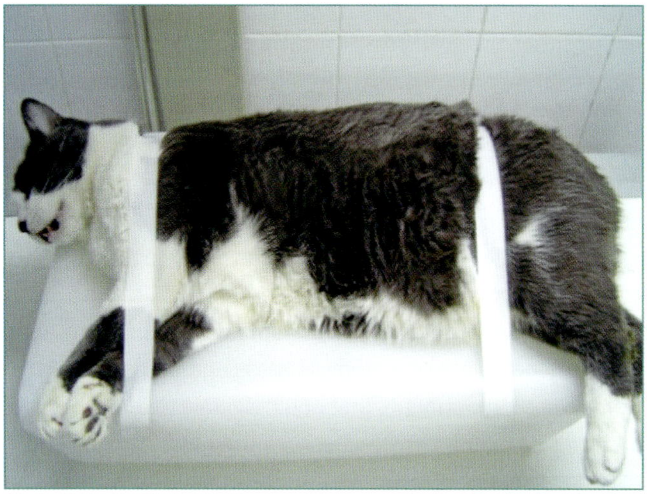

FIGURE 9. Immobilization of a cat with possible spinal trauma. The base of an X-ray positioning wedge is used as a rigid surface. Because the wedge is radiotransparent, it will not interfere with the radiographic images.

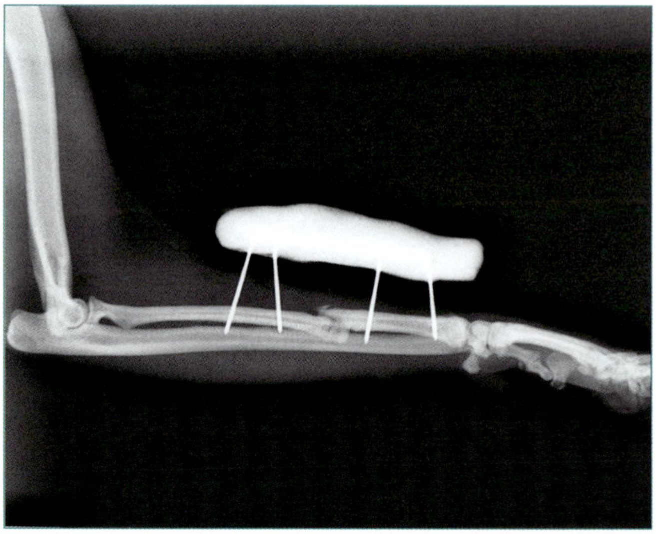

FIGURE 10. Type I external fixators for the temporary stabilization of a fracture of the radius and ulna.

immobilize the fracture (Fig. 10). With some practice, placing a type I external fixator is a fast and easy process.

> Always having sterilized standard material, as well as different gauge Kirschner wires and an epoxy resin to connect these wires in the form of a connecting bar, is advised.

This procedure results in stable fixation, which lowers the patient's pain, prevents displacement of bone fragments, and decreases damage to the surrounding tissue. This fixator can be used as the final treatment if good fracture reduction is achieved, along with enough stability to achieve ossification. If not, it can be used for temporary fixation until the patient's health status enables it to be replaced with more appropriate osteosynthesis materials in a scheduled surgery (Fig. 11). It can also complement another fracture fixation method.

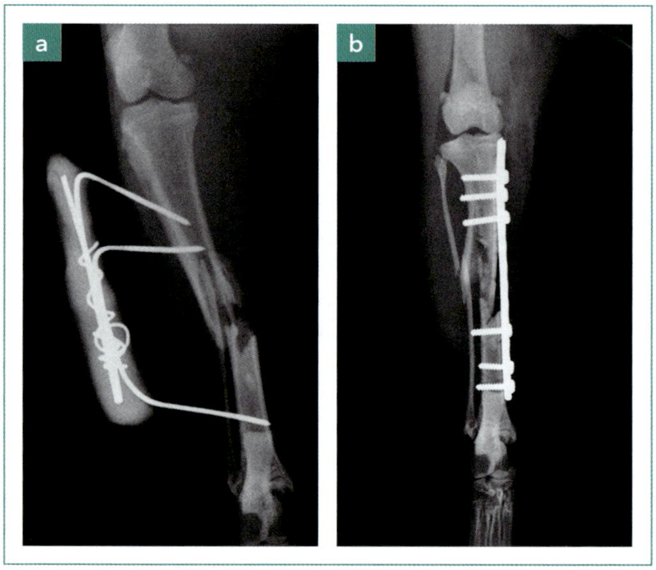

FIGURE 11. Open tibia fracture after fall from a height. (a) Temporary external fixator for use until the patient is completely stabilized. (b) Replacement of the external fixator by an osteosynthesis plate during a surgery scheduled several days after the trauma.

Bibliography

Adamantos S, Garosi L. Head trauma in the cat: 1. assessment and management of craniofacial injury. *J Feline Med Surg*, 2011; 13(11):806–814.

Bonner SE, Reiter AM, Lewis JR. Orofacial manifestations of high-rise syndrome in cats: a retrospective study of 84 cases. *J Vet Dent*, 2012; 29(1):10–18.

Corr S. Complex and open fractures: a straightforward approach to management in the cat. *J Feline Med Surg*, 2012; 14(1):55–64.

Crowe DT. Assessment and management of the severely polytraumatized small animal patient. *J Vet Emerg Crit Care*, 2006; 16(4):264–275.

Cruz-Arámulo R, Nykamp S. Acute intraparenchymal spinal cord injury in a cat due to high-rise syndrome. *Can Vet J*, 2012; 53(3):274–278.

Driessen B, Brainard B. Fluid therapy for the traumatized patient. *J Vet Emerg Crit Care*, 2006; 16(4):276–299.

Drobatz KJ, Costello MF. *Feline Emergency and Critical Care Medicine*. Iowa, USA: Wiley Blackwell, 2010.

Garosi L, Adamantos S. Head trauma in the cat: 2. assessment and management of traumatic brain injury. *J Feline Med Surg*, 2011; 13(11):815–823.

Goich M, Bascuñán A, Faúndez P, Valdés A. Multimodal analgesia for treatment of allodynia and hyperalgesia after major trauma in a cat. *JFMS Open Rep*, 2019; 5(1):2055116919855809.

Kerwin S. Orthopedic examination in the cat: clinical tips for ruling in/out common musculoskeletal disease. *J Fel Med Surg*, 2012; 14(1):6–12.

Knight R, Meeson RL. Feline head trauma: a CT analysis of skull fractures and their management in 75 cats. *J Feline Med Surg*, 2019; 21(12):1120–1126.

Liehmann LM, Dörner J, Hittmair KM et al. Pancreatic rupture in four cats with high-rise syndrome. *J Feline Med Surg*, 2012; 14(2):131–137.

Lisciandro G. The abdominal FAST (AFAST) exam. In: Lisciandro G (ed.). *Focused Ultrasound Techniques for the Small Animal Practitioner*. Iowa, USA: Wiley Blackwell, 2014; pp. 17–43.

Lisciandro G. The thoracic FAST (TFAST) exam. In: Lisciandro G (ed.). *Focused Ultrasound Techniques for the Small Animal Practitioner*. Iowa, USA: Wiley Blackwell, 2014; pp. 140–165.

Mahoney P. Musculoskeletal imaging in the cat. What's normal? What's abnormal? *J Feline Med Surg*, 2012; 14(1):13–22.

Mathews K, Kronen PW, Lascelles D et al. Guidlines for recognition, assessment and treatment of pain. WSAVA Global Pain Council members and co-authors of this document. *J Small Anim Pract*, 2014; 55(6):E10–E68.

Muir W. Trauma: physiology, pathophysiology and clinical implications. *J Vet Emerg Crit Care*, 2006; 16(4):253–263.

Nakladal B, vom Hagen F, Brunnberg M et al. Carpal joint injuries in cats—an epidemiological study. *Vet Comp Orthop Traumatol*, 2013; 26(5):333–339.

Popovitch CA, Nannos AJ. Emergency management of open fractures and luxations. *Vet Clin North Am Small Anim Pract*, 2000; 30(3):645–655.

Pratschke KM, Kirby BM. High rise syndrome with impalement in three cats. *J Small Anim Pract*, 2002; 43(6):261–264.

Robertson SA, Lascelles BD. Long-term pain in cats: how much do we know about this important welfare issue? *J Feline Med Surg*, 2010; 12(3):188–199.

Scott HW, McLaughlin R. Fractures and disorders of the skull and mandible. In: Scott HW, McLaughlin R (eds.). *Feline Orthopedics*. Boca Raton, FL: Taylor and Francis Group, 2006; pp. 261–278.

Taylor A, Cooper E, Ham K. Delayed intestinal perforation secondary to blunt force abdominal trauma in a cat. *JFMS Open Rep*, 2018; 4(1):2055116918763410.

Tundo I, Southerden P, Perry A, Haydock RM. Location and distribution of craniomaxillofacial fractures in 45 cats presented for the treatment of head trauma. *J Feline Med Surg*, 2019; 21(4):322–328.

Vnuk D, Pirkic B, Maticic D et al. Feline high-rise syndrome: 119 cases (1998–2001). *J Feline Med Surg*, 2004; 6(5):305–312.

Voss K, Langley-Hobbs SJ, Grundmann S, Montavon PM. Mandible and maxila. In: Montavon PM, Voss K, Langley-Hobbs SJ (eds.). *Feline Orthopedic Surgery and Musculoskeletal Disease*. St. Louis, MO: Elsevier Saunders, 2009; pp. 311–328.

Zacher AM, Marretta SM. Oral and maxillofacial surgery in dogs and cats. *Vet Clin North Am Small Anim Pract*, 2013; 43(3):609–649.

Zimmermann E, Hittmair KM, Suchodolski JS et al. Serum feline-specific pancreatic lipase immunoreactivity concentrations and abdominal ultrasonographic findings in cats with trauma resulting from high-rise syndrome. *J Am Vet Med Assoc*, 2013; 242(9):1238–1243.

COMMON FRACTURES OF THE FORELIMB IN POLYTRAUMATIZED CATS

31

Antonio Peña

Fractures of the humeral diaphysis

Fractures of the humeral diaphysis tend to be caused by a direct impact on the surface of the humerus rather than as a consequence of breaking a fall. They can also result from the limb twisting when caught in something, causing spiral fractures. These fractures are usually transverse or oblique, although there may be multiple fragments.

Surgical anatomy and approach

The approach can be craniolateral or medial. In the case of lateral approach (Fig. 1), damage to the radial nerve should be avoided in metaphyseal or distal diaphyseal fractures (Fig. 2). In the case of medial approach, the supracondylar foramen should be located, and the integrity of the median nerve and the brachial artery, which pass through it, should be verified. This nerve may exhibit damage caused by bone fragments. Likewise, it is important to locate these structures during the approach to avoid damaging them during dissection and when handling the bone fragments or implants to be placed.

The **craniolateral approach** is the most common:

- An incision is made in the skin over the craniolateral edge of the humerus, from the greater tubercle of the humerus to the lateral epicondyle.
- The fat and brachial fascia is incised and retracted. The cephalic vein is located. It may be necessary to ligate this vein to access the fracture site.
- Next, in order to visualize the laterocaudal surface of the bone, an incision is made in the fascia of the brachial muscle and in the insertion of the lateral head of the triceps

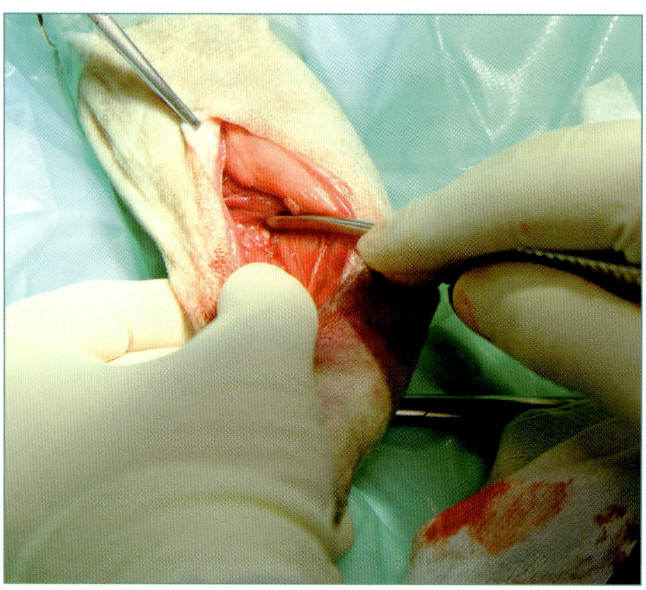

FIGURE 1. Lateral approach to the humerus. This is the most common approach for fractures of this anatomical region.

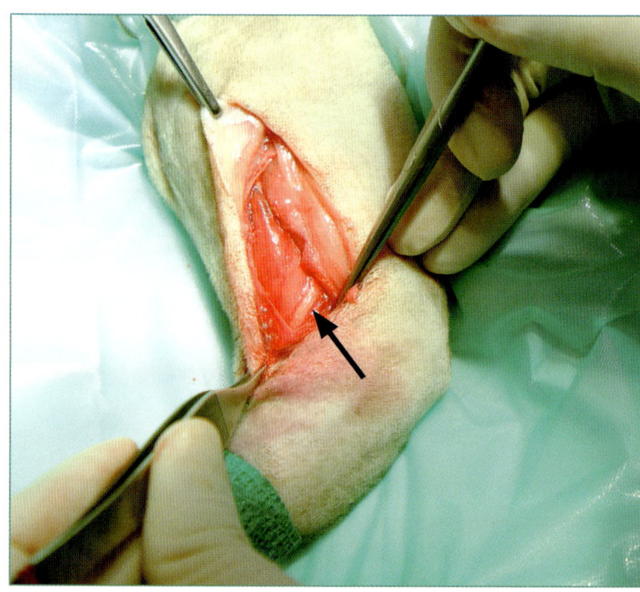

FIGURE 2. Lateral approach of the distal humeral diaphysis. Visualization of the radial nerve (arrow).

brachii muscle on the humerus. Damage to the radial nerve should be avoided during this incision. Another incision is made the same way in the insertions of the superficial pectoral muscle and the brachiocephalic muscle on the humerus.

- The muscle groups are elevated with a retractor, and the craniolateral surface of the humerus can be visualized.

To be able to properly access more proximal or more distal fractures, this approach can be extended proximally over the greater tubercle of the humerus or distally over the supracondylar surface, respectively.

For the **medial approach** to the humerus:

- The skin is incised medially from the greater tubercle of the humerus to the medial epicondyle, followed by the deep brachial fascia along the length of the brachiocephalic and superficial pectoral muscles.
- Care must be taken in the distal area to preserve the vascular and nervous structures (Fig. 3).
- The brachiocephalic muscle is retracted cranially to expose the insertion of the superficial pectoral muscle. This insertion is then incised, allowing this muscle to be retracted and the biceps brachii to be exposed.
- Next, the biceps brachii is retracted caudally to expose the medial surface of the humerus.

Stabilization of fractures

There are several ways to resolve this type of fracture. The use of bandages or external coaptation is not advised, since it does not enable proper immobilization of the humerus. The use of different types of implants is preferred, including intramedullary pins/nails, osteosynthesis plates, external fixators, interlocking nails, or combinations of these systems (Fig. 4).

Intramedullary pins or nails are useful and easy to place along the straight-edged humerus in cats (Fig. 5).

> When placing intramedullary pins or nails, keep in mind that the distal portion of the medullary cavity is narrow, and a single pin or nail may fill the whole space.

They can be placed in a normograde or retrograde fashion. In normograde placement, the fracture is reduced with the help of bone-holding forceps or cerclage wire. The first pin or nail is inserted at the greater trochanter, moving in the direction of the fracture site and ending up at the distal humerus, close to but not past the supracondylar foramen. This is to avoid damaging the median nerve or brachial artery, or penetrating the elbow joint. Next a second pin of equal length is placed. If smaller gauge pins are used, more than two pins may be needed to properly stabilize the fracture. After placing the pins, the elbow

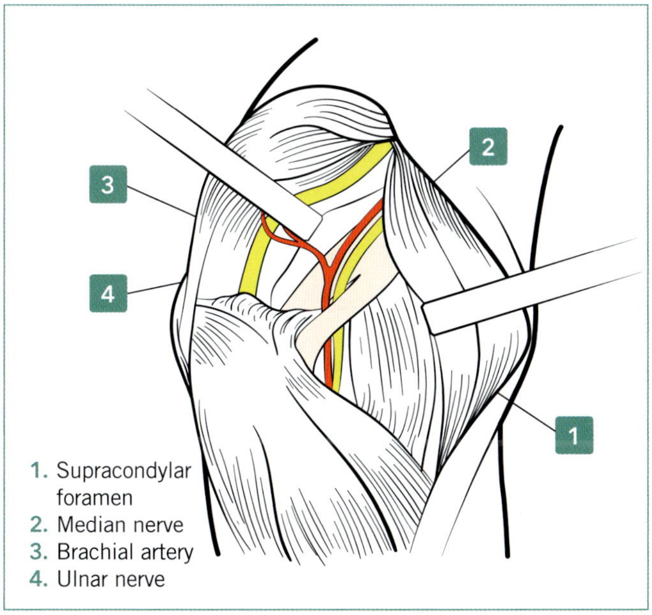

FIGURE 3. Anatomy of the distal medial region of the humerus in cats.

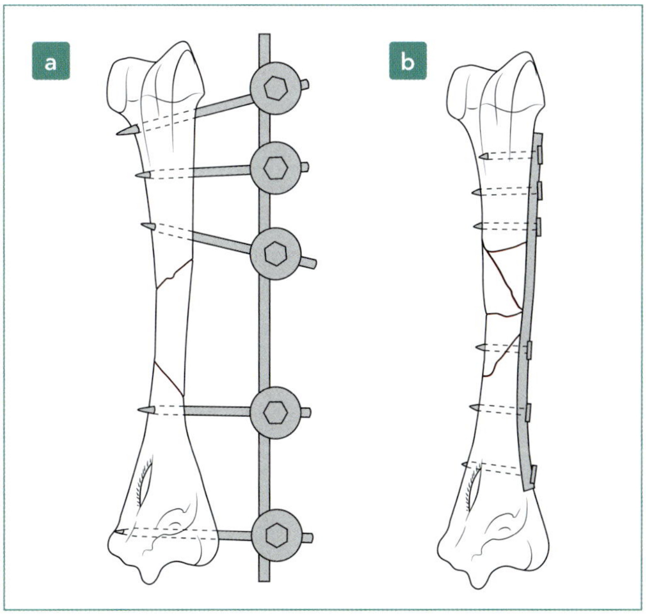

FIGURE 4. Resolution of humeral fractures in cats: (a) type I fixator and (b) osteosynthesis plate in a fracture of the diaphysis.

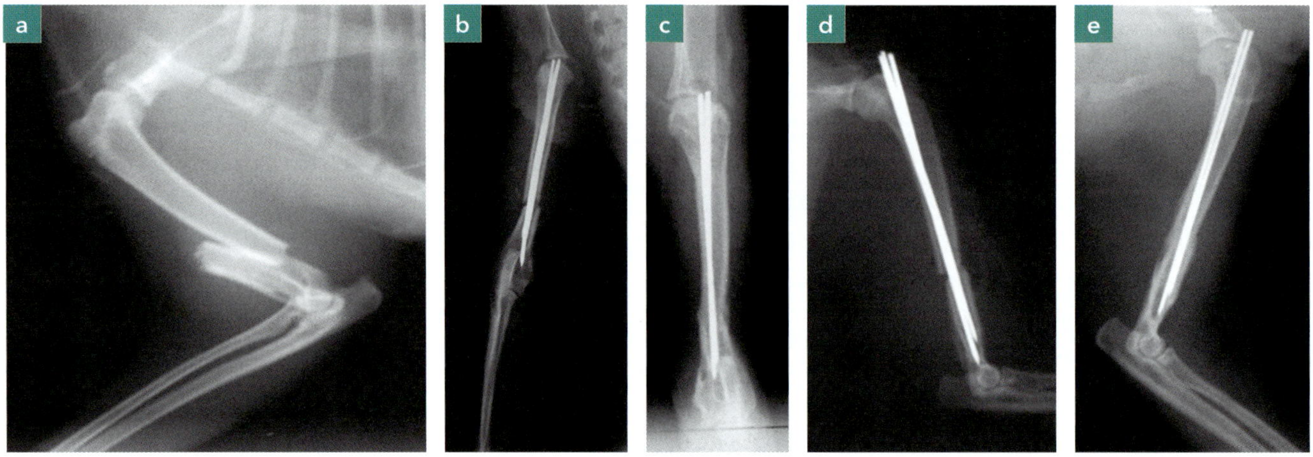

FIGURE 5. (a) Transverse fracture of the humerus in a cat. Fixation of the fracture by means of placement of intramedullary pins: (b,d) postoperative X-rays; (c,e) X-rays 2 months after surgery showing complete ossification.

is flexed and extended to ensure full range of motion (from maximum flexion to maximum extension) and to ensure that none of the pins or nails have penetrated inside the elbow joint. Proper reduction and placement of the material is confirmed with postoperative radiographic monitoring.

In retrograde placement, the pin is inserted at the fracture site, through the medullary canal, in a proximal direction and exiting at the greater tubercle. The pin is inserted until its distal part is close to the proximal line of the fracture. The fracture is subsequently reduced, and the pin is inserted in the distal fragment, leaving it near the supracondylar foramen (Fig. 6).

If these intramedullary pins or nails provide enough stability to the fracture, they suffice as the sole fixation method. However, this cannot always be achieved, and the additional use of cerclage wire, screws or half-pin external fixators (type I fixators) is needed to prevent rotational movement. This rotation can also be prevented by using several intramedullary pins.

If using a type I external fixator, it is placed in the craniolateral aspect of the humerus, whether as the sole fixation method or in combination with intramedullary pins or nails, as mentioned above.

Kirschner wires can be used alone, but better fixation is achieved if some of them have a positive-profile thread. Bars and clamps that connect the pins to the bars can be used as connectors. To give the structure more stability, different configurations of the fixator can be used, such as two connecting bars or a hybrid type I–II structure with a curved connecting bar or with a tie-in configuration.

For cats, and especially for small cats, this arrangement of pins, clamps, and connecting bars can be heavy. As such, an epoxy substance can be used to link the pins of the fixator.

Longer pins are used in this arrangement, and they are bent in such a way that they are proximal and parallel to the surface of the humerus. These pins are then fixed to each other with epoxy, making the structure rigid and much lighter. Before applying the epoxy, the pins are circled together with cerclage wire to give the epoxy more of a base for fixation. An advantage of this type of configuration is that it enables the use of different gauge pins that can be oriented in different directions. This is unlike straight connecting bars, for which the pins must lie on a single plane.

Closed fixation can be used if the fracture can be reduced manually or if intraoperative radiographic imaging is available to help with the reduction. However, open reduction of the fracture may often be required before placing the fixator.

The most distal pin can be placed through the humeral condyles from the lateral epicondyle, and it may exit through the medial epicondyle and the skin. This pin is used as the site of fixation for the bar in the hybrid type I–II structure. The other pin is placed in the proximal humerus. If opting for an intramedullary pin, this type of fixator, with two pins and a connecting bar, is the model used if wishing to avoid rotational forces. For sufficient stability in noncomplicated fractures, additional pins are placed on either side of the fracture line (at least two on each side of the fracture) and fixed to the connecting bar, or the

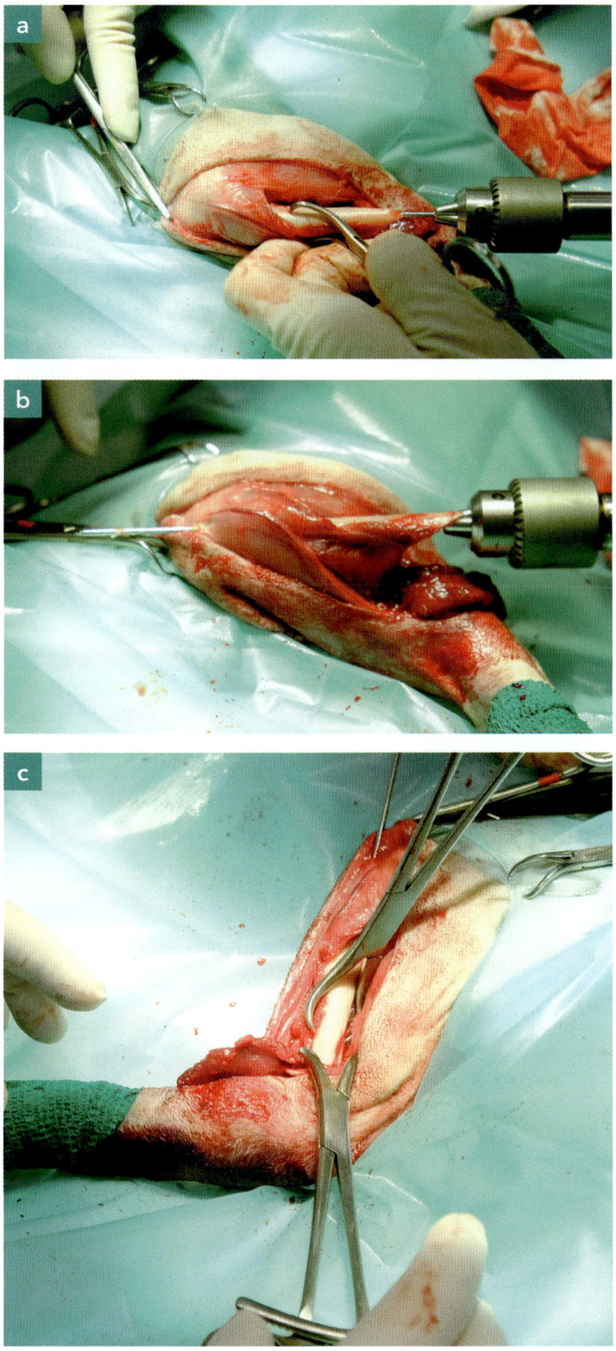

FIGURE 6. Retrograde placement of an intramedullary pin in a fracture of the humerus. (a) Insertion of the pin from the fracture site in a retrograde fashion. (b) Exit of the pin from the greater tubercle of the humerus. (c) Normograde insertion of the pin in the distal fragment of the fracture.

pins are fixed to each other with epoxy putty, for assembly of a type I fixator.

> The connecting bar can be given more stability if it is fixed to the proximal part of the intramedullary pin. This is called a tie-in configuration (Figs. 7 and 8).

In this case, the intramedullary pin may be left protruding and be connected to the bar with a clamp. Another option is to use a long intramedullary pin and bend it so it can act as a connecting bar.

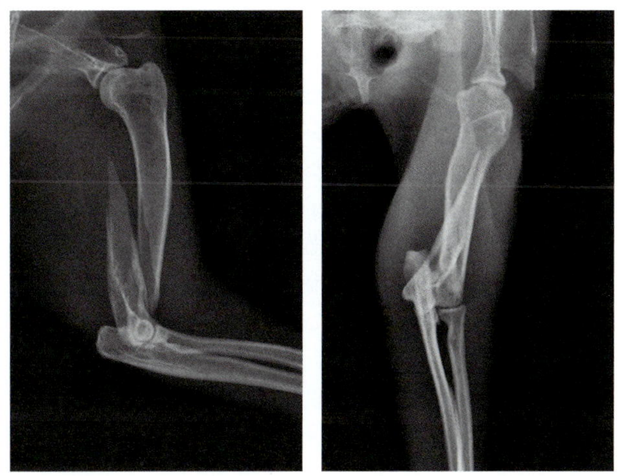

FIGURE 7. Spiral fracture of the humeral diaphysis.

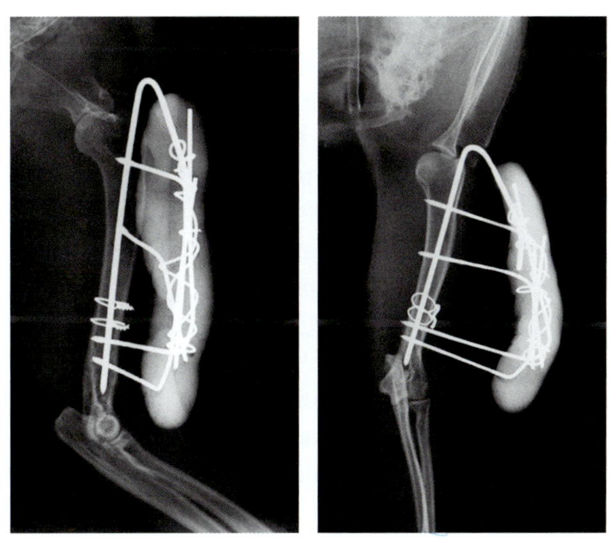

FIGURE 8. Resolution of the spiral fracture of the humeral diaphysis from the previous figure by using a hybrid tie-in fixator and cerclage wire. In lieu of a connecting bar, epoxy putty was used to attach the pins to each other.

Dynamic compression plates, cuttable plates, or locking plates can be used if choosing an osteosynthesis plate to resolve the fracture. In some cases an osteosynthesis plate can be combined with another fixation system, such as an intramedullary pin.

The plate can be placed on the cranial, lateral or medial surface of the humerus. If using lateral placement, the approach is craniolateral. Plate contouring is easier if placed on the medial surface of the humerus, since it is flatter. However, the approach is more complicated, and care must be taken to preserve the neurovascular structures that pass through the supracondylar foramen, as mentioned above.

Dynamic compression plates and at least three bicortical screws on each side of the fracture tend to be used for transverse diaphyseal fractures. If the fracture is oblique, a neutral plate is used, and this can be combined with a separate compression screw through the fracture line.

For comminuted fractures, a plate is placed which leaves the fragment area free of screws. Fixation is effectuated in the proximal and distal sections of the humerus. Plates can be used in which screws are not placed in the holes near the fragment area. Bridging plates can also be used to provide more rigidity and reduce stress on the material in this area of the plate. Plates can also be combined in such cases with an intramedullary pin to align the proximal and distal portions of the humerus. As an additional treatment, a cancellous bone graft is performed to activate ossification of the area and to shorten the healing time.

The relatively straight shape of the humerus means that interlocking nails are another good option for fixation of fractures. In the case of noncomplicated fractures, the approach is through the greater tubercle of the humerus, inserting an interlocking nail in the medullary cavity. In the case of comminuted fractures, this interlocking intramedullary nail allows for alignment of the proximal and distal fragments of the humerus; we may then opt not to reduce the fragments at the fracture site or to use cerclage wire for this purpose.

Locking plates are a suitable solution when the fracture is distal and not enough bicortical screws can be placed in that fragment, requiring the use of monocortical screws.

Complications

Careful dissection of the fracture site must be performed, by separating muscle groups or transecting muscles at their insertions, to avoid damaging soft tissue. The previously mentioned neurovascular structures should likewise be located and handled with care. These structures include the radial nerve in the lateral approach, and the ulnar nerve, the median nerve and the brachial artery in the medial approach.

If using intramedullary pins in a normograde fashion, make sure to reach an adequate distance in the distal fragment. If these pins do not reach far enough in the distal fragment, it may cause instability in the fracture and poor alignment of the fragments, resulting in abnormal angulation between them. The pin should not be inserted too deep into the distal fragment either, to avoid exiting at the joint line of the humeral condyles. A decreased range of motion when flexing and extending the elbow during the intervention indicates that the implant is passing through the joint line. Proper alignment of the humerus is aided by using bone prominences such as the greater tubercle and the humeral epicondyles as landmarks, and correcting any rotations during fracture reduction.

If the intramedullary pin is placed in a retrograde fashion, it is important to make sure that it comes out through the greater tubercle and to avoid damaging the joint surface of the humeral head, although this is less likely in cats due to the shape of the humerus itself.

If using a half-pin external fixator, edema and inflammation may present after the surgery. It is important to avoid damaging muscle groups during closed reduction and pin placement. The length of the fixator pins should also be considered to ensure that they do not protrude too much, thus damaging nearby soft tissues and causing discomfort when putting weight on the limb. It is important to avoid damaging the growth plate when placing pins in distal areas of the humerus, and also to avoid injuring the radial nerve, the median nerve and the brachial artery, especially if using threaded pins. These complications can be prevented if the approach is open and these anatomical structures are visualized.

Another common complication that can occur when using a fixator is drainage of serous or mucous fluid along the tract of the pins, where they pass through the skin. This can predispose the patient to an infection as well as the risk of osteomyelitis, with the consequent failure in proper fixation of the bone with pins. This complication should be discussed with the owner before surgery, so that they carry out the proper postoperative care. The pin site should be kept covered, and the caretakers should communicate if they see fluid coming out from any openings in the skin. Likewise, if there is excessive inflammation or edema of the soft tissues, the skin can make contact with the clamps, connecting bars or with the acrylic material used in place of these bars, causing ulcerations of the skin and increasing the risk of infection, the severity of which may vary.

For this reason, when assembling these structures during surgery, they should be sufficiently separated from the skin to prevent contact. However, it is important to keep in mind the fact that the further the fixator is from the surface of the skin, the less stability it will have to fix the fracture. A distance of approximately 1.5 cm between the skin and the clamps or bars is usually sufficient.

If a hybrid type I–II external fixator is used, it is important to make sure that the pin that protrudes from the medial epicondyle of the humerus is not very long. This pin should be properly covered so that it does not interfere with or damage the contralateral limb. This type of hybrid structure, along with the tie-in structure, should be completely covered by a bandage to prevent the fixator elements from being caught on objects, with the consequent risk of the pins shifting out of place.

If using osteosynthesis plates, complications can occur if the plate is not well contoured, which carries the risk of poor alignment and possibly breakage of a screw caused by stress on the material. In addition, the plate should be long enough to enable the screws to be placed such that they pass through the bone cortex a minimum of 6 times on each side of the fracture (if using bicortical screws, 3 on each side is enough).

As in the case of pins in a half-pin external fixator, screws should not protrude too much to avoid damaging nearby soft tissues. It is also important to monitor the orientation of screws near growth plates or joint surfaces. If errors in screw placement are detected during postoperative radiographic monitoring, an immediate reintervention may be necessary to correct them. This may sometimes not be necessary, however, if these screws do not interfere with any joints or vital structures.

In the case of comminuted fractures, the selection of material should be properly planned to avoid the chance of using implants of insufficient length, and thus shortening the limb. X-rays of the contralateral limb should be done to have a reference point for the length of the implants that are needed and prevent this error.

There may be delays in ossification if there is poor stability at the fracture site. However, this can also occur with too much stability, as the formation of bone callus is not stimulated quickly enough, risking nonunion. If there is excessive rigidity when using an external half-pin fixator, part of the structure can be removed to give slight mobility to the fracture site and stimulate ossification without the need for surgical reintervention. However, if using other fixation methods, such as screws, cerclage wire or plates, it will be necessary to reintervene for this purpose.

Fractures of the distal humeral epiphysis

Fractures of the distal humeral epiphysis occur frequently in polytraumatized cats that fall from a height. This is due to the pressure exerted by the head of the radius on the humeral condyles when the limb absorbs the impact of the fall.

Surgical anatomy

The anatomy of this area in cats is unique to them. **On the medial aspect**, caudal to the biceps muscle there is a neurovascular bundle that includes the median, musculocutaneous and ulnar nerves, as well as the brachial artery and vein. There is no supratrochlear foramen. The **supracondylar foramen** is situated on the **medial aspect**, and the **median nerve** and the **brachial artery** run through it (see Fig. 3). These structures should be visualized during surgical approach to avoid iatrogenic injury when stabilizing fractures in this region.

The radial nerve runs laterally at the middle third of the humerus, in an oblique position and in a caudocranial direction. It then divides into the different sensory and motor branches, over the epiphysis of the radius, superficial to the brachial muscle.

Fractures and stabilization methods

Fractures of the distal epiphysis of the humerus include supracondylar, lateral condyle and Salter-Harris fractures. Within the latter group of fractures, the most frequent in cats that fall from heights are type I (supracondylar), type III and the type IV T-fracture or Y-fracture.

Adult cats often have combined intercondylar and supracondylar fractures, and comminuted fractures of the metaphysis of the humerus are common. Stabilization is always through surgical treatment with internal fixation techniques alone or in combination with external fixators. Treatment with bandages and splints is never advised because the stabilization failure rate is very high. In very young kittens, nonsurgical treatment has been described using restraint in a cage. This, however, is also not advised given the inability to prevent movement of the fracture site, the chance that the fragments will not unite, and joint degeneration in the case of intercondylar fractures.

> Supracondylar fractures can be stabilized by angling two pins across each other from each of the humeral epicondyles. Better stabilization is obtained if these pins are anchored in the opposite cortical surface of the distal humeral diaphysis.

Fractures of a humeral condyle are fixed with an intercondylar screw combined with one or more pins placed in an angled direction to prevent rotation. As in the previous case, these pins should be anchored in the opposite cortical surface of the humerus for better stability. Instead of these pins, a second screw can be used for this purpose.

When dealing with intercondylar fractures, perfect reduction of the joint surface of the humerus must be achieved, given that poor alignment in this area will cause rubbing of the joint surfaces of the ulna and radius and subsequently joint degeneration, signs of osteoarthritis and pain.

There may be some cases in which a comminuted fracture of the distal diaphysis of the humerus is produced in addition to an intercondylar fracture. In these cases, an intercondylar screw can be combined with placement of a plate on the lateral aspect of the humerus, or also an intercondylar screw combined with a half-pin external fixator (type I) or with a tie-in configuration connecting the intramedullary pin to the bar of the fixator.

The surgical approach to resolve these fractures can be lateral, medial, caudal, or a combination. A **caudal approach** combined with an osteotomy of the olecranon of the ulna provides for full visualization of the articular surface of the humerus, and thus enables the reduction of intercondylar fractures. This is the most advised approach in these cases.

A **medial approach** is advised for the resolution of supracondylar fractures, since dissection is simpler. The supracondylar foramen and the vascular and nervous structures must be identified to avoid damaging them during dissection and placement of implants. The neurovascular bundle can be retracted cranially to prevent injury by the implants. It may also be necessary to free the median nerve and the brachial artery at the level of the supracondylar foramen by means of an osteotomy with a bone gouge, to be able to displace these structures and therefore prevent injury to them.

Salter-Harris fractures of the growth plate

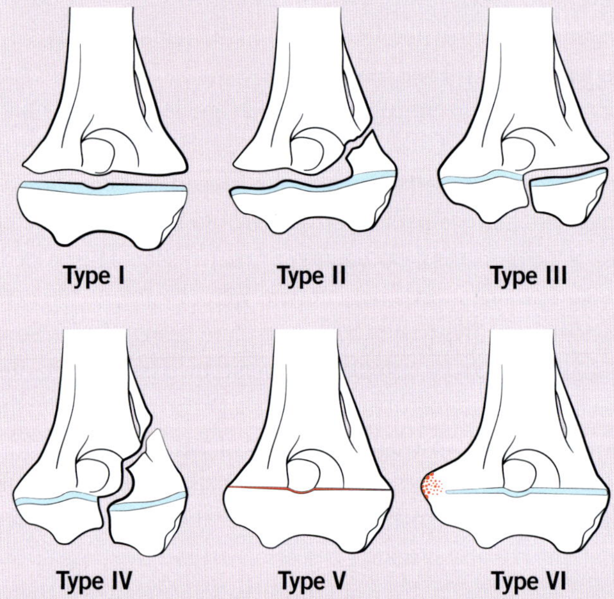

- **Type I:** physeal fracture with complete epiphyseal displacement.
- **Type II:** through the physis and metaphysis.
- **Type III:** through the physis with separation of a fragment from the epiphysis.
- **Type IV:** separation of a fragment from the physis and metaphysis.
- **Type V:** impaction or compression of the physis, with premature closure of the growth plate.
- **Type VI:** partial closure of the growth plate caused by trauma. Separation and subsequent repositioning can occur; therefore, although it appears that there is no displacement, blood vessels are damaged and there is premature closure.

Complications

The most important complication that should be avoided is an imperfect reduction of the joint surface. This is often achieved with proper planning of the surgery, correctly choosing the required fixation methods and, of utmost importance, using the most suitable approach, even if the procedure itself is more complex. In many cases, caudal access to the joint surface of the humerus is required, and this is achieved through ulnar osteotomy, which provides better visualization during fracture reduction and joint surface reconstruction.

Another complication that may arise is breakage of the implants. Often this is due to poor choice of material or improper fracture reduction, which stresses the material.

Movement of the intercondylar screw may also be observed. Therefore, care should be taken when placing it, using a suitable hole in the humeral condyles so that the threading of the screw is well anchored. Another complication can be that the screw penetrates too deeply, and the screw head sinks into the epicondyle. This can be prevented by using a washer, which serves as a stopper.

Fractures of the radius and ulna

These fractures often occur when cats fall from heights. Although both bones tend to fracture, stabilization of the radius is usually sufficient to enable the patient to recover functionality of the limb, since that is the bone that supports the most weight. Nevertheless, better results are obtained if the ulnar fracture is also fixed, especially if the fracture is proximal.

> Pronation and supination movements are important to cats, and therefore the fracture must be reduced properly. Reduction is more successful if both the radius and ulna are fixed, and if implants are well placed to prevent synostosis of the two bones, which would limit these movements.

Fractures of the distal half of the diaphysis and the distal metaphysis are most common, although fractures that are proximal to the head of the radius and of the olecranon may also occur. Distal ulnar fractures that include the styloid process are rare. Open fractures of this region are also rare.

Surgical anatomy and approach

Surgical approach to the diaphysis of the radius and ulna is relatively simple. In fractures of the radial head, it is important to take into account the radial nerve that runs laterally to cranially between the muscle groups.

The **lateral approach** is focused over the lateral edge of the radius:

- The incision is initiated near the radial head and extends to the distal end of the bone, incising the antebrachial fascia.
- The body of the radius is accessed by retracting the common digital extensor and lateral digital extensor muscles in a caudal direction, and the extensor carpi radialis muscle in a cranial direction.
- If a caudolateral approach is needed to resolve the ulnar fracture, the best access is obtained by making an incision through the long abductor muscle of the first digit.

Stabilization of fractures

In some cases, if the fractures of the diaphysis of the radius and/or ulna are not complex, the use of bandages or slings may have a good prognosis. Better results are obtained if the ulna is not fractured or if the animal is young, since less time is needed to achieve ossification. However, these patients should have their bandage changed weekly to avoid growth issues of the limb.

Intramedullary pins cannot be used in the radius, since they would have to be inserted from the radiocarpal joint surface. In contrast, the ulna does permit placement of such implants. For ulnar fractures, an intramedullary pin can be the sole stabilization method or it can be used in conjunction with an osteosynthesis plate or external fixators on the radius. This pin can be inserted in a normograde fashion from the olecranon, or in a retrograde manner from the fracture line. The gauge of the pin is selected based on the diameter of the intramedullary cavity of the distal ulna.

External fixators can be used in many cases, especially if the fracture is open or comminuted. A type I or a modified type I external fixator is usually sufficient to achieve good stability. If slower ossification is expected, type II or modified type II fixators will be required. Bars can be used to connect and stabilize the pins; alternately, epoxy putties can be used for this purpose to make the structure lighter.

These fixators can be placed using a closed approach in many cases. Other times, it will be necessary to effectuate an open approach to the fracture site to reduce it. An open approach is also required if an intramedullary pin will also be placed in the ulna in a retrograde fashion. Due to the flattened shape of the radius, it may be difficult to insert the fixator pins into the bone in a mediolateral manner. Often these pins can be inserted from a craniolateral to a caudomedial direction. This results in a larger surface of the radius on either side of the pins, giving them more stability. Threaded or unthreaded pins can be used to assemble the external fixator.

An osteosynthesis plate can be employed on the radius to fix the fragments of the fracture (Fig. 9). Usually it is placed in a dorsal position, although it can be placed in a medial position if the radial fracture is in the distal third of the bone. Cuttable plates of the appropriate length can be used on a case by case basis; however, these plates may provide poor stability if they are too thin. If more rigidity is needed for the implant, two plates can be placed one on top of the other ("sandwich plating"). Figure 10 shows different stabilization methods for radius and ulna fractures in cats.

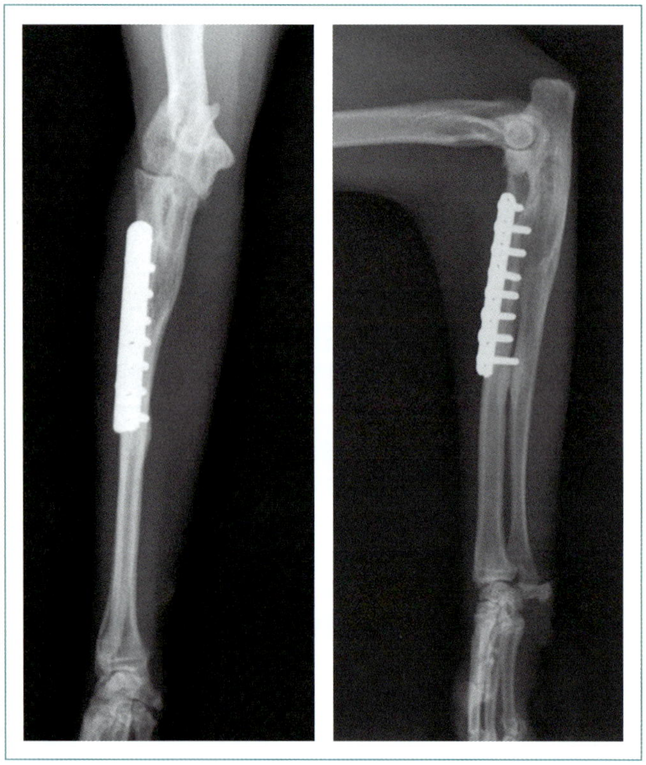

FIGURE 9. Osteosynthesis plate for fixation of a diaphyseal fracture of the radius.

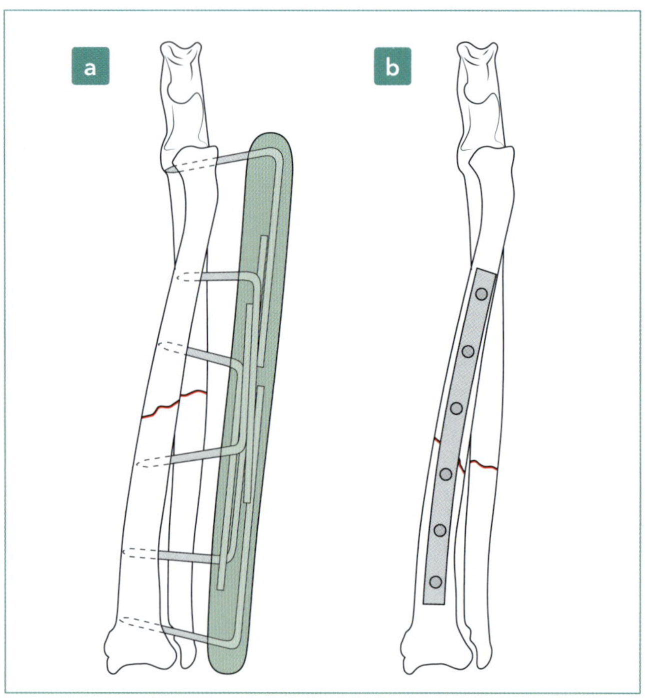

FIGURE 10. Stabilization of fractures of the radius and ulna in cats. (a) Modified type I external fixator, with a resin bar. (b) Osteosynthesis plate in the medial part of the radius.

Locking plates are especially useful for fractures near the elbow or carpal joints.

Fractures of the proximal radial diaphysis are usually accompanied by ulnar fractures, and there may also be luxation of the head of the radius. In such cases, osteosynthesis plates with 1.5–2.0 mm screws can be used, given the small diameter of this area of the radius. Placement of a transarticular fixator may be needed to ensure immobilization of the joint and to promote stability and ossification of the fracture. This fixator is removed after 3 weeks to prevent ankylosis of the elbow joint.

For fractures of the distal radius, it may be useful to place T-shaped plates with 1.5–2.0 mm screws. Cuttable plates can also be used. In some cases, placing crossed pins anchored in the contralateral cortical surface is sufficient.

Fractures of the proximal ulna that include the olecranon can be fixed with intramedullary pins and a tension band or via an osteosynthesis plate on the lateral or caudal surface of the ulna. In the case of distal ulnar fractures that affect the styloid process, there is instability in the carpal joint, since that is where the lateral collateral ligament of the carpus inserts; therefore, these fractures must be fixed, whether with two Kirschner wires that traverse the styloid process and anchor in the distal radius, or with a tension band.

Complications

Damage to the extensor muscle tendons must be avoided when using osteosynthesis plates. Another complication may arise when closing the skin; there may be more tension at the suture line because of the space occupied by the plate and screws.

The screws of a plate placed in a dorsal position should not protrude too much to prevent a reaction over the ulna, as this could give rise to synostosis and consequently a lessening of pronation and supination movements. This union between the radius and ulna occurs more frequently if the fracture is comminuted.

Due to rubbing of the pins, proximal ulnar fractures fixed with pins may produce ulceration of the skin over the olecranon. This complication can be prevented by bending the pins over the olecranon enough that the bent away section of pins no longer rubs against the skin. This fixation should always be accompanied by a tension band to prevent the fracture site from separating and to prevent the pins from moving in a proximal direction as a result of the traction force of the triceps muscle.

To prevent inflammation of the soft tissues after the surgery, a padded compression bandage is applied up to above the elbow. This bandage is removed 4–5 days later.

Carpal injuries

Cats that fall from high places often suffer carpal injuries, the most frequent being hyperextension of the carpometacarpal joint. Fractures of the carpal bones are rare, with the exception of accessory carpal bone fractures, which are seen with some frequency as a result of this hyperextension produced by the fall. Injuries of the carpal joint ligaments are also uncommon.

To diagnose these injuries, X-rays must be taken in a forced position (stress radiography) to confirm the instability of the joint. Tomography may also be required to be able to see certain fractures in these bones.

This section focuses on the most common injuries: fracture of the accessory carpal bone and injuries caused by hyperextension of the carpus.

Fracture of the accessory bone of the carpus

The accessory carpal bone is articulated to the palmar surface of the ulnar carpal bone and serves as a point of insertion of the ulnar carpal flexor muscle. The fragment that is fractured is usually small and is displaced proximally by the contraction of the muscle that inserts on it.

If the fracture does not affect the joint surface, and if the fragment is small and not greatly displaced, conservative treatment may be a good option. This involves a bandage and splint, with 20°–25° flexion of the carpus for 3–4 weeks.

If the fracture affects the joint surface, or if the fragment is larger or displaced, it must be fixated (Fig. 11). For the approach, an incision is made in the skin at the caudomedial edge of the distal ulna and continued towards the palmar part of the fifth metacarpal bone. When displacement of the fragment is considerable, the dissection must be prolonged proximally until the fragment is found and fixed in its place. Kirschner wires, small-gauge threaded pins or a 1.5 mm screw can be used for this purpose. As described above, the carpus is bandaged in flexion for 4 weeks after the surgery.

Injuries caused by hyperextension of the carpus

The structures that maintain stability during extension of the carpus are the palmar ligaments and the fibrocartilage. Hyperextension occurs when a cat breaks its fall from a high place with its forelimb, and the tension forces generated on the palmar side cause tears in these structures, along with possible injury to the antebrachiocarpal, intercarpal or carpometacarpal joints. Even if there is fibrosis of the palmar ligaments, palmigrade stance in the affected limb is observed during examination (Fig. 12). This is confirmed with forced-position X-rays, which also show which joint of the carpus is injured. In these images, any possible carpal fractures that may present concomitantly must be ruled out.

The treatment of choice for intercarpal or carpometacarpal joint injuries is partial carpal arthrodesis, and the treatment of choice for antebrachiocarpal joint injuries is pancarpal arthrodesis. Conservative treatment before considering arthrodesis is also an option. The carpus is bandaged in flexion in an attempt to encourage fibrosis of the palmar ligaments, resulting in an acceptable functionality to the limb. If this does not occur, surgical treatment is the next course of action.

Surgical approach

The incision in the skin is made from the distal metaphysis of the radius to the midway point of the metacarpus. The subcutaneous fascia is incised, while the accessory cephalic vein is retracted laterally and left intact. Next, the deep antebrachial fascia is incised between the extensor carpi radialis muscle and the common digital extensor muscle. Both muscles are retracted, and the distal periosteum of the radius is exposed and dissected for better muscle retraction. After this, the

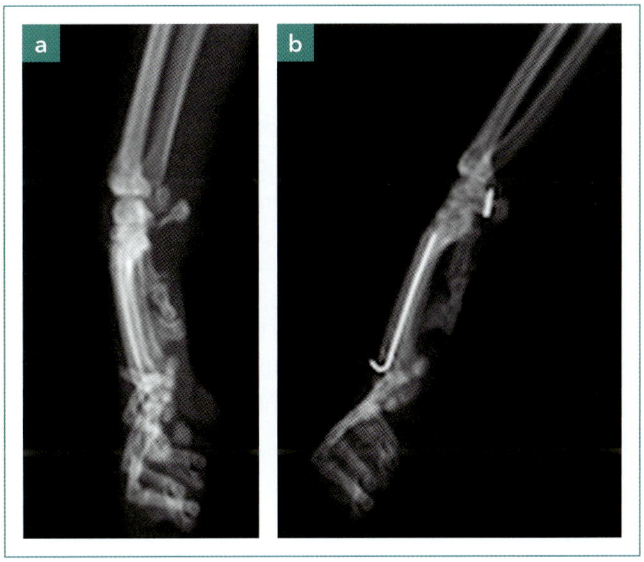

FIGURE 11. (a) Fracture of the accessory bone of the carpus and the fifth metacarpal bone. (b) Fixation of the accessory carpal bone fracture via a 1 mm threaded pin; fixation of the fifth metacarpal fracture via placement of an intramedullary pin.

synovial capsules around the bones of the carpus are incised to expose the joint surfaces. If the carpus is flexed, better visualization of these joint surfaces is achieved (Fig. 13).

Partial carpal arthrodesis

Partial arthrodesis of the carpus is indicated in hyperextension injuries of the intercarpal and carpometacarpal joints. This surgery enables the patient to preserve functional mobility of the antebrachiocarpal joint. A partial arthrodesis of this joint can also be performed (Fig. 14), but proper ossification and correct weight bearing on the limb may not be achieved.

A dorsal approach to these joints is made as described previously. The cartilage is removed from the joint surfaces with a burr, and the bones are fixed with Kirschner wires, which are inserted in an intramedullary position from the second, third and fourth metacarpal bones, continuing across the joints and inserting on the radiocarpal bone. To facilitate proper placement, the carpus is kept in full flexion while the wires are being inserted.

It may be difficult to insert these wires due to the small size and the hardness of the carpal bones and the narrow intramedullary space of the metacarpal bones. Crossed wires can also be placed: the medial wire from the dorsomedial area of the second metacarpal bone, and the lateral wire from the fifth metacarpal bone, anchoring both in the radiocarpal bone.

Another possible fixation method is to place a plate on the medial aspect, placing the first screw in the radiocarpal bone and the most distal screws in the metacarpal bones.

> Once the joint has been fixed, an autologous cancellous bone graft is placed between the affected articular spaces to promote ossification. Cancellous bone can be obtained from the intramedullary cavity of the greater tubercle of the humerus in the same limb.

Rather than using saline solution to preserve this graft, it is preferable to use some of the patient's blood from the surgical field until it is used. This way, the cancellous bone cells are not diluted (Fig. 15).

Pancarpal arthrodesis

Pancarpal arthrodesis is performed if the antebrachiocarpal joint is injured. This treatment allows the patient to bear weight on the limb without pain, but there is alteration in movement since the carpus cannot be flexed. Instead, the cat will compensate for this with a different movement of the shoulder joint.

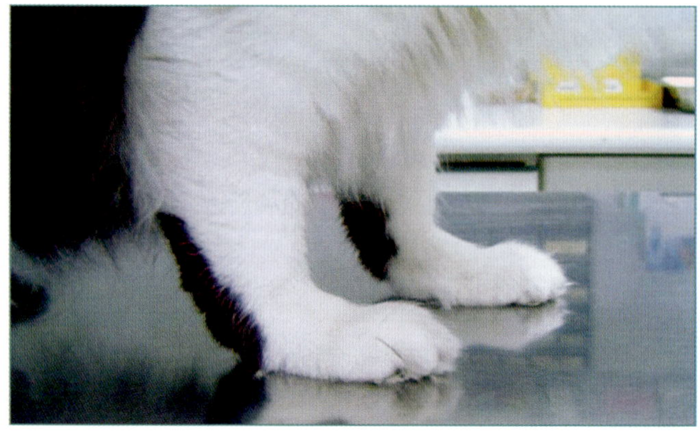

FIGURE 12. Palmigrade stance of both forelimbs as a result of hyperextension injuries of the carpi.

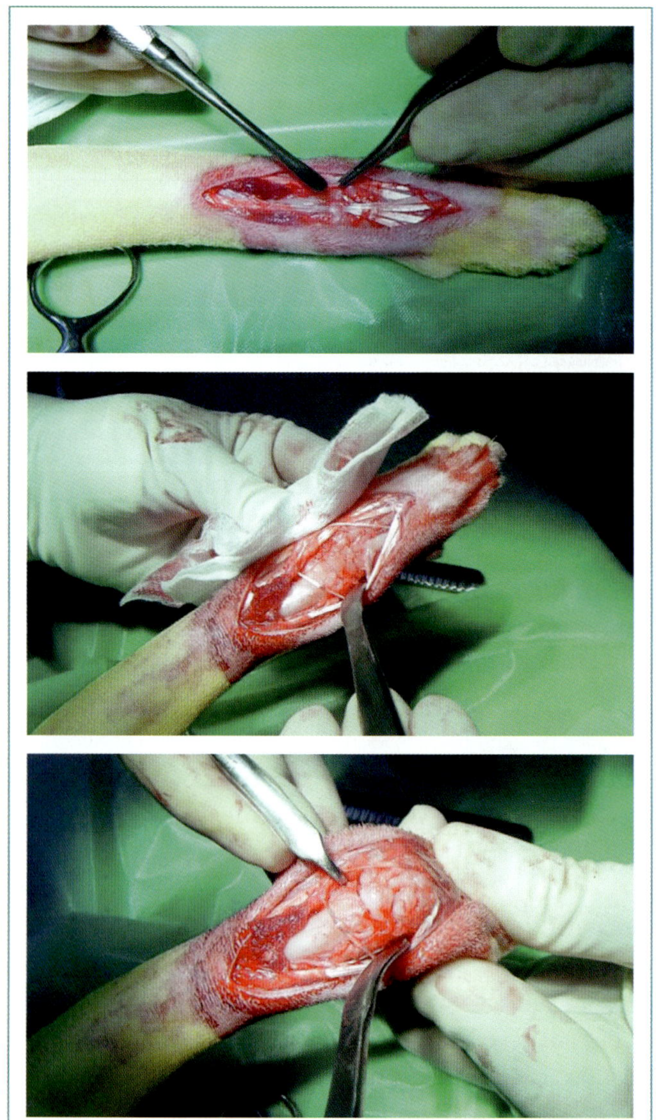

FIGURE 13. Dorsal approach to the carpal joint. Flexion of the joint enables better exposure of the carpal bones.

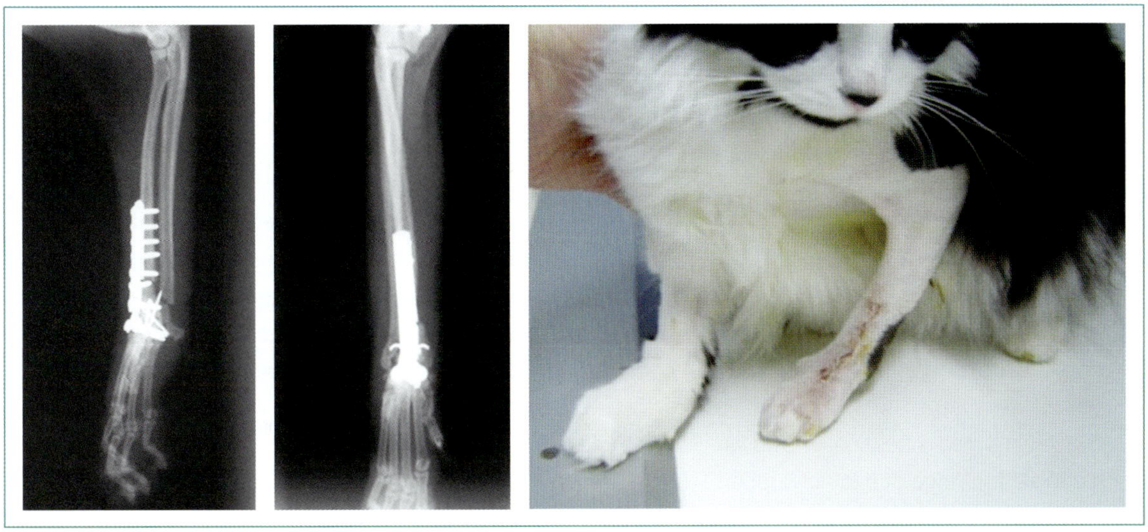

FIGURE 14. Partial arthrodesis of the carpus and resolution of a distal fracture of the radius and ulna. This female cat sustained two falls: the first caused hyperextension of the carpus and the second resulted in radial and ulnar fracture.

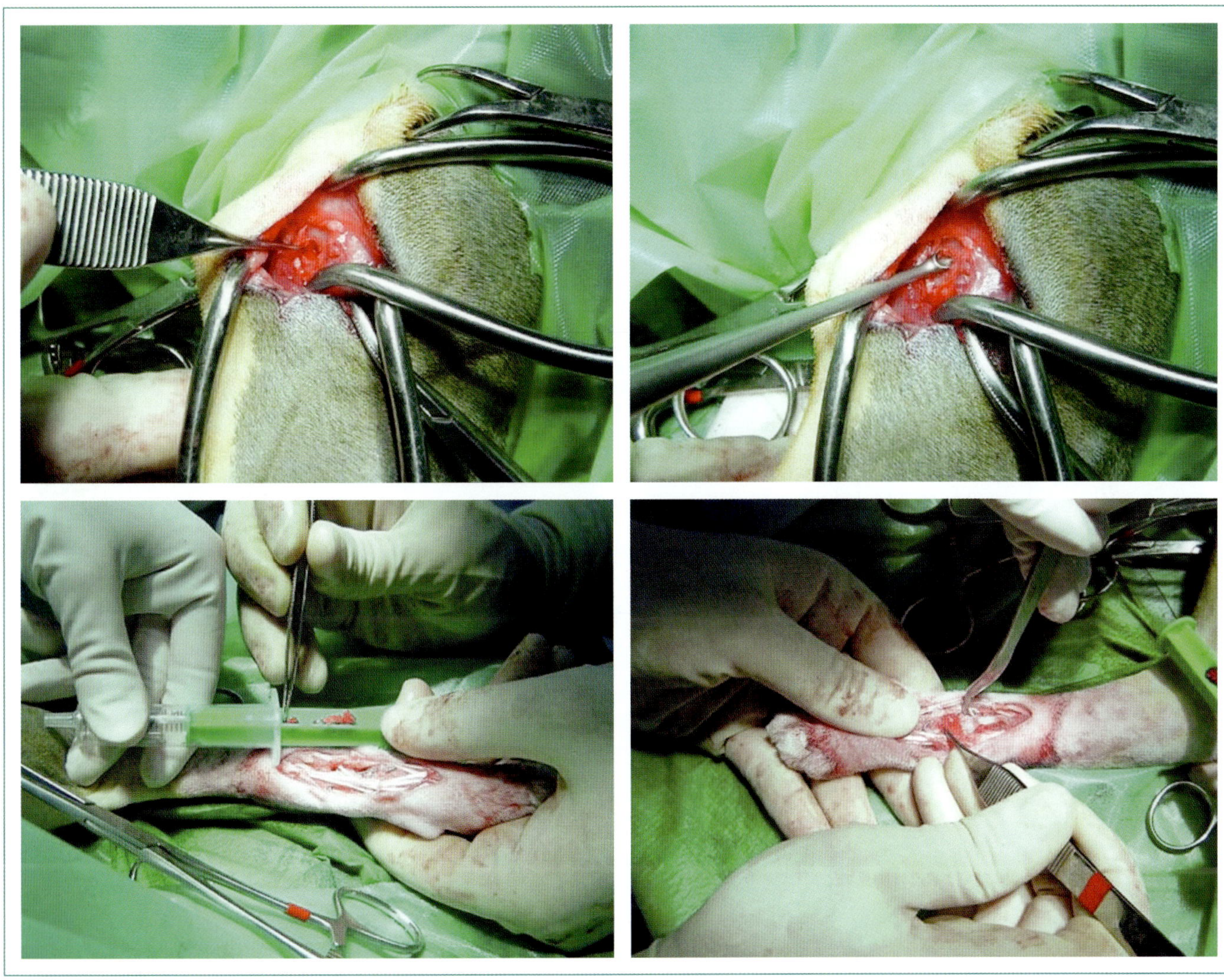

FIGURE 15. Harvesting a cancellous bone graft from the patient's humerus and placing it in the carpus. The cancellous bone graft is preserved inside a 5 ml syringe.

Pins, osteosynthesis plates on the dorsal surface, or external fixators can be used. The joint is fixed at an extension angle of 15°–20°, and this can be compared to the angle at which the patient bears weight on the contralateral carpus.

If using a dorsal plate, the size is chosen in accordance with the length of the metacarpal bones. In general, 1.5 mm screws are used along with a dynamic compression plate or a cuttable plate. Once the articular cartilage is removed from all the joints of the carpus, the plate is fixed with at least three screws in the radius, one in the radiocarpal bone, and another three in the third metacarpal bone (Fig. 16).

This plate can also be placed in a medial position. The advantages are a lower chance of plate breakage due to not supporting as much force, and more stability given that the screws have more bone surface for anchorage. In this case, approach is on the medial side of the carpus, and the first digit is removed so that the plate has a better contact surface. As described above, the articular cartilage is removed from the joint surfaces, and the plate is fixed with a first screw in the radiocarpal bone. Next, the remaining screws are placed in the radius and the metacarpal bones. Fixing the ulna with screws should be avoided in order to enable pronation and supination movements.

Crossed pins can cause more complications and are less stable, although their stability can be improved by anchoring threaded pins in the cortical surface of the radius. If this method is chosen, it can be combined with placement of a transarticular external fixator, although this method can also be used as the sole fixation method.

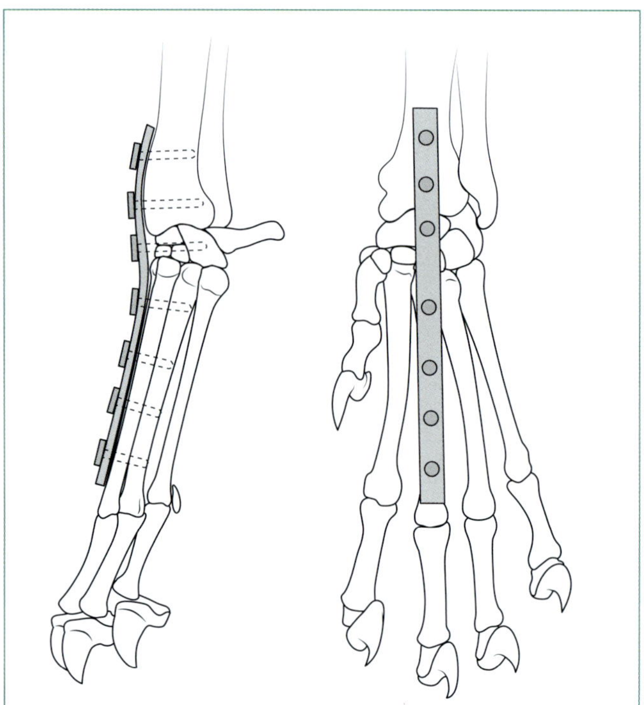

FIGURE 16. Pancarpal arthrodesis with an osteosynthesis plate.

If using an external fixator, a type II fixator is chosen, along with two pins that traverse the entirety of the area, one in the radius and the other at the base of the metacarpal bones. The connecting bars are then attached, enabling the carpus to be extended at 15°–20°. In addition, at least two more pins are added in the distal radius and two more in the metacarpal bones. These pins are attached to the bars. Acrylic or epoxy putty can be used in place of connecting bars to stabilize the structure.

Finally, irrespective of what fixation method is chosen, an autologous cancellous bone graft is added to the articular spaces, as described for partial arthrodesis.

Complications

The most common complication, considering all types of arthrodesis, is injury to the soft tissues caused by bandages or splints used to immobilize the extremity, followed by implant failure. Bandages should be sufficiently padded to prevent soft tissue compression. Action should be taken if there are signs such as inflamed or cold digits, erythema, inflammation or pain of the limb, decreased weight-bearing, or licking or biting the area. The first thing to do is to remove the bandage, warm the limb by submerging it in lukewarm water, massage the area from a distal to a proximal direction to facilitate drainage, administer enough analgesia to control the pain, and, if needed, rebandage with a much more padded bandage (Robert Jones type).

The arthrodesis may fail in approximately 33% of the cases. One of the reasons this may occur is that the joint cartilage is not fully removed from the joint that is to be fixed, as this impedes proper ossification. To avoid this, the articular cartilage must be burred away completely, making sure to reach the subchondral bone at all articular surfaces, but without creating defects when removing the bone. Any spaces left between the bones are filled with cancellous bone grafts or with demineralized bone matrix.

Another reason for failure is the improper immobilization of the carpus until ossification is achieved. This is due to an unsuitable choice of implants, or because these implants have broken or moved, creating instability. The use of crossed pins as the sole fixation method may also lead to improper immobilization. Fixation with a plate and screws or with a transarticular fixator are more reliable methods in that regard.

Fractures of the metacarpal bones

Metacarpal fractures are often observed in cats that fall from heights. Fractures in these bones can occur at their base, on the diaphysis or at the head. Many times, there may also be soft tissue damage, including blood vessels.

Surgical approach

An incision is made in the skin in the dorsal part of the metacarpus. This incision can be straight or curved to expose all the fractured metacarpal bones. Next, the tendons of the extensor muscles are carefully retracted, and an incision is made on the metacarpal bone that must be approached.

Treatment of fractures

These fractures can be treated with external bandages, but sometimes surgical intervention to stabilize them is required.

If one or two metacarpal bones are fractured, conservative treatment with bandages is often enough. The nonfractured metacarpals act as guide, facilitating fracture ossification. Surgical treatment is advised if more than two metacarpal bones are fractured or if the fracture fragments are highly displaced.

In general, surgical stabilization is done using intramedullary pins placed in a normograde fashion starting at the distal fragment (Fig. 17). A hole for the intramedullary pin is made in the distal diaphysis. This means a hole does not have to be made in the surface of the metacarpophalangeal joint, which would damage it. Fractures in which the distal fragment is small can be fixed by inserting the intramedullary pin from the fracture line and through the inside of the proximal fragment, leaving part of the pin exposed so that it can be attached to the distal fragment afterwards.

External fixators or 1.0–1.5 mm minifragment plates can also be employed if the fractures are comminuted. In such cases, to avoid healing complications, efforts should be made to ensure that the skin incision is not directly over the implants.

Complications

Postoperative edema occurs frequently, but the risk can be lowered or avoided altogether if a padded compression bandage is applied postoperatively. This bandage should be kept in place for 3–4 days.

Only small-gauge (0.8, 1.0 and 1.2 mm) intramedullary pins can be used due to the small size of the intramedullary cavity of the metacarpal bones. If larger-gauge pins are used, it could even cause an iatrogenic fracture of the bone.

The pins should not protrude proximally or distally in order to avoid damaging the articular surfaces of the carpometacarpal joint or the metacarpophalangeal joint, respectively. Likewise, the pins should not be inserted in a normograde fashion from the surface of the metacarpophalangeal joint in order to avoid damaging it. This would also decrease the extension of the digits since the pin over the joint would act as a physical impediment, resulting in poor weight-bearing.

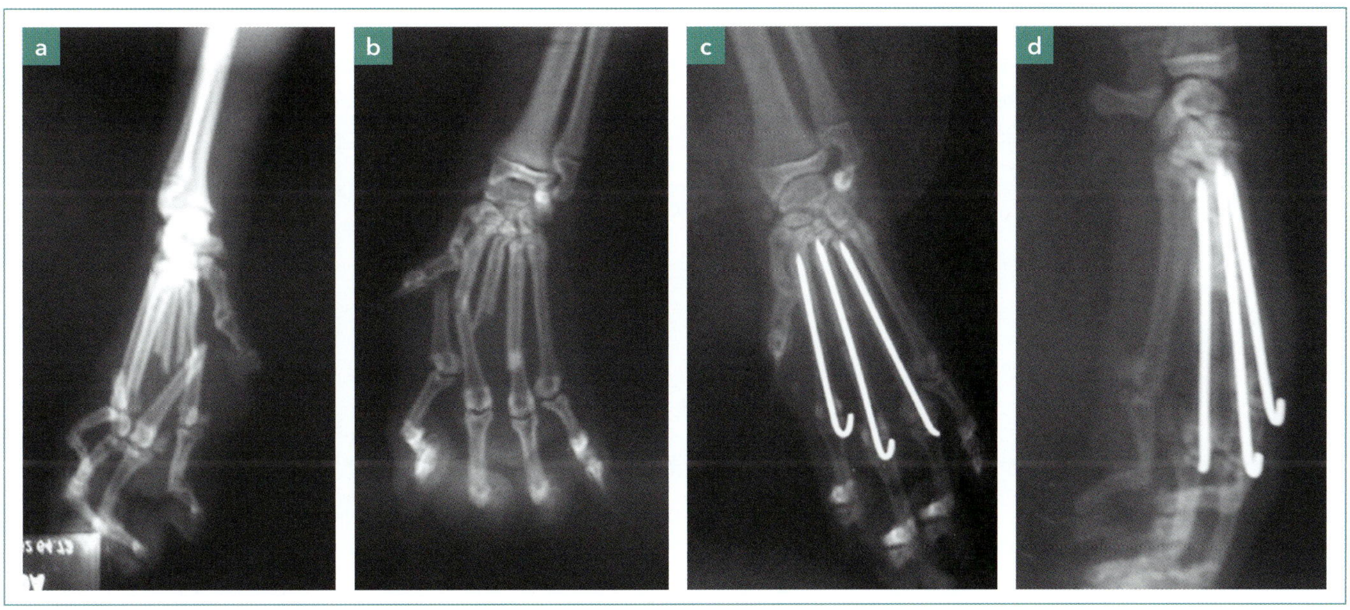

FIGURE 17. (a,b) Fracture of the second, third and fourth metacarpal bones. (c,d) Treatment with intramedullary pins placed in normograde fashion.

Bibliography

Beever L, Giles K, Meeson R. Postoperative complications associated with external skeletal fixators in cats. *J Feline Med Surg*, 2017; 19(7):727–736.

Calvo I, Farrell M, Chase D et al. Carpal arthrodesis in cats. Long-term functional outcome. *Vet Comp Orthop Traumatol*, 2009; 22(6):498–504.

Díaz-Bertrana MC, Durall I, Puchol JL et al. Interlocking nail treatment of long-bone fractures in cats: 33 cases (1995–2004). *Vet Comp Orthop Traumatol*, 2005; 18(3):119–126.

Greeff DR, Owen M, Bush M. Management of carpal hyperextension injury in a cat using temporary transarticular internal and external skeletal fixation. *J Feline Med Surg*, 2014; 16(10):842–845.

Griffon D, Hamaide A. *Complications in Small Animal Surgery*. Ames, IA: Wiley Blackwell, 2016; pp. 627–750.

Hulse D. MIPO techniques for the humerus in small animals. *Vet Clin North Am Small Anim Pract*, 2012; 42(5):975–982.

Johnson AL, Dunning D. *Atlas of Orthopedic Surgical Procedures of the Dog and Cat*. St. Louis, MO: Sanders/Elsevier, 2005.

Johnson KA. *Piermattei's Atlas of Surgical Approaches to the Bones and Joints of the Dog and Cat*, 5th ed. St. Louis, MO: Saunders, 2014.

Kraus KH, Toombs JP, Ness MG. *External Fixation in Small Animal Practice*. Malden, MA: Blackwell Science, 2003.

Langley-Hobbs SJ, Straw M. The feline humerus. An anatomical study with relevance to external skeletal fixator and intramedullary pin placement. *Vet Comp Orthop Traumatol*, 2005; 18(1):1–6.

Langley-Hobbs SJ, Voss K, Lapish JP. Orthopaedic implants. In: Montavon PM, Voss K, Langley-Hobbs SJ (eds.). *Feline Orthopedic Surgery and Musculoskeletal Disease*. St. Louis, MO: Elsevier Saunders, 2009; pp. 259–282.

Langley-Hobbs SJ, Voss K, Montavon PM. Metacarpus, metatarsus and phalanges. In: Montavon PM, Voss K, Langley-Hobbs SJ (eds.). *Feline Orthopedic Surgery and Musculoskeletal Disease*. St. Louis, MO: Elsevier Saunders, 2009; pp. 397–406.

Longley M, Chase D, Calvo I et al. A comparison of fixation methods for supracondylar and distal humeral shaft fractures of the dog and cat. *Can Vet J*, 2018; 59(12):1299–1304.

Mathis KR, Voss K. Partial carpal arthrodesis using a medially applied mini-plate in three cats with carpometacarpal hyperextension injury. *J Feline Med Surg*, 2015; 17(8):727–732.

Piermattei DLF, Gretchen L, DeCamp CE. *Brinker, Piermattei, and Flo's Handbook of Small Animal Orthopedics and Fracture Repair*, 4th ed. St. Louis, MO: Saunders/Elsevier, 2006.

Scott HW, McLaughlin R. Fractures and disorders of the forelimb. In: Scott HW, McLaughlin R. *Feline Orthopedics*. London, UK: Manson Publishing, 2007; pp. 107–166.

Unger M, Montavon PM, Heim UFA. Classification of fractures of long bones in the dog and cat: Introduction and clinical application. *Vet Comp Orthop Traumatol*, 1990; 3(2):5–14.

Voss K, Langley-Hobbs SJ, Montavon PM. Carpal joint. In: Montavon PM, Voss K, Langley-Hobbs SJ (eds.). *Feline Orthopedic Surgery and Musculoskeletal Disease*. St. Louis, MO: Elsevier Saunders, 2009; pp. 385–396.

Voss K, Langley-Hobbs SJ, Montavon PM. Humerus. In: Montavon PM, Voss K, Langley-Hobbs SJ (eds.). *Feline Orthopedic Surgery and Musculoskeletal Disease*. St. Louis, MO: Elsevier Saunders, 2009; pp. 343–358.

Voss K, Langley-Hobbs SJ, Montavon PM. Radius and ulna. In: Montavon PM, Voss K, Langley-Hobbs SJ (eds.). *Feline Orthopedic Surgery and Musculoskeletal Disease*. St. Louis, MO: Elsevier Saunders, 2009; pp. 371–384.

FRACTURES OF THE PELVIS AND COXOFEMORAL JOINT

32

Antonio Peña

Introduction

Pelvic fractures are common in cats that suffer trauma as a result of road traffic accident or falling from a height. They account for 20%–22% of all fractures and are more frequent in young cats. In most cases, the pelvic bones are broken in two or more places, although a single fracture accompanied by sacroiliac luxation is possible. These fractures may have displaced bone fragments and cause a narrowing of the pelvic canal.

Fractures of the different anatomical structures comprising the pelvis may be encountered:

- Fracture/luxation of the sacroiliac joint
- Iliac fractures
- Acetabular fractures
- Ischial fractures
- Pubic fractures or separation of the pubic symphysis

In 59%–72% of cases of pelvic fractures, other injuries may be found (Box 1). In order to identify these concurrent injuries, a complete physical examination, orthopedic examination and neurological examination should be performed. Diagnostic imaging of the thorax and abdomen by means of X-rays and ultrasound scans is equally important.

BOX 1. Injuries that may be present in cats with pelvic fracture

Orthopedic

- Sacroiliac luxation
- Sacral fracture
- Femoral head fracture
- Femoral neck fracture
- Hip luxation

Thorax

- Pneumothorax
- Hemothorax
- Rib fracture
- Diaphragmatic hernia

Nervous system

- Lumbosacral plexus injury
- Sciatic nerve injury

Abdomen

- Urinary tract injuries
- Gastrointestinal tract injuries
- Abdominal hernia
- Prepubic tendon rupture

Clinical signs

Cats with pelvic fractures are usually unable to remain standing or walk, but they can bear weight on the contralateral limb if the injuries are unilateral and involve only one hemipelvis. They may also be able to bear weight if the injuries are old or if the fractures only involve the ischium or pubis. Asymmetry in the pelvic region is noted, as well as inflammation and pain.

On examination, crepitus may be detected upon palpation of the fractured pelvic area, which is confirmed by radiography in laterolateral and ventrodorsal projections. Oblique projections may also be necessary to avoid overlapping bony structures. Computed tomography (CT), magnetic resonance imaging (MRI) and 3D images of these scans are very helpful in planning the most appropriate treatment in each case.

A neurological examination should always be performed to diagnose possible damage to the nervous system, which may influence the patient's treatment and prognosis (Box 2). This is also used to differentiate preoperative neurological damage caused by trauma from iatrogenic damage that may be seen in the postoperative period. It is important that this examination be performed before administering opioid analgesic medication, especially in the evaluation of deep sensation, as it may mask the response.

Sacroiliac luxation

Sacroiliac luxation occurs when the body of the ilium is displaced and separates from its attachment to the sacrum. The ilium is usually displaced in a craniodorsal direction. This luxation occurs in 24% of cats suffering trauma and in 60% of cats with pelvic fractures. It is usually accompanied by ischial and pubic fractures if the luxation is unilateral, but there may not be other pelvic fractures if it is bilateral.

The clinical signs are pain and a lack of weight-bearing on the affected limb, and may be accompanied by neurological deficit or dysfunction in urination due to damage to the sciatic nerve or the lumbosacral nerve trunk.

It is most easily diagnosed on a ventrodorsal X-ray of the pelvis (Fig. 1). It is common to find sacroiliac luxation as such or sacroiliac luxation with avulsion of the cranial part of the sacral wing.

Treatment

Treatment can be conservative if the displacement is small (displacement less than 50% of the joint length), if the cat can walk by bearing weight on the limb on the affected side and if there are no neurological deficits. It is necessary to administer analgesic treatment for a prolonged period of time. However, if surgical treatment is performed in these cases, improvement is faster and a return to normal physical activity is achieved sooner, in addition to avoiding the risk of causing damage to the lumbosacral nerves.

In cats with pain and lameness, bilateral luxation, neurological deficit or major displacement of the ilium, surgical treatment is required to stabilize the lumbosacral joint.

The surgical approach can be by two different routes: ventrolateral or dorsolateral. The **ventrolateral approach** is also useful if concurrent iliac wing fractures need to be repaired:

- The cat is positioned in lateral recumbency on the unaffected side. To facilitate placement of the wing of the ilium parallel to the table, a rolled towel or pad is placed under the cat's caudal abdomen.
- A skin incision is made from the iliac crest to the greater trochanter of the femur.
- The subcutaneous tissue and superficial fascia are dissected and the fascia between the gluteus medius muscle and the tensor fascia latae muscle is incised to access the ventral border of the wing of the ilium.

BOX 2. Neurological evaluation of a cat with pelvic fracture

Deep pain sensation

- Poor prognosis if absent.
- Ensure there is a pain sensation response (vocalization, turning the body, attacking) and no limb withdrawal reflex.

Pudendal nerve reflexes

- Anal sphincter reflex.
- Perineal reflex.
- Tone of the external urethral sphincter by manual compression of the bladder.

Sensory and motor functions of the tail

- Check the function of the coccygeal nerve by pinching the tail with hemostatic forceps at different levels.
- Evaluate movement and pain sensation.

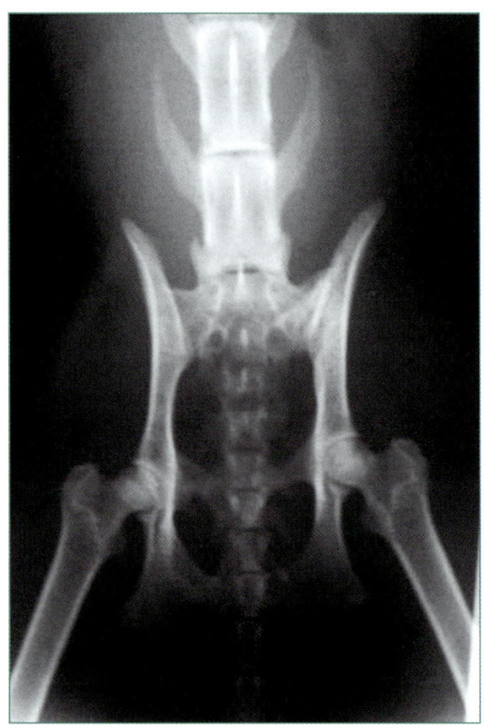

FIGURE 1. Ventrodorsal X-ray of a patient with right sacroiliac luxation.

- The gluteus medius muscle is retracted dorsally, separating it from its insertion in the wing of the ilium, prolonging this dissection in a cranial and dorsal direction.
- An incision is then made at the origin of the iliacus muscle along the ventral border of the ilium, and, by elevating it, the ventral part of the body of the sacrum is palpated (Fig. 2).

In the **dorsolateral approach**:

- The cat is placed in ventral recumbency, with a rolled towel or pad placed under the caudal abdomen to elevate the pelvis dorsally.
- The skin incision starts from the iliac crest and extends along the dorsal border of the wing of the ilium.
- The subcutaneous tissue is dissected and the origin of the gluteus medius muscle is incised to retract it ventrally away from the surface of the wing of the ilium.
- Next, the soft tissue between the wing of the ilium and the sacrum is dissected to gain access to the sacroiliac joint (Fig. 3).
- A retractor can be used to shift the wing of the ilium ventrally to facilitate visualization. Some of the fibrocartilaginous tissue may also be removed from the sacroiliac joint to improve its exposure.

Once one of the two approaches has been performed, reduction forceps or Kern bone-holding forceps are placed on the cranial border of the iliac crest in order to handle the ilium and move it in a caudoventral direction to reduce the sacroiliac luxation. Moving the sacrum with a blunt instrument facilitates the maneuver.

Once the luxation has been reduced, the wing of the ilium is fixed to the body of the sacrum by means of a long screw that compresses both bony structures. This screw should reach beyond the middle of the body of the sacrum (at least 60% of its width), and it is usually a 2.7 mm cortical screw (Fig. 4). Depending on the size of the sacral body, it may be necessary to use a thinner screw (2 mm). This screw must be correctly placed and not inserted in the wings of the sacrum, the lumbosacral joint space or the spinal canal. It may be useful to place a Kirschner wire before the screw as a landmark for where to place it. This wire can be left in place to avoid rotation of the wing of the ilium around the screw, as the body of the sacrum in cats is usually too small to accommodate two screws.

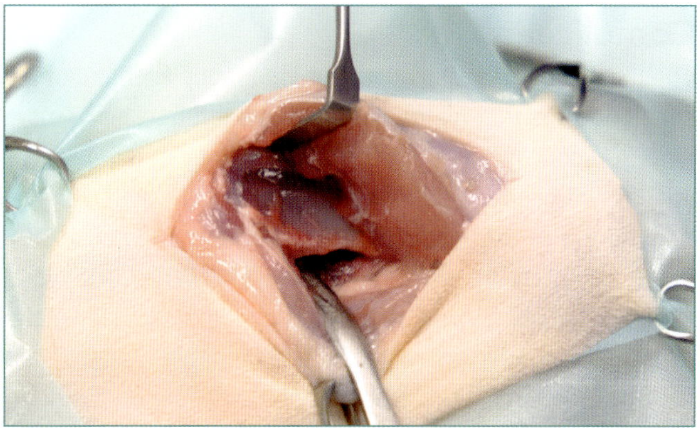

FIGURE 2. Ventrolateral approach to the wing of the ilium. The tip of the retractor indicates the area where the body of the sacrum is palpated. Cranial is to the left side of the image

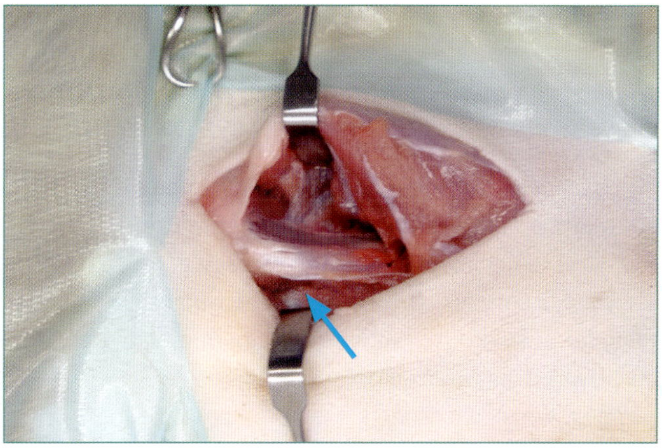

FIGURE 3. Dorsolateral approach to the wing of the ilium. The arrow indicates the location of the sacroiliac joint. Cranial is to the left side of the image.

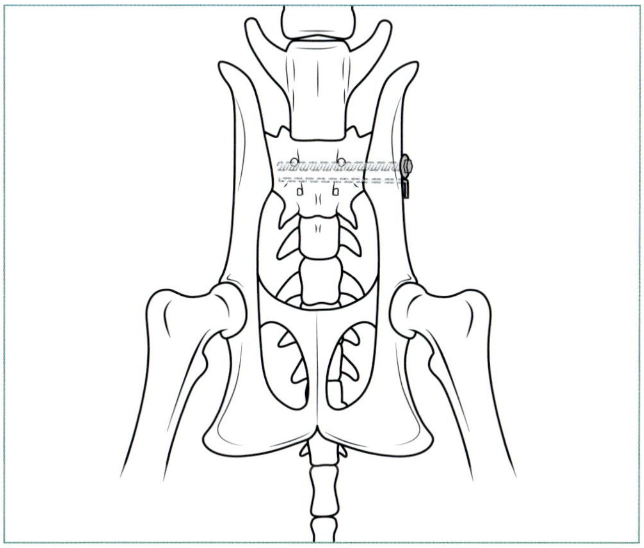

FIGURE 4. Placement of a screw and a Kirschner wire for the resolution of a sacroiliac luxation.

Complications

The most common complication is incorrect placement of the screw or wires that fix the ilium to the sacrum. This is more likely to occur if the sacroiliac luxation is bilateral, as there is a lack of properly positioned anatomical landmarks. The body of the sacrum is small in the cat and it is possible to incorrectly place the screw and insert it into the lumbosacral joint, into the spinal canal or fail to anchor into the body of the sacrum if directed ventrally to it. The probability of error can be reduced with good positioning of the patient on the operating table, an approach that allows the identification of anatomical structures, palpating the body of the sacrum and correct orientation when placing the screw or wire that attaches the ilium and sacrum.

Iliac fractures

Iliac fractures result in a significant inability to use the affected limb. In the cat, they are most frequently oblique, although transverse or comminuted fractures of the ilium may also occur. They are usually accompanied by pubic and ischial fractures that cause bone displacement and a narrowing of the pelvic canal, which may even collapse.

As previously mentioned, it is necessary to perform a neurological examination and evaluate the integrity of the sciatic nerve, which runs along the medial aspect of the body of the ilium.

Treatment

Surgical reduction and fixation of these fractures is necessary to recover the functionality of the limb and to avoid a narrowing of the pelvic canal and injury to the sciatic nerve due to bone fragments.

The **surgical approach** is performed with the animal placed in lateral recumbency on the uninjured side:

- The skin incision begins at the iliac crest and extends to the greater trochanter of the femur.
- The subcutaneous tissue is dissected to expose the muscles. An incision is made between the gluteus medius muscle and the tensor fascia latae muscle to separate them.
- The medial and deep gluteal muscles are then moved dorsally by separating their attachment to the periosteum of the iliac wing to expose the wing of the ilium. The circumflex femoral vessels and the cranial gluteal vessels and nerves should be preserved.
- The disinsertion of the gluteal muscles may be prolonged along the entire cranial border of the iliac crest. This allows further displacement of these muscles and greater exposure of the wing of the ilium (Fig. 5).
- To maintain this exposure, a Hohmann retractor can be placed over the dorsal border of the ilium, taking care not to damage the sciatic nerve.

Forceps are used to reduce the fracture fragments. One of the forceps is placed just cranial to the acetabulum and another forceps is placed on the cranial fragment of the ilium, so that both fragments can be handled to achieve fracture reduction. If there is no ischial fracture, reduction of the ilium fracture can also be achieved via traction of the caudal fragment (which is usually displaced cranially) from the ischial tuberosity by placing a forceps into the ischial tuberosity through a small surgical access.

There are various fixation methods for treating these fractures, although placement of osteosynthesis plates is the most commonly used. This plate should be contoured to fit the surface of the wing of the ilium. At least two or three screws should be placed on both sides of the fracture line. The part of the plate over the cranial fragment of the ilium should be positioned in such a way as to allow one of the screws to be inserted through the body of the sacrum, which allows for greater stability of that screw and better fixation of the plate.

Dynamic compression plates of 2.7 mm are usually used. Cuttable plates or reconstruction plates can also be utilized.

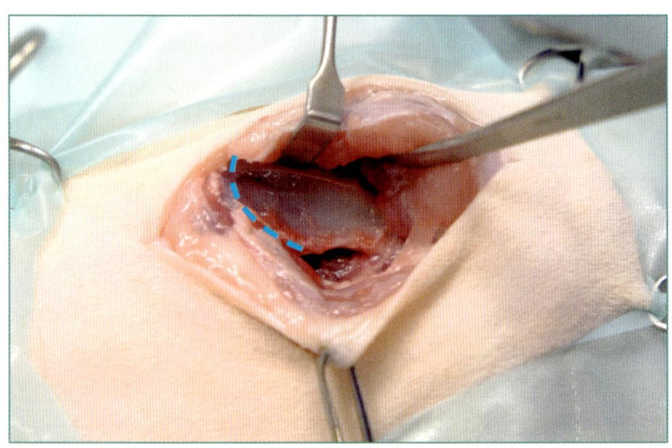

FIGURE 5. Approach to the wing of the ilium by extending the gluteal dissection along the edge of the iliac crest (dashed line).

T-plates, L-plates or locking plates can be used if it is not possible to place a minimum of two screws in one of the fragments using straight plates. In the case of fractures in which the caudal fragment of the ilium is small, it may be necessary to contour the plate over the dorsal edge of the acetabulum so that at least two screws can be placed in that fragment. If the caudal edge of the plate is very close to the coxofemoral joint, it must be prevented from contacting the joint capsule, as this causes pain and a lack of weight-bearing on the limb, and it may limit the movement of the joint.

Once the fracture has been reduced, forceps can be placed until the plate is in place. If it is not possible to stabilize the fracture in this manner, the plate is contoured to the shape of each fragment separately, or the intact iliac wing can be used as a model. The plate is fixed to the caudal fragment of the fracture, the greater trochanter is tractioned with forceps, and the most cranial area of the plate is pressed on the wing of the ilium until the plate is in contact with the bone. The screws are placed once fracture reduction is achieved.

In the case of comminuted fractures, 2 mm screws can be placed in each fragment and joined together with figure-8 cerclage wire, tightening it until the fractures are reduced. The entire construct is then covered with bone cement to add consistency and prevent the screws from moving. Care must be taken to prevent the cement from contacting the sciatic nerve, so as not to damage it. For this purpose, the nerve is located during surgery, moved aside by means of a manual retractor and covered to avoid said contact. The area should be irrigated with cold sterile saline to minimize the risk of thermal damage to the nerve.

Complications

Fractures of the ilium can be difficult to reduce, especially when there are more than two fragments or they are accompanied by sacroiliac luxation. Many times an attempt is made to make the approach as small as possible, resulting in inadequate visualization of the fragments and inadequate access to place reduction forceps or osteosynthesis material. This leads to longer surgery time, poor fracture reduction and possible damage to nearby nerve, vascular or soft tissue structures. It is easier to reduce these fractures by using an approach that is wide enough to correctly mobilize the fragments and to place the fixation material more easily. Dissection between muscle groups and their separation from the periosteum without damaging them makes exposure better and the cat's recovery faster, as there are no fibrillar ruptures that have to heal.

Another complication that can occur is screw mobilization. The wing of the ilium is a flat bone in which short screws can be placed, so it is important to place the plate so that at least one of the screws is fixed to the body of the sacrum. This stabilizes the plate on the iliac wing and considerably reduces the risk of implant mobilization. Another method of avoiding screw mobilization is to place the plate on the dorsal edge of the pelvis, since longer screws can be used.

Implant failure leads to faulty fracture ossification with consequences such as defective consolidation, nonunion or the formation of an exuberant (hypertrophic) callus, which can cause damage to the sciatic nerve and a narrowing of the pelvic canal due to displacement of the bone fragments. In one study, it was observed that half of the cats in which the screws had mobilized presented some degree of narrowing of the pelvic canal. In cases where constipation occurs secondary to this narrowing, pelvic osteotomies may be required in an attempt to widen the pelvic canal.

Acetabular fractures

Fractures of the acetabulum account for 17.5%–26% of pelvic fractures. They are usually unilateral in cats, and most are composed of two fragments (77%).

Diagnosis can be made by X-rays. The ventrodorsal projection is the most useful, as the laterolateral is of little help due to the overlapping image of the femoral trochanter or other anatomical structures. Currently, in many cases, CT scans can be used to obtain better images. This allows for a correct diagnosis of orthopedic alterations and a better planning of the necessary surgical treatment.

Treatment

Treatment can be conservative in cases in which there is no displacement of the fragments, the size of the pelvic canal is not compromised and the insertion area of the round ligament is not affected. Concerning the importance of fracture location in choosing between conservative or surgical treatment, the previous practice was that if the fracture was in the distal third of the acetabulum, the treatment could be conservative. However, current studies evaluating the topography of the coxofemoral joint suggest that all parts of the joint play some role in weight-bearing, so the location of the fracture should not influence the decision between conservative or surgical treatment.

In very young kittens, in which fracture of the acetabular growth plate often occurs, conservative treatment may be chosen under the right conditions. In kittens younger than 12 weeks, the complications of conservative treatment result from an ossification that causes a deformity of the acetabulum, which becomes flatter and a hip subluxation may occur. To reduce the convalescence time and the risk of these complications, surgical treatment is also usually indicated for these kittens. This prevents a narrowing of the pelvic canal and future defecation problems, which would require the cat to undergo surgery to correct the narrowing or digestive surgery to resolve chronic constipation.

In cases where joint stability is compromised due to a fracture with multiple fragments, or because conservative treatment has failed, **hip arthroplasty by osteotomy of the femoral head and neck** and resolution of the fracture without fixation may be chosen as a way to save the functionality of the limb. In many of these cases there will be gait abnormalities.

Open reduction for fracture stabilization is indicated when there is an obvious displacement of the fragments, there is crepitus between them and an adequate reconstruction of the articular surface is desired (Fig. 6). The purpose of this fixation is to reduce pain, obtain adequate functionality of the limb and reduce the probability of osteoarthritis development.

Various approaches can be performed depending on the need for exposure of the surgical field for fracture reduction and implant placement.

A dorsal approach can be performed between the gluteal muscles in the case of Kirschner wire placement. Also, if it is a caudal fracture of the acetabulum and a small plate is to be used for fixation.

The approach that allows the greatest exposure of the acetabulum is performed **dorsal to the coxofemoral joint, with osteotomy of the greater trochanter of the femur** to achieve visualization of the entire joint. The sciatic nerve must be located in order to protect it from being damaged by the manipulation of the bone fragments or by the instruments used. In young kittens, instead of an osteotomy of the greater trochanter of the femur, a tenotomy of the gluteal muscles should be performed to achieve this approach and avoid damaging the growth plate.

Once the fracture has been reduced, with the aid of fragment reduction forceps with curved tips, the fragments are held in place. Perfect anatomical reduction of the articular surface, with no steps or gaps, must be ensured prior to placement of the implants.

Fracture fixation with an osteosynthesis plate is the most common method and provides adequate stability. Acetabular plates, 2 mm straight plates or L-plates can be used. Locking plates can also be used in the case of fractures with multiple fragments that do not allow the use of bicortical screws. The plates are placed in the dorsal area of the acetabular ring and contoured to adopt the appropriate shape and avoid displacement. Screws should not be inserted into the acetabulum, to avoid rubbing against the femoral head.

Other forms of fixation of fractures of the acetabulum include the use of screws perpendicular to the fracture line, in cases of oblique fractures, or **screws in the acetabular rim and placing a tension band around their heads** (Fig. 7). This fixation method may be accompanied by one or two Kirschner wires across the fracture line to increase stability. This technique is also indicated in the case of young kittens. In kittens younger than 12 weeks, early removal of the screws and cerclage wire should be considered to avoid acetabular deformities due to the premature closure of the acetabular growth plate. In kittens 16 weeks or older, it is not necessary to remove these implants, as the development of the acetabulum is usually normal.

The figure-8 tension band with screws can also be combined with polymethylmethacrylate covering the implants to provide more stability to the construct, thus preventing mobilization of the screws.

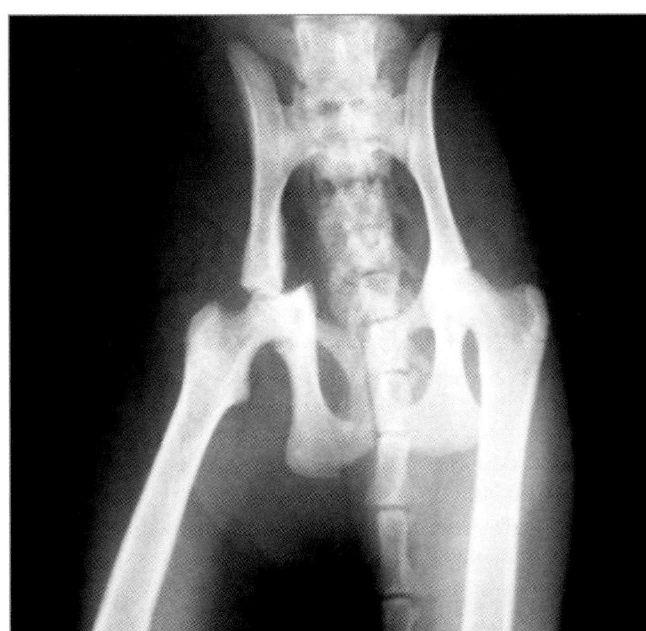

FIGURE 6. Acetabular fracture of the right hip.

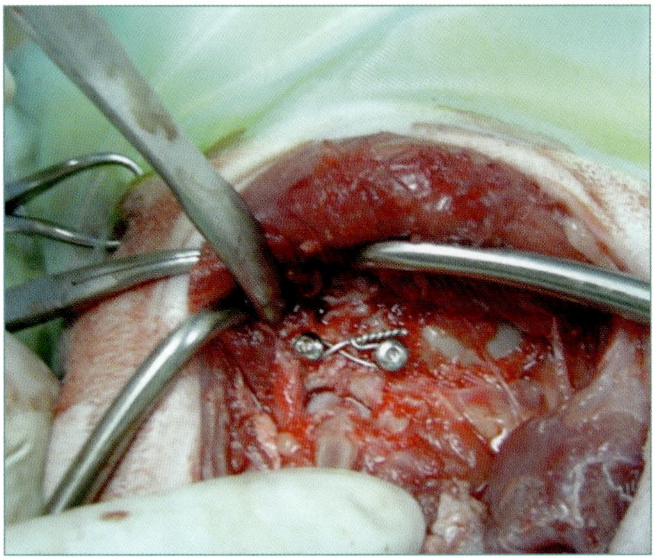

FIGURE 7. Resolution of an acetabular fracture with two screws in the dorsal acetabular rim and figure-8 cerclage wire. Approach with osteotomy of the greater trochanter of the femur.

Complications

The possible complications of conservative treatment in this type of fracture have already been discussed. Among the most common are pelvic canal deformity, which causes constipation and megacolon, long-term pain and muscle atrophy that result in a significant decrease in limb function.

When surgical treatment is performed and an adequate reduction of the fracture is not achieved or the fixation is not correct, the functionality of the joint will be impaired. There will be pain when bearing weight, joint degeneration and signs of osteoarthritis. It is therefore important, as in any joint fracture, to reduce the bone fragments as perfectly as possible to ensure stable internal fixation and interfragmentary compression.

> One of the causes of poor reduction is an approach that does not allow correct visualization of the bone fragments and the joint line.

In these fractures, it is advisable to resort to osteotomy of the greater trochanter of the femur in order to elevate the gluteal muscles and obtain a complete view of the joint. This also helps in locating and isolating the sciatic nerve, to avoiding damage to it during surgery.

Another complication can be the placement of implants that pass through the fragments and penetrate the acetabular joint. This probability is reduced by the proper orientation of the screws or wires to be placed. Again, complete visualization of the joint using a wide approach reduces the likelihood of this occurring.

There may be cases in which fracture ossification has not been correct due to an exuberant bony callus, misalignment of the articular surface, displacement of the fragments or the appearance of osteoarthritis. The patient presents pain when bearing weight on the limb and the functionality of the limb is not correct. These are the cases in which subsequent femoral head arthroplasty may be necessary to control pain and achieve adequate weight-bearing.

Ischial fractures

Fractures of the ischium in cats do not usually require fixation. Most occur at the same time as other fractures of the pelvis, and fixation of these fractures should be sufficient to achieve ischial alignment.

An ischial tuberosity fracture may occur, which is usually accompanied by an obvious displacement of the bone fragment due to the insertions of the biceps femoris, semitendinosus and semimembranosus muscles pulling on it (Fig. 8). Its repositioning and fixation results in a shorter recovery time and a significant reduction of the associated pain. It can be fixed by means of Kirschner wires, cerclage wire or a combination of both. However, there are cases in which, even if there is a large displacement, conservative treatment can allow the cat to recover its gait, even if it takes longer to do so.

Coxofemoral luxation

Coxofemoral luxation can occur as a result of direct trauma or falls from a great height. It may be accompanied by other orthopedic injuries and there may be various joint-associated soft tissue injuries. Parts of the joint capsule and round ligament may be torn, in addition to tears in the gluteal muscles. This may be accompanied by fractures of the acetabular ring and the greater trochanter of the femur, in addition to an avulsion of a fragment of the femoral head where the round ligament inserts.

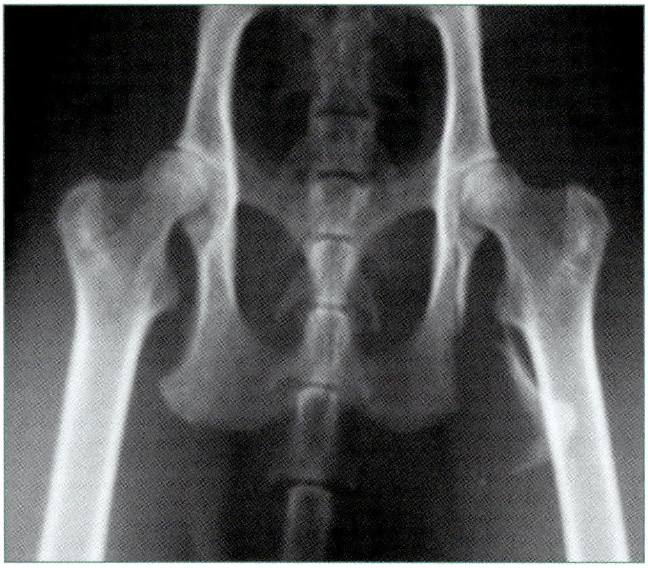

FIGURE 8. Fracture of the left ischial tuberosity with displacement.

> The femoral head may be displaced in various directions in relation to the acetabulum. Within this classification, craniodorsal luxation is the most common (72%), followed by caudodorsal luxation, while ventral luxation rarely occurs.

Clinical signs in cats with coxofemoral luxation include hip pain and lameness with a lack of weight-bearing on the limb, which is rotated and adducted. Asymmetry of the hips may be observed due to displacement of the femoral trochanter in the luxated hip. In normal animals, a triangle can be formed between three anatomical points: the cranial border of the iliac crest, the greater trochanter of the femur and the ischial tuberosity; the greater trochanter is closer to the ischial landmark than to the iliac landmark. In the case of craniodorsal luxation, the three points are aligned and the space between the ilium and the femoral trochanter is shortened due to the displacement of the trochanter.

Diagnosis by X-rays is necessary to confirm the suspicion of coxofemoral luxation during the examination (Fig. 9). The direction in which the luxation has occurred and whether it is accompanied by fractures of nearby structures can also be assessed. Another pathology to rule out via X-rays is the presence of hip dysplasia, which can predispose the cat to luxation even after only mild trauma, in addition to influencing the choice of treatment.

Treatment

In some cases, **closed reduction of the coxofemoral luxation** may be performed. This should be done as soon as possible to avoid damage to the articular cartilage and muscle fibrosis that will occur if luxation reduction is delayed. It must also be ensured that there are no fractures in the acetabulum or in the femoral head and that there is no hip dysplasia.

In the most common coxofemoral luxation, craniodorsal, the cat under general anesthesia is placed in lateral recumbency with the affected limb uppermost. A wide towel or bandage is wrapped around the groin of the luxated limb in order to manipulate and secure the cat's body when pulling on the limb to reposition the femoral head. For this, the femoral head is elevated to bridge the dorsal border of the iliac wing. Next, the limb is pulled distally and caudally to align the femoral head over the acetabulum. The limb is then rotated and abducted to fit the head into the acetabulum. Once the luxation is reduced, the trochanter is pushed medially and the limb is moved through its full range of motion. The purpose of this is to remove clots and debris of soft tissue and lacerated joint capsule from the acetabulum. The reduction must be confirmed by X-rays.

Subsequently, an Ehmer bandage is applied to prevent the limb from bearing weight and to keep the femoral head within

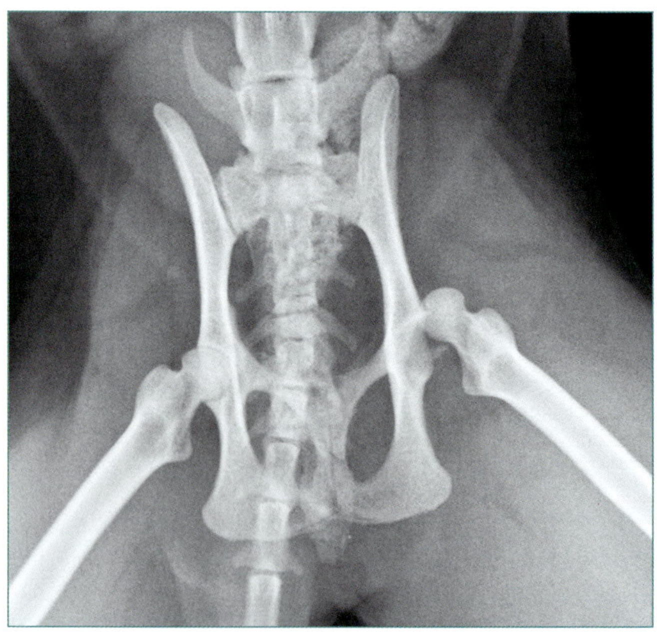

FIGURE 9. X-ray of a left coxofemoral luxation. A small intra-articular bone fragment due to avulsion of the insertion of the round ligament is observed. Image courtesy of Ayavet veterinary clinic.

the acetabulum until the joint capsule heals and the muscle groups recover. This should be maintained for 2 weeks, if possible, although many cats do not tolerate it well or it may cause complications such skin and soft tissue lesions. In addition, reluxation occurs in 50% of patients. In these cases, open reduction or arthroplasty of the femoral head should be performed.

In many cases, **open reduction and fixation of the coxofemoral luxation** may be necessary. This achieves a higher level of success than closed reduction. In addition, it allows the exploration of all the structures that make up the joint and permits the removal of soft tissue debris or clots from the acetabulum. There are different techniques described and the most appropriate one is selected depending on the damage to the bony structures and soft tissues that make up the joint.

The initial approach to the coxofemoral joint is **craniolateral**:

- The skin incision begins in the craniodorsal area of the greater trochanter and extends longitudinally along the cranial femoral border. Alternatively, a curvilinear incision can be made starting over the iliac wing cranial to the coxofemoral joint and continuing to the greater trochanter before running along the cranial edge of the femur.
- Next, the subcutaneous tissue is dissected and the superficial part of the fascia lata is incised until the fibers of the superficial gluteal, tensor fascia latae and biceps femoris muscles are visualized.
- The biceps femoris muscle is retracted caudally and the deep part of the fascia lata is incised between the three muscles described.
- Next, the tensor fascia latae is retracted cranially and the biceps femoris is retracted caudally with a Gelpi retractor. Care must be taken at this point not to damage the sciatic nerve with the retractor.
- The superficial and medial gluteal muscles are then moved dorsally to visualize the deep gluteus, whose insertion tendon on the greater trochanter may need to be partially sectioned for better exposure. This tenotomy should be performed leaving a few millimeters of its insertion into the trochanter, so that it can be sutured at closure. Once this is done, the joint capsule or its remnants attached to the acetabular rim and femoral neck can be visualized.
- If the entire joint cannot be visualized or if damage to the joint structures warrants further exposure, this approach can be combined with an osteotomy of the greater trochanter of the femur to retract the gluteal muscles dorsally, and can also be used as another method of joint stabilization, as described below.

If the joint is found to have capsular tissue remnants that can be reconstructed, **capsulorrhaphy** can be performed. Simple interrupted sutures can be placed in a U or cross shape using nonabsorbable monofilament material. Braided suture, absorbable or nonabsorbable, can also be used to make it more difficult to break. If this suture is properly performed, the success rate increases considerably.

> In the case of another open reduction technique, whenever possible, capsulorrhaphy should be added as a supplementary technique to achieve greater joint stability.

There may be cases in which the capsule remnants are badly damaged or have become detached from the acetabular rim, and some other additional technique should be used to achieve greater stability. In these cases, the **joint capsule can be replaced with prosthetic material**. This requires a craniolateral and dorsal approach to the joint, accompanied in many cases by an osteotomy of the greater trochanter of the femur. Two screws are placed in the dorsal acetabular rim (imagining a clock, at 10 o'clock and 1 o'clock in the left hip, and at 11 o'clock and 2 o'clock in the right hip) and a tunnel is made in a caudocranial direction in the femoral neck. Sutures are then placed at the heads of both screws, joining them together and passing through the perforated tunnel to achieve dorsal stabilization of the joint. Several sutures can be placed in a mesh-like fashion to provide greater stability and decrease the probability of the technique failing.

Transposition of the greater trochanter of the femur can be used in cases where trochanter osteotomy has been necessary in order to visualize the entire joint or to perform a capsulorrhaphy, although it can also be part of the initial surgical plan. The greater trochanter is transposed distally and caudally, approximately 1 cm from its original position. It should be fixed to the femur with two Kirschner wires and a tension band or with a long screw (Fig. 10). This technique uses the tendons of the gluteal muscles that insert into the trochanter to add stability.

Another technique is the placement of an **iliofemoral suture**, which keeps the femur internally rotated and adducted, in addition to maintaining ventromedial compression. This technique can be used if reluxation does not occur during surgery when the femur is placed in this position and if there are no avulsion fractures. Two tunnels are made, one in the greater trochanter of the femur using a drill bit from caudal to cranial and protruding at the base of the femoral neck, and the other in the ventral edge of the ilium cranial and as close as possible to the acetabulum. Several strands of braided suture in a figure of 8 are passed through these tunnels, and they are knotted while adduction and internal rotation of the extremity is performed. Capsulorrhaphy should also be performed to the extent possible to achieve greater success with the technique.

Temporary transarticular pinning may also be used, especially in cases where early weight-bearing on the limb is required, such as in cats with injuries to other limbs. A 1.5–2.0 mm Kirschner wire should be used. The pin is placed in a retrograde fashion from the femoral head fovea, passing through the femoral neck and exiting near the trochanter. It is then advanced until the tip is just at the level of the femoral head. The luxation is reduced with a slight abduction of the limb and the pin is inserted until it traverses the acetabular wall and penetrates the pelvic canal. The pin must be bent and cut at the level of the trochanter so that it can be removed later. This pin should be kept in place for 2–3 weeks while all the joint structures damaged by the luxation recover.

Another possible technique is the placement of a 2 mm **toggle rod** and associated suture material (monofilament nylon or braided polyester) in order to mimic the function of the round ligament, achieve early weight-bearing on the limb and allow the periarticular soft tissues to heal. For this, a routine approach to the coxofemoral joint is performed. The remains of the round ligament, clots and soft tissues still inside the acetabulum are removed and the remains of the joint capsule are maintained in order to perform a capsulorrhaphy. Taking care not to perforate the rectum, a hole is drilled in the acetabular fossa, with a diameter larger than that of the toggle rod to be used (in cats this usually requires a 2.7 mm drill bit). A tunnel is then drilled through the femur with a 2 mm drill bit, passing from the femoral head fovea to the lateral aspect of the femur at the level of the third trochanter, with a sufficient diameter for the two suture threads to pass through. The toggle rod is placed through the acetabular hole and the suture ends are pulled to position it on the medial aspect of the acetabulum. The suture ends are passed through the tunnel made in the femur until they protrude through the lateral aspect of the femur. The luxation is reduced and the threads are tightened, then the sutures are fixed with another toggle rod. Fixation can also be done by drilling another tunnel through the femur from its lateral cortical area (in the diaphysis, in a caudocranial direction). The suture ends are then passed through it and knotted or fixed with a metallic crimp tube. The system is tightened to prevent subluxation of the joint, but not so tight as to limit joint movement (Fig. 11).

As mentioned above, in cases in which reduction with closed or open techniques fails, there are fractures of the acetabular ring or femoral head or neck, the luxations are old or show signs of joint degeneration, or there is hip dysplasia, **arthroplasty of the femoral head and neck** (Fig. 12) or the

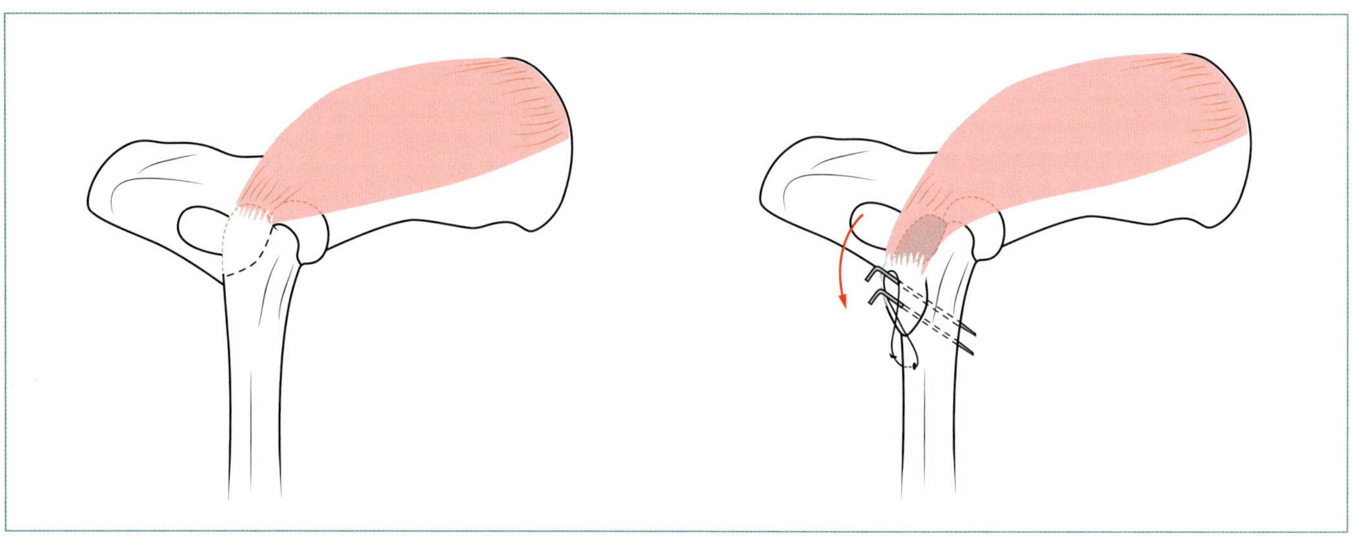

FIGURE 10. Transposition of the greater trochanter of the femur. Fixation with Kirschner wires and a tension band.

placement of a **hip prosthesis** may be chosen to achieve adequate functionality of the limb.

Hip replacements are not as well established as they are in dogs, partly because of the good prognosis for hip arthroplasty in cats, as they are light-weight animals that recover well and quickly.

The approach to the joint to perform an **osteotomy of the femoral head and neck** is craniolateral, as described above. An incision is made between the fascia lata and the biceps femoris muscle. The muscle groups are retracted until the coxofemoral joint is exposed. In cats, a more extensive exposure than in dogs is required to correctly visualize the entire femoral neck. For this purpose, a partial tenotomy of the deep biceps muscle can be performed and the dissection can be extended by retracting part of the vastus lateralis muscle. The limb is externally rotated and the patella is moved upwards until the cranial part of the femur can be seen. An osteotomy is then performed on the femoral neck from the intertrochanteric fossa to just in front of the lesser trochanter to ensure that there are no remnants of the femoral neck that could rub against the acetabulum and cause pain when bearing weight on the limb. The prognosis in these cases is usually very good, achieving good functionality at 4–5 weeks and a practically complete recovery in a period of about 5 months.

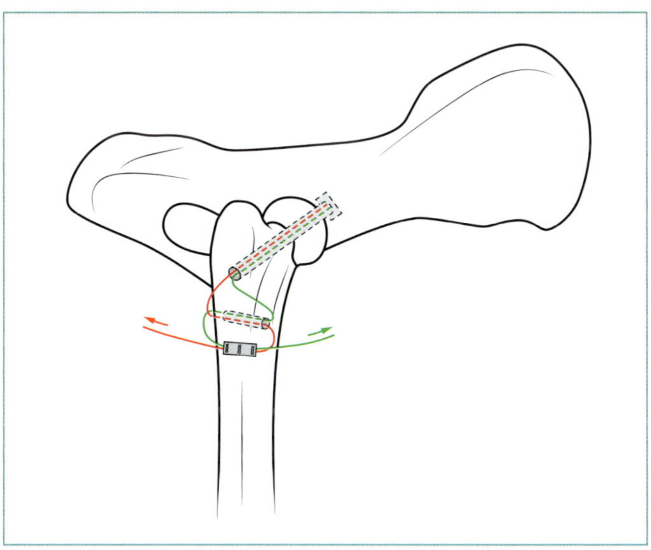

FIGURE 11. Diagram of the placement of a toggle rod to replace the function of the round ligament.

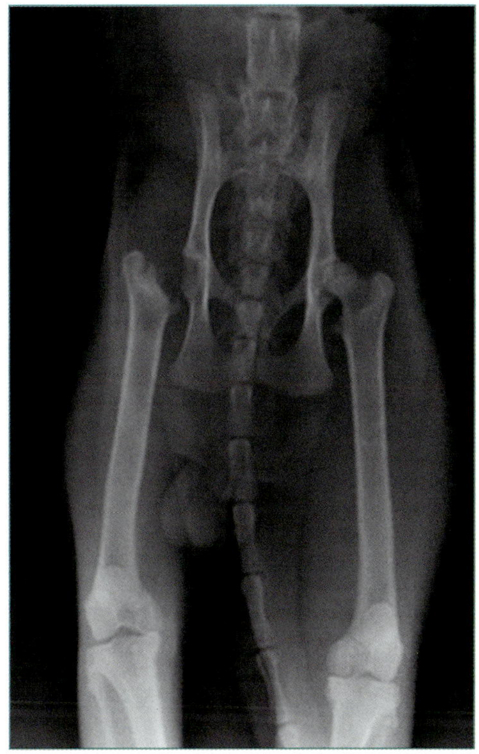

FIGURE 12. Right hip arthroplasty.

Complications

As mentioned above, reluxation is a common complication in these cases. Ehmer-type immobilizing bandages are usually not well tolerated by cats, so it is preferable to keep the animal's mobility reduced. Initially the cat should be kept in a carrier for approximately 10 days, although this may also complicate the patient's rest as it tries to escape from the carrier. Then, relative rest should be implemented for 2–3 weeks, restricting movements to walking only, with no climbing heights, jumping or playing. Correct femoral head placement should be confirmed 10 days after the reduction via X-ray. Instances in which the reduction is maintained may initially be as high as 85%, but in the long term this percentage decreases. If this has not been achieved, joint arthroplasty may be necessary.

If transarticular pinning is used, the complications observed include damage to the articular cartilage, subluxation of the femoral head if the pin is not correctly positioned, migration or breakage of the pin, bone resorption around the pin and perforation of the rectum with the tip of the pin.

The complications described associated with the use of the toggle rod include a reduction in pelvic diameter of approximately 16%, although no consequences of this reduction have been described. Severe bleeding can also occur if the acetabular fossa is perforated and the vessels just behind the acetabulum are damaged. Reluxation with this system has been described at an incidence of 14% in cats.

As for complications, if an osteotomy of the femoral head and neck is performed, one possibility is that a bony prominence may be left, which could rub against the acetabulum. This causes pain due to friction between the bony structures, so it is important to ensure no femoral neck remnants are left behind. If, after performing the osteotomy, any portion of the femoral neck remains, it can be removed using gouge forceps or a bone file.

Another possible complication of this technique is performing the osteotomy in the wrong direction, resulting in the fracture of part of the femoral diaphysis, the greater trochanter or the lesser trochanter of the femur. This results in the disinsertion of the muscles found in these bony prominences and their displacement and reduced function, with subsequent atrophy and decreased mobility of the limb.

These complications related to the direction of the osteotomy can be lessened with an adequate, wide approach to the joint and rotation of the extremity to visualize the cut line. Presurgical X-rays should also be obtained to facilitate planning the procedure and appropriate equipment should be used to perform the procedure, such as an oscillating saw with the appropriate blade for the size of the bone.

Postoperative pain should be controlled in an attempt for the cat to restore full function of the limb as soon as possible, in order to avoid muscle atrophy that delays weight-bearing or from which recovery is difficult. It may be necessary to administer analgesics for a long period of time to achieve earlier use of the limb. This also helps with rehabilitation, as the patient is more cooperative if they feel less pain. If possible, physiotherapy and rehabilitation should begin very early in order to recover the functionality of the limb faster. Hip extension and flexion movements are performed to recover as much range of motion as possible.

Bibliography

Bookbinder P, Flanders J. Characteristics of pelvic fracture in the cat. *Vet Comp Orthop Traumatol*, 1992; 5(3):122–127.

Burger M, Forterre F, Brunnberg L. Surgical anatomy of the feline sacroiliac joint for lag screw fixation of sacroiliac fracture-luxation. *Vet Comp Orthop Traumatol*, 2004; 17(3):146–151.

Burton NJ. Composite fixation of comminuted ilial wing fractures in cats: three cases. *J Feline Med Surg*, 2011; 13(5):376–382.

De Vicente F. Cadera. In: Calvo I, De Vicente F, Solano M, Aisa J (eds.). *Ortopedia en pequeños animales. El miembro posterior*. Zaragoza, Spain: Servet-Grupo Asís Biomedia, 2020; pp. 7–27.

Forterre F, Tomek A, Rytz U et al. Iatrogenic sciatic nerve injury in eighteen dogs and nine cats (1997–2006). *Vet Surg*, 2007; 36(5):464–471.

Haine DL, Parsons K, Barthelemy N et al. Outcome of surgical stabilisation of acetabular fractures in 16 cats. *J Feline Med Surg*, 2019; 21(6):520–528.

Han CK, Kang J, Lee H et al. Evaluation of a screw insertion landmark for a minimally invasive repair technique in induced bilateral sacroiliac luxation in feline cadavers. *J Feline Med Surg*, 2022; 24(2):152–159.

Johnson KA. *Piermattei's Atlas of Surgical Approaches to the Bones and Joints of the Dog and Cat*. St. Louis, MO: Saunders, 2014.

Langley-Hobbs SJ, Sissener TR, Shales CJ. Tension band stabilisation of acetabular physeal fractures in four kittens. *J Feline Med Surg*, 2007; 9(3):177–187.

LeFloch MD, Coronado GS. Outcome of coxofemoral luxation treated with closed reduction in 51 cats. *J Feline Med Surg*, 2022; 24(8):709–714.

Liska WD. Micro total hip replacement for dogs and cats: surgical technique and outcomes. *Vet Surg*, 2010; 39(7):797–810.

Meeson R, Corr S. Management of pelvic trauma: neurological damage, urinary tract disruption and pelvic fractures. *J Feline Med Surg*, 2011; 13(5):347–361.

Meeson RL, Geddes AT. Management and long-term outcome of pelvic fractures: a retrospective study of 43 cats. *J Feline Med Surg*, 2017; 19(1):36–41.

Parslow A, Simpson DJ. Bilateral sacroiliac luxation fixation using a single transiliosacral pin: surgical technique and clinical outcomes in eight cats. *J Small Anim Pract*, 2017; 58(6):330–336.

Philp H, Durand A, De Vicente F. Use of computed tomography to define a sacral safe corridor for placement of 2.7 mm cortical screws in feline sacroiliac luxation. *J Feline Med Surg*, 2018; 20(6):487–493.

Piermattei DLF, Gretchen L, DeCamp CE. *Brinker, Piermattei, and Flo's Handbook of Small Animal Orthopedics and Fracture Repair*, 4th ed. St. Louis, MO: Saunders/Elsevier, 2006.

Pratesi A, Grierson J, Moores AP. Toggle rod stabilisation of coxofemoral luxation in 14 cats. *J Small Anim Pract*, 2012; 53(5):260–266.

Pratesi A, Grierson JM, Moores AP. Single transsacral screw and nut stabilization of bilateral sacroiliac luxation in 20 cats. *Vet Comp Orthop Traumatol*, 2018; 31(1):44–52.

Scott HW, McLaughlin R. Fractures and disorders of the hindlimb. In: Scott HW, McLaughlin R. *Feline Orthopedics*. London, UK: Manson Publishing, 2007; pp. 167–191.

Shales C, Moores A, Kulendra E et al. Stabilization of sacroiliac luxation in 40 cats using screws inserted in lag fashion. *Vet Surg*, 2010; 39(6):696–700.

Shales CJ, White L, Langley-Hobbs SJ. Sacroiliac luxation in the cat: defining a safe corridor in the dorsoventral plane for a screw insertion in lag fashion. *Vet Surg*, 2009; 38(3):343–348.

Sissener TR, Whitelock RG, Langley-Hobbs SJ. Long-term results of transarticular pinning for surgical stabilisation of coxofemoral luxation in 20 cats. *J Small Anim Pract*, 2009; 50(3):112–117.

Voss K, Langley-Hobbs SJ, Borer L, Montavon PM. Pelvis. In: Montavon PM, Voss K, Langley-Hobbs SJ (eds.). *Feline Orthopedic Surgery and Musculoskeletal Disease*. St. Louis, MO: Elsevier Saunders, 2009; pp. 423–441.

Voss K, Langley-Hobbs SJ, Montavon PM. Hip joint. In: Montavon PM, Voss K, Langley-Hobbs SJ (eds.). *Feline Orthopedic Surgery and Musculoskeletal Disease*. St. Louis, MO: Elsevier Saunders, 2009; pp. 443–454.

Yap FW, Dunn AL, Farrell M, Calvo I. Trans-iliac pin/bolt/screw internal fixation for sacroiliac luxation or separation in cats: six cases. *J Feline Med Surg*, 2014; 16(4):354–362.

Yap FW, Dunn AL, Garcia-Fernandez PM et al. Femoral head and neck excision in cats: medium- to long-term functional outcome in 18 cats. *J Feline Med Surg*, 2015; 17(8):704–710.

COMMON FRACTURES OF THE HIND LIMB IN POLYTRAUMATIZED CATS 33

Antonio Peña

Femoral fractures

Femoral fractures account for 30% of fractures in cats, making it the bone that is broken most often in this species, with this occurring most frequently in the diaphysis and the distal area. These are usually closed fractures because of the muscle tissue surrounding the femur. They are common after falls from heights and are usually accompanied by injuries to the abdomen, thorax or head and fractures in other areas such as the pelvis and spine.

> Femoral fractures must be repaired surgically in all cases, as stabilization with bandages or splints is not possible.

Conservative treatment with confinement in a very restricted space, such as a carrier, can only be considered for some diaphyseal greenstick fractures that occur in very young kittens.

TABLE 1. Types of femoral fractures according to anatomical region

Anatomical region	Bone location
Proximal femoral fractures	■ Proximal epiphysis ■ Proximal physis ■ Subcapital ■ Femoral neck ■ Trochanteric and subtrochanteric
Diaphyseal femoral fractures	—
Distal femoral fractures	■ Supracondylar ■ Distal physis ■ Condylar

But this can also cause more nervousness as the kitten tries to get out, which would be counterproductive to the proper ossification of the femur. In addition, surgery should be performed as soon as possible to prevent contracture of the quadriceps. This injury is more frequent in diaphyseal fractures and when there is damage to this muscle, such as hematomas or tears.

Implants should be chosen taking into account the forces that this bone withstands, i.e., rotational, torsional, axial and bending forces.

To facilitate their description, femoral fractures can be classified according to the area where they occur: proximal region, femoral diaphysis and distal region (Table 1).

Fractures of the proximal femur

The most common fractures in this area are in the femoral head at the level of the growth plate and in the femoral neck.

Fractures in the physis of the femoral head may be due to traumatic causes in young animals, less than 12 months of age, in which the growth plate is not yet closed (Fig. 1). This growth plate closes at about 30–40 weeks of age. They can also be found in animals older than 1 year of age without being related to trauma. It is thought that in these cats there has been a delay in the closure of this physis as a consequence of metaphyseal alterations and growth plate dysplasia. This delay in closure has been observed more frequently in males sterilized before reaching puberty, and in the physis of the greater trochanter, in the distal area of the femur and in the growth plate of the tibial tuberosity. It occurs more frequently in large cats, such as the Maine Coon, Ragdoll and Norwegian Forest breeds, but it can also occur in nonpurebred cats; no statistically significant breed predisposition has been found.

Most of these cats are lame and do not bear weight on the affected limb, although some patients may show only mild lameness. On examination, pain, crepitus and decreased range of motion of the hip joint are observed.

The definitive diagnosis will be obtained via X-rays. It can be difficult to diagnose these fractures in the ventrodorsal projection with the extremities extended, as the fragment may move to a normal position, so it is necessary to also take X-rays with the hips flexed (frog-leg position) to make the diagnosis.

It is important to know whether there is a history of trauma as a possible cause of the fracture, since treatment differs according to its etiology. In cats that have not suffered trauma, lameness is usually progressive and often bilateral. Two possible causes have been described for femoral head fracture to occur without a history of trauma:

- One of them is physeal dysplasia, possibly due to a multicentric alteration in the chondrocytes (in different growth plates), leading to their separation. These are also called spontaneous fractures of the femoral head physis. It may be difficult to differentiate these cases from a traumatic fracture on X-rays, although spontaneous femoral capital physeal fractures usually occur in cats older than 2 years of age.
- The other cause is a metaphyseal osteopathy of the femoral neck that occurs in older animals, with the radiographic appearance of an older fracture due to the signs of remodeling that occur.

Treatment

Conservative treatment is not recommended in these fractures, since in many cases it leads to malunions and the consequent appearance of hypertrophic pseudarthrosis and chronic lameness (Fig. 2).

Surgical treatment offers better and shorter recoveries, with minimal complications. Even with less than perfect fracture reduction, good results can be achieved. As discussed above, treatment options will differ depending on whether there is a history of trauma, with the goal of restoring the original anatomy of the femoral head and neck in cases of traumatic fractures. This is not recommended in nontraumatic fractures, or old traumatic fractures, due to the remodeling that the fracture fragments will have undergone. In these cases, the most appropriate option is to perform an arthroplasty via osteotomy of the femoral head and neck.

A **craniolateral approach** to the hip joint is performed to reach the femoral head and neck, both to reduce and fix the fracture and to perform the hip arthroplasty. If access to the greater trochanter or third trochanter is required, the incision is extended laterally to the femoral diaphysis, identifying and protecting the sciatic nerve during dissection. It may be necessary to perform a partial tenotomy of the deep gluteal muscle tendon

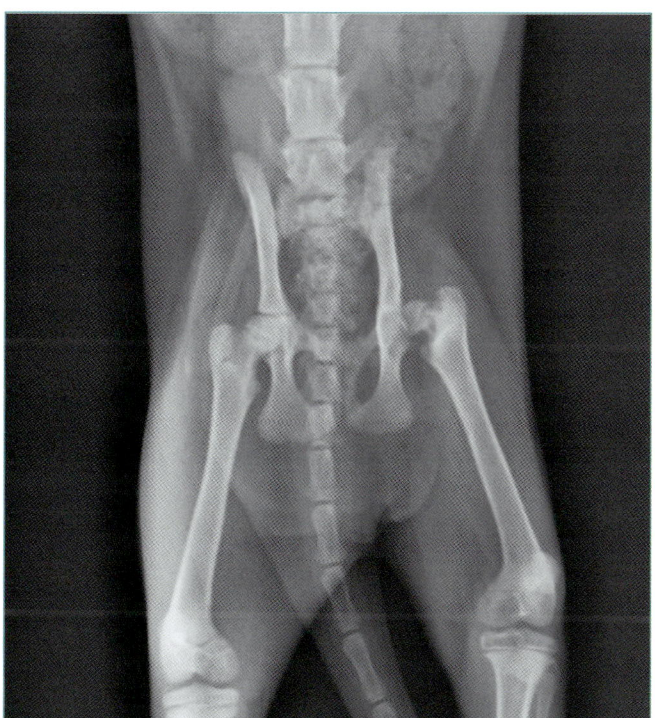

FIGURE 1. Fracture of the femoral head physis.

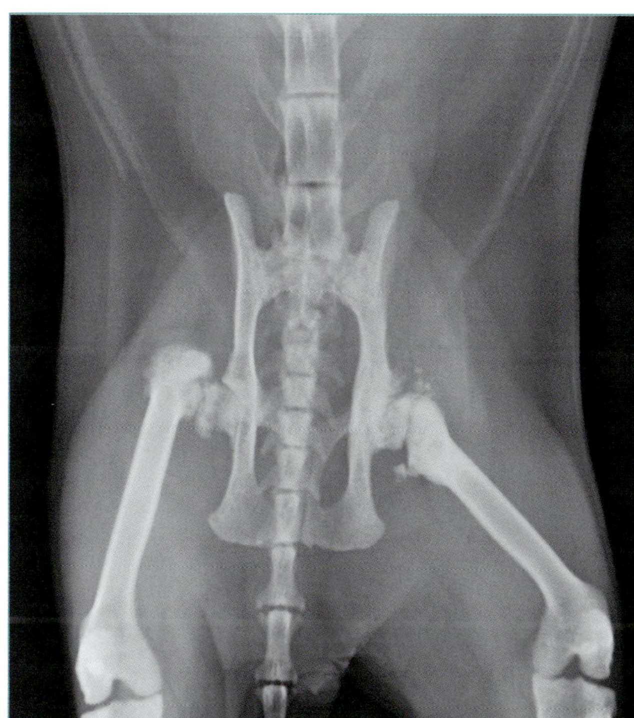

FIGURE 2. Old fractures of both femoral necks, with signs of severe osteoarthrosis and decreased range of motion in both hips.

to better access the joint. A longitudinal incision is then made in the joint capsule to access the fracture of the femoral head and neck.

A **ventral approach** to the coxofemoral joint can also be performed, with the cat lying on its back and the hind limbs abducted. A pectinectomy may be necessary. This approach is much more complicated, as care must be taken not to damage important structures during dissection, such as the femoral artery and vein, the saphenous nerve and the medial circumflex femoral vein and artery.

In the case of traumatic fractures, attempts may be made to reduce the fracture and fix the femoral head using two 1–1.2 mm Kirschner wires. These wires should be placed parallel to each other to avoid damaging the vascularization of the growth plate (Fig. 3). The parallel position of the Kirschner wires also confers more stability than if they are placed divergently. In animals younger than 7 months of age, there is a large blood supply to the femoral head through a vessel in the round ligament (unlike in dogs), so all structures must be handled carefully so as not to damage that vascularization. For this reason, normograde rather than retrograde placement is recommended to reduce fragment manipulation and avoid vessel damage. The Kirschner wires are placed from the caudolateral area of the third trochanter through the femoral neck and inserted into the femoral head without protruding to avoid damaging the coxofemoral joint. It can be ensured that they do not protrude by passing a blunt instrument over the surface of the femoral head. In addition, full flexion and extension movements are performed to check that the range of motion is correct without detecting friction. Finally, the Kirschner wires are bent before cutting to prevent them from migrating.

In large cats, a combination of a cortical screw together with a Kirschner wire to prevent rotation can be used to fix these fractures. This method is not advised in young animals, as it may further damage vascularization in the growth plate.

After surgery, a 4-week rest period should be provided, limiting the patient's movement until correct ossification is achieved.

In the case of avulsion of a femoral head fragment, this fragment may be too small to be fixed. In these cases, Kirschner wires can be placed in a retrograde fashion, cut at the level of the head and pushed so that they do not rub in the acetabular cavity. If surgery is unsuccessful or the fragment is too small, **hip arthroplasty via osteotomy of the femoral head and neck** (described in Ch. 32) must be performed, as well as in cases of old fractures or fractures not due to trauma. For many authors, due to the good functionality obtained without noteworthy complications in cats, it is the treatment of choice for fractures of this type, regardless of whether or not the cause is traumatic, or whether the fracture is old or recent (Fig. 4).

Another treatment option, although less frequent in part because of the good results of hip arthroplasty in cats, is the placement of a hip prosthesis, with increasingly better results.

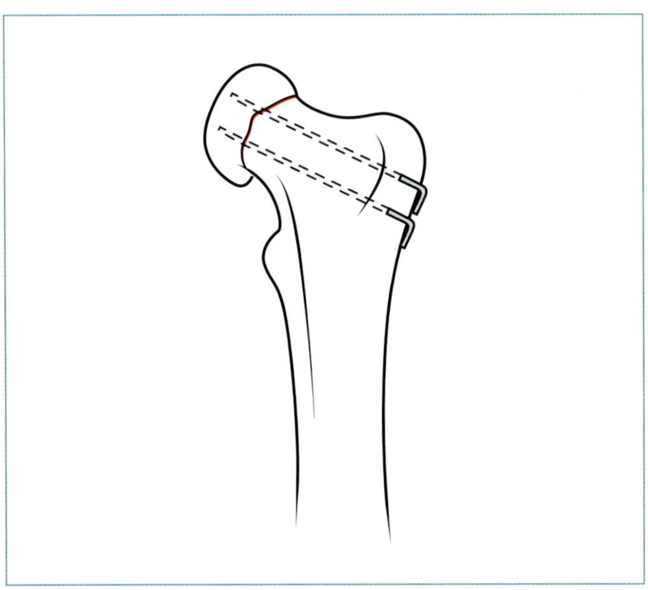

FIGURE 3. Placement of two Kirschner wires to fix a fracture of the femoral head physis.

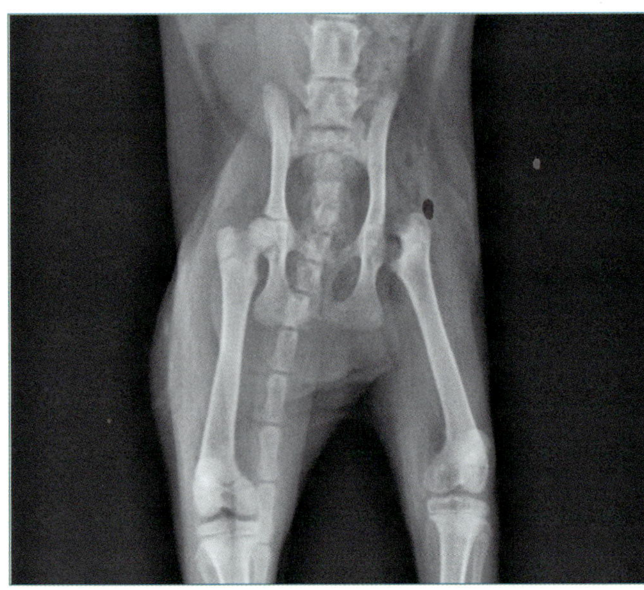

FIGURE 4. Resolution of the case in Figure 1 via osteotomy of the femoral head and neck.

Complications

One complication in this type of fracture is the tips of the Kirschner wires rubbing in the acetabular cavity. This is more likely when the wires need to be placed in a normograde fashion. This risk is reduced by correctly measuring the length of the wires. Measures can be taken from the X-ray of the contralateral femur, if it is not fractured. Otherwise, it should be verified that the tips of the Kirschner wires do not protrude by palpating the surface of the femoral head with a blunt instrument.

Kirschner wire migration may occur, either protruding through the femoral head or coming out at the level of its insertion in the third trochanter. In these cases, it may be necessary to remove the Kirschner wires or reposition them if ossification of the fracture has not yet been achieved.

In these fractures, there is always a risk for avascular necrosis of the femoral head and neck, both because of the fracture itself and because of the implants used for fixation. In such cases, there is a narrowing of the femoral neck and a displacement of the femoral head, which are visible on X-rays starting 4 weeks after surgery. If the necrosis does not progress further, it can be considered part of the normal remodeling process of these fractures, with a thickening of the femoral neck to its normal thickness being seen later.

In cases where fixation fails, femoral head and neck osteotomy or prosthesis placement, as mentioned previously, may be required to preserve limb function. As discussed in the previous chapter, one of the complications when performing femoral head and neck osteotomy is making the femoral neck cut in the wrong direction. Figures 5 and 6 show an example of this complication, in which osteotomy of the greater trochanter of the femur was caused in a case with spontaneous fracture of both femoral heads, appearing at different times.

Fractures of the femoral diaphysis

Diaphyseal femoral fractures require fixation in virtually all cases. Clinical signs include severe pain with a complete lack of weight-bearing on the affected limb.

Many of these fractures are comminuted and there may be significant damage to nearby soft tissues. Open fractures are not frequent, but large hematomas and significant muscle damage may be found as the fragments pass through the muscles surrounding the femur (Fig. 7). The reduction of diaphyseal femoral fractures is performed in an open manner, since closed reduction is difficult to achieve due to the muscles surrounding the femur. The integrity of the quadriceps femoris muscle should be checked for lacerations, edema or hemorrhages under its fascia, which can lead to fibrosis of this muscle and the consequent risk of contracture.

Treatment

The **surgical approach** is performed laterally with a straight incision over the craniolateral border of the femur:

- The skin and subcutaneous tissue is incised and then the fascia is incised over the cranial aspect of the biceps

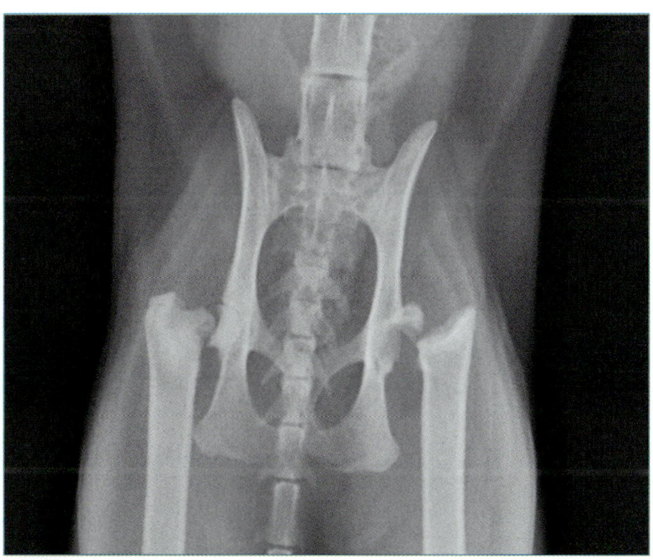

FIGURE 5. Complication of a left femoral neck osteotomy, in which the greater trochanter was affected by an incorrect cutting direction. Fracture of the right femoral head physis appeared later.

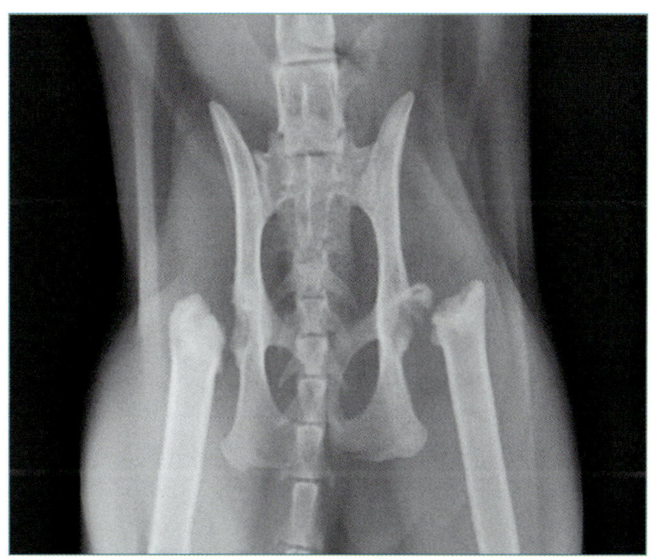

FIGURE 6. Right femoral neck osteotomy with correct orientation.

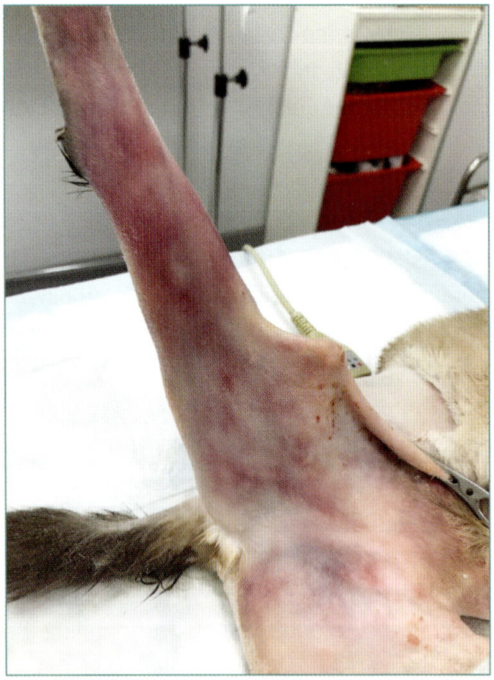

FIGURE 7. Displaced diaphyseal femoral fracture and secondary hematoma.

femoris muscle. This muscle is retracted caudally to expose the femur. Retraction must be performed carefully so as not to damage the sciatic nerve with the instruments, as this nerve runs parallel to the caudal edge of the femur.

- The vastus lateralis muscle is then retracted cranially, exposing the femoral diaphysis.
- Care must also be taken when reducing the fracture, avoiding damage to the soft tissues surrounding the femoral diaphysis.

There may be a large overlap of fracture fragments and significant retraction is necessary to achieve reduction. One technique can be to stretch the limb manually to relax the muscle contracture once the patient has been anesthetized. Also, after approaching the fracture, the bone fragments can be held by forceps to separate them by exerting continuous and progressive traction. In uncomplicated fractures, the fragments can be aligned by means of an intramedullary pin and the muscles can be stretched. In addition, this intramedullary pin can be part of the fracture fixation system; for example, by combining it with an osteosynthesis plate. In more complex cases, where it is difficult to stretch the muscle contracture to align the fragments, a distractor, similar to a fixator, can be used, which by means of a screw mechanism helps stretch the musculature and achieve fracture reduction.

There are different methods for fixing these fractures (Fig. 8), depending on the type. In general, being a relatively straight bone in the cat, the use of osteosynthesis plates and intramedullary pins or nails is indicated. An external fixator with different compositions can also be used to stabilize these fractures, especially in comminuted fractures and in young animals.

Precisely because of the straight shape of the femur in cats, minimally invasive techniques have been described for the treatment of diaphyseal femoral fractures. If used, special attention should be paid to the alignment of the proximal and distal femur to avoid rotated positions. Fracture reduction and stabilization is performed by placing the implants without using an approach that exposes the fracture site. This reduces the iatrogenic damage that may be caused to the soft tissues. It is very helpful to have an intraoperative imaging system (fluoroscopy), which is not possible in many veterinary centers.

An alternative to this would be a traditional approach to the femoral diaphysis and an open reduction, but in this case the anatomical alignment of the bone would be performed without removing the hematoma or separating the soft tissue insertions of the fragments. This method respects the vascularization of the fragments as much as possible and favors fracture ossification, without the need for fluoroscopy.

Different osteosynthesis plate models can be chosen to fix the fracture, depending on the type. In uncomplicated transverse diaphyseal fractures, a dynamic compression plate can

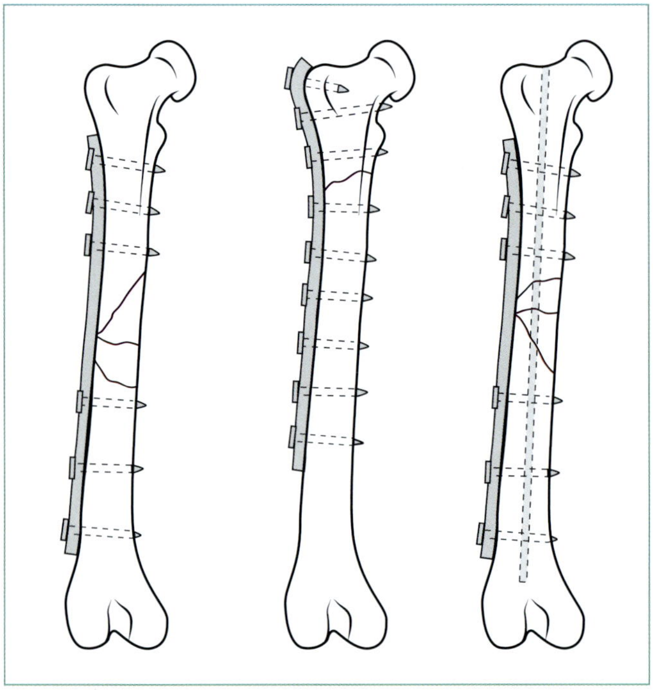

FIGURE 8. Fixation with osteosynthesis plate in different types of diaphyseal femoral fractures.

be used to achieve better fixation. In oblique fractures, compression of the fracture site cannot be performed, so a neutralization plate, a reconstruction plate or also a compression plate, but using it as a neutralization plate, can be placed. In comminuted fractures, a bridging plate or a neutralization or compression plate is used, but placed as a bridging plate. Locking plates can also be used in all these fractures. Another possibility, especially in small animals, is to use cuttable plates in all these types of fractures to accommodate the size of the femur. These are used as a neutralizing or a bridging plate, not as a compression plate. In addition, they allow more screws to be placed than is possible with a compression plate of the same length, as they have more holes.

As for intramedullary pins, they can also be used as the sole fixation system, although more stability can be gained if they are combined with an osteosynthesis plate or a type I external fixator. It is advisable to place the pin in a normograde fashion from the trochanteric fossa and introduce it as far as the distal femur until anchoring it in the metaphysis. It can be placed in a retrograde fashion, but this is not indicated as often, since there is a greater risk of injuring the sciatic nerve.

Another option is the use of 2.5–4.7 mm interlocking nails. Again, this is a suitable system due to the straight shape of the feline femur. These nails have a number of advantages, such as preserving the periosteal vascularization or preserving the hematoma at the fracture site to improve ossification.

An external fixator can be used in any type of fracture of the femoral diaphysis (Figs. 9 and 10), but it is indicated more for fractures with several fragments that are difficult to reconstruct. Ideally, 1.5–2 mm positive-profile threaded pins should be used, placing three pins in each fragment of the fracture, although depending on the size of the fragment, it may be possible to place only two. In comminuted fractures, these pins are placed in the proximal and distal fragments of the femur to align them and achieve the appropriate length of the femur, which is calculated on an X-ray image of the contralateral femur. Special attention must be paid to the alignment of the proximal and distal areas of the femur to avoid rotations and, consequently, poor weight-bearing and lateral or medial luxation of the patella.

> To correctly orient the fragments, the greater trochanter of the femur must be positioned laterally and the femoral condyles must be placed in the same position.

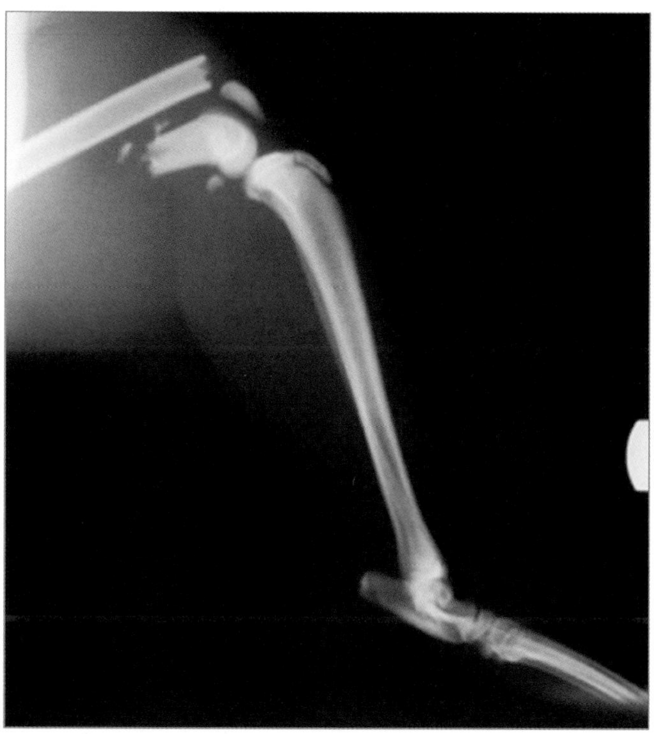

FIGURE 9. Distal diaphyseal femoral fracture.

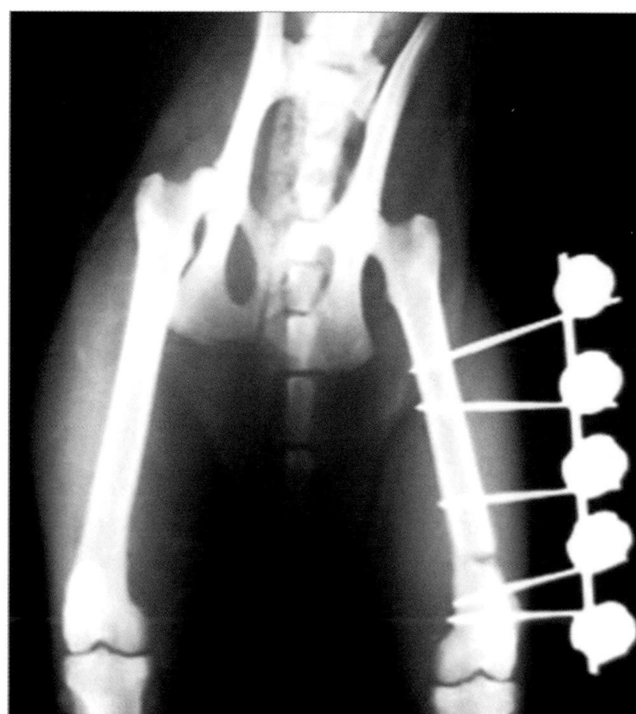

FIGURE 10. Type I external fixator with 2 mm positive-profile threaded pins for resolution of the fracture in Figure 7.

In adult cats, with harder cortical surfaces, it is better to make a hole with a diameter smaller than the threaded pin (0.1 mm less) beforehand and then place the pin at a low speed to avoid excessive heat in the bone. In young cats, it is not necessary to perforate the bone cortex beforehand, as the bone is softer. If nonthreaded pins are used, they should be angled so that they do not slip out. Once the pins are in place, they are attached to the connecting bar. To give more stability to the construct, two connecting bars can be placed together and the pins can be fixed to both bars. Instead of connecting bars, epoxy putty can be used to fix the pins together. Another option is to combine the fixator with an intramedullary pin attached to the connecting bar (tie-in configuration).

All of these fixation methods generally have a good success rate in the treatment of diaphyseal femoral fractures. In the case of external fixators, more care is required to avoid complications in the pin tracts and additional radiographic examinations are needed. The use of interlocking nails is a system with very few complications and good results.

Complications

The sciatic nerve and other soft tissues surrounding the femur may be damaged by the fracture itself (by the bone fragments), by the surgical approach or by the implants placed to fix the fracture. The last two cases can be prevented during surgery, so a careful approach must be taken to identify and protect these structures.

In this type of fractures, external fixators are the method with the most complications, followed by osteosynthesis plates. The combination of a plate with an intramedullary pin is the technique that causes the least complications; however, although there are fewer complications, they are more serious. On the other hand, although complications in fractures treated with external fixators are more numerous, they are less severe. This is influenced by the fracture type, patient characteristics and the surgeon's choice of fixation method, which may result in a bias in this data.

The complications observed with the placement of external fixators include patellar luxation due to rotation of the femoral longitudinal axis, irritations and seromas in the area where the pins exit through the skin, loss of fixation of the pins and fractures after removal of the implants.

When using interlocking nails, care should be taken not to insert them too cranially into the distal fragment, as they may damage the intercondylar area of the femur along their tract. This can also occur with intramedullary pins or nails.

Rotation of the femur due to misalignment of the proximal and distal fragments can occur with any fixation method. It is more common for this error to be made in comminuted fractures in which these fragments are not reconstructed and only the proximal and distal femur are fixed. As previously mentioned, the greater trochanter of the femur and the femoral condyles must be correctly oriented to prevent this rotation from occurring.

Contracture of the quadriceps is another complication that can occur in this type of fracture. This can lead to hip subluxation and patellar luxation. Extensive bruising and tears in the fasciae and muscle fibers of the quadriceps can lead to fibrosis and contracture. Likewise, contracture can occur in the absence of correct ossification of the fracture. It can also occur due to not correctly bearing weight on the limb because of bandages or pain, which causes a sustained extension of the limb and the appearance of a contracture. This complication can be prevented with an atraumatic approach, proper fixation and preoperative and postoperative pain management, which will allow the cat to use and bear weight on the limb. Adequate analgesia must be administered for the period of time required for each patient. Another recommended practice to prevent this injury is to perform passive flexion and extension movements of the stifle as soon as possible after surgery.

Fractures of the distal femur

Distal femoral fractures are common in cats that fall from heights. Most of them are Salter–Harris type I and II fractures (see Ch. 31). Intercondylar and supracondylar fractures may also be found. These fractures must be differentiated from instability of the stifle joint and, to do so, attention must be paid to the presence of crepitus and proper palpation must be performed.

Treatment

Surgical access is performed based on the location of the fracture within that area. In many cases, a craniolateral parapatellar approach to the stifle joint is used, as most of these fractures are in an intracapsular location. But there are other cases of supracondylar fractures above the joint capsule, in which the approach is extended laterally to the distal femoral diaphysis. In many cases of intercondylar fractures, it is necessary to combine the lateral and medial approaches to properly place the implants to be used. Therefore, positioning the cat in dorsal recumbency facilitates the surgical accesses needed during surgery.

After incising the skin and subcutaneous tissue, the incision is extended over the fascia lata along the cranial edge of the biceps femoris muscle and then distally and parallel to the patellar ligament. Sufficient fascia should be left over the patella so that closure can be performed later. If necessary, access to the stifle joint is gained by incising the joint capsule.

Supracondylar fractures (Fig. 11) can be difficult to stabilize, especially if they are comminuted. Rotation or misalignment, which could cause patellar luxation, should be avoided. For this reason, the use of osteosynthesis plates or external fixators, instead of intramedullary pins, is recommended to obtain greater stability in the fracture, especially if the distal fragment is short. Ideally, an attempt should be made to place a sufficient number of screws or pins in the distal fragment.

Due to the inclination of the femoral condyle, J-shaped or "hockey stick" plates can be used, allowing three screws to be placed in the distal fragment. Plates of this type are commercially available for both the right and left femur. Reconstruction plates of 2.7 mm can also be used, which can be molded to adapt to the curvature of the distal femur and allow a few more screws to be placed than is possible in straight plates. If no more than two screws can be placed in the distal fragment, the plate should be accompanied by, for example, an intramedullary pin reaching that fragment. Another option, especially in comminuted fractures, is to place two plates, one lateral and one medial. Locking plates can also be used in all these fractures, with the advantage of being able to place monocortical screws and obtain great stability.

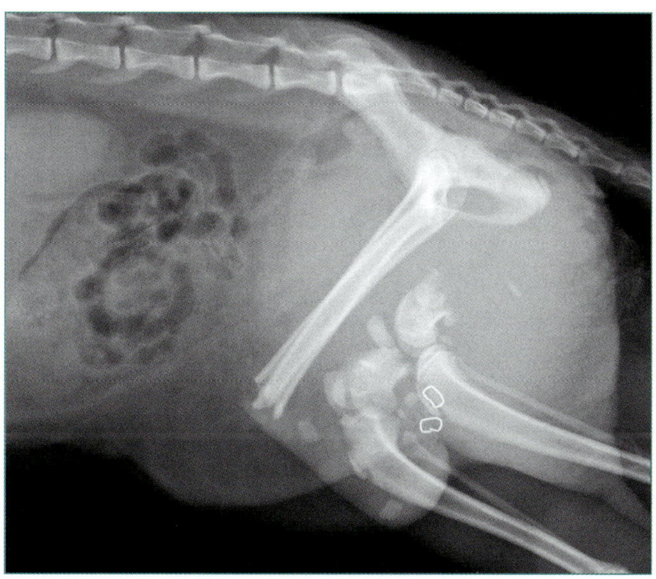

FIGURE 11. Bilateral supracondylar femoral fracture.

An alternative is the use of a modified type I or type II external fixator. An intramedullary pin attached to the connecting bar can be added (tie-in configuration). The placement of circular fixators has also been described.

The prognosis for this type of fracture is good with proper management and when anatomical reduction of the stifle is achieved.

Another type of fracture affecting this area of the femur is **distal physeal fractures**. Most are Salter–Harris type I (in cats around 9 months of age) or type II (in cats around 6 months of age) fractures. This physis closes between 54 and 76 weeks of age and, as with the femoral head physis, a delay in the closure of this growth plate is observed in young cats that have undergone early neutering, delaying its closure beyond 24 months of age.

Achieving the most correct reduction and fixation possible is paramount in these fractures to ensure adequate functionality of the stifle and promote subsequent growth in the physis. There is usually caudal displacement of the distal fragment due to the forces exerted by the gastrocnemius muscles, so the fragments must be tractioned and compressed for proper reduction. This is more easily achieved with the stifle extended. If double-point fragment reduction forceps are used to facilitate repositioning, care must be taken in young animals as the bone is softer.

The fixation method can be two cross pins or dynamic intramedullary pins. In the case of cross pins, these would be 1–1.5 mm Kirschner wires inserted cranial to the lateral and medial ligaments in the direction of the opposite cortical surface of the proximal fracture fragment, to anchor in the cortex. This fixation system has been found to be the strongest to counteract torsional forces. Such pins can also be placed so that they slide inside the diaphysis as dynamic intramedullary pins, instead of being anchored to the opposing cortical surfaces. Attempting to place a cross pin in order to anchor it in the opposite cortical surface may not be successful, and it may instead be placed in an intramedullary fashion. In such cases, the pin should be long enough to reach the greater trochanter of the femur. This system can also be used in supracondylar fractures (Figs. 12 and 13).

Regardless of the method of fixation, there should be no compression of the physis so as not to cause inadequate growth of the femur. In cats under 6 months of age, follow-up X-rays should be taken more frequently (every 2–4 weeks) to see if the implants need to be removed. However, in cases where premature closure of the growth plate occurs, it is not known whether this is due to the pins used for fracture fixation or as a direct consequence of trauma to the growth plate. In these patients, it is not necessary to remove the implants unless they cause a problem in the tissues or move out of place.

Femoral condyle fractures may involve one condyle, usually the medial condyle, or both condyles, usually referred to as T-fractures or Y-fractures. In bicondylar fractures, the meniscus and cruciate ligaments may be damaged, and there may also be a comminuted supracondylar fracture. All of these fractures require the most perfect anatomical reduction possible to restore the articular line and provide stable fracture fixation. This reduces the risk of joint degeneration in the stifle.

The surgical approach is performed with a lateral or medial parapatellar incision in the stifle, prolonging it as necessary on the lateral or medial aspect of the femoral diaphysis. In fractures involving one condyle, the fragment is usually not very displaced, as this is prevented by the cranial cruciate ligament and the medial collateral ligament.

Monocondylar fractures are usually fixed with a 2–2.7 mm intercondylar screw to produce interfragmentary compression, combined with a 0.8–1.2 mm transcondylar pin to prevent rotation of the fractured condyle. This pin can also be directed towards the diaphysis, anchoring it on the opposite cortical surface.

In **bicondylar fractures**, the intercondylar fracture is fixed in the same way, and then the condyles are fixed to the femoral diaphysis as explained for distal femoral physeal fractures or supracondylar fractures (Fig. 14).

Complications

In fractures that affect the growth plate, it is important to achieve good reduction and to use implants that do not hinder the correct development of the bone. In the event of uneven ossification along the femoral physis, corrective osteotomies should be performed at a later date to correct any deviations that may occur.

> The occurrence of complications is considerably reduced with the use of specific plates for this type of distal femoral fracture (hockey stick plates), reconstruction plates or locking plates.

The use of external fixators in distal femoral fractures may present certain complications such as secretions through the pin tracts. This is due to the mobility that the skin and soft tissue surrounding the stifle and the muscles surrounding the femur have around the pin.

As in all articular fractures, one possible complication is the development of osteoarthritis due to incorrect reduction or unstable fixation of the intra-articular fracture. Special attention

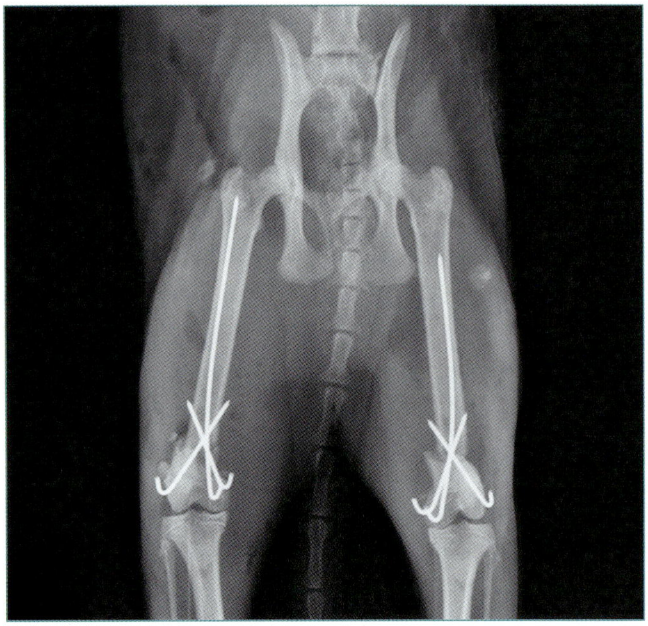

FIGURE 12. Craniocaudal X-ray showing the resolution of a bilateral supracondylar femoral fracture with cross pins and a dynamic intramedullary pin.

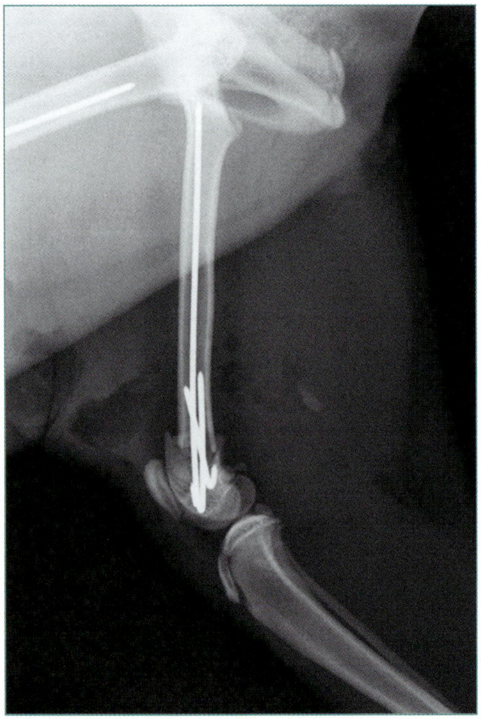

FIGURE 13. Mediolateral X-ray showing the resolution of a supracondylar femoral fracture with cross pins and a dynamic intramedullary pin.

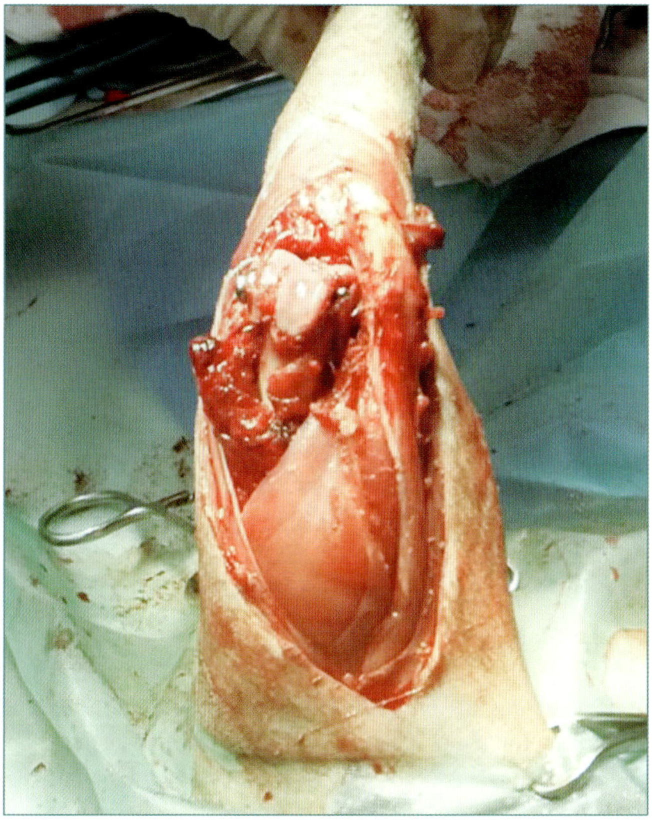

FIGURE 14. Resolution of a bicondylar fracture using a compression screw with a washer and cross pins. The muscle damage caused by the exit of the proximal fragment of the femur through the quadriceps muscle is observed.

should be paid to ensure correct alignment of the articular surface and to achieve compression of the fracture line. In young animals, in which the bone is softer, it may be necessary to add a washer when placing the intercondylar screw to prevent its head from penetrating the condyle and causing instability in the fixation.

Tibial and fibular fractures

Tibial and fibular fractures are frequent in cats, accounting for 5%–19% of all fractures. They are common in animals that are involved in road traffic accidents or fall from heights. Open fractures (Fig. 15) often occur, in up to 46% of cases, as the tibia has little soft tissue coverage on its medial aspect, and they occur frequently in cats that fall from heights, more so than with other types of trauma. There may be complications in the ossification of tibial fractures (delayed ossification, nonunion, osteomyelitis) due to several factors: due to the high frequency of open fractures, because in many cases they are comminuted fractures and also as a consequence of the low extraosseous vascular supply and the little soft tissue that covers the tibia.

Forms of stabilization

There are different forms of stabilization for fractures affecting the tibia, depending on the type of fracture and its location. Due to the anatomy of the area, in many cases a closed reduction and the placement of external fixators can be performed. However, placement of osteosynthesis plates using a minimal approach can also be performed.

External stabilization with bandages/splints may be performed in young kittens with greenstick fractures, transverse fractures or tibial fractures in which the fibula is intact. In these cases, the prognosis can be good. As these are growing kittens, the bandages should be changed every 7–10 days to avoid disturbing normal bone growth.

As the tibia is a straight bone, it allows the placement of an **intramedullary nail or pins** to stabilize fractures, but this is not used as much as in the femur or humerus. The pin must always be inserted in a normograde fashion, since the pin will exit through the tibial plateau and cross the patellar ligament if it is inserted in a retrograde fashion. The normograde insertion is performed on the medial aspect of the tibial plateau, between the insertion of the patellar ligament and the medial collateral ligament, cranial to the intermeniscal ligament (Fig. 16). The pin/nail gauge should be chosen according to the diameter of the medullary canal of the distal tibial diaphysis. The intramedullary pin is introduced up to the fracture site and, after reduction, the pin is further advanced to the distal diaphysis. Care should be taken not to insert the pin into the tibiotarsal joint. The proximal part of the pin/nail should be cut as short as possible to avoid rubbing against the patellar ligament or surrounding soft tissue.

Intramedullary pins/nails can also be used **in combination with other fixation systems**, such as osteosynthesis plates or external fixators. The intramedullary pin must leave enough space inside the medullary canal of the tibia to be able to place the screws or pins of the other fixation system; otherwise, fissures in the bone could occur when the different materials collide with each other.

External fixators on the tibia are used in many cases, as they are a form of fixation that is simple to place on this bone, with open or closed techniques. This type of fixation is especially indicated in open fractures, fractures with multiple fragments and fractures located in the distal diaphysis or metaphysis. The

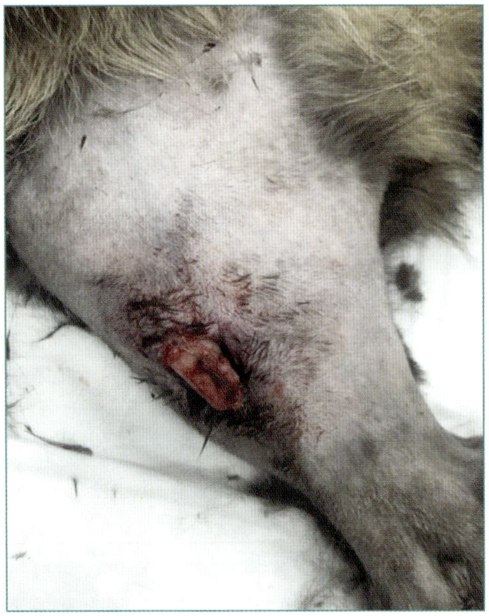

FIGURE 15. Open tibial fractures with exposure of the proximal fragment through the skin.

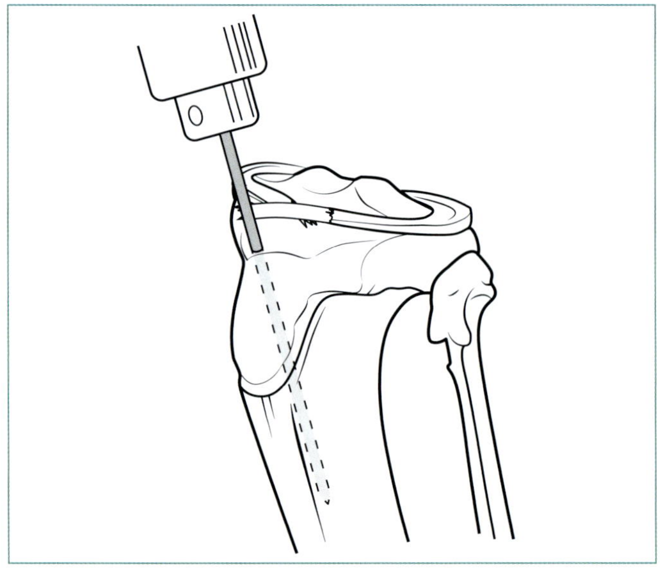

FIGURE 16. Normograde insertion of the intramedullary pin in the tibia.

entire medial aspect of the tibia has only skin and subcutaneous tissue as soft tissues, which facilitates pin insertion. These fixators can be type I or II. Type I will only penetrate from the medial aspect of the tibia to the lateral cortex, thus avoiding damage to the extensor muscles. Type II (Fig. 17) are used more commonly in fractures that are expected to need more time for ossification, since they confer greater stability and there is less risk of implant failure. Kirschner wires and positive-profile threaded pins can be used. The gauge of the pins to be placed should be taken into account to avoid iatrogenic fractures, especially if threaded pins of a larger gauge than necessary are used. Usually, 2 mm pins are used in the proximal tibia, while 1.6 mm pins are used in the distal tibia. To provide greater stability to the type I fixator, two bars can be placed side by side in parallel. Epoxy resin can also be used to fix the pins to each other to make the structure lighter.

Another fixation system is **osteosynthesis plates**. These can be placed in an open manner or with miniapproaches in the proximal and distal metaphysis of the caudomedial area of the tibia. The plate is slid over the medial aspect of the tibia from the proximal approach to the distal approach and then screws are placed through both approaches to fix the plate to the tibia. This system is useful especially in comminuted fractures, to avoid the open approach to the fracture site and to facilitate ossification by not damaging vascularization. The placement of two orthogonal plates, one on the medial aspect and the other on the cranial edge of the tibia, using miniapproaches in the proximal and distal areas, has also been described.

The plates can be 2 mm cuttable plates or 2 or 2.7 mm dynamic compression plates (in simple transverse fractures) or neutralization plates (in oblique or comminuted fractures). The 2.7 mm screws may be too wide a gauge for use in some cats, so in many cases 2 mm screws are preferred. Locking plates can also be used in these fractures, especially in cases where one of the fragments is small and does not allow at least three bicortical screws to be placed.

Another option is the combination of an osteosynthesis plate with a small-gauge intramedullary pin. This system provides adequate stability in many cases.

The most appropriate fixation method must be chosen depending on the area of the tibia that has been fractured.

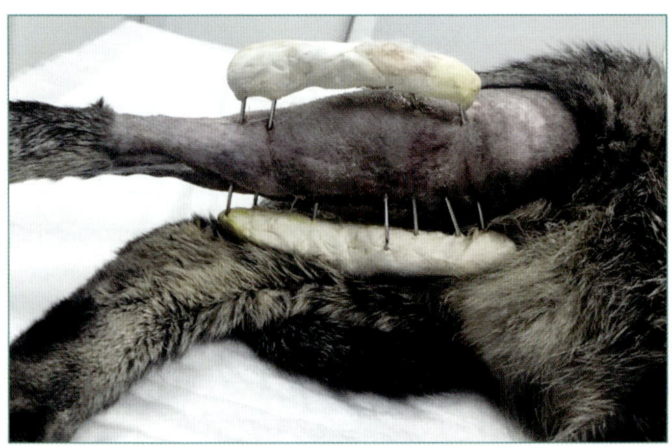

FIGURE 17. Type II external fixators for the resolution of an open tibial fracture.

Fractures of the proximal tibia and fibula

Proximal tibial and fibular fractures are not common in cats. They are usually Salter–Harris tibial fractures in the case of young kittens, or metaphyseal fractures in cats that have finished growing.

The approach is performed medially with an incision in the skin and fascia near the medial aspect of the patellar ligament. The incision is continued along the craniomedial border of the tibia in order to retract the soft tissues in a caudal direction. Care must be taken not to damage the medial collateral ligament of the stifle.

Fibular head fractures may involve lateral instability of the stifle, but treatment is not necessary in all cases, since stability is restored by fixing the tibial fracture.

The growth plates in the proximal tibia are located in the tibial plateau and tibial tuberosity. Salter–Harris type I and II fractures may occur in kittens under 10 weeks of age. **Tibial tuberosity fractures** do not usually occur in adult cats. This fracture is fixed with two Kirschner wires introduced through the tibial tuberosity and placed parallel to the surface of the tibial plateau to counteract the force of the quadriceps and prevent the pins from mobilizing. A tension band can be added to hold them in place, but only in cats that have finished growing.

In the case of **proximal tibial epiphysis fractures**, the proximal fragment is usually displaced caudally with respect to the tibia. Failure to properly reduce these fractures results in tibial tuberosity angulation changes that impact stifle function. These fractures can be fixed with cross pins from the lateral and medial areas and anchored to the opposite cortical surfaces of the tibial metaphysis. A third pin may be added to give greater stability to the structure, placed from the tibial tuberosity and anchored in the caudal diaphyseal cortex of the tibia (Fig. 18).

Proximal tibial metaphyseal fractures are common in adult cats. In these cases, fracture fixation may be difficult if the proximal fragment is very small. Cross pins, as explained for fractures at the level of the physis, a combination an intramedullary pin with a Kirschner wire to avoid rotation, external fixators or osteosynthesis plates can be used. These plates can be straight if they allow at least two screws to be placed in the proximal fragment. Otherwise, T-plates or L-plates should be used to achieve the placement of two screws. If an osteosynthesis plate is used, it should be contoured so that it fits as much as possible the shape of the tibial metaphysis.

Fractures of the tibial and fibular diaphysis

Diaphyseal tibial and fibular fractures should be considered fractures with possible complications in their ossification. Blood supply to the area should be preserved as much as possible and the fragments and surrounding soft tissue should be handled appropriately.

The surgical approach is simple in this area, through an incision in the medial area of the tibia, taking care not to damage the saphenous vein, which runs obliquely in the distal area.

As mentioned above, the most common methods of fixation of diaphyseal tibial fractures are external fixators and osteosynthesis plates (Figs. 19–22). External fixators are especially useful in open fractures, comminuted fractures and in cases of nonunion. Type I or II fixators can be used, and connecting bars or acrylics can be used to fix the pins to each other. It is not usually necessary to use a double connecting bar. In some cases they can be combined with an intramedullary pin. They can be placed using a closed technique in the case of reduced fractures or via a small approach if manual reduction is needed.

Diaphyseal fibular fractures usually do not require treatment, as fixation of the tibial fracture is sufficient.

> Fibular fractures only need to be fixed if they affect the fibular head or the lateral malleolus, as these are the origin of the stabilizing ligaments of the stifle and tibiotarsal joints, respectively.

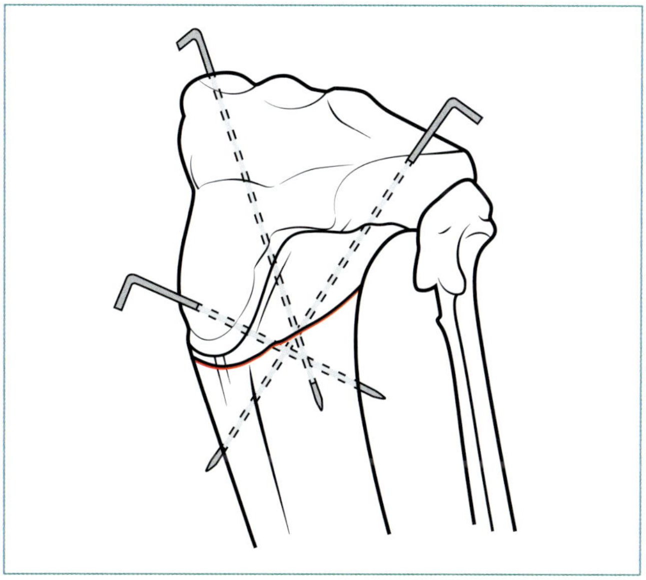

FIGURE 18. Placement of three Kirschner wires to fix a proximal tibial epiphyseal fracture.

Fractures of the distal tibia and malleolus of the fibula

These fractures are frequent in cats that fall from heights and in many cases they are open fractures, in which the most appropriate method of fixation is the placement of external fixators. The small size of the distal fragment may preclude the performance of any fixation, as there would be insufficient space to insert pins to adequately fix the fracture. Osteosynthesis plates, alone or in combination with an intramedullary pin to correctly align the fragments, can also be used as internal fixation.

In the case of Salter–Harris fractures in this area (Figs. 23–26), cross pins can be used that are anchored on the opposing cortical surfaces. In these cases, if the distal fragment is very small, it may be necessary to use a transarticular external fixator that immobilizes the tibiotarsal joint to prevent flexion and extension of the joint and allows ossification of the fracture. In young animals, this fixator can be removed after 3–4 weeks.

As mentioned above, fractures of the fibula should be treated when they involve the lateral malleolus. Once the fracture is reduced, the malleolus is fixed to the tibia with Kirschner wires anchored to the cortical surfaces. Cerclage wire can also be added as a tension band to attach it to the fibula. These implants can ulcerate the skin over time, given the scarcity

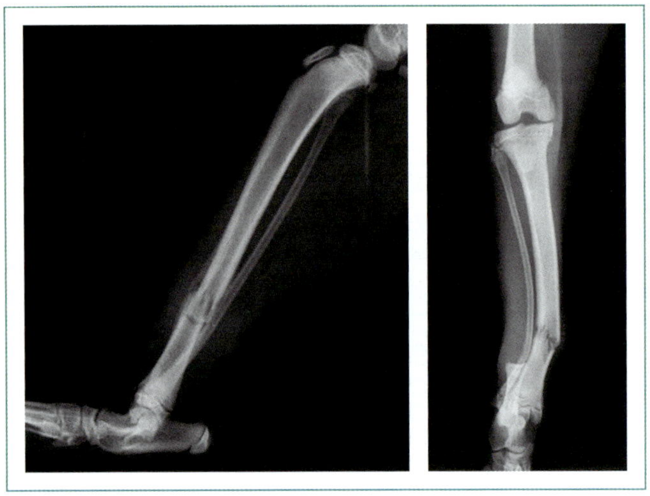

FIGURE 19. Diaphyseal tibial fracture.

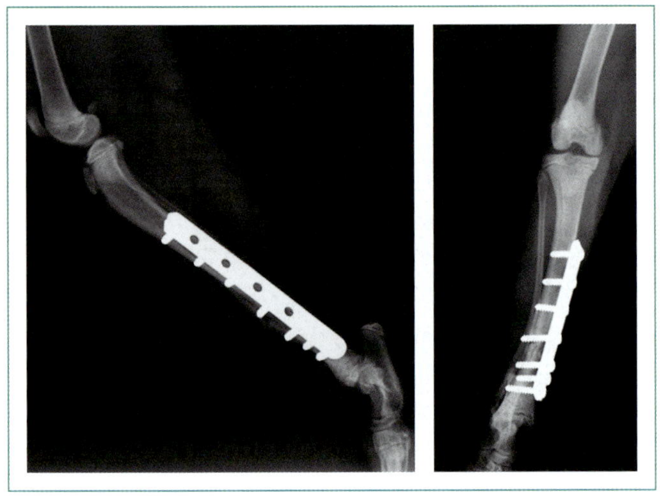

FIGURE 20. Placement of an osteosynthesis plate in the diaphyseal fracture from the previous figure.

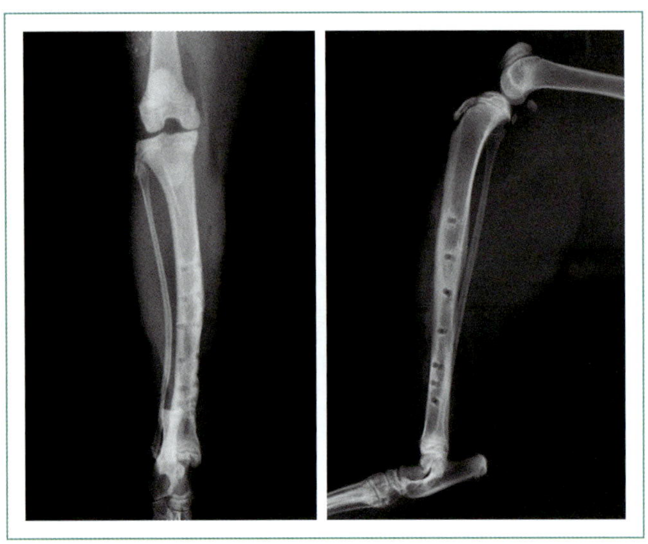

FIGURE 21. Follow-up X-ray after removal of the osteosynthesis plate in the case shown in the previous figures.

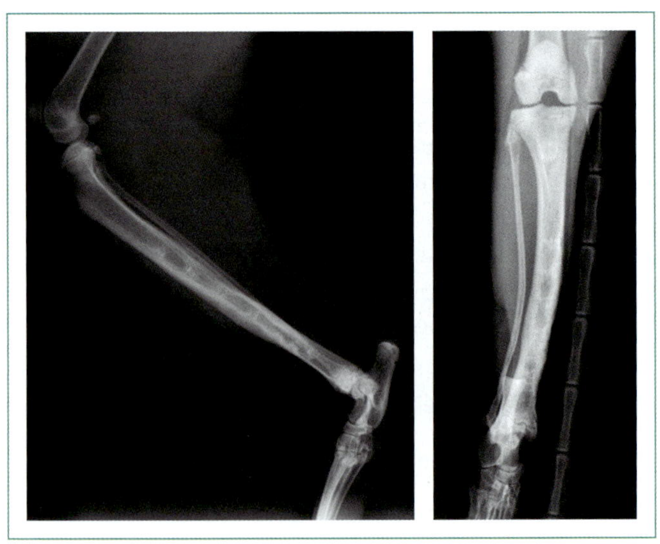

FIGURE 22. Follow-up X-ray 2 months after removal of the osteosynthesis plate in the case shown in the previous figures.

of soft tissue over the area, so it may be necessary to remove them once ossification of the fracture is achieved or if complications occur.

Complications

The approaches to all these anatomical areas are simple to perform because the medial aspect of the tibia is associated with very little soft tissue; therefore, complications involving vascular and neural structures do not usually occur. However, care must be taken when approaching the distal diaphysis of the tibia to avoid damaging the saphenous vein. Likewise, in approaches performed close to the stifle or tarsal joint, caution must be exercised to avoid injury to the collateral ligaments.

As with other fractures, the placement of external fixators involves a greater number of complications and follow-ups.

If osteosynthesis plates are used for internal fixation, when closing the skin the suture should not be placed directly over the plate or screws so as not to hinder healing.

Fixation methods are usually efficient in metaphyseal fractures and ossification is usually rapid, so the prognosis is often favorable. On the contrary, as previously mentioned, ossification may be slower in diaphyseal tibial fractures, and it may take at least 2 months to achieve ossification.

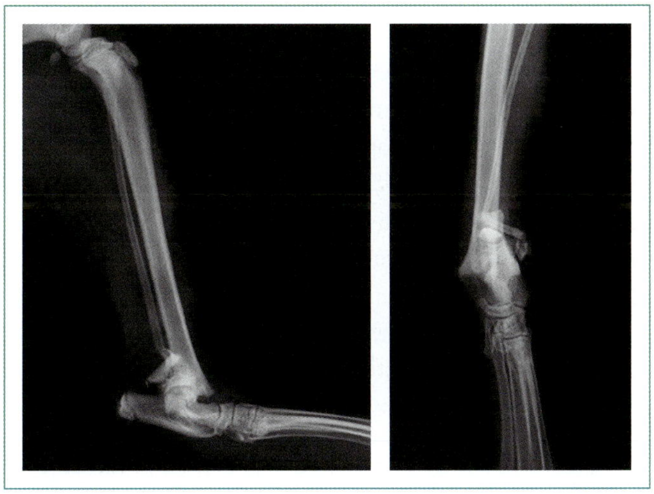

FIGURE 23. Fracture of the distal tibia and the distal diaphysis of the fibula.

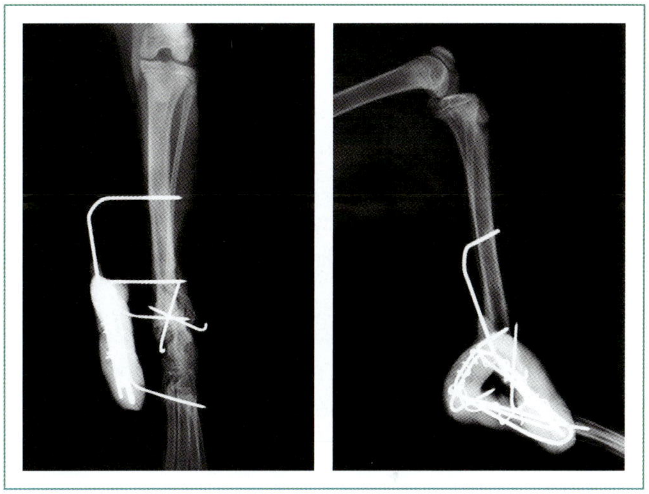

FIGURE 24. Fixation of the tibial fracture shown in the previous figure by placing two cross pins in the malleoli and a type I external fixator to immobilize the tarsal joint.

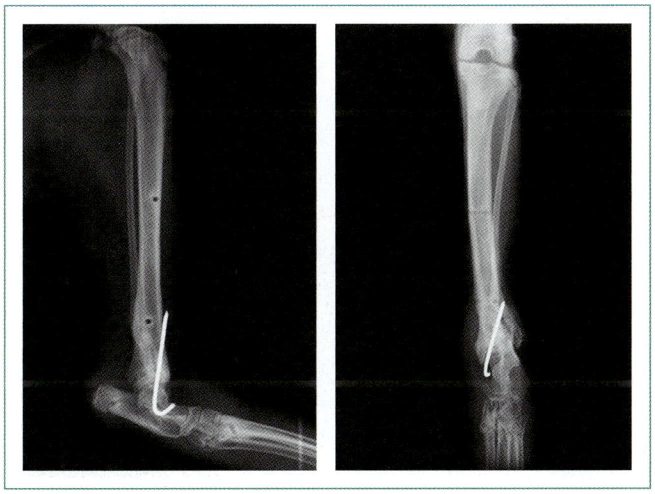

FIGURE 25. Removal of the external fixator and the pin from the lateral malleolus in the case from the previous figures.

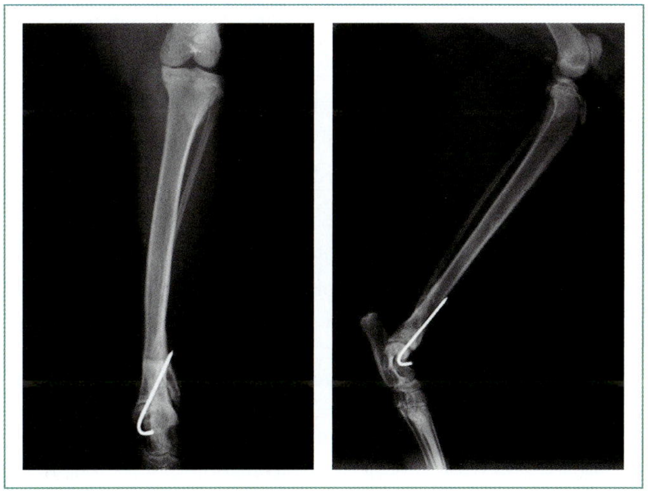

FIGURE 26. Follow-up of the fracture in the case shown in Figure 23, 2 months after removal of the external fixator.

It is estimated that bone nonunion occurs in approximately 15% of cases and is more frequent in patients with open fractures, comminuted fractures, in older animals and in those that are overweight.

In distal tibial and fibular fractures, with very small fragments or comminuted fractures, in which proper immobility of the fracture line is not achieved, there will be instability of the tarsal joint. In these cases, pantarsal arthrodesis may be necessary.

Tarsal injuries

Tarsal injuries include fractures and luxations, which usually occur as a result of trauma. Although in many cases these injuries are caused by falls from heights, in some patients they occur indoors, such as from jumping from furniture or when introducing the limb somewhere where there is a lever movement; for example, when the hind limb is caught between the wall and a radiator.

They are often open injuries, especially in the case of calcaneal fractures. In some cases, it may be necessary to resolve the skin defect via skin plasty at the same time that the fracture is resolved.

In the case of fractures of the central, first, second, third and fourth tarsal bones, conservative treatment with a bandage and splint may be sufficient. In cases where this does not work, a partial or total tarsal arthrodesis must be performed.

Ligament injuries can affect the tibiotarsal, intertarsal and tarsometatarsal joints. To diagnose these lesions, it is important to understand the anatomy of these joints. The distal tibia and the fibula are joined together by the inferior tibiofibular ligament. Both malleoli, lateral and medial, are the insertion zone for the collateral ligaments, which, unlike in dogs, are short ligaments. They are straight and oblique fibers. Between the bones that make up the tarsus, there are many short ligaments in dorsal, plantar, lateral and medial locations. In addition, there is a long ligament in a plantar position that extends from the distal aspect of the calcaneus to the base of the fourth metatarsal bone.

Clinical signs in cats suffering from tarsal ligament injuries usually include pain, lameness, swelling and crepitus, which are due to the instability caused by these injuries. Diagnosis is made by X-ray. It is always helpful to compare it to the X-ray image of the tarsus of the contralateral extremity. In addition, it may be necessary to perform X-rays with the joint placed in the varus and valgus positions for diagnosis, since in the neutral position signs of joint gaping or malposition of the tarsal bones may not be evident.

In cats bearing weight on the plantar aspect of the limb, the possibility of tendon injury should be considered. The common calcaneal tendon should be palpated to assess for inflammation and tension, which may be lost in cases of calcaneal fractures or avulsions of the tendon from its insertion in the calcaneus bone. In these cases, when forced flexion of the tarsus is performed, this flexion is more pronounced due to the lack of tendon tension.

Calcaneal fractures

In these cases, the proximal fragment is displaced when the common calcaneal tendon pulls the fragment in a proximal direction (Fig. 27), making internal fixation of the fracture necessary. For this purpose, there are various methods of fixation. Typically, one or two intramedullary pins are used in conjunction with a tension band (Fig. 28), which is necessary to counteract the force exerted by the common calcaneal tendon so that the pins do not slip out. This tension band can be placed differently depending on the size of the proximal fracture fragment:

- In the case of a small fragment, a hole is drilled at the base of the distal fragment, from lateral to medial, through which cerclage wire is passed. Then, in a figure of eight, the portion of the pins protruding from the calcaneal tuberosity is encircled with this cerclage wire.
- If both fragments of the fracture are larger because the fracture is in a medial area of the calcaneus, two holes are drilled as explained in the previous case: one in the proximal fragment and one at the base of the distal fragment. In this case, the figure-of-eight cerclage wire is passed through both holes instead of around the pins, which are cut flush at the level of the bone so they do not protrude. This configuration will prevent the osteosynthesis material from rubbing against soft tissue, thus avoiding irritation.

Another form of fixation, in large cats with an adequate calcaneal size, may be the placement of a cuttable osteosynthesis plate with 2 mm screws, although this is not usually necessary in cats.

Tibiotarsal joint luxation

This injury is caused by a rupture or avulsion of the collateral ligaments or, more frequently, by a fracture of the lateral and/or medial malleoli.

Diagnosis is established radiographically, by identifying the malleolus fractures or, thanks to X-rays in a forced position, by seeing separation of the joints.

Treatment in the case of malleolus fractures has been explained above, in the discussion of distal tibial fractures. In cases of ligament rupture or avulsion, due to the small size of the fragments, collateral ligament prostheses are usually placed. For this purpose, a monofilament suture placed in a figure-of-eight pattern is used to replace the two components of the collateral ligament. This suture can be passed through perforated tunnels at the points of origin and insertion of the ligaments, thus replacing the function of the collateral ligament. Alternatively, screws with washers can be used to anchor the suture around them, although this is difficult to do in small cats.

If the latter technique is used:

- In the case of **injuries to the lateral collateral ligament**, the screws are fixed: one in the lateral malleolus, one in the dorsal area of the base of the calcaneus and one in the coracoid process of the calcaneus.
- In the case of **injuries to the medial collateral ligament**, the screws are fixed: one in the medial malleolus, one in the body of the talus and one in its base (Fig. 29).

After placing the prosthetic material, the joint must be immobilized. For this purpose, an additional transarticular external fixator is placed temporarily. This fixator can be type I, or type II if greater stability is required. The pins are placed as follows: one in the proximal tibia, one at the level of the distal metaphysis of the tibia, one in the calcaneus bone and, finally, one across the head of all the metatarsal bones (see Fig. 24).

Tarsal arthrodesis

Tarsal arthrodesis may be necessary in the case of comminuted fractures of the tarsal bones, or when previous fracture fixation treatments have failed. In this cases, the consequent pain, lameness and osteoarthritis may warrant arthrodesis.

As explained in Chapter 31, in the discussion of carpal arthrodesis, it is necessary to remove all cartilage from the joints to be fused, perform a cancellous bone graft in that area and place a stable fixation system so that ossification can occur between the bones that make up that joint.

In the case of the tarsus, two types of arthrodesis can be performed depending on the joints affected: partial or pancarpal when it includes the tibiotarsal joint.

Partial tarsal arthrodesis

Partial arthrodesis is performed to fix the proximal and distal intertarsal joints and the tarsometatarsal joints (Fig. 30). It is indicated in hyperextension injuries when subluxation of the

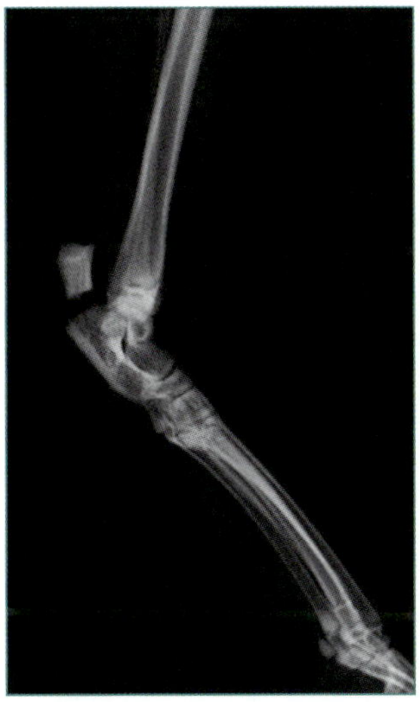

FIGURE 27. Calcaneal fracture.

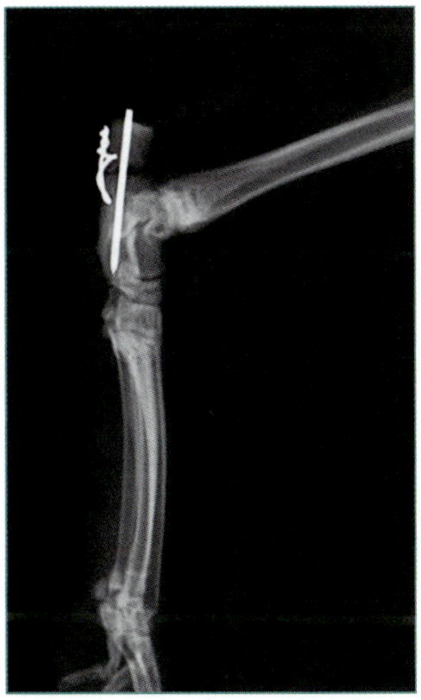

FIGURE 28. Intramedullary pin and tension band as fixation of the calcaneal fracture.

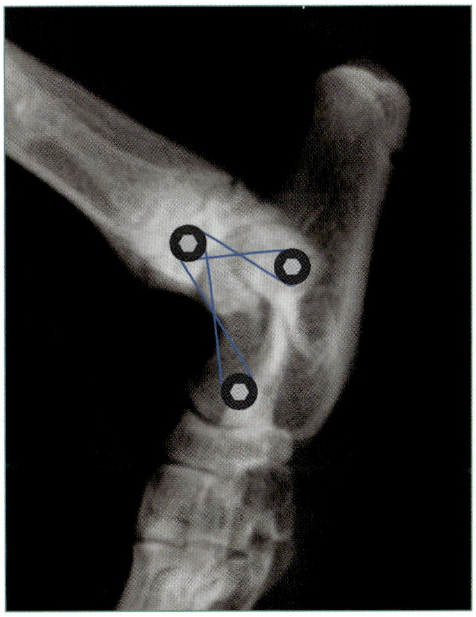

FIGURE 29. Diagram of the placement of screws and ligament prostheses in the medial aspect of the tibiotarsal joint.

intertarsal and tarsometatarsal joints has occurred. It is also indicated for comminuted fractures of these tarsal bones.

Different methods can be used for fixation. In some cases, an intramedullary pin can be placed through the calcaneus and anchored in the fourth metatarsal bone. This method can be accompanied by cross pins placed from the lateral aspect of the joint, from the fourth tarsal bone to the second metatarsal bone and from the head of the fifth metatarsal bone to the central tarsal bone. A figure-of-eight tension band can also be used, passing cerclage wire through a lateral tunnel in the calcaneus and through another tunnel encompassing all the metatarsal heads.

Another method of fixation is the placement of an osteosynthesis plate on the lateral aspect of the tarsus, from the calcaneus to the fifth metatarsal bone. For this purpose, cuttable plates are useful because they allow the required plate size to be obtained. In most cases, 2 mm screws are used. Ideally, the screws should be inserted as follows: three in the calcaneus, one at the level of the intertarsal bones and another three in the fifth metatarsal bone, reaching the fourth and even the third metatarsal bone. Another screw placement is to insert three screws proximal and three distal to the tarsometatarsal joints.

The plate can also be placed on the medial aspect of the tarsal joint (Figs. 31 and 32), with one or two screws in the talus, one screw in the central tarsal bone and three screws in the second metatarsal bone.

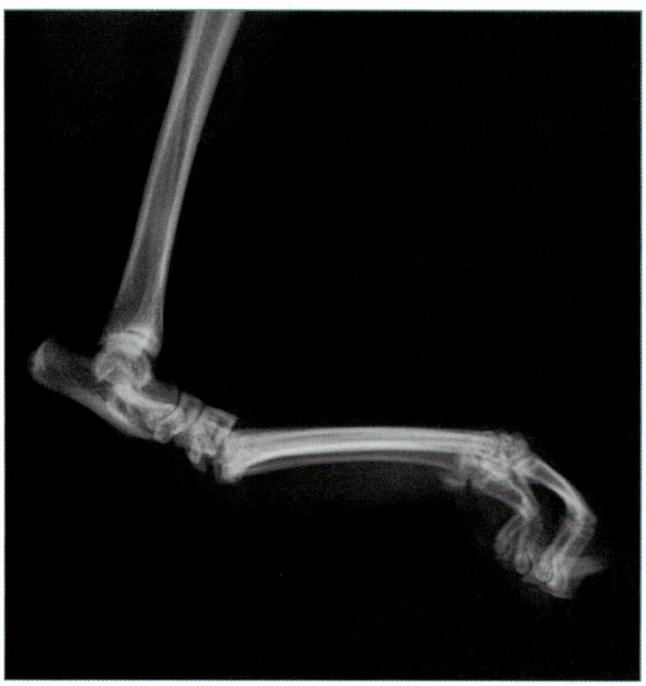

FIGURE 30. Tarsometatarsal luxation.

Pantarsal arthrodesis

Pantarsal arthrodesis is performed in cases in which the tarsus needs to be immobilized due to injuries affecting the tibiotarsal joint, since it has better results than immobilizing only this joint.

A plate placed in a dorsal position is usually used for this purpose. A dorsal approach is made from the distal tibia to the end of the metatarsal bones. Cuttable plates of 1.5–2 mm, specially designed plates for pantarsal arthrodesis of 2.0–2.7 mm or locking plates can be used. After contouring the plate, it is fixed to the third metatarsal bone with three or four 1.5–2 mm screws. The plate is then attached to the tibia with forceps and four screws are placed in the distal tibia. Finally, two screws are placed in the medial area of the plate to be fixed through the talus and calcaneus.

Another possible location for placing the plate is the medial or lateral aspect of the tarsus. The approach is the same as for the dorsal plate. In this case, a reconstruction plate, which allows for lateral contouring, or plates specially designed for pantarsal arthrodesis—the shape of which is chosen according to which tarsus is being treated, right or left—can be used. For the application of the latter, the surface of the medial malleolus of the tibia or the lateral malleolus and the proximal part of the metatarsal bone must be removed to obtain a flat surface and properly place the plate.

This plate location may be subject to forces that can lead to complications, such as the bending or breaking of the plate or the mobilization of the screws. To prevent these complications, an intramedullary pin can be placed through the tibiotarsal joint from the tibia, anchoring into the talus.

The combination of pins and an external fixator can also be used, especially in cases of open fractures or joint infections. In this case, an intramedullary pin is introduced through the joint from the base of the calcaneus to the proximal metaphysis of the tibia. Two cross pins are then inserted through the tarsus: one from the fourth tarsal bone to the second metatarsal bone, and one from the fifth metatarsal bone to the central tarsal bone. Finally, a type II transarticular external fixator is placed.

Complications

In open calcaneal fractures, contamination of the fracture site may occur, which causes the proximal fragment to devitalize, complicating its ossification. In these cases, the existing skin defect must be covered by a skin plasty so that the bone is not exposed. Attention should be paid to the placement of the implants so that they do not interfere with skin healing.

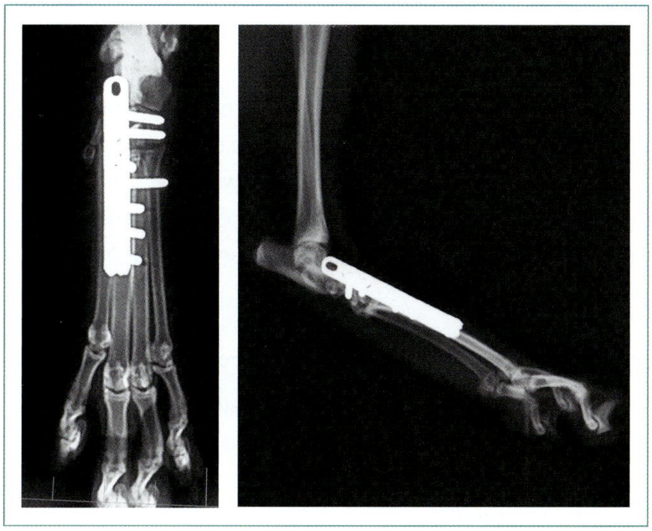

FIGURE 31. Partial tarsal arthrodesis with the placement of an osteosynthesis plate on the medial aspect of the tarsus.

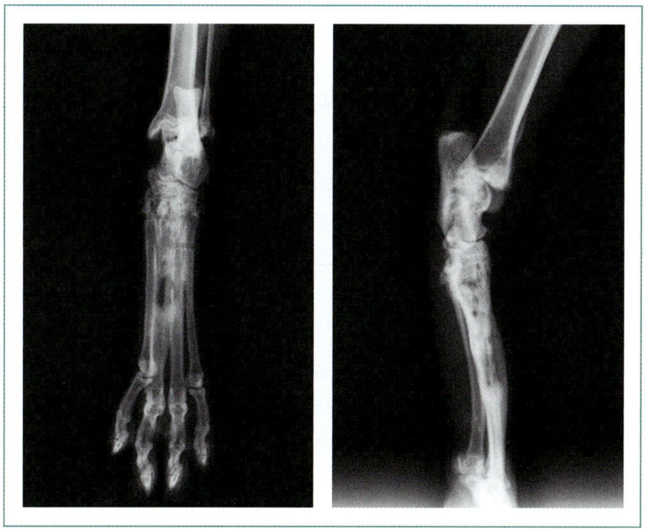

FIGURE 32. Partial tarsal arthrodesis achieved after the placement of an osteosynthesis plate with ossification of the tarsometatarsal joints.

In tarsal arthrodesis, like in other arthrodeses, the main complication is lack of ossification. This may be due to not having removed all the articular cartilage from the bone surfaces that make up the joint to be fused, or due to a mobilization of the area because of the failure of the implants or an incorrect placement or choice of implants. A cancellous bone graft should always be used to facilitate this ossification.

The choice of arthrodesis fixation method depends on various patient factors. Their age, body condition, where they live and their living habits should be taken into account. In addition, their movement must be limited long enough for ossification to occur.

Metatarsal fracture

Metatarsal fractures are treated in a manner very similar to that described for metacarpal fractures in Chapter 31.

In cases of closed and reduced fractures, conservative treatment with padded bandages or splints usually has an adequate result, especially if one of the metatarsal bones is not fractured and serves as stabilization for the others. These bandages and splints should be maintained for 4–6 weeks.

In cases of open fractures or when the bone fragments are displaced, surgical intervention is required to reduce and fix the fracture with intramedullary Kirschner wires (Fig. 33).

Rupture of the cranial cruciate ligament of the stifle

Cranial cruciate ligament rupture (CCLR) is rare in cats. One reason for this is that the length of this ligament is longer in cats than in dogs or humans. CCLR usually occurs as a result of trauma, such as a fall from heights or jumping indoors. However, there are cats that suffer this injury without evidence of trauma, without going outdoors and without falling. This suggests that it occurs due to a degeneration of the ligament that eventually leads to its rupture. Signs of meniscal calcification and joint degeneration are usually present in these cats at the time of diagnosis and precede CCLR. It occurs more commonly in animals 7.5–8.5 years of age that are overweight.

The clinical signs are pain, inflammation and lameness, the latter being usually very evident in the first few days after CCLR. Progressively greater weight-bearing may then be seen, although the patients do not usually bear their full weight on the affected hind limb. Partial ligament ruptures may also occur, which may go unnoticed by owners as the clinical signs are mild or because the cat completely recovers within a few days.

Diagnosis is made by clinical examination, with a positive anterior drawer movement and a positive tibial compression test. There are cases in which cranial displacement of the tibia is not evident when performing the anterior drawer movement test, but it does occur when the cat is sedated. In the mediolateral X-ray of the stifle (Fig. 34), cranial displacement of the tibia can be observed when performing tarsal flexion (positive tibial compression test).

Another radiographic finding that can be seen in these patients is calcification or mineralization of the meniscus (Fig. 35). This is found in a small number of cats, sometimes as an incidental finding when performing X-rays of the stifle, since in many animals there are no clinical signs suggestive of discomfort or pain. Some studies put the incidence at 37%. It may appear in older cats with poor body condition and signs of joint degeneration, which are common in older animals. In some studies, these mineralizations are graded on a scale from 0 (normal radiographic image) to 4 (severe).

These calcifications usually occur in the cranial horn of the menisci (most frequently in the medial meniscus), but they can also be seen in the intermeniscal ligament, at the insertion of the cranial cruciate ligament, in the synovial membrane and in the infrapatellar fat. There are studies that suggest that these calcifications are secondary to CCLR, but there are other studies that demonstrate the presence of calcifications at the time of the radiographic diagnosis of CCLR. It is even considered possible that the mineralized meniscus loses its characteristics and this predisposes to CCLR. A relationship has also been found between the mineralization of the meniscus and the presence of degenerative signs in the cartilage of the medial femoral condyle and the medial area of the tibial plateau. No data is available on the incidence of medial meniscus lesions in cases of CCLR. If lameness does not significantly decrease within 3 weeks, the menisci should be explored during surgery and treatment considered.

Other clinical signs that may be found include alterations due to osteoarthritis in cats with an unstable stifle that have not undergone surgery for stabilization, with the appearance of signs 3 months after the injury. This joint degeneration can also appear in cats that have undergone surgery, although it occurs later and is less severe.

Treatment

Regarding the treatment of CCLR in cats, conservative treatment or surgical treatment can be chosen.

Conservative treatment of CCLR in cats is usually effective. Weight loss and relative rest should be implemented, avoiding going outdoors, climbing or descending from places that could force the limb to bear weight. Nonsteroidal anti-inflammatory and other analgesic drugs should also be administered for the first few days after the injury. Improvement of clinical signs can usually start to be observed after the fourth week, but many cats remain uncomfortable upon weight-bearing due to joint laxity and muscle atrophy. The onset of osteoarthritis progresses slowly in cats and radiographic signs of this degeneration can be observed in the medium to long term.

Surgical treatment is performed in cats in which conservative treatment has been unsuccessful. It is also performed in cats that, due to their life habits, body condition or injuries in other extremities, need stabilization of the stifle for faster

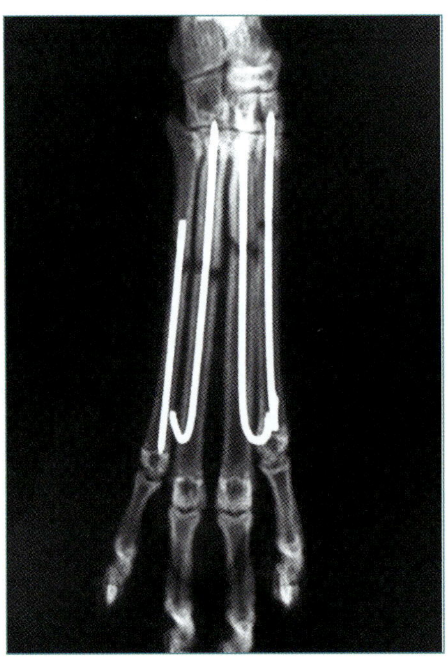

FIGURE 33. Reduction of fractures in all four metatarsal bones, with normograde placement of pins in metatarsals II, III and IV and an intramedullary pin for metatarsal V alignment.

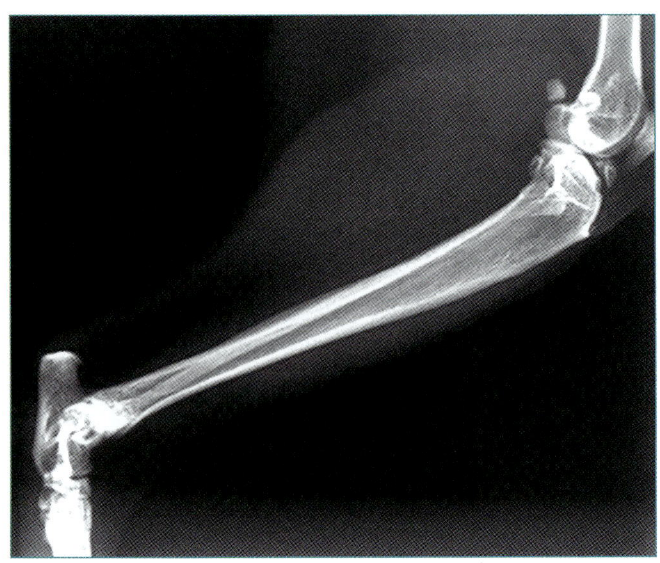

FIGURE 34. Positive tibial compression test: cranial displacement of the tibia as a consequence of the rupture of the cranial cruciate ligament of the stifle. Calcification of the meniscus is also present.

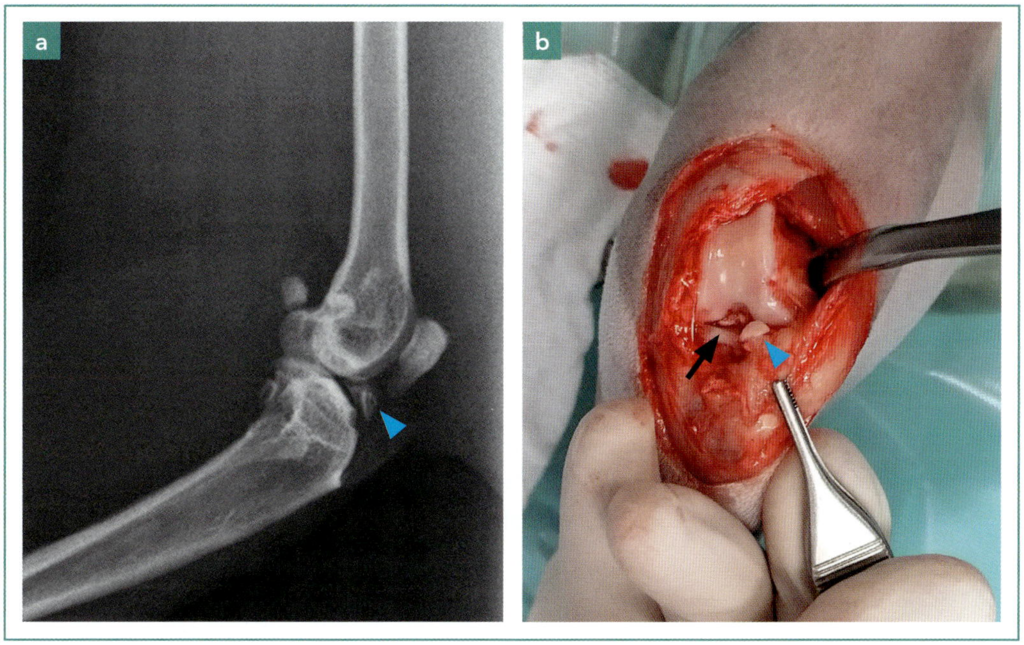

FIGURE 35. (a) X-ray of a patient with meniscus calcification. (b) Approach to the stifle joint, showing meniscal calcification (arrowhead) and cranial cruciate ligament rupture (arrow).

recovery. Surgical stabilization of the stifle has also been shown to improve proprioception and muscle activity in the limb, in addition to reducing or delaying the onset of osteoarthritis.

> Surgery should not be considered if only meniscal calcification is present, as many of these cats have no clinical signs, but such mineralization should be removed if lameness persists after conservative treatment.

Intracapsular, extracapsular and corrective osteotomy techniques (tibial plateau leveling osteotomy—TPLO—or tibial tuberosity advancement—TTA—) have been described, but due to its simplicity and the good results it offers in most cases, extracapsular stabilization using a lateral suture technique is the most widely used and is the one explained below. This technique decreases anterior drawer movement and internal rotation of the tibia. TPLO and TTA techniques may be more appropriate in cases involving very obese cats in which the extracapsular technique has not been successful.

Extracapsular lateral suture stabilization

Extracapsular lateral suture stabilization technique is also described as lateral retinacular imbrication suture or lateral fabellotibial suture. The suture material used to perform it can be multifilament or monofilament. In general, multifilament suture provides greater resistance to breakage but may present more complications due to postoperative infections. Nonabsorbable monofilament suture is the most indicated because it causes fewer complications. Either 0 gauge nylon suture that is then knotted or commercially available 0.7 mm monofilament suture systems (50 lb; for animals up to 25 kg) with a swaged needle and a 10 mm metal crimp tube that can be crimped to secure the suture can be used (Fig. 36). The crimp tube allows for stronger fixation and avoids suture elongation problems, which can occur if the suture is knotted.

To perform the extracapsular technique:

- Using a lateral parapatellar approach, the stifle joint is accessed and explored to assess the condition of the menisci and remove remnants of the cranial cruciate ligament and meniscal calcification, if present. When removing remnants of the cruciate ligament or mineralization, care should be taken not to damage the intermeniscal ligament.
- The joint capsule is then closed with a monofilament suture in a continuous or simple interrupted pattern.
- After this, a bone tunnel is made in the tibial tuberosity below the insertion of the patellar ligament (Fig. 37a). This tunnel should be made perpendicular to the long axis of the tibia or slightly inclined from medial to lateral. If this is done too obliquely or too far away from the insertion point of the patellar ligament, there is a risk that the suture may break due to increased friction and tension on the suture.

- Next, the lateral sesamoid bone of the femur is located (Fig. 37b) and the suture is passed around it. The stability and strength of the suture are checked by pulling on its ends (Fig. 37c).
- The suture is then passed through the tunnel created in the tibia and under the patellar ligament (Fig. 37d). This suture can be made in the shape of a 0 or 8. Once in place, its two ends are passed through the crimp tube and tensioned, avoiding cranial movement and internal rotation of the tibia (Fig. 37e) until stifle stability is achieved, without locking the joint.
- Once the suture has been tensioned, the central area of the crimp tube is crimped, without applying full pressure (Fig. 37f). Then, stifle flexion and extension movements are performed to check for suture elongation and prevent joint locking. The central area of the crimp tube is then fully squeezed and the tube is crimped on both sides of this first pressure zone, without reaching its edges (Fig. 38).
- The next step is to close the lateral fascia over the suture. A fascial imbrication may also be performed to provide additional stability to the stifle. Afterwards, routine closure in layers is performed.

Postoperative follow-up X-rays should be taken (Fig. 39), which will help us, in the event of complications, to know if the position of the radiopaque crimp tube has changed. If, in subsequent revisions, the tube is misplaced with respect to that X-ray, this could indicate suture breakage.

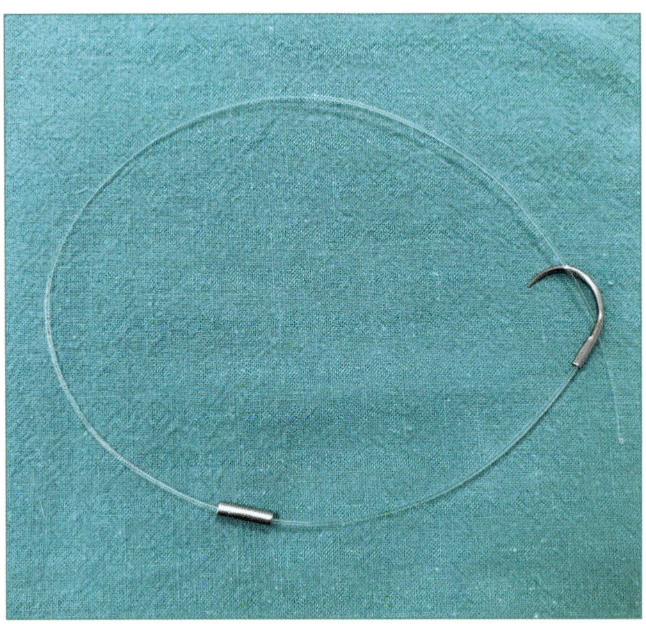

FIGURE 36. Nylon suture with a swaged needle and a crimp tube for the extracapsular technique for cranial cruciate ligament rupture repair.

A compressive bandage can be applied for the first 3–5 days postoperatively, although quite a few cats do not tolerate it and will try to remove it, which many of them succeed in doing. In aggressive cats, when the animal would have to be sedated again to remove it after a few days, the author prefers not to place this bandage. In such cases, the owner/caregiver should be advised that there may be swelling in the distal area that disappears after a few days.

The patient should rest for the first 2–3 months; they should not be allowed to climb and movement should be limited to walking on the floor. Adequate analgesia should be administered for a sufficient length of time. For the first few days, it may be necessary to combine a nonsteroidal anti-inflammatory drug with an opioid and then maintain the nonsteroidal drug for a prolonged period of time, with the aim of using the minimum effective dose in that patient.

> The prognosis is usually good, with recovery of normal gait in approximately 5 weeks, although normal or near normal weight-bearing is achieved 3-4 months after surgery.

Complications

Cats undergoing this surgery may show signs of pain for the first 24–48 hours postoperatively. They may find the bandage uncomfortable and may bite at it if in enough pain. Owners should be warned that the animal may complain and experience discomfort when trying to change position during this period. This discomfort can be greatly reduced with adequate analgesia in the immediate postoperative period.

Some complications are due to the surgical technique. Excessive tension may have been applied to the suture and this may cause further twisting of the tibia and result in lateral patellar luxation. Conversely, if the suture has been tightened too little, it may not be sufficient to stabilize the stifle and may not prevent the anterior drawer movement of the tibia or its medial rotation.

In virtually all cases, the suture used to perform this technique eventually breaks down, but the result is adequate if there has been enough time to build up fibrous tissue to stabilize the stifle. If it breaks before that tissue is produced, stability will not be sufficient. It is important to consider certain technical factors to prevent this. Attention must be paid to the direction and location of the

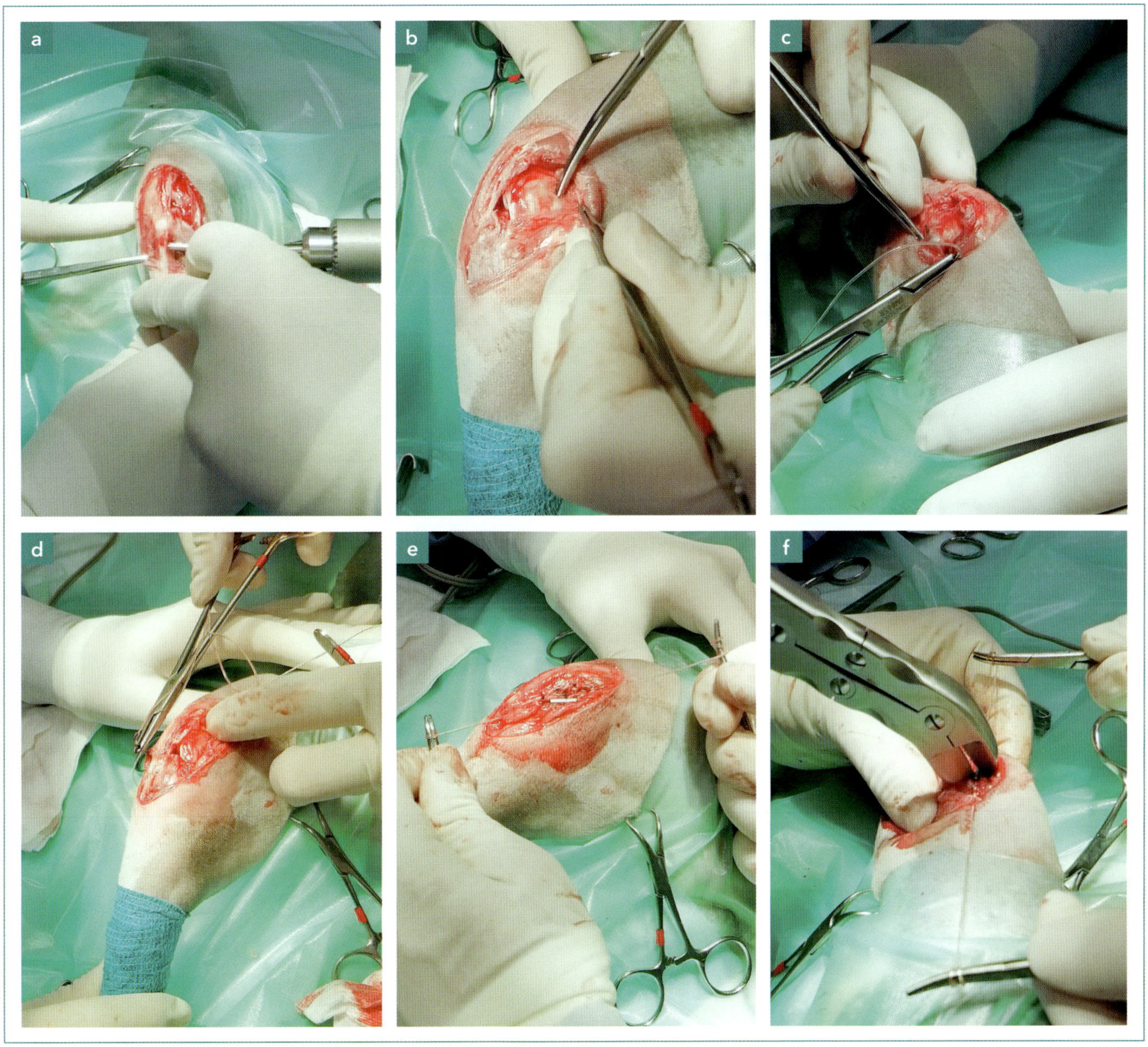

FIGURE 37. Repair of cranial cruciate ligament rupture via the extracapsular technique. (a) Drilling of a hole in the tibial tuberosity. (b) Location of the lateral sesamoid bone of the stifle. (c) Suture passage around the lateral sesamoid bone. (d) Passage of the suture through the perforated tunnel in the tibial tuberosity and under the patellar ligament. (e) Tightening of the sutures and placement of the crimp tube. (f) Pressure on the crimp tube to close it and secure the suture.

tibial tuberosity tunnel, because if it is too oblique or too far away from the insertion of the patellar ligament in the tibial tuberosity, tension and friction are caused to the suture upon contact with the bone and the suture may break. In some cases the suture does not break, but it may loosen if knotting has been done or may slip in the crimp tube if crimping has not been correctly performed.

Care must be taken when passing the suture around the lateral sesamoid bone of the femur to avoid damaging the peroneal nerve. Likewise, care must be taken not to put pressure on the patellar ligament when passing the suture under it or through the tunnel created in the tibia.

Another possible complication is related to injuries to the medial meniscus. Failure to remove the damaged area of the meniscus results in continued pain and lameness, even if stability is adequate. In addition, this predisposes to the appearance of joint degeneration.

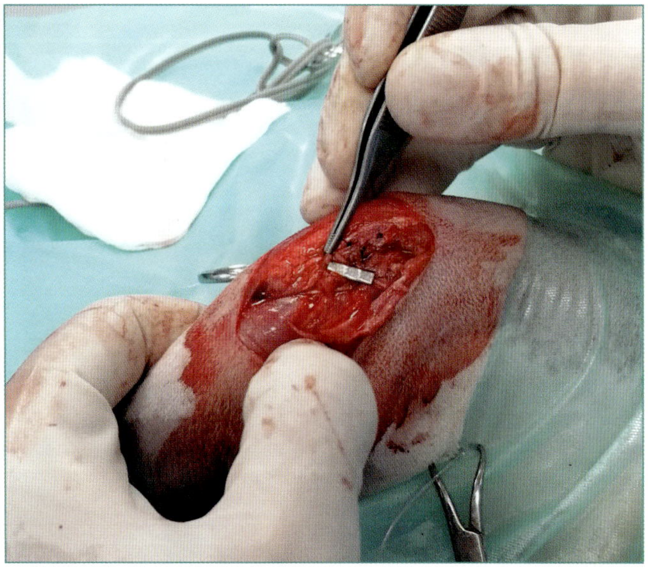

FIGURE 38. Crimp tube placed as fixation of the extracapsular suture.

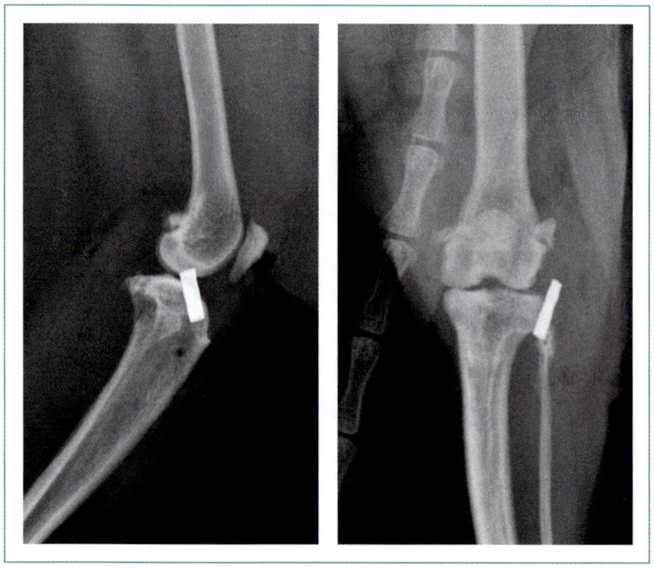

FIGURE 39. Postoperative follow-up X-ray after placement of the lateral extracapsular suture.

Bibliography

ALZA SALVATIERRA DN, WITTE PG, SCOTT HW, CATCHPOLE C. Pantarsal arthrodesis in cats using orthogonal plating. *J Feline Med Surg*, 2018; 20(1):45–54.

BULA E, PERRY KL. Tibial tuberosity transposition advancement for treatment of concomitant cranial cruciate ligament rupture and medial patellar luxation in four feline stifles. *JFMS Open Rep*, 2021; 7(2):20551169211044695.

COOK JL. Extracapsular stabilization. In: MUIR P (ed.). *Advances in the Canine Cranial Cruciate Ligament*. Iowa, USA: Wiley-Blackwell, 2010; pp. 163–168.

COPPOLA M, DAS S, MATTHEWS G et al. Traumatic stifle injury in 72 cats: a multicentre retrospective study. *J Feline Med Surg*, 2022; 24(6):587–595.

CORR S. Complex and open fractures. A straightforward approach to management in the cat. *J Feline Med Surg*, 2012; 14(1):55–64.

CRAIG A, WITTE PG, MOODY T et al. Management of feline tibial diaphyseal fractures using orthogonal plates performed via minimally invasive plate osteosynthesis. *J Feline Med Surg*, 2018; 20(1):6–14.

CULVENOR JA, BLACK AP, LORKIN KF, BRADLEY WA. Repair of femoral capital physeal injuries in cats—14 cases. *Vet Comp Orthop Traumatol*, 1996; 9(4):182–185.

DEGASPERI B, GRADNER G, DUPRÉ G. Intramedullary pinning of metacarpal and metatarsal fractures in cats using a simple distraction technique. *Vet Surg*, 2007; 36(4):382–388.

FITZPATRICK N, PRATOLA L, YEADON R et al. Total hip replacement after failed femoral head and neck excision in two dogs and two cats. *Vet Surg*, 2012; 41(1):136–142.

FREIRE M, BROWN J, ROBERTSON ID et al. Meniscal mineralization in domestic cats. *Vet Surg*, 2010; 39(5):545–552.

GÓMEZ-BARRENA E, NUÑEZ A, BALLESTEROS R et al. Anterior cruciate ligament reconstruction affects proprioception in the cat's knee. *Acta Orthop Scand*, 1999; 70(2):185–193.

GRIERSON J. Hips, elbows and stifles: common joint diseases in the cat. *J Feline Med Surg*, 2012; 14(1):23–30.

GRIFFON D. Avascular necrosis. In: GRIFFON D, HAMAIDE A (eds.). *Complications in Small Animal Surgery*. Ames, IA: Wiley Blackwell, 2016; pp. 655–657.

GUERRERO TG, KOCH D, MONTAVON PM. Fixation of a proximal femoral physeal fracture in a dog using a ventral approach and two Kirschner wires. *Vet Comp Orthop Traumatol*, 2005; 18(2):110–114.

HARASEN GL. Feline cranial cruciate rupture. 17 cases and a review of the literature. *Vet Comp Orthop Traumatol*, 2005; 18(4):254–257.

HOOTS EA, PETERSEN SW. Tibial plateau leveling osteotomy and cranial closing wedge ostectomy in a cat with cranial cruciate ligament rupture. *J Am Anim Hosp Assoc*, 2005; 41(6):395–399.

KALIS RH, LISKA WD, JANKOVITS DA. Total hip replacement as a treatment option for capital physeal fractures in dogs and cats. *Vet Surg*, 2012; 41(1):148–155.

KAPATKIN AS, HOWE-SMITH R, SHOFER F. Conservative versus surgical treatment of metacarpal and metatarsal fractures in dogs. *Vet Comp Orthop Traumatol*, 2000; 13(3):123–127.

KNEIFEL W, BORAK D, BOCKSTAHLER B, SCHNABL-FEICHTER E. Use of a custom-made limb-press model to assess intra- and extracapsular techniques for treating cranial cruciate ligament rupture in cats. *J Feline Med Surg*, 2018; 20(4):271–279.

KÖNNING T, MAARSCHALKERWEERD RJ, ENDENBURG N, THEYSE LF. A comparison between fixation methods of femoral diaphyseal fractures in cats—a retrospective study. *J Small Anim Pract*, 2013; 54(5):248–252.

KRAUS KH, TOOMBS JP, NESS MG. *External Fixation in Small Animal Practice*. Malden, MA: Blackwell Science, 2003.

LAFUENTE P. Young, male neutered, obese, lame? Non-traumatic fractures of the femoral head and neck. *J Fel Med Surg*, 2011; 13(7):498–507.

LARIN A, EICH CS, PARKER RB, STUBBS WP. Repair of diaphyseal femoral fractures in cats using interlocking intramedullary nails: 12 cases (1996–2000). *J Am Vet Med Assoc*, 2001; 219(8):1098–1104.

LECHNER B, HANDSCHUH S, BOCKSTAHLER B et al. Comparison of a novel extracapsular suture technique with a standard fabellotibial suture technique for cranial cruciate ligament repair using a custom-made limb-press model in cats. *J Feline Med Surg*, 2020; 22(10):1016–1024.

LISKA WD, DOYLE N, MARCELLIN-LITTLE DJ, OSBORNE JA. Total hip replacement in three cats: surgical technique, short-term outcome and comparison to femoral head ostectomy. *Vet Comp Orthop Traumatol*, 2009; 22(6):505–510.

LISKA WD, DOYLE ND, SCHWARTZ Z. Successful revision of a femoral head ostectomy (complicated by postoperative sciatic neurapraxia) to a total hip replacement in a cat. *Vet Comp Orthop Traumatol*, 2010; 23(2):119–123.

McCartney WT, Carmichael S. Talar neck fractures in five cats. *J Small Anim Pract*, 2000; 41(5):204–206.

McLaughlin RM. Surgical diseases of the feline stifle joint. *Vet Clin North Am Small Anim Pract*, 2002; 32(4):963–982.

McNicholas WT Jr, Wilkens BE, Blevins WE et al. Spontaneous femoral capital physeal fractures in adult cats: 26 cases (1996–2001). *J Am Vet Med Assoc*, 2002; 221(12):1731–1736.

Millis D. Quadriceps contracture. In: Griffon D, Hamaide A (eds.). *Complications in Small Animal Surgery*. Ames, IA: Wiley Blackwell, 2016; pp. 692–696.

Montavon PM, Pohler OEM, Olmstead ML, Wendelburg KL. The mini instrument and implant set and its clinical application. *Vet Comp Orthop Traumatol*, 1988; 1(1):44–51.

Owen MA. Use of contoured bar transhock external fixators in 17 cats. *J Small Anim Pract*, 2000; 41(10):440–446.

Payne J, McLaughlin R, Silverman E. Comparison of normograde and retrograde intramedullary pinning of feline tibias. *J Am Anim Hosp Assoc*, 2005; 41(1):56–60.

Perez-Aparicio FJ, Fjeld TO. Femoral neck fractures and capital epiphyseal separations in cats. *J Small Anim Pract*, 1993; 34(9):445–449.

Piermattei DL, Johnson KA. *An Atlas of Surgical Approaches to the Bones and Joints of the Dog and the Cat*, 4th ed. Philadelphia, PA: WB Saunders, 2004.

Prackova I, Paral V, Kyllar M. Safe corridors for external skeletal fixator pin placement in feline long bones. *J Feline Med Surg*, 2021; 1098612X211057329.

Queen J, Bennett D, Carmichael S et al. Femoral neck metaphyseal osteopathy in the cat. *Vet Rec*, 1998; 142(7):159–162.

Rahal SC, Fillipi MG, Mamprim MJ et al. Meniscal mineralisation in little spotted cats. *BMC Vet Res*, 2013; 9:50.

Roberts VJ, Meeson RL. Feline femoral fracture fixation. What are the options? *J Feline Med Surg*, 2022; 24(5):442–463.

Rubinos C, Meeson RL. Traumatic physeal fractures in cats: a review of 36 cases (2010–2020). *J Fel Med Surg*, 2022; 24(2):98–106.

Schiller TD. BioMedtrix total hip replacement systems: an overview. *Vet Clin North Am Small Anim Pract*, 2017; 47(4):899–916.

Scott HW, McLaughlin R. Stifle disorders. In: Scott HW, McLaughlin R (eds.). *Feline Orthopedics*. Boca Raton, FL: Taylor and Francis Group, 2006; pp. 222–225.

Şen I. Clinical and radiological evaluation of the treatment of cranial cruciate ligament rupture in cats with the musculus biceps femoris transposition technique. *Acta Veterinaria*, 2019, 69(3):300–311.

Tamburro R, Collivignarelli F, Falerno I et al. Clinical outcomes and stifle osteoarthritis assessment of nine cats before and after tibial plateau levelling osteotomy. *Acta Veterinaria*, 2020, 70(3):346–354.

Von Werthern CJ, Bernasconi CE. Application of the maxillofacial mini-plate Compact 1.0 in the fracture repair of 12 cats/2 dogs. *Vet Comp Orthop Traumatol*, 2000; 13(2):92–96.

Voss K, Langley-Hobbs SJ, Montavon PM. Stifle joint. In: Montavon PM, Voss K, Langley-Hobbs SJ (eds.). *Feline Orthopedic Surgery and Musculoskeletal Disease*. St. Louis, MO: Elsevier Saunders, 2009; pp. 475–490.

Witte PG, Scott HW, Tonzing MA. Preliminary results of five feline total hip replacements. *J Small Anim Pract*, 2010; 51(7):397–402.